reproduction
in
farm animals

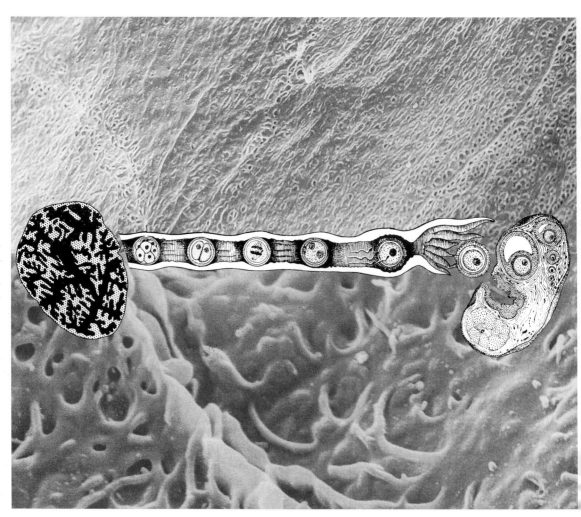

Frontispiece: The beginning of life. The oviduct: spermatozoa and eggs are transported, simultaneously, in opposite direction; sperm hyperactivation and final maturation of eggs are completed before sperm binding to the zona pellucida and fertilization.

reproduction

in

farm animals

Edited by

E.S.E. HAFEZ

Executive Director
Reproductive Health Center
IVF/Andrology International
Kiawah Island, South Carolina, USA

6th Edition

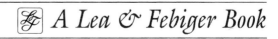 *A Lea & Febiger Book*

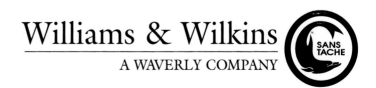

Williams & Wilkins
A WAVERLY COMPANY

BALTIMORE • PHILADELPHIA • LONDON • PARIS • BANGKOK
HONG KONG • MUNICH • SYDNEY • TOKYO • WROCLAW

Williams & Wilkins
Rose Tree Corporate Center, Building II
1400 North Providence Road, Suite 5025
Media, PA 19063-2043 USA

Executive Editor—Carroll C. Cann
Developmental Editor—Susan Hunsberger
Project Editor—Lisa Stead
Production Manager—Samuel A. Rondinelli

First Edition, 1962
    Japanese translation, 1965
    Spanish translation, 1967
Second Edition, 1968
    Japanese translation, 1971
Third Edition, 1974
Fourth Edition, 1980
    Reprinted, 1982
    Portugese translation, 1982
    Italian translation, 1985
Fifth Edition, 1987
    Japanese translation, 1992
    Spanish translation, 1992

Library of Congress Cataloging-in-Publication Data

Reproduction in farm animals / edited by E.S.E. Hafez. — 6th ed.
    p.   cm.
  Includes bibliographical references and index.
  ISBN 0-8121-1534-1
  1. Livestock—Reproduction. 2. Veterinary physiology. I. Hafez,
E. S. E. (Elsayed Saad Eldin), 1922-
SF871.R47 1993
636.089′26—dc20

92-32846
CIP

PRINTED IN THE UNITED STATES OF AMERICA

Print number: 5 4

Dedicated to M.C. Chang
*(The Worcester Foundation of Experimental Biology,
Shrewsbury, Massachusetts, USA)*

preface

The first edition, published in 1962, covered the basic and comparative aspects of reproductive physiology in a simplified manner to meet the needs of students in reproductive biology, veterinary medicine, and animal sciences. This objective is maintained in the sixth edition, which represents a condense, concise treatise on the physiology and biochemistry of reproduction of farm animals. The book is divided into major sections and these, in turn, are loosely arrayed into two domains: the components of the reproductive system and the regulation of the reproductive process, from the control of ovulation to the initiation of parturition. The reader will note the profound differences among the various animal species. To address this issue we provided separate coverage of the major species, where this seemed appropriate so that the student of reproduction could ascertain the similarities and differences among them.

During the past decade there were significant advances in the main concepts of animal reproduction as a result of modern biotechnology such as the use of immunology and radioimmunoassay; andrology; biochemistry; cryobiology; tissue, organ, and cell culture; and gonadotropin releasing hormones and their analogs. Modern techniques of bioengineering of farm animals involves microinsemination, recombination of DNA, and in vitro manipulation, transfer and expression of genes. These techniques were greatly improved with the use of computers, microcomputers, and commercially available diagnostic and analytical kits. A wide variety of techniques have been employed for the evaluation of semen, such as evaluation of sperm fertilizability using zona-free hamster egg (fresh or frozen); motility pattern as viewed by videotape microscopy; in vitro penetrability of sperm in bovine cervical mucus; and cryopreservation of embryos and semen using computerized freezers. Most of the investigations reviewed in this edition are based more on holistic research than on research at the submicroscopic or molecular level. However, the excitement generated by recent advances in molecular biology and development tend to downgrade the value of whole-animal research. No attempt was made to provide a detailed bibliography, but a selected number of classic papers and review articles are listed at the end of each chapter.

This edition could not have been revised without the cooperation of the contributing authors and their willingness to follow the editorial guidelines. The chapters have been concisely edited, and the major concepts have been summarized in tables supplemented by line drawings and scanning electron micrographs. All chapters have been completely revised and condensed. There have been numerous deletions from the fifth edition, as well as integration of new and modern concepts such as "growth factors," molecular biology and genetics, and in vitro and micromanipulation of gametes and embryos.

Some tabulated appendices include: chromosome numbers and reproductive ability of bovine, caprinae and equinae species and some of their hybrids; reproductive disease of viral, protozoan, or bacterial origin; and preparation of physiologic solutions, sperm stains, tissue culture media, and cryoprotectants. These appendices proved to be helpful for staging demonstrations, laboratory exercises, and training workshops for teachers, laboratory technicians, and students. It is hoped that the sixth edition will be of some help to serious students in animal sciences and veterinary medicine, as well as researchers and teachers.

E.S.E. Hafez
Kiawah Island, South Carolina, USA

acknowledgments

Included in the sixth edition, the contribution and the valuable information provided in the fifth edition by Ms. Marie-Claire Levasseur, and Professors C. Thibault; I. G. White, G. Alexander, A. McLaren, T. Sugie, G. E. Seidel, Jr. and J. P. Signoret. Special thanks are due to them for their continuous contributions. Professor M. R. Jainudeen, my friend and long time associate, has contributed greatly to the improvement of the table of contents and detailed structure of several chapters.

The critical remarks of Professor R. Foote have been extremely helpful.

Sincere thanks are due to Carroll C. Cann and Ms. Susan Hunsberger of Lea & Febiger for their meticulous and painstaking efforts during the preparations of the book. Special thanks are also due to Mrs. Dorothy DiRienzi, Samuel Rondinelli, Ms. Lisa Stead, and Tom Colaiezzi for their editorial skills, excellent cooperation, and continued interest in the development of animal and veterinary sciences.

contributors

Anderson, L.L.:
Department of Animal Science
11 Kilde Hall
Iowa State University
Ames, Iowa

Ashdown, R.R.:
"Downlands"
East Dean
Chichester, West Sussex
PO1805A, United Kingdom

Bahr, J.M.:
Department of Animal Science/
Physiology
University of Illinois
Urbana, Illinois

Bakst, M.R.:
United States Department of Agriculture
Agricultural Research Service
Germplasm and Gamete Physiology
Laboratory
Beltsville, Maryland

Bazer, F.W.:
Editor-in-Chief
442D Kleberg Center
Animal Science Department
Texas A&M University
College Station, Texas

Garner, D.L.:
Department of Animal Science
College of Agriculture
University of Nevada
Reno, Nevada

Geisert, R.D.:
Department of Animal Science
Oklahoma State University
Stillwater, Oklahoma

Hafez, E.S.E.:
Reproductive Health Center
IVF/Andrology International
Kiawah Island, South Carolina

Jainudeen, M.R.:
Department of Clinical Studies
Faculty of Veterinary Medicine
University of Pertanian Malaysia
Serdang, Selangor, West Malaysia

Zavy, M.T.:
Department of Obstetrics and
Gynecology
University of Oklahoma
Health Sciences Center
Oklahoma City, Oklahoma

contents

I. functional anatomy of reproduction

1. Anatomy of Male Reproduction 3
   R.R. Ashdown and E.S.E. Hafez

2. Anatomy of Female Reproduction 20
   E.S.E. Hafez

II. physiology of reproduction

3. Hormones, Growth Factors, and Reproduction 59
   E.S.E. Hafez

4. Reproductive Cycles 94
   E.S.E. Hafez

5. Folliculogenesis, Egg Maturation, and Ovulation 114
   E.S.E. Hafez

6. Transport and Survival of Gametes 144
   E.S.E. Hafez

7. Spermatozoa and Seminal Plasma 165
   D.L. Garner and E.S.E. Hafez

8. Fertilization, Cleavage, and Implantation 188
   F.W. Bazer, R.D. Geisert and M.T. Zavy

9. Gestation, Prenatal Physiology, and Parturition 213
   M.R. Jainudeen and E.S.E. Hafez

10. Reproductive Behavior 237
    E.S.E. Hafez

III.   reproductive failure

11. Reproductive Failure in Females.. 261
M.R. Jainudeen and E.S.E. Hafez

12. Reproductive Failure in Males 287
M.R. Jainudeen and E.S.E. Hafez

13. Genetics of Reproductive Failure 298
M.R. Jainudeen and E.S.E. Hafez

IV.   reproductive cycles

14. Cattle and Buffalo 315
M.R. Jainudeen and E.S.E. Hafez

15. Sheep and Goats... 330
M.R. Jainudeen and E.S.E. Hafez

16. Pigs.. 343
L.L. Anderson

17. Horses 361
E.S.E. Hafez

18. Poultry 385
J.M. Bahr and M.R. Bakst

V.   techniques for improving reproductive efficiency

19. Semen Evaluation... 405
E.S.E. Hafez

20. Artificial Insemination 424
E.S.E. Hafez

21. X- and Y-Chromosome–Bearing Spermatozoa 440
E.S.E. Hafez

22. Pregnancy Diagnosis.. 446
    M.R. Jainudeen and E.S.E. Hafez

23. Ovulation Manipulation, *In Vitro* Fertilization and Embryo Transfer, and
    Genetic Engineering.. 461
    E.S.E. Hafez

24. Preservation and Cryopreservation of Gametes and Embryos 503
    E.S.E. Hafez

    Glossary of Reproductive Biology 527

    Glossary of Common Abbreviations 536

    Appendices 539

    Index 557

I. functional anatomy of reproduction

1
Anatomy of Male Reproduction

R.R. ASHDOWN and E.S.E. HAFEZ

The male gonads, the testes, lie outside the abdomen within the scrotum, which is a purselike structure derived from the skin and fascia of the abdominal wall. Each testis lies within the vaginal process, a separate extension of the peritoneum, which passes through the abdominal wall at the inguinal canal. The deep and superficial inguinal rings are the deep and superficial openings of the inguinal canal. Blood vessels and nerves reach the testis in the spermatic cord, which lies within the vaginal process; the *ductus deferens* accompanies the vessels but leaves them at the orifice of the vaginal process to join the urethra. Besides permitting the passage of the vaginal process and its contents, the inguinal canal also gives passage to vessels and nerves supplying the external genitalia.

The spermatozoa leave the testis by efferent ductules that lead into the coiled duct of the epididymis, which continues as the straight ductus deferens. Accessory glands discharge their contents into the ductus deferens or into the pelvic portion of the urethra.

The urethra originates at the neck of the bladder. Throughout its length it is surrounded by cavernous vascular tissue. Its pelvic portion, which is enclosed by striated urethral muscle and receives secretions from various glands, leads into a second penile portion at the pelvic outlet. Here it is joined by two more cavernous bodies to make up the body of the penis, which lies beneath the skin of the body wall. A number of muscles grouped around the pelvic outlet contribute to the root of the penis. The apex or free part of the penis is covered by modified skin—the penile integument; in the resting condition it is enclosed within the prepuce. The topographic features of the organs of the important farm species are shown in Figure 1–1. Detailed descriptions of the organs are given by Nickel et al. (1973).

The testis and epididymis are supplied with blood from the testicular artery, which originates from the dorsal aorta near the embryonic site of the testes. The internal pudendal artery supplies the pelvic genitalia and its branches leave the pelvis at the ischial arch to supply the penis. The external pudendal artery leaves the abdominal cavity via the inguinal canal to supply the penis, scrotum, and prepuce. Lymph from the testis and epididymis passes to the lumbar aortic lymph nodes. Lymph from the accessory glands, urethra, and penis passes to the sacral and medial iliac nodes. Lymph from the scrotum, prepuce, and peripenile tissues drains to the superficial inguinal lymph nodes.

Afferent and efferent (sympathetic) nerves accompany the testicular artery to the testis. The pelvic plexus supplies autonomic (sympathetic and parasympathetic) fibers to the pelvic genitalia and to the smooth muscles of the penis. Sacral nerves supply motor fibers to the striated muscles of the penis and sensory fibers to the free part of the penis. Afferent fibers from the scrotum and prepuce travel mainly in the genitofemoral nerve.

3

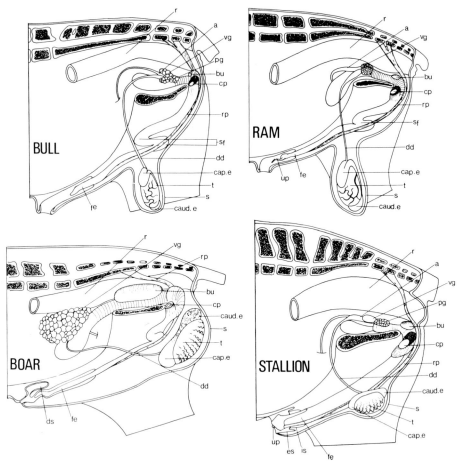

FIG. 1–1.   Diagram of the male reproductive tracts as seen in left lateral dissections.
a, Ampulla; *bu*, bulbourethral gland; *cap. e*, caput epididymidis; *caud. e*, cauda epididymidis; *cp*, left crus of penis, severed from the left ischium; *dd*, ductus deferens; *ds*, dorsal diverticulum of prepuce; *es*, prepenile prepuce; *fe*, free part of penis; *is*, preputial fold; *pg*, prostate gland; *r*, rectum; *rp*, retractor penis muscle; *s*, scrotum; *sf*, sigmoid flexure; *t*, testis; *up*, urethral process; *vg*, vesicular gland. (Adapted from Popesko (1968). Atlas der topographischen Anatomie der Haustiere. Vol. 3, Jena, Fischer.)

DEVELOPMENT

Prenatal Development

The testes develop in the abdomen, medial to the embryonic kidney (mesonephros). The plexus of ducts within the testis becomes connected to mesonephric tubules and so to the mesonephric duct, to form the epididymis, ductus deferens, and vesicular gland. The prostate and bulbourethral glands form from the embryonic urogenital sinus and the penis forms

by tubulation and elongation of a tubercle that develops at the orifice of the urogenital sinus.

Two agents produced by the fetal testis are responsible for this differentiation and development (Gondos, 1980). Fetal androgen causes development of the male reproductive tract. "Müllerian inhibiting substance," a glycoprotein, is responsible for suppression of the paramesonephric (Müllerian) ducts from which the uterus and vagina develop (Vigier et al., 1983). Abnormalities in differentiation and development of gonads and ducts can result in varying degrees of intersexuality (Hare and Singh, 1979).

Descent of the Testis

During testicular descent (Wensing, 1986), the gonad migrates caudally within the abdomen to the deep inguinal ring. It then traverses the abdominal wall to emerge at the superficial inguinal ring, which is, in fact, the much-enlarged foramen of the genitofemoral nerve (L3, L4). The testis completes its migration by passing fully into the scrotum. Descent is preceded by the formation of the vaginal process, a peritoneal sac extending through the abdominal wall and enclosing the inguinal ligament of the testis. The inguinal ligament of the gonad is often called the *gubernaculum testis,* and it terminates in the region of the scrotal rudiments. Descent follows the line of the *gubernaculum testis.* The time of descent varies (Table 1–1). In the horse, the epididymis commonly enters the inguinal canal before the testis, and that part of the inguinal ligament connecting testis and epididymis (proper ligament of testis) remains extensive until after birth.

Sometimes the testis fails to enter the scrotum. In this condition (cryptorchidism), the special thermal needs of testis and epididymis are not met, although the endocrine function of the testis is unimpaired. Bilaterally cryptorchid males therefore show more or less normal sexual desire but are sterile. Occasionally some of the abdominal viscera pass through the orifice of the vaginal process and enter the scrotum; scrotal hernia is particularly common in pigs.

Postnatal Development

Each component of the reproductive tracts of all farm animals grows in size relative to overall body size and undergoes histologic differentiation, but functional competence is not achieved simultaneously in all components of the reproductive system. Thus, in the bull, the capacity

TABLE 1–1. **Chronology of Development of the Male Reproductive Tract in Farm Animals**

	Bull	Ram	Boar	Stallion
Testicular descent	Enters scrotum half-way through fetal life	Enters scrotum half-way through fetal life	Enters scrotum in last quarter of fetal life	Enters scrotum just before or just after birth
Primary spermatocytes in seminiferous tubules	24 weeks	12 weeks	10 weeks	Variable throughout seminiferous tubules of each testis
Spermatozoa in seminiferous tubules	32 weeks	16 weeks	20 weeks	56 weeks (variable)
Spermatozoa in cauda epididymidis	40 weeks	16 weeks	20 weeks	60 weeks (variable)
Spermatozoa in the ejaculate	42 weeks	18 weeks	22 weeks	64–96 weeks
Completion of separation between penis and penile part of prepuce	32 weeks	> 10 weeks	20 weeks	4 weeks
Age at which animal can be considered sexually "nature"	150 weeks	> 24 weeks	30 weeks	90–150 weeks (variable)

for erection of the penis precedes the appearance of spermatozoa in the ejaculate by several months. In rams, the terminal segment of the epididymis is morphologically "adult" at 6 weeks, but the initial segment is not so until 18 weeks (Nilnophakoon, 1978). At puberty all the components of the male reproductive system have reached a sufficiently advanced stage of development for the system as a whole to be functional. The period of rapid development that precedes puberty is known as the prepubertal period, although this period is itself sometimes referred to as "puberty." During the postpubertal period, development continues and the reproductive tract reaches full sexual maturity months or even years after the age of puberty. In horses, significant increases in testicular weight, daily sperm production, and epididymal sperm reserves occur at 15 years of age. Some important anatomic changes that occur during postnatal development are summarized in Table 1–1.

TESTIS AND SCROTUM

The testis is secured to the wall of the vaginal process along the line of its epididymal attachment (Fig. 1–2). The position in the scrotum and the orientation of the long axis of the testis differ with the species (Fig. 1–1). The arrangement of tubules and ducts within the testis in the bull is shown in Figure 1–3. The histologic and cytologic characteristics of the cellular components of the seminiferous tubules are summarized in Table 1–2 and illustrated in Figure 1–11. (see also Hafez, 1975). The rete testis is lined by a nonsecretory cuboidal epithelium (Goyal/Williams, 1987).

Testicular size varies throughout the year in seasonal breeders (ram, stallion, camel). Removal of one testis results in considerable enlargement of the remaining gonad (up to 80% increase in weight). In the unilateral cryptorchid, removal of the descended testis may be followed by descent of the abdominal testis as it enlarges.

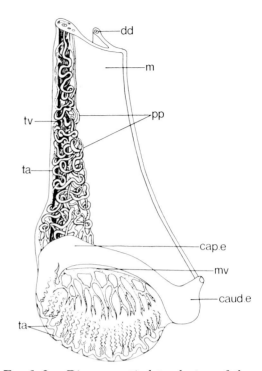

FIG. 1–2. Diagrammatic lateral view of the left testis of a stallion to show arrangement of arteries and veins. *cap. e,* Caput epididymidis; *caud. e,* cauda epididymidis; *dd,* ductus deferens; *m,* mesorchium; *mv,* marginal vein of testis; *pp,* pampiniform plexus of veins; *ta,* testicular artery; *tv,* testicular vein. (Adapted from Tagand and Barone (1956). Anatomie des Équidés Domestiques. 2, iii, Lyons, École Nat. Vet.)

The interstitial (Leydig) cells, which lie between the seminiferous tubules, secrete male hormones into the testicular veins and lymphatic vessels. The spermatogenic cells of the tubule divide and differentiate to form spermatozoa. Just before puberty, the sustentacular (Sertoli) cells of the tubule form a barrier (Vazama et al., 1988), which isolates the differentiating germ cells from the general circulation. These sustentacular cells contribute to fluid production by the tubule and may produce the Müllerian-inhibiting factor found in the rete fluid of adult males (Vigier et al., 1983). The sustentacular cells do not in-

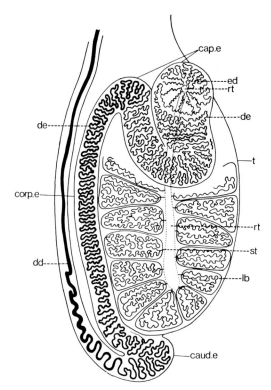

FIG. 1–3.   Schematic drawing of the tubular system of the testis and epididymis in the bull (for clarity the duct system of the rete testis is omitted).
cap. e, Caput epididymidis; *caud. e,* cauda epididymidis; *corp. e,* corpus epididymidis; *dd,* ductus deferens; *de,* duct of the epididymis; *ed,* efferent ductule; *lb,* lobule with seminiferous tubules; *rt,* rete testis; *st,* straight tubule; *t,* testis. (Simplified from Blom and Christensen (1960). Nord. Vet. Med. *12,* 453.)

crease in numbers after puberty is attained. This may limit spermiogenesis (Hochereau-de-Reviers et al., 1987; Johnson and Tatum, 1989). Daily sperm production varies between species but is about 15 to 30 $\times$ 10^6g of testicular tissue. Sperm production increases with age in the postpubertal period and is subject to seasonal changes in many species. Castration of prepubertal males suppresses sexual development. Regressive changes in behavior and structure take place following castration of adult males. Castration is a standard procedure in animal husbandry

to modify aggressive male behavior and to eliminate undesirable carcass qualities, e.g., boar taint. Testosterone exerts some sparing effects on protein metabolism and there is now a trend toward the use of intact males for meat production.

Thermoregulation of the Testis

For effective functioning, the mammalian testes must be maintained at a temperature lower than that of the body. Anatomic features of the testis and scrotum permit the regulation of testicular temperature. Temperature receptors in the scrotal skin can elicit responses that tend to lower *whole* body temperature and provoke panting and sweating (Robertshaw and Vercoe, 1980). The scrotal skin is noticeably lacking in subcutaneous fat. It is richly endowed with large adrenergic sweat glands, and its muscular (dartos) component enables it to alter the thickness and surface area of the scrotum and vary the closeness of the contact of the testes with the body wall. In the horse, this action may be supported by the smooth muscle within the spermatic cord and tunica albuginea, which can lower or raise the testis. In cold conditions, these smooth muscles contract, elevating the testes and wrinkling and thickening the scrotal wall. In hot conditions the muscles relax, lowering the testes within the thin-walled pendulous scrotum. The advantages offered by these mechanisms are enhanced by the special relationship of the veins and arteries.

In all farm animals, the testicular artery is a convoluted structure in the form of a cone, the base of which rests on the cranial or dorsal pole of the testis (Fig. 1–2). These arterial coils are intimately enmeshed by the so-called pampiniform plexus of testicular veins (Hees et al., 1990). In this countercurrent mechanism, arterial blood entering the testis is cooled by the venous blood leaving the testis. In the ram, blood in the testicular artery falls 4 °C in its course from the superficial inguinal ring to the surface of the testis; the blood in

TABLE 1–2. Functional Histology of the Testis

Segment	Histologic Characteristics
Tunica albuginea	A thick, white capsule of connective tissue surrounding the testis; made primarily of interlacing series of collagenous fibers with elongated and flattened nuclei of the fibroblasts.
Seminiferous tubules	Appear as large isolated structures, round or oblong in outline; varying appearance due to the complex coiling of the tubules at many different angles and levels. Between the tubules are blood vessels of variable diameter (smaller than tubules) packed with erythrocytes and embedded in small masses of interstitial (Leydig) cells, which produce the male sex hormones. Strands of connective tissue form a thin layer around each tubule.
Spermatogonia	Lie in the outermost region of the tubule; round nuclei appear as an irregular layer just within surrounding connective tissue. Nuclei may be recognized by small size and dark stain due to presence of large numbers of chromatin granules.
Primary spermatocytes	Located just inside an irregular layer of spermatogonia and Sertoli cells; nuclei are noticeably larger than those of the spermatogonia and stain lighter, although they still contain a considerable amount of granular chromatin.
Secondary spermatocytes	Maturation divisions and secondary spermatocytes are not seen in the average tubule owing to the short duration of these stages.
Spermatids	Located internally to primary spermatocytes. Cells are small and round with light-staining nuclei. Layer of spermatids may be several cells in thickness. Spermatozoa lie along the border of the lumen; their long tails extending into the cavity as filamentous structures, their heads appearing as dark-staining small points or short lines. The sperm heads are lodged in deep indentations of the surface of the Sertoli cell but never actually within the cytoplasm.
Sertoli cells	Large and relatively clear except for the prominent, dark-staining nucleolus. Cytoplasm is diffuse, and its limits are indefinite.

the veins is warmed to a similar degree between the testis and the superficial ring. The position of the arteries and veins close to the surface of the testis tends to increase direct loss of heat from the testis. In the boar, the scrotum is less pendulous (Fig. 1–1) and sweating is less efficient; this may explain the smaller difference between scrotal and rectal temperatures (2.3 °C) (Stone, 1981). Relatively short periods of high temperature and humidity can cause significant increases in abnormal spermatozoa ejaculated by bulls, rams, and boars.

EPIDIDYMIS AND DUCTUS DEFERENS

Three anatomic parts of the epididymis are recognized (Fig. 1–3). The *caput epididymidis* (head), in which a variable number of efferent ductules (13 to 20) (Hemeida et al., 1978) join the duct of the epididymis, forms a flattened structure applied to one pole of the testis. It continues as the narrow *corpus epididymidis* (body),

which terminates at the opposite pole in the expanded *cauda epididymidis* (tail). The contour of the cauda epididymidis is a visible feature in a live animal. The caput, corpus, and cauda epididymidis are less clearly differentiated in the stallion than in other farm species, and in the foal the attachment to the testis is very loose.

The middle region of each efferent duct shows marked secretory activity (Goyal et al., 1988). The convoluted duct of the epididymis is very long (bull, 36 m; boar, 54 m). Histologic features are shown in Figure 11–4. The wall of the duct of the epididymis has a prominent layer of circular muscle fibers and a pseudostratified epithelium of columnar cells. Three segments of the duct of the epididymis can be distinguished histologically; these do not coincide with the gross anatomic regions (Amann, 1987).

There is a progressive decrease in the height of the epithelium and stereocilia

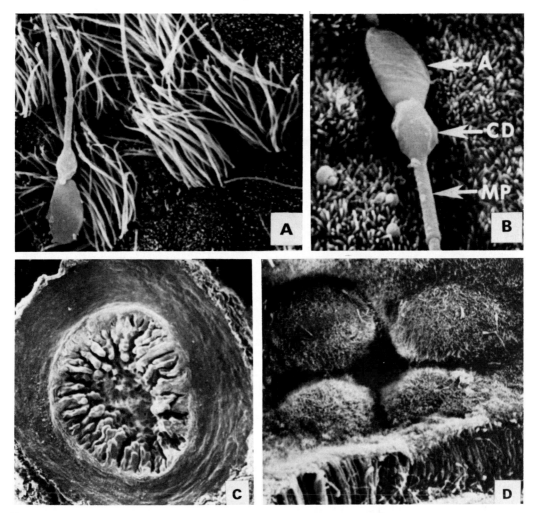

FIG. 1–4. *A*, Luminal surface of an efferent duct with ciliated and nonciliated cells and a spermatozoon. *B*, Short microvilli on the luminal surface of nonciliated cells in the *efferent ducts.* The spermatozoal cytoplasmic droplet (CD), acrosome (A), and middle piece (MP) are distinguishable by SEM (6,500×). *C*, Cross section of the distal cauda epididymidis. Thick layers of smooth muscle surround the highly infolded epithelium (25×). *D*, Sagittal section of the corpus epididymidis. Columnar cells covered with stereocilia. Undulations are due to differences in cell height (276×). (Johnson, L. et al. (1978). Am. J. Vet. Res. Courtesy of Dr. Larry Johnson.)

and a widening of the lumen throughout the three segments. The first two segments are concerned with sperm maturation, whereas the terminal segment is for sperm storage. The epithelial lining of the epididymis consists of different kinds of cells; principal columnar cells, small basal cells on basal membrane, and some lymphocytes.

The lumen of the epididymal tubules is lined with epithelium made of a basal layer of small cells and a surface layer of tall columnar ciliated cells. Masses of sperm are often found in the lumen. Spaces between tubules are filled with a loose connective tissue.

The ductus deferens leaves the cauda epidymidis and is supported in a separate fold of peritoneum; it is readily separable from the rest of the spermatic cord (Figs. 1–2, 1–3).

The mucosa of the ductus deferens is thrown into longitudinal folds. Near the epididymal end, the epithelium resembles

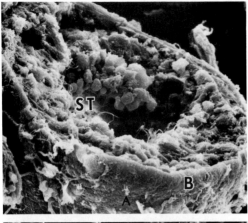

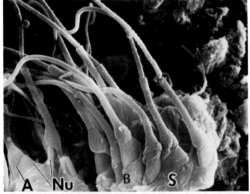

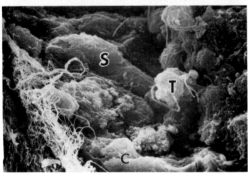

FIG. 1–5.   Scanning electron micrographs of testicular components. *A,* Cross section of a seminiferous tubule (ST). Note several "stages" of spermatogenesis, encased in a muscular boundary tissue (B) composed of myoid cells, collagen fibers, and glycoprotein matrix (438×). *B,* Clone of mid-late elongated spermatids from a canine testis. Note their insertion into the cytoplasm of Sertoli cells (S). The spermatids on the left side of the micrograph clearly show the relationship of the nucleus (Nu) and the cytoplasmic attachment (A) of the spermatid to the Sertoli cell (2,640×). *C,* Conical Sertoli cells (S) extend from the basement membrane, where they are obscured by collagen fibers, to the lumen of the tubule; round spermatids with flagellae are shown at the right (T). (930×). (C.J. Connell (1978). Spermatogenesis. *In* Scanning Electron Microscopy of Human Reproduction. E.S.E. Hafez (ed.). Ann Arbor, MI, Ann Arbor Science Pubs.)

that of the epididymis: The nonciliated cells have little secretory activity. The lumen is lined with pseudostratified epithelium. The ampulla of the ductus deferens is furnished with branched tubular glands, which, in the stallion, are highly developed and contribute ergothioneine to the ejaculate. The ejaculatory duct enters the urethra; in ruminants and the horse, it is formed by union with the duct of the vesicular gland. Fluid uptake and spermiophagy take place in the epithelium of the ejaculatory duct (Abou-Elmagd and Wrobel, 1990). Scanning electron microscopy has been used to evaluate functional ultrastructure of male reproductive organs (Fig. 1–4) with emphasis on spermatogenesis (Fig. 1–5). Large volumes of fluid (up to 60 ml in the ram) leave the testis daily, and most of this is absorbed in the caput epididymidis by the initial segment of the duct of the epididymis. Transport of spermatozoa through the epididymis takes about 9 to 13 days for the farm species and is thought to be due to flow of rete fluid, activity of the ciliated epithelium of the efferent ductules, and contractions of the muscular wall of the duct of the epididymis. Maturation of spermatozoa occurs during transmit through the epididymis; motility increases as spermatozoa enter the corpus epididymidis. The environment of the spermatozoa in the cauda epididymidis provides factors that enhance fertilizing ability; spermatozoa from this region give higher fertility than those from the corpus epididymidis (Amann, 1987).

Spermatozoa stored in the epididymis retain fertilizing capacity for several weeks; the cauda epididymidis is the principal storage organ, and it contains about 75% of the total epididymal spermatozoa. The special ability of the cauda epididymidis to store sperm depends on low scrotal temperatures and on the action of male sex hormone (Foldesy and Bedford, 1982). Spermatozoa stored in the ampullae constitute only a small part of the total extragonadal sperm reserves. Small numbers of nonmotile spermatozoa appear in ejaculates collected weeks or even months after castration; these are mainly derived from the ampullae.

ACCESSORY GLANDS

The prostate, vesicular, and bulbourethral glands pour their secretions into the urethra, where, at the time of ejaculation, they are mixed with the fluid suspension of spermatozoa and ampullary secretions from the ductus deferens (Fig. 1–6). All the accessory glands are essentially lobular branched tubular glands with smooth muscle prominent in the interstitial tissue. Weber et al. (1990) have demonstrated volumetric changes in the accessory glands of the stallion resulting from sexual stimulation (increased volume) and ejaculation (reduced volume). Anatomic

differences between farm species are shown in Figure 1–7.

Comparative Anatomy

The Vesicular Glands. These lie lateral to the terminal parts of each ductus deferens. In ruminants, they are compact lobulated glands. In the boar, they are large and less compact. In the stallion, they are large pyriform glandular sacs. The duct of the vesicular gland and the ductus deferens may share a common ejaculatory duct that opens into the urethra.

Prostate Gland. A distinct lobulated external part of body lies outside the thick urethral muscle, and a second internal or disseminated part surrounds the pelvic urethra deep to the urethral muscle. The disseminate prostate extends caudally as far as the ducts of the bulbourethral glands. The body of the prostate is small in the bull and large in the boar, while in the smaller ruminants, no body is visible. In the stallion, the prostate gland is wholly external.

The Bulbourethral Glands. These are dorsal to the urethra near the termination of its pelvic portion. In the bull they are almost hidden by the *bulbospongiosus muscle*, and in all species they are covered by a thick layer of striated bulboglandularis muscle. They are large in the boar and contribute the gel-like component of boar semen. In ruminants and the boar, the ducts of the bulbourethral glands open into urethral recesses, situated dorsally (Garrett, 1987), which may prevent passage of a catheter in these species.

Urethral Glands. The bull lacks urethral glands comparable with those found in man (Kainer et al., 1969). Glands of this name in the horse have been considered comparable to the disseminate prostate of ruminants, but in the boar, the disseminate prostate and the urethral glands are histologically distinct (McKenzie et al., 1938).

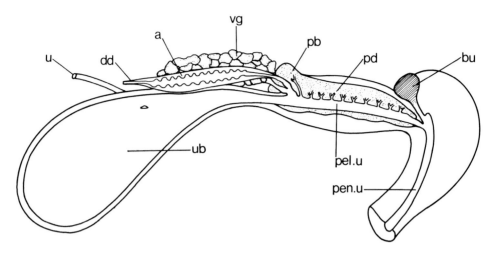

FIG. 1–6. Diagram to show the disposition of the glands that discharge into the pelvic urethra of the bull. *a*, Ampulla; *bu*, bulbourethral gland; *dd*, ductus deferens; *pb*, body of prostate gland; *pd*, disseminate part of prostate gland; *pel. u*, pelvic urethra; *pen. u*, penile urethra; *u*, ureter; *ub*, urinary bladder; *vg*, vesicular gland.

Function

Apart from providing a liquid vehicle for the transport of spermatozoa, the function of the accessory glands is obscure although much is known about the specific chemical agents contributed by the glands to the ejaculate (Spring-Mills and Hafez, 1979, 1980). Fructose and citric acid are important components of vesicular gland secretions of domestic ruminants. Citric acid alone is found in stallion vesicular glands; boar vesicular glands also contain little fructose and are characterized by a high content of ergothioneine and inositol.

Spermatozoa from the cauda epididymidis are capable of fertilization when inseminated without the addition of accessory gland secretions. The gel-like fraction of the boar ejaculate forms a plug in the vagina of mated females, but in commercial insemination practice, this fraction is removed from the semen by filtration.

In large animals, rectal palpation of some of the accessory glands is possible. The positions of these glands relative to the bony pelvis are shown in Figure 1–7.

In the pig, the size of the bulbourethral glands can be used to differentiate the cryptorchid from the castrated state. After prepubertal castration, the bulbourethral glands are small; at 100 kg body weight, each gland is about 5 cm long and weighs less than 1 g. In boars with retained testes, the glands are of normal size; each is over 10 cm long and weighs 45 g at 100 kg body weight (Lauwers et al., 1984). These differences can easily be felt, ventral to the rectum, with a finger inserted through the anus (Fig. 1–7).

PENIS AND PREPUCE

Structure

In the mammalian penis, three cavernous bodies are aggregated around the penile urethra (Figs. 1–8 and 1–9). The *corpus spongiosum penis*, which surrounds the urethra, is enlarged at the ischial arch to form the penile bulb. This bulb is covered by the striated *bulbospongiosus* muscle. The *corpus cavernosum penis* arises as a pair of *crura* from the ischial arch, which are covered by *ischiocavernosus* muscles. The corpus cavernosum penis continues to the apex of the penis as a more or less paired dorsal cavernous body. A thick covering (tunica albuginea) encloses the cav-

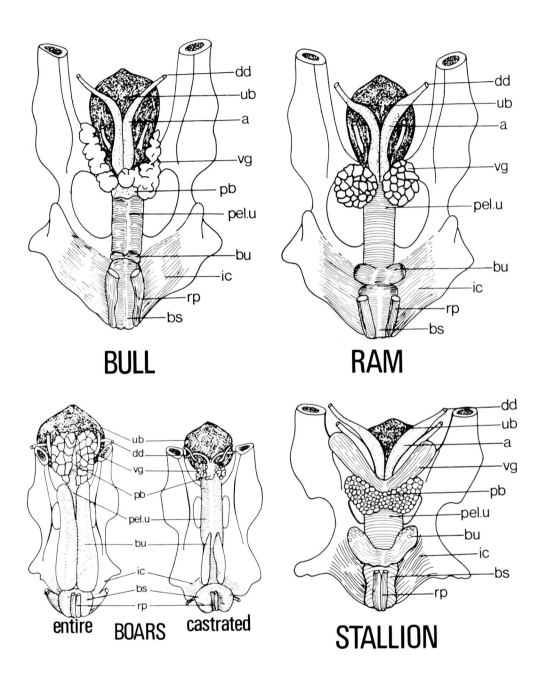

FIG. 1–7. Diagrams of the pelvic genitalia, within the pelvic bones, as seen from a dorsal view. (The cranial parts of the ilium have been removed.)
a, Ampulla; *bs*, bulbospongiosus muscle; *bu*, bulbourethral gland; *dd*, ductus deferens; *ic*, ischiocavernosus muscle; *pb*, body of prostate gland; *pel. u*, pelvic urethra; *rp*, retractor penis muscle; *ub*, urinary bladder; *vg*, vesicular gland. (Diagrams of bull, boar and stallion redrawn from Nickel (1954). Tierärztl. Umschau *9*, 386.)

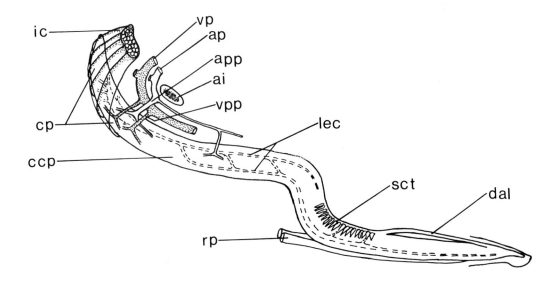

FIG. 1–8. Diagram to show mechanisms of erection in the penis of a ruminant. (1) Vasodilatation of penile artery (*ap*) increases blood flow to cavernous spaces of crus penis (*cp*) via deep artery of penis (*app*). (2) "Pumping" contractions of ischiocavernosus muscle (*ic*) pull crus penis craniodorsally against ischiatic arch (*ai*), occluding deep vessels (*app, vpp*), and compressing crus penis. (3) Compression of crus penis forces blood out of crus into body of corpus cavernosum penis (*ccp*) through longitudinal cavernous spaces ("erection canals"; *lec*), raising intracorporeal pressure to very high levels. (4) Filling of special dorsal cavernous tissue (*sct*) in distal bend of sigmoid flexure eliminates flexure as retractor penis muscle (*rp*) relaxes. (5) Cessation of "pumping" contractions of ischiocavernosus muscle allows blood to flow back into cavernous spaces of crus penis and so to drain through deep penile veins (*vpp*) into penile vein (*vp*).
The diagram also shows the dorsal apical ligament (dal).

ernous bodies. The *retractor penis* muscles in ruminants and swine control the effective length of the penis by their action on the sigmoid flexure.

In the stallion, the cavernous bodies contain large cavernous spaces; during erection, considerable increases in size result from accumulation of blood in these spaces. In bull, ram, and boar, the cavernous spaces of the corpus cavernosum penis are small, except in the crura and at the distal bend of the sigmoid flexure. The cavernous spaces of the corpus spongiosum penis are large, but distention is limited by the tunica albuginea. In ruminants and swine, erection results from the inflow of a relatively small volume of blood.

The subcutaneous tissues of the free part of the penis in some species form a well-developed cavernous body, the *cor-pus spongiosum glandis*, which is the erectile body of the glans penis. It is large in the stallion, poorly developed in the bull, and indistinct in the boar.

In ruminants and swine, the orifice of the prepuce is controlled by the cranial muscle of the prepuce; a caudal muscle may also be present. In the boar there is a large dorsal diverticulum in which urine and epithelial debris accumulate (see Fig. 1–1). The penile (inner) prepuce of the stallion is enclosed in a voluminous prepenile (outer) prepuce by the formation of a distinct and permanent preputial fold. Eversion of the prepuce can expose the epithelium to injury and infection.

Erection and Protrusion

Sexual stimulation produces dilatation of the arteries supplying the cavernous

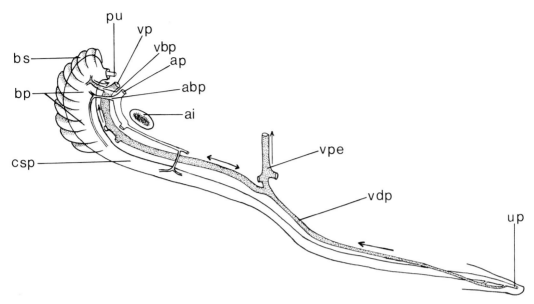

FIG. 1–9. Diagram to show mechanisms of ejaculation in the penis of a ruminant. (Arrows show direction of venous flow.) (1) Vasodilatation of penile artery (*ap*) increases blood flow to cavernous spaces of penile bulb (*bp*) via artery of penile bulb (*abp*). (2) "Pumping" contractions of bulbospongiosus muscle (*bs*) compress penile bulb and force blood from it into body of corpus spongiosum penis (*csp*), producing pressure waves along length of cavernous body. (3) Each pressure wave passing down corpus spongiosum penis results in venous drainage from distal cavernous spaces into dorsal vein of penis (*vdp*) and so to external pudendal (*vpe*) and/or penile (*vp*) veins. Note: bulbus penis is drained by veins of penile bulb (*vbp*). (4) The penile urethra (*pu*) runs through corpus spongiosum penis to terminate at urethral process (*up*) and is therefore compressed in a "peristaltic" fashion by waves of pressure in this cavernous body. Contents of the urethra are emptied, and ejaculation occurs.

bodies of the penis (especially the crura). In farm animals, parasympathetic fibers in the pelvic nerve (n. erigens) are probably responsible for this vasodilatation, but the neurotransmitter involved has not been identified, and a vasoactive polypeptide may be important (Dixson et al., 1984). Adrenergic reduction in motor control may also play a part in vasodilation (Domer et al., 1978). Stiffening and straightening of the penis in ruminants is caused by the ischiocavernosus muscle, which pumps blood from the cavernous spaces of the crura into the rest of the corpus cavernosum penis by way of special longitudinal cavernous spaces (erection canals) (Ashdown et al., 1979). High peak pressures have been recorded from the cavernous body of many species during erection (Beckett 1983).

In the normal adult bull, ram, billy goat, boar, and stallion there are no veins draining the distal levels of the corpus cavernosum penis (Ardalani and Ashdown, 1988), and this facilitates development of the erection pressure in the organ. Erection failures (impotence) arise from structural defects affecting the mechanisms outlined in Figure 1–8 rather than from psychological causes (Glossop and Ashdown, 1986). Rising pressure in the corpus cavernosum penis produces considerable elongation of the ruminant and porcine penis with little dilatation (Ashdown et al., 1981). Distention of the cavernous spaces of the corpus cavernosum penis, especially those at the distal bend of the sigmoid flexure, eliminates the flexure as the retractor muscles of the penis relax. When the penis of the bull is protruded, the prepuce is everted and stretched over the protruded organ. The fibrous architecture of the penile integument causes the penis to spiral when the integument is stretched (Fig. 1–10A$_2$); the urethral orifice turns in a counterclockwise direction through 300 ° as ejaculation occurs (Ashdown and Smith, 1969; Seidel and Foote, 1969). In normal service, this occurs after intromission. If it occurs before the penis enters the vestibule, intromission cannot be achieved.

Intromission in the bull lasts for about 2 seconds, and straightening of the penis after withdrawal often occurs abruptly as the dorsal apical ligament reasserts its action in keeping the penis straight. Withdrawal into the prepuce follows as the pressure in the cavernous spaces subsides. The fibrous architecture of the corpus cavernosum penis in the region of the sigmoid flexure tends to reform the flexure; this is assisted by shortening of the retractor penis muscle. The terminal 5 cm or so of the boar penis are spiralled (see Fig. 1–10), and during erection the whole visible length of the free end of the penis becomes spiralled around its long axis like a twisted rope. This spiralling results from the fibrous architecture of the corpus cavernosum penis (Ashdown et al., 1981). Intromission lasts for up to 7 minutes, during which time a large volume of semen is ejaculated. Spiral deviation does not occur in the ram or goat, and intromission is of short duration. In the horse intromission lasts for several minutes.

Emission and Ejaculation

Emission consists of movement of the spermatic fluid along the ductus deferens to the pelvic urethra, where it is mixed with secretions from the accessory glands. Ejaculation is the passage of the resultant semen along the penile urethra. Emission is brought about by smooth muscles, under the control of the autonomic nervous system. Ejaculation is brought about by striated muscles, under the control of somatic efferent components in the sacral nerves (deep perineal nerve). Electrical stimulation of ejaculation in farm animals is a crude imitation of the complex natural mechanisms. During natural service, the sensory nerve endings in the penile integument and the deeper penile tissues are essential to the process of ejaculation. The afferent nerves travel in the dorsal nerve of the penis.

Passage of semen along the ductus deferens is continual during sexual inactivity. Prinz and Zaneveld (1980) suggest that during sexual rest a complex random or cyclic process of sperm removal from the cauda epididymidis may aid the regulation of sperm reserves. Sexual excitement and ejaculation are accompanied by contractions of the cauda epididymidis and ductus deferens, which increase the rate of flow, but this is followed by movement of

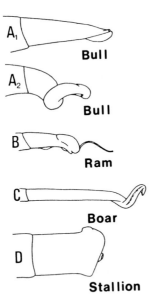

FIG. 1–10. Diagrams to show the shape of the free end of the penis. A_1 shows the shape of the penis just before intromission, and A_2 shows the shape after intromission when spiral deviation has occurred. *B* shows the shape of the penis during natural service. *C* does not show the full degree of spiralling that occurs during service. *D* was drawn after injection and shows enlargement of the erectile bodies (A_1, A_2 *and B from photographs. C and D from fixed specimens. Not drawn to scale.*)

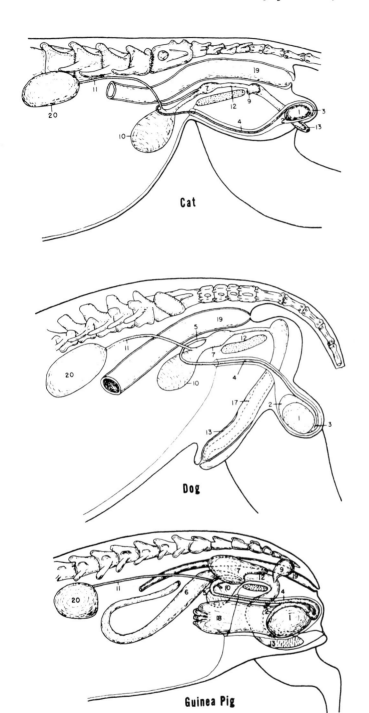

Cat

Dog

Guinea Pig

FIG. 1–11. Reproductive structures, *in situ*, of the cat, the dog, and the guinea pig. *1*, Testis; *2*, caput epididymidis; *3*, cauda epididymidis; *4*, ductus deferens; *5*, ampullary gland; *7*, prostate gland; *9*, bulbourethralgland; *10*, urinary bladder; *11*, ureter; *12*, urethera; *13*, penis; *17*, baculum; *18*, fat body; *19*, rectum; *20*, kidney. (From S. McKeever (1970). Male reproductive organs. *In* Reproduction and Breeding Techniques for Laboratory Animals. Hafez, E.S.E. (ed.). Philadelphia, Lea & Febiger.)

TABLE 1–3. Age and Weight of First Breeding and Semen Characteristics

Species	Beginning of Breeding Life Age (months)	Body Weight	Volume of Ejaculate Range	Mean	Sperm Concentration 10^8 per ml Range	Mean
Cat	9	3.5 kg	0.01–0.3	0.04	1.5–28	14
Dog	10–12	varies	2–25	9.0	0.6–5.4	1.3
Guinea pig	3–5	450 gm	0.4–0.8	0.6	0.05–0.2	0.1
Rabbit	4–12	varies	0.4–6	1.0	0.5–3.5	1.5

(From Hamner, C.E., 1970. The semen. In *Reproduction and Breeding Techniques for Laboratory Animals.* E.S.E. Hafez [ed.], Philadelphia, Lea & Febiger.)

spermatic fluid back into the epididymis and by a reduction in rate of flow for 10 to 20 hours after ejaculation. Overall, the number of spermatozoa passing through the ductus deferens is not increased by sexual activity.

Muscular contraction of the wall of the duct is controlled by sympathetic autonomic nerves of the pelvic plexus derived from the hypogastric nerves. In normal stallions, α-receptor stimulation and β-receptor blockade increase the sperm concentration in the ejaculate (Klug et al., 1982). Emission of semen from the duct into the urethra is accompanied by muscular contraction of the ampullae of the ductus deferens.

During ejaculation (see Fig. 1–9), the bulbospongiosus muscle compresses the penile bulb and so pumps blood from the penile bulb into the remainder of the corpus spongiosum penis. Unlike the corpus cavernosum penis, this cavernous body is normally drained by distal veins; peak pressures recorded during ejaculation are much lower than those in the corpus cavernosum penis (Beckett, 1983). The waves of pressure passing down the penile urethra may help to transport the ejaculate. Pressure changes in the corpus spongiosum penis during ejaculation are transmitted to the corpus spongiosum glandis; the glans penis enlarges in the ram, goat, and stallion but not in the bull.

LABORATORY ANIMALS

Species differences in the male reproductive organs are shown in Figure 1–11.

The relatively large inguinal canal and vaginal process in rodents and lagomorphs is associated with great mobility of the adult testis and epididymis. These organs can move from a wholly scrotal to a wholly abdominal position. Differences in relative sizes of the accessory glands are reflected in the semen characteristics (Table 1–3).

REFERENCES

Abou-Elmagd, A. and Wrobel, K.H. (1990). The epithelial lining of the bovine ejaculatory duct. Acta Anat. *139*, 60.

Amann, R.P. (1987). Function of the epididymis in bulls and rams. J. Reprod. Fertil. Suppl. *34*, 115.

Ardalani, G. and Ashdown, R.R. (1988). Venous drainage of the bovine corpus cavernosum penis in relationship to penile dimensions and age. Res. Vet. Sci. *45*, 174.

Ashdown, R.R., Barnett, S.W. and Ardalani, G. (1981). Impotence in the boar. (1): Angioarchitecture and venous drainage of the penis in normal boars. Vet. Rec. *109*, 375.

Ashdown, R.R., Gilanpour, H., David, J.E. and Gibbs, C. (1979). Impotence in the bull. (2): Occlusion of the longitudinal canals of the corpus cavernosum penis. Vet. Rec. *104*, 598.

Ashdown, R.R. and Smith, J.A. (1969). The anatomy of the corpus cavernosum penis of the bull and its relationship to spiral deviation of the penis. J. Anat. *104*, 153.

Beckett, S.D. (1983). Circulation to male reproductive organs. *In* Handbook of Physiology—The Cardiovascular System III. S.T. Shepherd and F.M. Aboud (eds.). Washington, D.C., American Physiological Society.

Dixson, A.F., Kendrick, K.H., Blank, M.A. and Bloom, S.R. (1984). Effects of tactile and electrical stimuli upon release of vasoactive intestinal polypeptide in the mammalian penis. J. Endocrinol. *100*, 249.

Domer, F.R., Wessler, G., Brown, R.L. and Charles, H.C. (1978). Involvement of the sympathetic nervous system in the urinary bladder internal sphincter and in penile erection in the anaesthetized cat. Invest. Urol. *15*, 404.

Foldesey, R.G. and Bedford, J.M. (1982). Biology of the scrotum (1): Temperature and androgen as determinants of the sperm storage capacity of the rat cauda epididymidis. Biol. Reprod. *26*, 673.

Garrett, P.D. (1987). Urethral recess in male goats, sheep, cattle and swine. J. Am. Vet. Med. Assoc. *191*, 689.

Glossop, C.E. and Ashdown, R.R. (1986). Cavernosography and differential diagnosis of impotence in the bull. Vet. Rec. *118*, 357.

Gondos, B. (1980). Development and differentiation of the testis and male reproductive tract. *In* Testicular Development: Structure and Function. A. Steinberger and E. Steinberger (eds.). New York: Raven Press.

Goyal, H.O., Eljack, A. and Mobini, C. (1988). Regional differences in the morphology of the ductuli efferentes of the goat. Anat. Histol. Embryol. *17*, 369.

Goyal, H.O. and Williams, C.S. (1987). The rete testis of the goat, a morphological study. Acta Anat. *130*, 151.

Hafez, E.S.E. (1975). Scanning electron microscopic atlas of mammalian reproduction. New York, Springer.

Hare, W.C.D. and Singh, E. (1979). Cytogenetics in animal reproduction. Farnham Royal, Commonwealth Agricultural Bureaux.

Hees, H., Kohler, T., Leiser, R., Hees, I. and Lips, T. (1990). Gefäss-Morphologie des Rinderhodens. Licht-und rasterelektron-mikroskopische Studien. Anat. Anz. *170*, 119.

Hemeida, N.A., Sack, W.O. and McEntee, K. (1978). Ductuli efferentes in the epididymis of boar, goat, ram, bull and stallion. Am. J. Vet. Res. *39*, 1892.

Hochereau-de-Reviers, M.T., Monet-Kunz, C. and Courot, M. (1987). Spermatogenesis and Sertoli cell numbers and function in rams and bulls. J. Reprod. Fertil. Suppl. *34*, 101.

Hoffer, A.P. and Hinton, B.T. (1984). Morphological evidence for a blood–epididymis barrier and the effects of gossypol on its integrity. Biol. Reprod. *30*, 991.

Johnson, L. and Tatum, M.E. (1989). Temporal appearance of seasonal changes in numbers of Sertoli cells, Leydig cells and germ cells in stallions. Biol. Reprod. *40*, 994.

Kainer, R.A., Faulkner, L.C. and Abdel-Raouf, M. (1969). Glands associated with the urethra of the bull. Am. J. Vet. Res. *30*, 963.

Klug, E., Deegen, E., Lazarz, B., Rojem, I. and Merkt, M. (1982). Effect of adrenergic neurotransmitters upon the ejaculatory process in the stallion. J. Reprod. Fertil. Suppl. *32*, 31.

Lauwers, J., Nicaise, M., Simoens, O. and de Vos, N.R. (1984). Morphology of the vesicular and bulbourethral glands in barrows and the changes induced by diethyl stilboestrol. Anat. Histol. Embryol. *13*, 50.

McKenzie, F.F., Miller, J.C. and Baugess, L.C. (1938). The reproductive organs and semen of the boar. Res. Bull. Mo. Agric. Exp. Sta. No. 279.

Nickel, R., Schummer, A. and Seiferle, E. (1973). The viscera of the domestic mammals. W.O. Sack (trans. and ed.). Berlin, Parey.

Nilnophakoon, N. (1978). Histological studies on the regional postnatal differentiation of the epididymis in the ram. Anat. Histol. Embryol. *7*, 253.

Prinz, G.S. and Zaneveld, L.J.D. (1980). Radiographic study of fluid transport in the rabbit vas deferens during sexual rest and after sexual activity. J. Reprod. Fertil. *58*, 311.

Robertshaw, D. and Vercoe, J.E. (1980). Scrotal thermoregulation of the bull. (*Bos* sp). Aust. J. Agric. Res. *31*, 401.

Seidel, G.E., Jr. and Foote, R.H. (1969). Motion picture analysis of ejaculation in the bull. J. Reprod. Fertil. *20*, 313.

Spring-Mills, E. and Hafez, E.S.E. (eds.)(1979). Accessory glands of the male reproductive tract. Ann Arbor, Ann Arbor Science Pubs.

Spring-Mills, E. and Hafez, E.S.E. (eds.) (1980). Male accessory organs. New York, Elsevier.

Stone, B.A. (1981). Thermal characteristics of the testis and epididymis of the boar. J. Reprod. Fertil. *63*, 551.

Vazama, F., Nishida, T., Kurohmara, M., and Hayashi, Y. (1988). The fine structure of the blood–testis barrier in the boar. Jap. J. Vet. Sci. *50*, 1259.

Vigier, B., Tran, D., duMesuil du Brusson, F., Heyman, Y. and Josso, N. (1983). Use of monoclonal antibody techniques to study the ontogeny of bovine anti-Müllerian hormone. J. Reprod. Fertil. *69*, 207.

Weber, J.A., Geary, R.T. and Woods, G.L. (1990). Changes in accessory sex glands of stallions after sexual preparation and ejaculation. J. Am. Vet. Med. Assoc. *196*, 1084.

Wensing, C.J.G. (1986). Testicular descent in the rat and a comparison of this process in the rat with that in the pig. Anat. Rec. *214*, 154.

2
Anatomy of Female Reproduction

E.S.E. HAFEZ

The female reproductive organs are composed of ovaries, oviducts, uterus, cervix uteri, vagina, and external genitalia. The internal genital organs (the first of four components) are supported by the broad ligament. This ligament consists of the mesovarium, which supports the ovary; the mesosalpinx, which supports the oviduct; and the mesometrium, which supports the uterus. In cattle and sheep, the attachment of the broad ligament is dorsolateral in the region of the ilium, so that the uterus is arranged like a ram's horns, with the convexity dorsal and the ovaries located near the pelvis (Fig. 2–1). The ovary, oviduct, and uterus are supplied primarily by autonomic nerves. The pudic nerve supplies sensory fibers and parasympathetic fibers to the vagina, vulva, and clitoris.

EMBRYOLOGY

The fetal reproductive system consists of two sexually nondifferentiated gonads, two pairs of ducts, a urogenital sinus, a genital tubercle, and vestibular folds (Fig. 2–2). This system arises primarily from two germinal ridges on the dorsal side of the abdominal cavity, and it can differentiate into a male or a female system, a condition referred to as *embryonic bisexuality*. The developmental fates of the sexual rudiments in the male and in the female fetus are shown in Table 2–1.

The sex of the fetus depends on inherited genes, gonadogenesis, and the formation and maturation of accessory reproductive organs. The expression of the genetic sex is a developmental process that depends on the functioning of the fetal gonads and, occasionally, on the functioning of the adrenal cortex.

Estrogen and androgen can cause sex reversal in male and female embryos, respectively, during only a brief period early in sexual differentiation. The age at which this bisexual potential is completely lost varies with the species.

Gonads

The gonads are formed from a group of large granulated yolk sac cells that invade the germinal ridges. Two invasions occur in the female. The initial one is abortive, but the second results in the formation of sex cords, which later spread upward into primordial germ cells (oogonia). The sex cords of the female are called *medullary cords*; those of the male are the *seminiferous tubules*.

The testis develops predominantly from the medulla of the sexually undifferentiated gonad, whereas the ovary arises primarily from its cortex.

Reproductive Ducts

Wolffian Müllerian ducts are both present in the sexually undifferentiated embryo. In the female, the Müllerian ducts develop into a gonaductal system and the wolffian ducts atrophy. The opposite is true in the male. The female Müllerian ducts fuse caudally to form a uterus, a cervix, and the anterior part of a vagina.

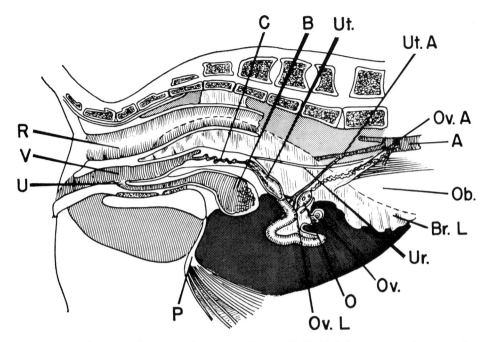

FIG. 2–1. Sagittal section through pelvic region (view of left side) showing attachments of rectum and urogenital tract, the pouches of the pelvic peritoneum, and attachments of the abdominal muscles to the prepubic tendon in the ewe.

A, Aorta; *B*, bladder; *Br.L*, broad ligament of uterus; *C*, cervix; *O*, ovary; *Ob.*, internal oblique muscle; *Ov.*, oviduct; *Ov. A*, ovarian artery; *Ov. L*, ovarian ligament; *P*, prepubic tendon; *R*, rectum; *U*, urethra; *Ur*, ureter; *Ut. A*, uterine artery; *V*, vagina.

In the male fetus, testicular androgen plays a role in the persistence and development of the wolffian ducts and the atrophy of the Müllerian ducts.

Urogenital Sinus

The urogenital sinus gives rise to the vestibule. The folds of skin that border the sinus form the lips of the vulva. The female phallus, or clitoris, homologous to the male penis, grows little in size.

THE OVARY

The ovary, unlike the testis, remains in the abdominal cavity. It performs both an exocrine (egg release) and endocrine function (steroidogenesis).

Prenatal Development

The predominant tissue of the ovary is the cortex. The primordial germ cells arise extragonadally and migrate through the yolk sac mesentery to the genital ridges. During fetal development, the oogonia are produced by mitotic multiplication. This is followed by the first meiotic division to form several million oocytes, a process that is arrested in the prophase. Subsequent atresia reduces the number of oocytes at the time of birth, a further reduction occurs at puberty, and only a few hundred are present during reproductive senescence. All ova arise from the original germ cell population of the genital ridge.

At birth, a layer of follicular cells surrounds the primary oocytes in the ovary to form the primordial follicles. At first these are scattered throughout the ovary, but during early neonatal life, they become localized in the peripheral cortical zone, beneath the tunica albuginea and surrounding the vascular medulla.

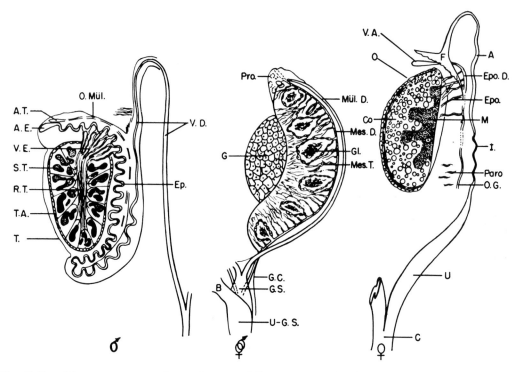

FIG. 2–2. Diagram representing embryonic differentiation of male and female genital systems. (*Center*) The undifferentiated system with its large mesonephros, mesonephric duct, müllerian duct, and undifferentiated gonad. Note that the müllerian and mesonephric ducts cross before they enter the genital cord. (*Right*) The female system, in which the ovary and müllerian ducts differentiate while the remnants of the mesonephros and mesonephric ducts atrophy into the epoophoron, paroophoron and Gartner's duct. (*Left*) The male system in which the testes and mesonephric (wolffian) ducts differentiate; the sole remnants of the müllerian ducts are the testicular appendix and prostatic utricle (vagina masculinus).

A	Ampulla	*G.C.*	Genital cord	*Paro*	Paroophoron
A.E.	Appendage of epididymis	*Gl.*	Glomerulus	*Pro.*	Pronephros
A.T.	Appendage of testis	*G.S.*	Genital sinus	*R.T.*	Rete tubules
B	Bladder	*I.*	Isthmus	*S.T.*	Seminiferous tubules
C	Cervix	*M*	Ovarian medulla	*T.*	Testis
Co	Ovarian cortex	*Mes. D.*	Mesonephric duct	*T.A.*	Testicle artery
Ep.	Epididymis	*Mes. T.*	Mesonephric tubules	*U*	Uterus
Epo.	Epoophoron	*Mul. D.*	Müllerian duct	*U-G.S*	Urogenital sinus
Epo. D.	Duct of epoophoron	*O*	Ovary	*V.A.*	Vesicular appendage
F	Fimbriae	*O.G.*	Obliterated Gartner's duct	*V.D.*	Vas deferens
G	Gonad (undifferentiated)	*O. Mul.*	Obliterated müllerian duct	*V.E.*	Vasa efferentia

The functional structure and ultrastructure of the ovary in farm animals are summarized and illustrated in Tables 2–2 and 2–3; and Figures 2–1 through 2–7. The shape and size of the ovary vary both with the species and the stage of the estrous cycle (Table 2–2). In cattle and sheep, the ovary is almond-shaped, whereas in the horse it is bean-shaped owing to the presence of a definite ovulation fossa, an indentation in the attached border of the ovary. The porcine ovary resembles a cluster of grapes because the protruding follicles and corpora lutea obscure the underlying ovarian tissue.

The part of the ovary that is not attached to the mesovarium is exposed and bulges into the abdominal cavity. The ovary,

TABLE 2–1. Developmental Fate of the Sexual Rudiments in the Male and the Female Mammalian Fetus

Sexual Rudiment	Male	Female
Gonad		
Cortex	Regresses	Ovary
Medulla	Testis	Regresses
Müllerian ducts	Vestiges	Uterus, oviducts, parts of vagina
Wolffian ducts	Epididymis, vas deferens	Vestiges
Urogenital sinus	Urethra, prostate, bulbourethral glands	Part of vagina, urethra
Genital tubercle (phallus)	Penis	Clitoris
Vestibular folds	Scrotum	Labia

(Frye, 1967. *Hormonal Control in Vertebrates.* New York, Macmillan.)

TABLE 2–2. Comparative Anatomy of the Ovary in the Adult Female of Farm Mammals

Organ	Animal			
	Cow	Ewe	Sow	Mare
Ovary				
Shape	Almond-shaped	Almond-shaped	Berry-shaped (cluster of grapes)	Kidney-shaped; with ovulation fossa
Weight of one ovary (g)	10–20	3–4	3–7	40–80
Mature graafian follicles				
Number	1–2	1–4	10–25	1–2
Diameter of follicle (mm)	12–19	5–10	8–12	25–70
Diameter of egg without zona pellucida (μ)	120–160	140–185	120–170	120–180
Mature corpus luteum				
Shape	Spheroid or ovoid	Spheroid or ovoid	Spheroid or ovoid	Pear-shaped
Diameter (mm)	20–25	9	10–15	10–25
Maximum size attained (days from ovulation)	10	7–9	14	14
Regression starts (days from ovulation)	14–15	12–14	13	17

composed of the medulla and cortex, is surrounded by the superficial epithelium, commonly known as *germinal epithelium* (Fig. 2–3). The ovarian medulla consists of irregularly arranged fibroelastic connective tissue and extensive nervous and vascular systems that reach the ovary through the hilus (attachment between ovary and mesovarium). The arteries are arranged in a definite spiral shape. The ovarian cortex contains ovarian follicles and/or corpora lutea at various stages of development or regression. (Table 2–3) The connective tissue of the cortex contains many fibroblasts, some collagen and reticular fibers, blood vessels, lymphatic vessels, nerves, and smooth muscle fibers.

Ovarian Blood Flow. The vascular pattern of the ovary changes with different hormonal states. Variations in the ar-

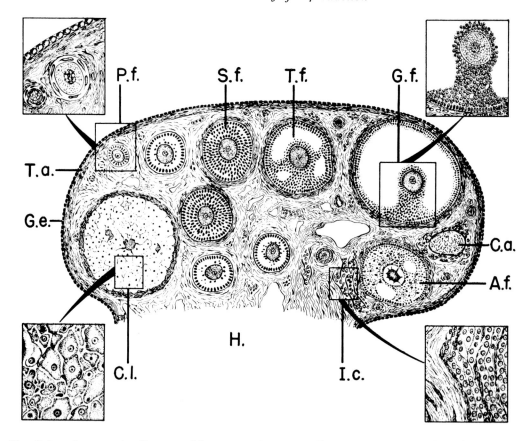

FIG. 2–3.   A composite diagram of the mammalian ovary. Progressive stages in the differentiation of a graafian follicle are indicated (*upper left to upper right*). The mature follicle may become atretic (*lower right*) or ovulate and form a corpus luteum (*lower left*).
A.f., Atretic follicle: *C.a.,* corpus albicans; *C.l.,* corpus luteum; *G.e.,* germinal epithelium; *G.f.,* graafian follicle; *H,* hilus; *I.c.,* interstitial cells; *P.f.,* primary follicle; *S.f.,* secondary follicle; *T.a.,* tunica albuginea; *T.f.,* tertiary follicle. (Partly adapted from Turner (1948). General Endocrinology. Philadelphia, W.B. Saunders.)

chitecture of the vessels allow adaptation of the blood supply to the needs of the organ. The relative distribution of the blood among the various compartments of the ovary is altered without affecting the total ovarian blood supply.

The intraovarian distribution of blood undergoes remarkable changes during the preovulatory period. In sheep, ovarian venous flow drops from about 8 ml/min 73 days before ovulation to 2 ml/min at estrus. A corresponding drop in ovarian arterial blood flow per minute is paralleled by a sharp decline in the flow of lymph from the ovary (Moor et al., 1975).

Arterial blood flow to the ovary varies in proportion to luteal activity. Hemodynamic changes seem to be important in regulating corpus luteum (CL) function and lifespan. Thus, changes in blood flow precede the decline in progesterone secretion, whereas restriction of ovarian blood flow causes premature CL regression. At the time of luteolysis in ewes, there is a reduction in ovarian blood flow as well as an increase in arteriole-venule shunting within the ovary (Niswender et al., 1976).

Blood flow to the bovine ovary is highest during the luteal phase, decreases with lu-

TABLE 2–3.　Functional Histology of the Mammalian Ovary

Anatomic Functional Unit	Histologic Characteristics
Superficial epithelium	A surface layer of flattened epithelium (commonly and incorrectly known as *germinal epithelium*) with abundant microvilli.
Tunica albuginea	Dense, fibrous connective tissue covering the whole ovary just beneath the superficial epithelium. Connective tissue cells near the surface are arranged roughly parallel to the ovarian surface and are somewhat denser than the cells lying toward the medulla.
Ovarian cortex	Contains several primary follicles (with oocytes in a quiescent state) and a few large follicles. During each estrous cycle, variable numbers of follicles undergo rapid growth and development, culminating in the process of ovulation.
Ovarian medulla	Loose connective tissue that contains nerves, lymphatics, and tortuous thin-walled blood vessels, collagen and elastic fibers, fibroblasts, and scattered smooth muscle cells.
Ovarian stroma	Poorly differentiated, embryonal-mesenchymal-like cells capable of undergoing complex morphologic alterations during the reproductive life; stromal cells can give rise to theca interna cells or interstitial cells.
Smooth muscle	Smooth muscle cells are present throughout the ovary, especially in the cortical stroma, where they intermingle with the cells of the theca. Ovarian myoid cells are similar to smooth muscle cells of other tissues. These cells contain large numbers of microfilaments arranged in characteristic bundles and also micropinocytotic vesicles located just beneath the plasmalemma. The cholinergic receptors on smooth muscle cells may mediate the contraction of the graafian follicle. Thus, smooth muscle cells and neural elements may be directly involved in ovulation. The presence of smooth muscle cells, especially in the perifollicular regions, may be involved in "squeezing the follicle" during ovulation.
Ovarian follicles 　Primary follicle	An oocyte enclosed by a single layer of flattened or cuboidal follicular cells and surrounded by interstitial tissue.
Growing follicle	Oocyte with increased diameter and increased number of layers of follicular cells; zona pellucida is present around the oocyte.
Secondary follicle	Flattened granulosa cells of the primordial or unilaminar follicle proliferate, assuming an irregular, polyhedral appearance.
Tertiary (vesicular) follicle	Under the influence of pituitary gonadotrophins, the granulosa cells of multilayered follicles secrete a fluid, the liquor folliculi, which accumulates in the intercellular spaces. The continued secretion and accumulation of liquor folliculi result in the dissociation of granulosa cells, which causes the formation of a large, fluid-filled cavity—the antrum. The zona pellucida is surrounded by a solid mass of radiating follicular cells, forming the corona radiata.
Graafian follicle	Follicular cells increase in size; the antrum is filled with follicular fluid (liquor folliculi). The oocyte is pressed to one side, surrounded by an accumulation of follicular cells (cumulus oophorus); elsewhere in the follicular cavity an epithelium of fairly uniform thickness called the *membrana granulosa* has formed. The theca interna and theca externa have formed.
Preovulatory follicle	A blister-like structure protruding from the ovarian surface due to rapid accumulation of follicular fluid and thinning of the granulosa layer. The viscous liquor folliculi is formed from the secretions of granulosa cells and plasma proteins transported into the follicle by transudation. The cumulus oophorus is detached from the thinned and extensively dissociated stratum granulosum. The oocyte lies free in the liquor folliculi, surrounded by an irregular mass of cells. Dramatic changes are noticeable at the subcellular level, particularly in the Golgi complex, which is involved in the formation of the zona pellucida and cortical granules. The oocyte, in the prophase of meiosis (dictyate stage), re-

TABLE 2–3. **Functional Histology of the Mammalian Ovary (*Continued*)**

Anatomic Functional Unit	Histologic Characteristics
	sumes meiosis several hours before ovulation. The first meiotic (maturational) division is associated with extrusion of the first polar body, which may briefly remain attached to the oocyte by a cytoplasmic bridge.
Corpus hemorrhagicum	The follicular cavity is filled with lymph and blood from broken thecal vessels, blood from follicular fluids, and blood from small vessels that hemorrhaged at ovulation. It acts as a "stopper," sealing the residual cavity after discharge of oocyte. Intact vessels and connective tissue cells from the surrounding theca begin to proliferate.
Corpus luteum	The transformation of a ruptured follicle into a corpus luteum involves characteristic folding of the granulosa layer toward the central portion of the residual cavity; luteinization of the granulosa cells occurs under the influence of LH. Lutein cells, polyhedral in form or without definite cell walls, are arranged in irregular masses. The cytoplasm may be clear or granular according to the secretory and functional activity.
Corpus albicans	White fibrous tissue that forms from the corpus luteum of previous ovulations.

teal regression, and reaches a nadir just before ovulation. Ovarian blood flow increases with the newly developing CL. The decline in blood flow seems to follow the abrupt decline at the time of regression of the CL (Wise et al., 1982). Uterine lymphatics may play a role in the transport of estrogens from a uterine horn to the ipsilateral ovary.

Ovariectomy

Unilateral ovariectomy (ULO) in the adult cyclic rats may lead to functional compensation of follicle growth and ovulation in the remaining ovary during the ongoing cycle. This compensatory mechanism involves increased FSH secretion 6 to 18 hours after unilateral ovariectomy.

Removal of one ovary causes a compensatory increase in the weight of the remaining ovary (compensatory ovarian hypertrophy) in the guinea pig. Ovarian nerves may participate in the development of compensatory hypertrophy after unilateral ovariectomy. Ovarian adrenergic nerves may normally exert a tonic inhibitory influence on the selection of follicles for maturation and/or ovulation (Curry, T.E., Jr., et al., 1984).

Corpus Luteum

The CL develops after the collapse of the follicle at ovulation. The inner wall of the follicle develops into macro- and microscopic folds that penetrate the central cavity. These folds consist of a central core of stromal tissue and large blood vessels, which become distended. The cells develop a few days before ovulation. They regress quickly, and within 24 hours after ovulation all remaining thecal cells are in an advanced stage of degeneration. Hypertrophy and luteinization of the granulosa cells commence after ovulation. The luteal tissue enlarges mainly through hypertrophy of the lutein cells.

Progesterone is secreted by the lutein cells as granules. In the ewe, this process appears to be maximal at day 10 of the cycle and begins to taper off noticeably at day 12. The secretory activity declines gradually until day 14.

In aged animals, the functions of the CL decline as a result of (a) an inability of follicular cells (granulosa and theca interna) to respond fully to hormonal stimuli, (b) changes in the quantity and/or quality of hormone secretion, and (c) a reduced stimulus for hormone secretion.

Development. The increase in the weight of the CL is initially rapid. In general, the period of growth is slightly longer than half the estrous cycle. In the cow, the weight and progesterone content of the CL increase rapidly between days 3 and 12 of the cycle (Fig. 2–4) and remain relatively constant until day 16, when regression begins. In the ewe and sow, corpora lutea increase rapidly in weight and progesterone content from day 2 to day 8, and remain relatively constant until day 15, when regression begins (Erb et al., 1971).

The diameter of the mature CL is larger than that of a mature graafian follicle except in the mare, in which it is smaller (Table 2–2).

The CL stimulates follicular development and ovulation through a local intraovarian mechanism. For example, the presence of a previously formed CL increases the efficacy of pregnant mare serum gonadotrophin (PMSG) in inducing ovulation in sheep.

Regression. If fertilization does not occur, the CL regresses, allowing other larger ovarian follicles to mature. As these cells degenerate, the whole organ decreases in size, becomes white or pale brown, and is known as the *corpus albicans*. Regressive changes include thickening of the walls of the arteries in the CL, a decrease in cytoplasmic granulation, a rounding of the cell outline, and peripheral vacuolation of the large luteal cells (Figs. 2–5 to 2–7). After two or three cycles, a barely visible scar of connective tissue remains. Remnants of the bovine corpus albicans persist during several

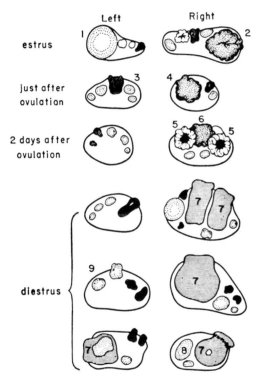

FIG. 2–4. Diagrammatic illustration of the morphologic changes in the estrous cycle of bovine ovary. *1*, Ripe follicle; *2*, regressing corpus luteum (brick brown); *3*, collapsed follicle—surface wrinkled and walls bloodstained; *4*, regressing corpus luteum (bright yellow); *5*, twin corpora lutea—some hemorrhage; *6*, regressing corpus luteum (*bright yellow*); *7*, corpus luteum of diestrus; *8*, largest follicle; *9*, corpus albicans. (Redrawn from Arthur (1964). Wright's Obstetrics. London, Bailliere, Tindall & Cox.)

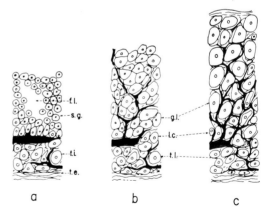

FIG. 2–5. Diagram showing the organization of cells in the corpus luteum of the ewe. *a*, Corpus haemorrhagicum; *b*, corpus luteum of the second day following estrus; *c*, corpus luteum of the fourth day following estrus. Blood vessels are shown with heavy black lines. *f.l.*, Lake of follicular fluid; *g.l.*, lutein cells from the membrana granulosa; *t.i.*, theca interna; *t.e.*, theca externa. (Adapted from Warbritton (1934). J. Morphol. *56*, 181.)

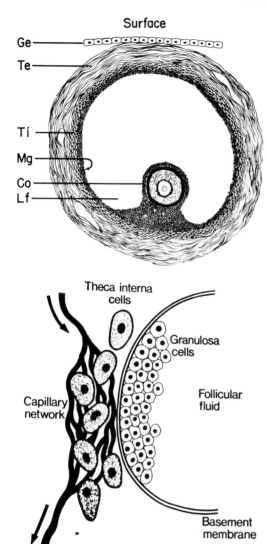

Surface

Ge

Te

Ti

Mg

Co

Lf

Theca interna cells

Capillary network

Granulosa cells

Follicular fluid

Basement membrane

FIG. 2–6. (*Top*) Illustration of a graafian follicle. *Co*, Cumulus oophorus; *Ge*, germinal epithelium; *Lf*, liquor folliculi; *Mg*, membrana granulosa; *Te*, theca externa; *Ti*, theca interna. (*Bottom*) The structure of the wall of the graafian follicle showing how the granulosa cells are deprived of a blood supply by the basement membrane. (Baird (1972). *In* Reproduction of Mammals. C.R. Austin and R.V. Short (eds.). Cambridge, Cambridge University Press.)

successive cycles. The bovine CL of the estrous cycle begins to regress 14 to 15 days after estrus, and its size may decrease by half within 36 hours.

Luteolysis. Estrogen-induced luteolysis, probably mediated through stimulation of uterine prostaglandin $F_{2\alpha}(PGF_{2\alpha})$ during the estrous cycle of the ewe, is responsible for the normal regression of the CL. An embryo must be in the uterus of ewes on days 12 and 13 after mating in order for the CL to be maintained. This time represents the state at which the uterus initiates steps leading to luteolysis.

$PGF_{2\alpha}$ is a potent, naturally occurring luteolysin in sheep. Various doses and routes of administration of exogenous $PGF_{2\alpha}$ are effective in producing complete luteal regression. Injection of $PGF_{2\alpha}$ into a large follicle in the ovary with CL is one of the more effective routes. Indomethacin [1-(*p*-chlorobenzoyl)-5-methoxy-2-methylindole-3-acetic acid] blocks the estrogen-induced release of $PGF_{2\alpha}$ from the ovine uterus. Intrauterine injections of indomethacin prevent estrogen-induced luteal regression in cattle and sheep.

The main uterine vein and the ovarian artery are the proximal and distal components of a local venoarterial pathway involved in the luteolytic and antiluteolytic effects. Hysterectomy abolishes the luteolytic effect and causes persistence of the CL. Luteolysis in the pig is associated with increased plasma prostaglandin PGF in the utero-ovarian vein (Guthrie and Rexroad, 1981).

Changes in Blood Flow to Corpus Luteum. The presence of a functional CL greatly increases blood flow to the ovary (Niswender et al., 1976); the regional blood flow within the CL uses 15μ radioactive microspheres. In the ewe, blood flow to the luteal ovary increases from less than 1 ml/min to 3 to 7 ml/min as the CL develops (Niswender et al., 1976). During regression, blood flow to the luteal ovary declines sharply (Fig. 2–8).

The changes in blood flow to the luteal tissue can be attributed to changes in flow to the CL, which receives most of the blood supply. Blood flow to the CL plays a role in the regulation of this gland and in regulating the activity of gonadotropins at the luteal cell level. A secondary action

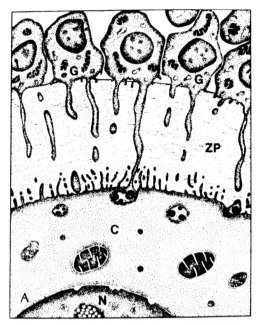

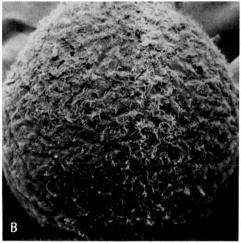

FIG. 2-7. *A*, Structure of fully formed zona pellucida (*ZP*) around an oocyte in a graafian follicle. Microvilli arising from the oocyte interdigitate with processes from the granulosa cells (*G*). These processes penetrate into the cytoplasm of the oocyte (*C*) and may provide nutrients and maternal protein; (*N*) oocyte nucleus. (Baker (1972). *In* Reproduction in Mammals. C.R. Austin and R.V. Short (eds.). Cambridge, Cambridge University Press.) *B*, Egg after removal of zona pellucida.

of LH may be to increase blood flow to the CL. $PGF_{2\alpha}$ affects the vascular component of the CL.

Corpus Luteum and Pregnancy. Progestogens are necessary for the maintenance of pregnancy. They act in part by altering the ionic permeability across the myometrial muscle cell membrane, resulting in an increased resting membrane potential and lowered cellular conduction and excitability. Some progestogens serve as immediate precursors to other steroids that are also necessary during pregnancy.

Except in the mare, there is an obligatory requirement for continued secretory activity of the CL throughout pregnancy because the placenta does not secrete progesterone in these species. Ovariectomy of the gilt at any time during pregnancy results in abortion within 2 to 3 days. After removing one ovary or the corpora lutea from each ovary on day 40 of gestation, a minimum of five corpora lutea is needed to maintain gestation.

Maternal Recognition of Pregnancy. Blastocysts must be present by day 12 after ovulation in ewes and day 13 in gilts to extend the lifespan of the CL. Maternal recognition of pregnancy in cattle occurs between the fifteenth and seventeenth days of gestation. Plasma concentrations of progesterone are higher in pregnant than in nonpregnant cows within 8 days after breeding. However, little is known about the physiologic mechanisms that control maintenance of the CL and synthesis of progesterone during early pregnancy.

The CL of pregnancy is known as the *corpus luteum verum* and may be larger than the *corpus luteum spurium* (false yellow body) of the estrous cycle. In cattle it increases in size for 2 to 3 months of gestation, regresses for 4 to 6 months, and thereafter remains relatively constant until calving, when it degenerates within 1 week postpartum.

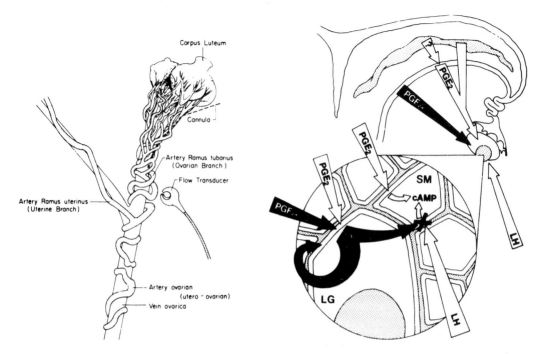

FIG. 2–8.   (*Left*) Anatomy of the bovine ovarian vasculature and location of the venous catheter in the anastomosing ovarian vein and ovarian artery blood flow transducer. (Wise, J.H. et al. (1982). Ovarian function during the estrous cycle of the cow. J. Anim. Sci. *55*: 627–637.) Ovarian blood flow and progesterone release rate. (*Right*) A hypothetical model depicting the interaction of the embryo, uterus and corpus luteum during luteolysis and early pregnancy. Large luteal cells (LG); small luteal cells (SM). (Silva et al. (1984). Cellular and molecular mechanisms involved in luteolysis and maternal recognition of pregnancy in the ewe. Anim. Reprod. Sci. *7*: 57–74.)

THE OVIDUCT

There is an intimate anatomic relationship between the ovary and the oviduct. In farm mammals, the ovary lies in an open ovarian bursa in contrast to some species (e.g., rat, mouse) in which it lies in a closed sac. This bursa in farm animals is a pouch consisting of a thin peritoneal fold of mesosalpinx, which is attached to a suspended loop at the upper portion of the oviduct (Fig. 2–9). In cattle and sheep, the ovarian bursa is wide and open. In swine it is well-developed, and although open, it largely encloses the ovary. In horses it is narrow and cleft-like and encloses only the ovulation fossa.

Anatomy

The morphology and functional anatomy of the mammalian oviduct are sum-marized and illustrated in Tables 2–4 and 2–5 and Figures 2–10 through 2–17. The oviducts are suspended in the mesosalpinx, a peritoneal fold that is derived from the lateral layer of the broad ligament. The length and degree of coiling of the oviduct vary in farm mammals. The oviduct may be divided into four functional segments: the fringe-like *fimbriae;* the funnel-shaped abdominal opening near the ovary—the *infundibulum;* the more distal dilated *ampulla;* and, the narrow proximal portion of the oviduct connecting the oviduct with the uterine lumen— the *isthmus* (Fig. 2–10).

The size of the infundibulum varies with the species and age of the animal; the surface area is 6 to 10 cm^2 in sheep, and 20 to 30 cm^2 in cattle. The opening of the infundibulum, the ostium abdominale, lies

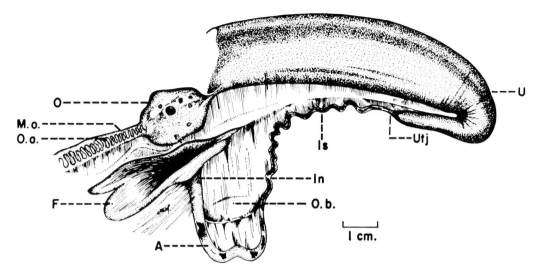

FIG. 2–9. Anatomic relationship between the ovary and the oviduct in the ewe. *A,* Ampulla; *F,* fimbriae; *In,* infundibulum; *Is,* isthmus; *M.o.,* mesovarium; *O,* ovary; *O.a.,* ovarian artery; *O.b.,* ovarian bursa; *U,* uterus; *Utj,* uterotubal junction. Note the suspended loop to which the ovarian bursa is attached. The oviduct in the ewe is pigmented.

in the center of a fringe of irregular processes that form the extremity of the oviduct, the fimbriae. The fimbriae are unattached except for one point at the upper pole of the ovary. This ensures close approximation of the fimbriae and the ovarian surface.

The ampulla, accounting for about half of the oviductal length, merges with the constricted section known as the *isthmus.* The anatomic and physiologic significance of this ampullary–isthmic junction is still unknown. The isthmus is connected directly to the uterus; it enters the horn in the form of a small papilla in the mare. No well-defined sphincter muscle is present at this point, the uterotubal junction. In the sow, however, this junction is guarded by long finger-like mucosal processes. In the cow and ewe, there is a flexure at the uterotubal junction, especially during estrus.

Muscle also extends from these layers into the connective tissue of the mucosal folds, permitting coordinated contractions of the entire wall. The thickness of the musculature increases from the ovarian to the uterine end of the oviduct.

Oviductal Mucosa

The oviductal mucosa is made of primary, secondary, and tertiary folds. The mucosa in the ampulla is thrown into high, branched folds that decrease in height toward the isthmus and become low ridges in the uterotubal junction. The complex arrangement of these mucosal folds in the ampulla almost completely fills the lumen so that there is only a potential space. Fluid is at a minimum; thus, the cumulus mass is the intimate contact with the ciliated mucosa (Figs. 2–11 to 2–14).

The mucosa consists of one layer of columnar epithelial cells. The underlying submucosa of smooth muscle fibers and connective tissue is permeated by fine blood and lymph vessels. The epithelium contains ciliated and nonciliated cells.

Ciliated Cells. The ciliated cells of the oviductal mucosa have a slender motile cilia (kinocilia) that extend into the lumen. The rate of beat of cilia is affected by the levels of ovarian hormones, activity being maximal at ovulation or shortly afterward when the stroke of the cilia in the fimbriated portion of the oviducts is closely synchronized and directed toward the os-

TABLE 2–4. **Comparative Anatomy of the Reproductive Tract in the Adult Nonpregnant Female of Farm Mammals**

Organ	Cow	Ewe	Sow	Mare
		Animal		
Oviduct				
Length (cm)	25	15–19	15–30	20–30
Uterus				
Type	Bipartite	Bipartite	Bicornuate	Bipartite
Length of horn (cm)	35–40	10–12	40–65	15–25
Length of body (cm)	2–4	1–2	5	15–20
Surface of lining of endometrium	70–120 Caruncles	88–96 Caruncles	Slight longitudinal folds	Conspicuous longitudinal folds
Cervix				
Length (cm)	8–10	4–10	10	7–8
Outside diameter (cm)	3–4	2–3	2–3	3.5–4
Cervical lumen				
Shape	2–5 Annular rings	Several annular rings	Corkscrew-like	Conspicuous folds
Os uteri				
Shape	Small and protruding	Small and protruding	Ill-defined	Clearly-defined
Anterior vagina				
Length (cm)	25–30	10–14	10–15	20–35
Hymen	Ill defined	Well developed	Ill defined	Well developed
Vestibule Length (cm)	10–12	2.5–3	6–8	10–12

The dimensions included in this table vary with age, breed, parity, and plane of nutrition.

tium. The action of ciliary beat seems to enable the egg within the surrounding cumulus cells to be stripped from the surface of the collapsing follicles toward the ostium of the oviduct. The percentage of ciliated cells decreases gradually in the ampulla toward the isthmus and reaches a maximum in the fimbriae and infundibulum. Ciliated cells are noted in large numbers at the apices of the mucosal folds. Variations in the percentage of ciliated and secretory cells along the length of the oviduct have some functional significance. Ciliated cells are most abundant where the egg is picked up from the ovarian surface, whereas secretory cells are abundant where luminal fluids are needed as a medium for the interaction of eggs and sperm.

The cilia beat toward the uterus. Their activity, coupled with oviductal contractions, keeps oviductal eggs in constant rotation, which is essential for bringing egg and sperm together (fertilization) and preventing oviductal implantation. Ciliation of the oviduct is hormonally controlled in the rhesus monkey: Cilia disappear almost completely after hypophysectomy and develop in response to administration of exogenous estrogens. The oviducts atrophy and deciliate during anestrus, hypertrophy and become reciliated during proestrus and estrus, and atrophy and deciliate during pregnancy.

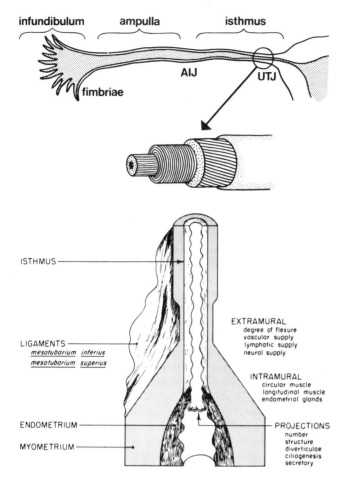

FIG. 2–10. (*Top*) Major segment of the oviduct. (*Bottom*) Anatomic variability of the uterotubal junction in different species.

Infections of the female reproductive tract are associated with dramatic changes in cell morphology. Infection is usually associated with the loss of ciliated cells. Inflamed oviductal epithelium has ciliated cells devoid of cilia that retain a certain number of ciliary basal bodies, the precursors of ciliary shafts. A decrease in the number of cilia may lead to the accumulation of tubal fluid and inflammatory exudate, which contributes to the agglutination of tubal plicae and subsequent development of salpingitis.

Nonciliated Cells. The secretory cells of the oviductal mucosa are nonciliated and characteristically contain secretory granules, the size and number of which vary widely among species and during different phases of the estrous cycle. The apical surface of the nonciliated cells is covered with numerous microvilli. Secretory granules accumulated in epithelial cells during the follicular phase of the cycle are released into the lumen after ovulation, causing a reduction in epithelial height.

Vasculature. The vasculature of the oviduct is derived from the uterine and ovarian arteries, which together supply arcades of vessels along the length of the oviduct. The remarkable increase in the prominence of the vasculature, largely regulated by ovarian estrogens, is partly associated with the enhanced secretory function of the oviduct.

Innervation. As with other segments of the female reproductive tract, the oviduct is partially supplied by "short" adrenergic neurons, which are physiopharmaco-

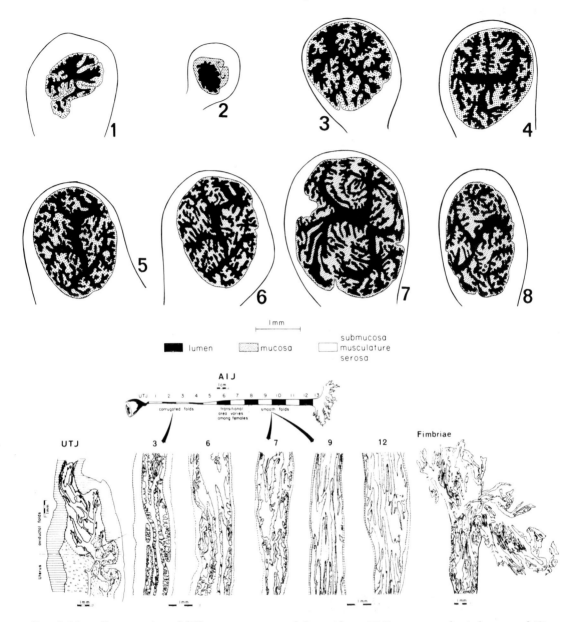

FIG. 2–11. Cross section of different segments of the oviduct. (1) Represents the isthmus and (8) represents the infundibulum. Note the variability in the degree of complexity of the mucosal folds.

logically different from those of the more common "long" adrenergic neurons. In addition to receiving nerves from pre- and paravertebral ganglia (long adrenergic neurons), the oviduct receives a portion from ganglionic formations in the utero-vaginal area (short adrenergic neurons).

The degree of innervation varies in the different muscle layers and in different regions of the oviduct. Adrenergic innervation is particularly prominent in the circular musculature of the isthmus and at the ampullary–isthmic junction, where adrenergic nerve terminals are in close contact

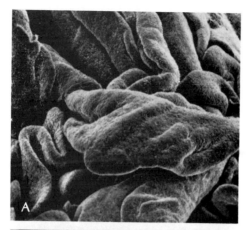

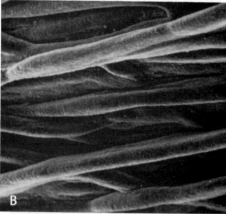

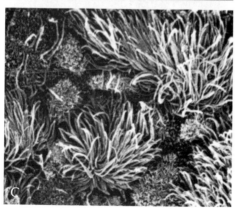

FIG. 2–12.   Scanning electron micrographs of the oviductal epithelium. *A*, Mucosal folds that protrude in the lumen of ampulla (37×). *B*, Mucosal folds that protrude in the lumen of the isthmus (40×). *C*, Micrograph of the oviductal epithelium in the isthmus (6,000×).

with individual smooth muscle cells. The dense adrenergic innervation permits the isthmus to act as a physiologic sphincter, which may be important for regulating egg transport.

Function of the Oviduct

Several in vivo and in vitro techniques have been used to study the function of the oviduct (Table 2–5). The oviduct has the unique function of conveying the eggs and spermatozoa in opposite directions, almost simultaneously. The structure of the oviduct is well adapted to its multiple functions. The fringe-like fimbriae transport ovulated eggs from the ovarian surface to the infundibulum. The eggs are transported through the mucosal folds to the ampulla, where fertilization and early cleavage of fertilized eggs take place. The embryos remain in the oviduct for 3 days before they are transported to the uterus. The mesosalpinx and oviductal musculature coordinate ovarian hormones, estrogen, and progesterone. The uterotubal junction controls, in part, the transport of sperm from the uterus to the oviducts.

The oviduct provides an optimal environment for union of the gametes and for early embryo development. This environment is both nutritive and protective for the sperm, oocyte, and subsequent embryo. Sperm and embryos possess foreign antigens that can be recognized and attacked by the maternal humoral immune system (Oliphant et al., 1984).

Oviductal Fluid.   The oviductal fluid provides a suitable environment for fertilization and cleavage of fertilized eggs. The rate of accumulation of oviductal fluid is regulated by ovarian hormones. By using different methods of cannulation for continuous collection of oviductal secretions, it has been shown that the volume of fluid secreted by both oviducts varies during the estrous cycle. The volume is low during the luteal phase, increases at the onset of estrus, reaches a maximum a day later,

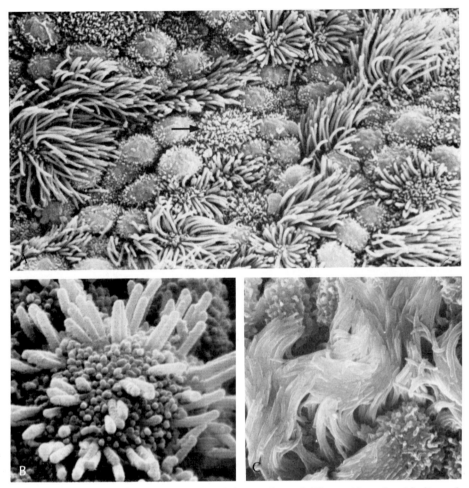

FIG. 2–13. Scanning electron micrographs of the oviduct. *A,* The oviductal epithelium showing secretory (arrow) cells heavily coated with microvilli and ciliated cells. Note that some cells are fully ciliated while others have cilia on the periphery. *B,* Rosette-like structure of a ciliated cell ciliogenesis, a process that occurs at random, culminating in complete ciliation as shown in *B. C,* Fully ciliated cells in the fimbriae that assist in the pick-up of ova after its release from the Graafian follicle.

and then declines to characteristic luteal phase levels (Fig. 2–17).

The direction of flow of a large part of the oviductal fluid is toward the ovary, since the isthmus blocks or partially blocks the flow of fluids into the uterus.

Several physiologic factors may be involved in creating currents and countercurrents: (a) quantitative and qualitative changes in oviductal secretions throughout the menstrual cycle and in response to contraceptives, (b) beat of kinocilia in oviductal compartments may vary in size

and shape, and (c) constant change in the diameter of the oviductal lumen in different segments as a result of muscle contraction and reorientation of mucosal folds.

The directional movement of oviductal secretions may contribute to ovum transport to the uterus. In sheep, most of the oviductal secretions pass out of the oviductal ostium early in the estrous cycle. On day 4, however, when ova usually enter the uterus, fluid flow through the uterotubal junction increases remarkably.

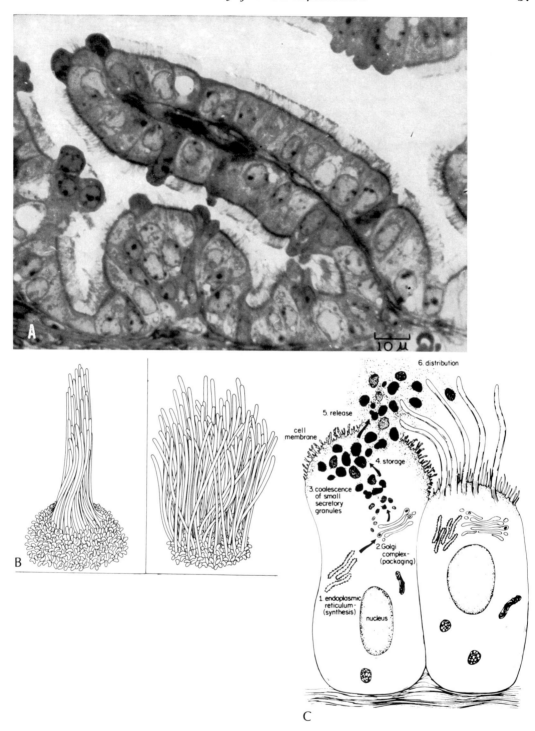

FIG. 2–14. Histology and cytology of the oviductal epithelium. *A*, Secretory cells with bulging secretory material and ciliated cells with kinocilia, toluidine blue staining. (Photo by Professor S. Reinius.) *B*, Ciliated cells from the oviduct (*right*) and uterus (*left*). Note the presence of microvilli on the apical surface of cell. *C*, Secretory cell showing the biosynthesis, packaging, storage, release and distribution of secretory material, which is the main component of the luminal fluid in the oviduct and uterus. The action of kinocilia facilitates the release of secretory granules from the surface of cells.

TABLE 2–5.   **In Vivo and In Vitro Techniques Used to Study Functions of the Oviduct**

Function Under Study	Techniques
Structure and ultrastructure of epithelium, secretory activity, and cilia	Scanning and transmission electron microscopy Culture of fragments of oviductal mucosa and transfer of growth to rose chambers Histochemical observations of frozen section
Identification of adrenergic or cholinergic receptors	Fluorescence histochemical technique Physiopharmacology of oviductal contractility (e.g., response to autonomic drugs)
Contractility of oviductal musculature	Visual observation of oviduct through abdominal wall or abdominal window Direct kymography Intraluminal catheter or microballoon placed in lumen to record intratubular pressure of oviduct Cineradiography
Biochemical composition of oviductal fluid	Extra-abdominal or intra-abdominal device to collect fluid Ligature of oviduct at the uterotubal junction and fimbriae to collect fluid Radioisotopes
Detection of protein uptake in oviductal epithelium	Immunofluorescence Pharmacology and neuropharmacology
Egg transport in oviduct	Effects of prostaglandins, steroid hormones, and oral contraceptives Segmental flushing of oviduct after salpingectomy Use of surrogate eggs Recovery of eggs from uterus *in vivo*
Sperm transport in oviduct	Segmental flushing of oviduct after salpingectomy at intervals following previous artificial insemination Flushing of oviduct from fimbriae, by laparoscopy, at intervals following breeding or artificial insemination
Kinetics of cilia beat	High-speed cinematography Photo probe to measure ciliary beat optically Laser photo correlation spectroscopy to study cilia beat in cultured ciliated cells

The oviductal fluid has several functions, including nourishing the freshly ovulated oocyte and allowing sperm capacitation, fertilization, and early preimplantation development. The oviductal fluid is composed of a selective transudate of serum and secretory products of the granules from the secretory cells of the oviductal epithelium (Oliphant et al., 1984). Oviductal secretions are regulated by steroid hormones.

Several protein components are common to oviductal fluid and serum. Some of these, however, are present in different proportions in these two body fluids; for example, the quantity of transferrin and prealbumin in oviductal fluid is far greater relative to albumin than is the quantity of these proteins in the serum. Many serum proteins have no counterparts in oviductal fluid and conversely, several proteins are unique to oviductal fluid. The presence of unique proteins in oviductal fluid implies that oviductal cells may be engaged in specific secretory activity. The oviductal fluid has a direct effect on the hyperactivation of sperm, a recently recognized phenomena that is essential for sperm–egg interaction.

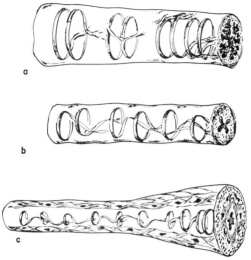

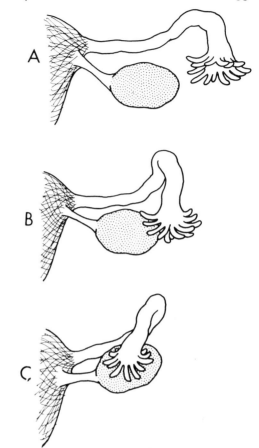

FIG. 2–15. Diagrammatic illustration of the musculature in the oviduct of ungulates. *A*, Ampulla: the musculature consists of spiral fibers arranged almost circularly. *B*, Isthmus: Note differences in morphology of muscle fibers. *C*, Uterotubal junction: Note the longitudinal muscle coat of uterine origin, as well as peritoneal fibers. (Schilling (1962). Zentralbl. Veterinaermed. *9*, 805.)

Oviductal Musculature and Related Ligaments

Oviductal contractions facilitate mixing of oviductal contents, help to denude the ova, promote fertilization by increasing egg–sperm contact, and partly regulate egg transport. Unlike intestinal peristalsis, oviductal peristalsis tends to delay slightly the progression of the ovum instead of transporting it.

Patterns of Oviductal Contractions. The oviductal musculature undergoes various types of complex contractions: localized peristalsis-like contractions originating in isolated segments or loops and traveling only a short distance; segmental contractions; and worm-like writhings of the entire oviduct. Contractions in an abovarian direction are more common than those in an adovarian direction. In general the ampulla is less active than the isthmus (see Figs. 2–15, 2–16).

FIG. 2–16. Contraction of fimbria in relation to ovarian surface, a mechanism by which eggs are picked up into the infundibulum.

Because longitudinal muscle fibers, which cause shortening, and circular muscle fibers, which cause annular constriction, are constantly activated, the contractile pattern of the oviduct is complex. Additional complicating factors are the contractile activities of the mesosalpinx, the myometrium, and the supporting ligaments, and ciliary movement.

Oviductal muscular contractions are stimulated by contractions of two major membranes that contain smooth musculature and are attached to the fimbriae, ampulla, and ovary: the mesosalpinx and the mesotubarium superius. The frequency and amplitude of spontaneous contrac-

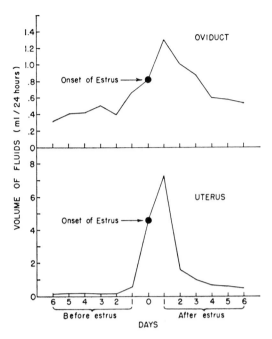

FIG. 2–17.   Fluctuations in the volume of secretions of the oviduct and the uterus during
the estrous cycle of sheep. Maximal secretion
rates occur one day following the onset of estrus; this period coincides with the time of ovulation and reception of the ovum by the fimbriae. During estrus the volume of uterine
fluids exceeds that of the oviduct, whereas the
reverse is true during the luteal phase. (Perkins
et al. (1965). J. Anim. Sci. *24,* 383.)

tions vary with the phase of the estrous
cycle. Before ovulation, contractions are
gentle with some individual variations in
the rate and pattern of contractility. At
ovulation, contractions become most vigorous. At this time, the mesosalpinx and
mesotubarium superius contract vigorously, independently, and intermittently;
the mesotubarium contracts more vigorously than the mesosalpinx. These contractions draw the oviduct into the form of a
crescent, slide the fimbriae over the surface of the ovary, and cause continuous
change in the contour of the oviduct. At
ovulation, the fringe-like folds contract
rhythmically and "massage" the ovarian
surface.

The pattern and amplitude of contraction vary in different segments of the ovi-

duct. In the isthmus, peristaltic and anti-
peristaltic contractions are segmental,
vigorous, and almost continuous. In the
ampulla, strong peristaltic waves move in
a segmented fashion toward the midportion of the oviduct. The varying patterns
of oviductal contraction may be associated
with cyclic changes in glycogen content
of oviductal musculature. Glycogen in the
oviduct is more abundant in the inner circular musculature than in the outer longitudinal musculature.

**Prostaglandins and Oviductal Contrac-
tility.** PGE_1 and PGE_2 exert a characteristic effect on the longitudinal musculature of the oviduct: an increase in tonus of
the proximal part and relaxation of the rest
of the organ. PGE_3, however, relaxes the
whole oviduct. On the other hand, PGF_1
and PGF_2 act as stimulators, the strongest
effect being exerted by PGF_2 with no apparent change in sensitivity or action
throughout the menstrual cycle. PGF_2 has
a relaxing effect on the whole oviduct.

**Utero-Ovarian   and   Related   Liga-
ments.**   The utero-ovarian ligament contains smooth muscle cells arranged primarily in longitudinal bundles, which
continue into the myometrium but not
into the ovarian stroma. The smooth muscles in the mesovaria and the various ligaments of the mesenteries attached to the
ovaries and the fimbriae contract intermittently. These rhythmic muscular contractions ensure that the fimbriae remain
in a constant position relative to the surface of the ovaries.

THE UTERUS

The role of the uterus during the estrous
cycle, pregnancy, and reproductive failure in farm animals is illustrated in Figures
2–18 through 2–22. The uterus consists of
two uterine horns (cornua), a body, and
a cervix (neck) (Fig. 2–18). The relative
proportions of each, as well as the shape
and arrangement of the horns, vary according to species (Table 2–4). In swine,
the uterus is of the bicornuate type (uterus
bicornis). The horns are folded or convo-

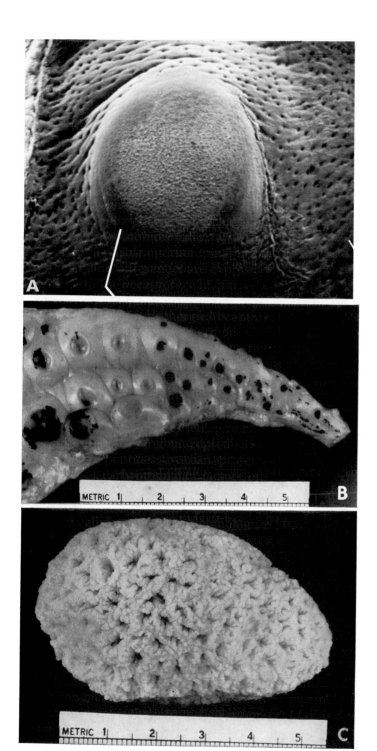

FIG. 2–18. *A*, Scanning electron micrograph of the endometrium in the ewe. Caruncle surrounded by openings of endometrial glands. *B*, Mucosa of uterine horn of the nonpregnant ewe. Note caruncles and pigmentation of the endometrium. *C*, Maternal caruncle from a pregnant cow. Note the spongy-like crypts to which the chorionic villi were embedded.

luted and may be as long as 4 to 5 feet, while the body of the uterus is short (Fig. 2–19). This length is an anatomic adaptation for successful litter bearing. In cattle, sheep, and horses, the uterus is of the bipartite type (uterus bipartitus). These animals have a septum that separates the two horns and a prominent uterine body (the horse has the largest). In ruminants the uterine epithelium has several caruncles (Fig. 2–18). Superficially, the body of the

uterus in cattle and sheep appears larger than it actually is because the caudal parts of the horns are bound together by the intercornual ligament.

Both sides of the uterus are attached to the pelvic and abdominal walls by the broad ligament. In multiparous animals the uterine ligaments stretch, allowing the uterus to drop into the pelvic cavity. In the mare this may hinder the removal of endometrial fluids or even allow small

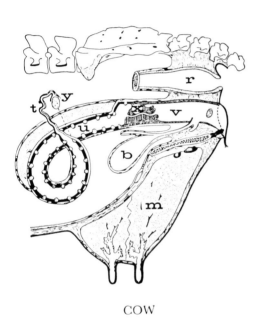

COW

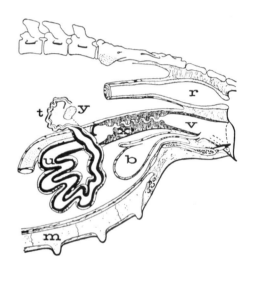

SOW

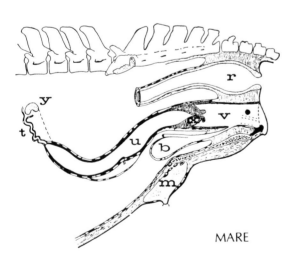

MARE

FIG. 2–19. Comparative anatomy of the reproductive organs in the female. *b*, Bladder; *m*, mammary gland; *r*, rectum; *t*, oviduct; *u*, uterus; *v*, vagina; *x*, cervix; *y*, ovary. Note species differences in anatomy of cervix, uterus and mammary gland. (Redrawn from Ellenberger and Baum (1943). Handbuch der vergleichenden Anatomie der Haustiere, 18th ed. Zietzschmann, Ackernecht and Grau (eds.). Berlin, Springer.)

amounts of urine to flow through the cervix during estrus, resulting in mild catarrhal inflammation.

Like most other hollow internal organs, the walls of the uterus consist of a mucous membrane lining, an intermediate smooth muscle layer, and an outer serous layer, the peritoneum. From the physiologic standpoint, only two layers are recognized—the endometrium and the myometrium.

Vasculature of the Uterus

The uterus receives its blood and nerve supply through the broad ligament (Fig. 2–20). The blood vessels are numerous, thick-walled and tortuous. The middle uterine artery, a branch of either the internal iliac artery or the external iliac artery, provides the chief blood supply to the uterus in the region of the developing fetus, and thus it enlarges greatly with advancing gestation. The cranial uterine artery, a branch of the utero-ovarian artery, supplies blood to the ovary by the ovarian artery and to the anterior extremity of the uterine horn by the cranial uterine artery.

The utero-ovarian artery runs closely along the surface of the corresponding vein and shows only a minor degree of tortuosity. This artery terminates by giving rise to a small branch to the tip of the uterine horn and oviduct, one or more highly convoluted ovarian branches, and a branch to the broad ligament.

Constriction of the uterine artery with a resultant reduction in blood flow is attributed to the response of vascular smooth muscle to norepinephrine liberated from innervating adrenergic nerves. The regulatory actions of ovarian steroids on the ovine uterine artery may also be potentiated by prostaglandin $F_{2\alpha}(PGF_{2\alpha})$, which is synthesized and released by the uterus.

Endometrial Glands and Uterine Fluid

The endometrial glands are branched, coiled, tubular structures lined with columnar epithelium. They open onto the

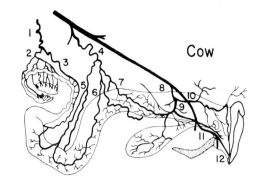

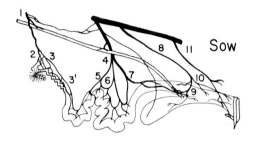

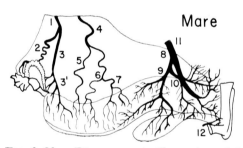

FIG. 2–20. Diagrammatic illustration of the arterial blood supply in the female reproductive tract.
1, utero-ovarian artery; *2*, ovarian artery; *3*, uterotubal artery; *3′*, anterior cornual artery or anterior artery of uterine horn; *4*, uterine artery; *5*, middle cornual artery; *6*, posterior cornual artery; *7*, artery of corpus uterii; *8*, vaginal artery; *9*, cervicouterine artery; *10*, vaginorectal artery; *11*, internal pudic artery; *12*, artery of the clitoris. (Barone and Pavaux (1962). Bull. Soc. Sci. Vet. Lyon No. 1, 33–52.)

endometrial surface, except in the caruncular areas (in ruminants). The glands are relatively straight at the time of estrus; they grow, secrete, and become more coiled and complex as the level of progesterone produced by the developing CL rises. They begin to regress when the first signs of luteal regression are also noted. The endometrial surface epithelial cells are relatively tall during estrus; following a period of active secretion during estrus, they become low and cuboidal at 2 days postestrus.

The volume and biochemical composition of the uterine fluid show consistent variation during the estrous cycle (Fig. 2–17). In sheep the volume of the fluid in the uterus exceeds that of the oviduct during estrus, whereas during the luteal phase, the reverse is true.

Uterine Proteins. The endometrial fluid contains mainly serum proteins but also small amounts of uterine-specific proteins. The ratio and amounts of these proteins vary according to the reproductive cycle. Differences in concentration as well as distribution of components in the uterine fluids compared to the blood serum provide evidence that secretion as well as transudation occurs. In the rabbit, a protein named *blastokinin* (uteroglobulin) can influence blastocyst formation from morulae, whereas uterine fluid in the mouse contains a factor that initiates implantation. Uterine secretions provide an optimal environment for the survival and capacitation of spermatozoa and the cleavage of the early blastocyst before implantation.

Glycerylphosphorylcholine diesterease (GPC) in the uterine secretions reaches a maximum concentration around the time of ovulation as a result of estrogen action. This enzyme hydrolyzes glycerylphosphorylcholine releasing glycerol of phosphoglycerol for use by the spermatozoa. The proestrous uterine secretions are responsible for the initiation of capacitation as well as the stimulation of sperm metabolism. In addition to these secretory proteins, the high levels of estrogen associated with ovulation are responsible for inducing the synthesis of a number of proteins—including stromal mucopolysaccharides, steroid hormone receptors, and enzymes—that

perform important functions within the endometrium itself.

The secretions may continue to be an important source of nourishment to the growing fetus during the postimplantation phase of gestation. This is particularly true in farm animals that exhibit either an epitheliochorial or a syndesmochorial type of placentation. In the form of receptors, for example, proteins are responsible for establishing the sensitivity of the uterus toward ovarian steroids. Estrogen secreted during the preovulatory phase appears to be responsible for inducing the synthesis of both progesterone and estrogen receptors, and it is through the synthesis of the progesterone receptors that preovulatory estrogen primes the uterus for its subsequent progestational proliferation.

Specific proteins of uterine and/or conceptus origin have been identified and characterized during early pregnancy in the ewe; however, it is unknown whether any of these proteins can influence cell-mediated immune responses. One of the proteins, a purple-colored, iron-containing glycoprotein named *uteroferrin* has been purified (Basha et al., 1980). Uterine secretions play a part in the control of embryonic growth and implantation.

The uterine fluid has two important functions, namely, to provide a favorable environment for sperm capacitation and to provide nutrition for the blastocyst until implantation is completed. In the cow, the embryo lies free in the medium for approximately 30 days, during which time extensive embryonic differentiation takes place before the conceptus becomes firmly attached to the endometrium.

Uterine Contraction

The contraction of the uterus is coordinated with the rhythmic movements of the oviduct and ovary. There is considerable variation in the origin, direction, amplitude degree, and frequency of contractions in the reproductive tract. In the estrous rabbit, contractions in the uterus are continuations of contractions of the oviducts and move along the uterine horn from the uterotubal junction toward the cervix. In general the greatest number of uterine contractions moves toward the oviducts during early estrus but toward the cervix after the end of estrus.

Uterine vascular dynamics and contractility are modulated by ovarian steroid hormones and biogenic amines. The uterine vascular plexus receives a rich, vasomotor innervation that alters both uterine blood flow and blood volume. Thus uterine vasculature has both a vasodilatory (cholinergic) and vasoconstrictive (adrenergic) innervation that are modulated by cyclic (hormonal) conditions (Garris et al., 1984).

During the estrous cycle, the frequency of myometrial contractions is maximal at and immediately after estrus. At estrus, uterine contractions originate in the posterior part of the reproductive tract and more predominantly toward the oviduct. During the luteal phase, the frequency of contractions is reduced and only a small percentage moves toward the oviducts. Estradiol increases the frequency of uterine contractions in ovariectomized ewes, where progesterone reduces the frequency. High levels of progesterone are noted when contractile activity is relatively quiescent. High levels of progestogen binding at estrus play a role in progesterone-induced quiescence during the luteal phase of the estrous cycle.

Uterine Metabolism

The endometrium metabolizes carbohydrates, lipids, and proteins to supply the necessary requirements for cell nutrition, rapid proliferation of the uterine tissue and development of the conceptus. Cyclic metabolic variations in this tissue consist of changes in the rate of nucleic acid synthesis, the availability of glucose, and the amount of glycogen reserves. These reactions depend on four phenomena: (a) the enzymatic reactions involved in glucose metabolism; (b) the increase in circulation through the spiral arterioles; (c) the mor-

phologic changes that occur in the endometrium and myometrium; and (d) the stimulating action of the ovarian and other hormones.

Ovarian hormones play a substantial role in regulating uterine metabolism. Growth of the uterus (both protein synthesis and cell division) is induced by estrogen; in the process it uses a large amount of energy in the form of ATP. Progestational responses in the endometrium involve major growth, a striking increase in DNA and RNA and a loss of water. A rapid change occurs in the metabolism of the endometrium about the time the egg passes through the uterotubal junction.

Function of the Uterus

The uterus serves a number of functions. The endometrium and its fluids play a major role in the reproductive process: (a) sperm transport from the site of ejaculation to the site of fertilization in the oviduct; (b) regulation of the function of the CL; and (c) initiation of implantation, pregnancy, and parturition.

Sperm Transport. At mating, the contraction of the myometrium is essential for the transport of spermatozoa from the site of ejaculation to the site of fertilization. Large numbers of spermatozoa aggregate in the endometrial glands; the physiologic and immunologic significance of this phenomenon is not known. As spermatozoa are transported through the uterine lumen to the oviducts, they undergo "capacitation" in endometrial secretions.

Luteolytic Mechanisms. There is a local utero-ovarian cycle whereby the CL stimulates the uterus to produce a substance that in turn destroys the CL. The uterus plays an important role in regulating the function of the CL. Corpora lutea are maintained in a functional state for long periods following hysterectomy of cattle, sheep, and swine. If small amounts of uterine tissue remain in situ, luteal regression occurs and cycles are resumed after variable periods. Following unilateral hysterectomy, corpora lutea adjacent to the excised uterine horn are usually better maintained than those adjacent to the remaining horn (Fig. 2–21).

It appears that the uterus produces or participates in the production of some luteolytic substance, and this uterine luteolysin may be selectively transferred from the utero-ovarian vein to the closely adherent ovarian artery and thus reaches the ovary in much greater concentrations than that in peripheral blood.

Intramuscular or intrauterine administration of prostaglandin causes complete luteal regression in the cow and ewe. Infusions of $PGF_{2\alpha}$ into the utero-ovarian vein in ewes also causes rapid regression of the corpora lutea and a decline in plasma progesterone levels. $PGF_{2\alpha}$ appears to be the uterine luteolysin in the ewe, transmitted by way of a venoarterial pathway directly from the uterus to the CL, where it causes luteal regression.

The gravid uterine horn exerts an antiluteolytic effect at the level of the adjacent ovary. This effect is exerted through a local utero-ovarian venoarterial pathway.

In the nonpregnant ewe, the uterus causes regression of the CL through a direct or local pathway between the uterine horn and the adjacent ovary. The local pathway between a uterine horn and adjacent ovary in sheep is venoarterial in nature, involving the main uterine vein (uterine branch of ovarian vein) as the uterine component and the ovarian branch of the ovarian artery as the ovarian component.

Uterine dilation and irritation inhibit the normal development and function of the cyclic corpora lutea of cows and ewes. This mechanism may play a role in reproductive failure. Infusions of large numbers of nonspecific bacteria into the uterus and insemination of heifers with semen containing a virus cause lateal inhibition and induce precocious estrus.

Implantation and Gestation. The uterus is a highly specialized organ that is adapted to accept and nourish the products of conception from the time of im-

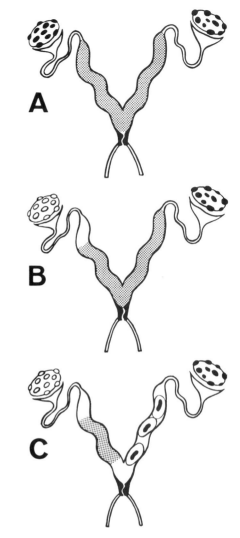

 PART OF UTERUS REMOVED

 REGRESSING CORPORA LUTEA

 PERSISTENT CORPORA LUTEA

FIG. 2–21. Diagram showing the effect of partial hysterectomy on persistence of corpora lutea in the pig. *A*, Total hysterectomy during the luteal phase causes retention of the corpus luteum for a period similar to gestation. *B*, Unilateral hysterectomy and partial removal of the other horn, retaining only a fragment 20 cm in length, causes asymmetric functioning of the two ovaries. *C*, The corpora lutea on the intact side are normally maintained, whereas those on the other side regress before the twenty-second day of gestation. (Data from Du Mesnil du Buisson (1961). Ann. Biol. Anim. Bioch. Biophys. *1*, 105.)

plantation until parturition. A well-described though obscurely defined uterine "differentiation" occurs, governed by the ovarian steroid hormones. This process must evolve to some critical stage when the uterus is prepared to selectively accept the blastocyst. Unless such differentiation occurs, the uterus is unsuited to permit implantation.

After implantation, the embryo depends on an adequate vascular supply within the endometrium for its development. Throughout gestation, the physiologic properties of the endometrium and its blood supply are important for the survival and development of the fetus. The uterus is capable of undergoing tremendous changes in size, structure, and position to accommodate the needs of the growing conceptus.

Parturition and Postpartum Involution. The contractile response of the uterus remains dormant until the time of parturition, when it plays the major role in fetal expulsion. Following parturition, the uterus almost regains its former size and condition by a process called *involution* (Fig. 2–22). In the sow, the uterus continuously declines in both weight and length for 28 days after parturition; thereafter it remains relatively unchanged during the lactation period. However, immediately after the young are weaned, the uterus increases in both weight and length for 4 days.

During the postpartum interval, the destruction of endometrial tissue is accompanied by the presence of large numbers of leukocytes and the reduction of the endometrial vascular bed. The cells of the myometrium are reduced in number and size. These rapid and disproportional changes in the uterine tissue are a possible cause of low postpartum conception rate. Neither the presence of suckling calves nor anemia delays uterine involution. Caruncular tissues are sloughed off and expelled from the uterus 12 days after calving. Regeneration of the surface epithelium over the caruncles occurs by growth from the sur-

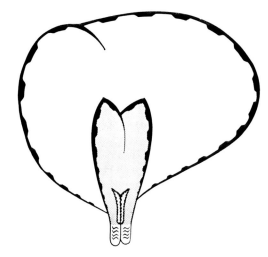

FIG. 2–22. Diagrammatic illustration of the changes taking place in size and shape of the ruminant uterus during pregnancy. Three uteri are shown in the diagram; the inner one represents a nonpregnant uterus; the outer one represents a gravid uterus prior to delivery, and the middle one represents a uterus after delivery in the process of involution.

rounding tissue and is completed 30 days after calving.

Effects of Foreign Bodies and IUDs. - The stimulation of the uterus during the early stages of the estrous cycle hastens regression of the CL and causes precocious estrus. Uterine stimulation can be initiated by placing a small foreign body in the lumen. The subsequent estrous cycle will be either shortened or prolonged, depending on when the foreign body was inserted and on the nature and size of the material introduced. The fact that the estrous cycle is unaffected when the uterine segment containing the foreign body is denervated implies that the nervous system is responsible for this effect.

Although intrauterine devices (IUDs) have an antifertility effect in several domestic animals, their apparent mode of action varies widely. The major antifertility effect of IUDs seems to be exerted between the time the embryo enters the uterus and the time of implantation. For example, the insertion of large-diameter (uterus-distending) IUDs in sheep and cattle results in an alteration of the estrous cycle by shortening the functional lifespan of the CL. In sheep, large-diameter IUDs inhibit sperm transport and fertilization.

CERVIX UTERI

The cervix is a sphincter-like structure that projects caudally into the vagina (Fig. 2–23). The cervix is a fibrous organ composed predominantly of connective tissue with only small amounts of smooth muscle tissue present. Since the properties of connective tissues depend on the type, concentration, and interactions of the molecules that make up the extracellular matrix, the functional characteristics of the cervix are altered dramatically by changes in these parameters (Fig. 2–24).

The cervix is characterized by a thick wall and constricted lumen. Although the structure of the cervix differs in detail among farm mammals, the cervical canal has various prominences. In ruminants these are in the form of transverse or spi-

rally interlocking ridges known as *annular rings*, which develop to varying degrees in the different species (Figs. 2–25 and 2–26). They are especially prominent in the cow (usually four rings) and in the ewe, where they fit into each other to close the cervix securely. In the sow, the rings are in a corkscrew arrangement that is adapted to the spiral twisting of the tip of the boar's penis. Distinguishing features of the mare's cervix are the conspicuous folds in the mucosa and the projecting folds into the vagina.

The cervix is tightly closed except during estrus, when it relaxes slightly, permitting sperm to enter the uterus. Mucus discharged from the cervix is expelled from the vulva.

Cervical Stroma and Physiologic Changes

The connective tissue of the cervical stroma is made of ground substance, fibrous constituents, and cellular elements. The ground substance contains proteoglycan, and hyaluronic acid, chondroitin-4,6

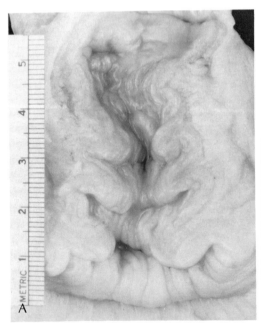
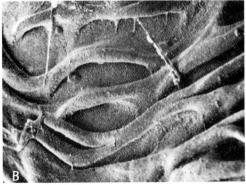

FIG. 2–23. Morphology and histology of the cervix. *A*, Cervix (cut open) of a heifer 4 days after estrus. Note the annular rings around the cervical canal. *B*, Scanning electron micrograph of bovine cervix. Note complexity of cervical crypts (59×).

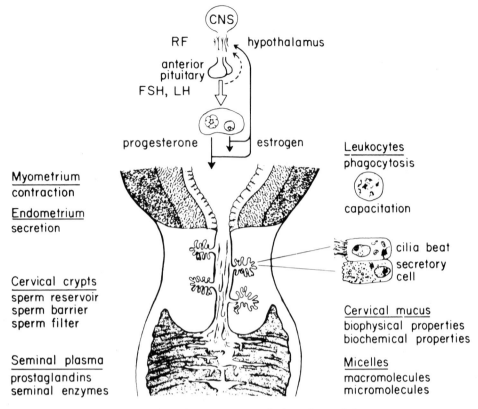

FIG. 2–24. Comparative aspects of the anatomy and physiology of the cervix.

sulfate, dermatan sulfate, heparan sulfate, and keratan sulfate associated with proteins. The fibrous constituents include collagen, elastin, and reticulin. Cellular elements comprise mast cells, fibroblasts, and wandering cells. Collagen is made of chains of several amino acids such as glycine, proline, hydroxyproline, lysine or hydroxylysine. The patterns of reticulin, elastin, and interfibrous ground substances facilitate the dilation of the cervix at delivery. The dissociation of the collagen fibers, which become widely separated from one another, causes the loosening of cervical tissues and increases clear spaces between collagen bundles.

Gross changes in the biochemical composition of the cervix during pregnancy indicate that the cervix is preparing for a change in its functional properties by alterations in the parameters that regulate the physical properties of connective tis-

sue matrices. Morphologically, these pregnancy-related changes do not become apparent until quite late during gestation, when tissue breakdown and destruction of the collagen network become apparent.

During the course of pregnancy, the cervix may show as much as an eightfold increase in mass. The enhanced growth and the decreased concentrations of the matrix components may be a consequence of several factors, including increased vascularization coupled with an influx of inflammatory cells and an increase in stromal cellularity as a result of active fibroblast mitosis. Smooth muscle hypertrophy increases in plasma proteins entering connective tissues during edema and increases concentrations of glycoproteins.

Cervical softening and ripening are not due exclusively to enzymatic activity involving only matrix degradation. The dynamic nature of the cervix at the time of

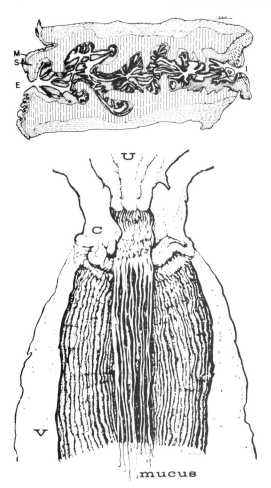

FIG. 2–25. (*Top*) Tracing of a longitudinal section of the bovine cervix showing the complexity of the cervical crypts which attract massive numbers of spermatozoa. *E,* external, or *I,* internal, or *M,* mucus-secreting mucosa; *S,* cervical stroma. (*Bottom*) Diagrammatic illustration showing how the strands of cervical mucus flow from the crypts of the cervix (C) to the epithelium of the vagina (V). The biophysical characteristics of cervical mucus and arrangement of the macromolecules of mucus facilitate sperm transport from the vagina to the uterus (U).

parturition may provide an anabolic basis by which a new matrix with altered physical properties is produced. The major characteristics of the parturient cervix include (a) increased rates of proteoglycan and hyaluronate synthesis with a concomitant decrease in hexuronate concentration, (b) the appearance of a new type of proteoglycan, and (c) a breakdown in the structure and organization of the collagen network.

Cervical Mucus

Cervical mucus consists of macromolecules of mucin of epithelial origin (Fig. 2–27) which are composed of glycoproteins (particularly of the sialomucinous type) that contain about 25% amino acids and 75% carbohydrates. The mucin is composed of a long, continuous polypeptide chain with numerous oligosaccharide side chains. The carbohydrate portion is made of galactose, glucosamine, fucose, and sialic acid. The proteins of cervical mucus include prealbumin, lipoprotein, albumin, and β- and γ-globulins. The cervical mucus contains several enzymes, including glucuronidase, amylase, phosphorylase, esterase, and phosphatases.

Owing to its unique biophysical characteristics, the cervical mucus has several rheologic properties such as ferning, elasticity, viscosity, thixotropy, and tack (stickiness). The cervical mucus during estrus shows a fern pattern of crystallization on drying on a glass slide. This fern pattern, associated with the high chloride content of the mucus, does not occur with drying of mucus obtained at stages of the cycle when progesterone levels are high or during pregnancy. The phenomenon may have some value, when combined with other observations, for early pregnancy diagnosis. The secretion of cervical mucus is stimulated by ovarian estrogen and inhibited by progesterone. Cyclic qualitative changes in the cervical mucus throughout the estrous cycle and cyclic variations in the arrangement and viscosity of these macromolecules cause periodic changes in the penetrability of spermatozoa in the cervical canal. Optimal changes of cervical mucus properties—such as an increase in quantity, viscosity, ferning, and pH, and decrease in viscosity and cell content—occur during estrus and ovulation, and these are reversed during the luteal phase when sperm penetration in the cervix is inhib-

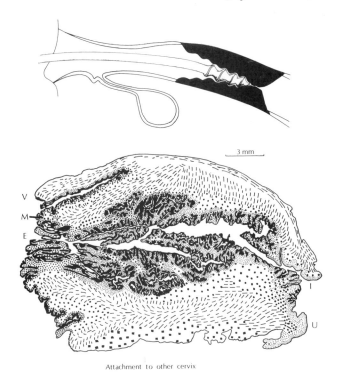

3 mm

V
M
E

I

U

Attachment to other cervix

FIG. 2–26. (*Top*) Corkscrew structure of the cervical canal to accommodate similar structure of the penis. (Hunter, 1983.) (*Bottom*) Cervix of the rabbit. Note the complexity of cervical canal of the double cervix.

ited. Under the influence of estrogens, the macromolecules of glycoprotein of the mucus are oriented so that the spaces between them measure 2 to 5 μ. In the luteal phase, the spaces of the meshwork of macromolecules become increasingly smaller. Thus at the time of estrus and ovulation, the large size of the meshes allows the transport of spermatozoa through the meshwork of filaments and through the cervical canal.

Functions

The cervix plays several roles in the reproductive process: (a) It facilitates sperm transport through the cervical mucus to the uterine lumen; (b) it acts as sperm reservoir (see Chapter 6); and (c) it may play a role in the selection of viable sperm, thus preventing the transport of nonviable and defective sperm.

Sperm Transport. Upon ejaculation, spermatozoa are oriented toward the internal os. As the flagellum beats and vibrates, the sperm head is propelled forward in the channels of least resistance. The macro- and microrheologic properties of cervical mucus play a major role in sperm migration. Sperm penetrability increases with the cleanliness of mucus, since cellular debris and leukocytes delay sperm migration. The aqueous spaces between the micelles permit the passage of sperm as well as diffusion of soluble substances. Proteolytic enzymes may hydrolyze the backbone protein or some of the crosslinkages of the mucin and reduce the network to a less resistant mesh with more open channels for the migration of sperm. When cervical mucus and semen are placed in apposition *in vitro,* phase lines immediately occur between the two fluids. Sperm phalanges soon appear and develop high degrees of arborization, the terminal aspects of which consist of channels through which one or two spermatozoa can pass.

After mating or artificial insemination, massive numbers of spermatozoa are lodged in the complicated cervical crypts.

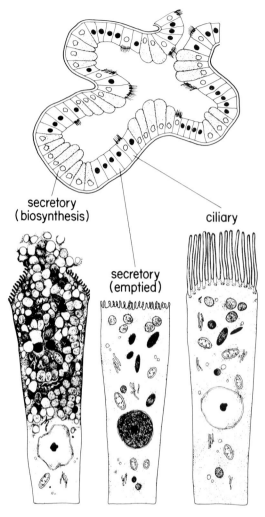

secretory
(biosynthesis)

ciliary

secretory
(emptied)

FIG. 2–27.   Cervical crypt (*top*) and secretory cells before and after secretion of mucus (*bottom*). The ciliated cells on the right may assist in releasing the mucus from the surface of adjacent secretory cells through the active beating of kinocilia.

The cervix might act as a reservoir for spermatozoa, thus providing the upper reproductive tract with subsequent releases of sperm. It is also possible that spermatozoa that are trapped in the cervical crypts are never released, thus preventing excessive numbers of spermatozoa from reaching the site of fertilization.

In ruminants prolonged survival of sperm in the cervix relative to other parts of the reproductive tract suggests that the cervix acts as a sperm reservoir. In the cervices of cattle and goats, most sperm are not randomly distributed but are located between cervical crypts. Penetration of sperm to these sites in the cervix depends on sperm viability and on the structure and, consequently, the rheologic properties of the cervical mucus.

The Cervix During Pregnancy. During pregnancy, a highly viscid, nonferning, thick and turbid mucus occludes the cervical canal, acting as an effective barrier against sperm transport and invasion of bacteria in the uterine lumen, thus preventing uterine infections. The only other time the cervix is open is before parturition. At this time the cervical plug liquefies and the cervix dilates to permit the expulsion of the fetus and fetal membranes.

THE VAGINA

The vaginal wall consists of surface epithelium, muscular coat, and serosa. The muscular coat of the vagina is not as well developed as the outer parts of the uterus. It consists of a thick inner circular layer and a thin outer longitudinal layer; the latter continues for some distance into the uterus. The muscularis is well supplied with blood vessels, nerve bundles, groups of nerve cells, and loose and dense connective tissue. The cow is unique in possessing an anterior sphincter muscle in addition to the posterior sphincter (at the junction of the vagina and vestibule) found in the other farm mammals.

The surface epithelium is composed of glandless, stratified, squamous epithelial cells, except in the cow, in which some mucous cells are present in the cranial part next to the cervix and the epithelial surface fails to cornify, probably because of low levels of circulating estrogens.

There are species differences in vaginal changes during the estrous cycle. These differences probably reflect different secretion rates for estrogen and progesterone and ultimately for the gonadotrophins. Vaginal smears, however, are not useful in diagnosing the stage of the cycle or hormonal abnormalities.

The surface of the vaginal cells is made of numerous microridges that run longitudinally or in circles (Fig. 2–28). In this multilayered stratified epithelium, the cells are wedged on each other by interlocking opposed microridges, thus forming a firm surface. The morphology and pattern of these microridges, which affect the firmness of the epithelium, vary throughout the reproductive cycle. The microridges exhibit a regular pattern during pregnancy, whereas pores appear within the microridges of the cells during the estrous cycle.

Physiologic Responses

Vaginal Contractions. Vaginal contractility plays a major role in psychosexual responses and possibly sperm transport. The contraction of the vagina, uterus, and oviducts is activated by fluid secreted into the vagina during precoital stimulation.

Immunologic Responses. The vagina appears to be one of the major sites for sperm antigen–antibody reaction since the vagina is more exposed to sperm anti-

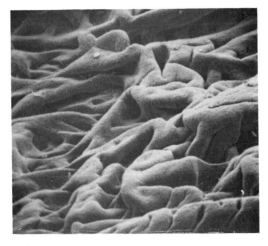

FIG. 2–28. Scanning electron micrograph of a rabbit's vagina showing the rugae of the vaginal epithelium to all expansion of the vagina during copulation and parturition.

gen than are the uterus and oviduct. Local production of antibodies to sperm antigens may occur within the vaginal tissues.

Immature and mature plasma cells, located beneath the epithelium, seem to be under endocrine control since these cells increase in number during the luteal phase, following ovariectomy and during the postmenopausal stage. These plasma cells seem to be involved in the secretion of immunoglobulins A and G, which seem to prevent bacterial infection and produce antibodies against spermatozoa.

Vaginal Fluid. The vaginal fluid is composed primarily of transudate through the vaginal wall, mixed with vulvar secretions from sebaceous glands and sweat glands and contaminated with cervical mucus, endometrial, and oviductal fluids and exfoliated cells of the vaginal epithelium. As estrus approaches, the vascularity of the vaginal wall increases and the vaginal fluid becomes thinner.

A specific and distinct odor is present in the urogenital tract of cows during estrus. This odor apparently disappears or is greatly attenuated during diestrus. Dogs can be trained to detect and respond to the odors associated with estrus in cattle (Kiddy et al., 1978).

Microbiologic Flora. The vaginal flora is made of a dynamic mixture of aerobic, facultatively anaerobic, and strictly anaerobic microorganisms with new strains constantly being introduced. The flora of microorganisms varies throughout the life cycle. The various populations of microorganisms are equipped enzymatically to survive and replicate under a given vaginal environment. Only those most suited to replicate and compete for nutrients can become established and join the flora or even replace other microorganisms. During periods of high glycogen content, acidophilic organisms predominate, but other organisms are present among the heterogeneous group making up the normal flora.

Functions of the Vagina

The vagina has multiple functions in reproduction. It is a copulatory organ in which semen is deposited and coagulated until spermatozoa are transported through the macromolecules of the cervical mucous column. The dilated bulbous vagina provides a postcoital semen pool to supply spermatozoa for cervical reservoirs. The rugae vaginales and the fence-like, rhomboidshaped arrangement of the musculature allow distention of the vagina during mating and parturition. Although the vagina contains no glands, its walls are moistened by transudates through the vaginal epithelium (incorrectly called *mucosa*), by cervical mucus, and by endometrial secretions.

Following ejaculation, the seminal plasma is not transported into the uterus; most of it is expelled or absorbed through the vaginal walls. Some of the biochemical components of the seminal plasma, when absorbed in the vagina, exert physiologic responses in other parts of the female reproductive tract.

The pH of the vaginal secretion is unfavorable to spermatozoa. A complex interaction of the cervical mucus, vaginal secretion, and seminal plasma induces a buffering system that protects spermatozoa until they are transported through the micelles of cervical mucus. Pathologic conditions resulting in insufficient buffering of the seminal pool (e.g., low volume of ejaculate, scanty amounts of thick cervical mucus, and leakage of semen) may cause rapid immobilization of spermatozoa. The vagina serves as an excretory duct for secretions of the cervix, endometrium, and oviduct; it also serves as the birth canal during parturition. These functions are accomplished through various physiologic characteristics, namely, contraction, expansion, involution, secretion, and absorption.

EXTERNAL GENITALIA

The vestibule, the labia majora, the labia minora, the clitoris, and the vestibular glands compose the external genitalia.

Vestibule. The junction of the vagina and vestibule is marked by the external urethral orifice and frequently by a ridge (the vestigial hymen). In some cattle, the hymen may be so prominent that it interferes with copulation.

The vestibule of the cow extends inward for approximately 10 cm, where the external urethral orifice opens into its ventral surface. Just posterior to this opening lies the suburethral diverticulum, a blind sac (Fig. 2–19). Gartner's tubes (remnants of the wolffian ducts) open into the vestibule posteriorly and laterally to Gartner's ducts. The glands of Bartholin, which secrete a viscid fluid, most actively at estrus, have a tuboalveolar structure similar to the bulbourethral glands in the male.

Labia Majora and Labia Minora. The integument of the labia majora is richly endowed with sebaceous and tubular glands. It contains fat deposits, elastic tissue, and a thin layer of smooth muscle and has the same outer surface structure as the external skin. The labia minora have a core of spongy connective tissue. The surface contains many large sebaceous glands.

Clitoris. The ventral commissure of the vestibule conceals the clitoris, which has the same embryonic origin as the male penis. It is composed of erectile tissue covered by stratified squamous epithelium, and it is well-supplied with sensory nerve endings. In the cow, the greater part of the clitoris is buried in the mucosa of the vestibule. In the mare, however, it is well developed, and in the sow it is long and sinuous, terminating in a small point or cone.

REFERENCES

Basha, S., Bazer, F.W., Geiser, R.D. and Roberts, R.M. (1980). Progesterone-induced uterine secretions in pigs. Recovery from pseudopregnant and unilaterally pregnant gilts. J. Anim. Sci. *50,* 113–123.

Curry, T.E., Jr., Lawrence, I.E., Jr. and Burden, H.W. (1984). Effect of ovarian sympathectomy on follicular development during compensatory ovarian hypertrophy in the guinea pig. J. Reprod. Fertil. *71*, 39–44.

Erb, R.E., Randel, R.D. and Callahan, C.J. (1971). Female sex steroid changes during the reproductive cycle. J. Anim. Sci. Suppl. 1, *32*, 80. (IX Biennial Symposium on Animal Reproduction).

Garris, D.R., Ingenito, A.J., McConnaughey, M.M. and Dar, M.S. (1984). Regulation of estrogen-induced uterine hyperemia and contractility in guinea pig: cholinergic modulation of an alpha-adrenergic response. Biol. Reprod. *30*, 863–868.

Guthrie, H.D. and Rexroad, C.E., Jr. (1981). Endometrial prostaglandin F release in vitro and plasma 13, 14-Dihydro-15-KETO Prostaglandin F_2 in pigs with luteolysis blocked by pregnancy estradiol bensoate or human chorionic gonadotrophin. J. Anim. Sci. *52*, 330–339.

Hunter, F. (1983). Reproduction of Farm Animals. London, Longman.

Kiddy, C.A., Mitchell, D.S., Bolt, D.J. and Hawk, H.W. (1978). Detection of estrus-related odors in cows by trained dogs. Biol. Reprod. *19*, 389.

Moor, R.M., Hay, M.R. and Seamark, R.F. (1975). The sheep ovary: regulation of steroidogenic, haemodynamic and structural changes in the largest follicle and adjacent tissue before ovulation. J. Reprod. Fertil. *45*, 595.

Niswender, G.D., Reimers, T.J., Diekman, M.A. and Nett, T.M. (1976). Blood flow: a mediator of ovarian function. Biol. Reprod. *13*, 381.

Oliphant, G., Cabot, C., Ross, P. and Marta, J. (1984). Control of the humoral immune system within the rabbit oviduct. Biol. Reprod. *31*, 205–212.

Oliphant, G., Reynolds, A.B., Smith, P.F., Ross, P.R. and Marta, J.S. (1984). Immunocytochemical localization and determination of hormone-induced synthesis of the sulfated oviductal glycoproteins. Biol. Reprod. *31*, 165–174.

Silvia, W.J., Fitz, T.A., Mayan, M.H. and Niswender, G.D. (1984). Cellular and molecular mechanisms involved in luteolysis and maternal recognition of pregnancy in the ewe. Anim. Reprod. Sci. *7*, 57–74.

Wise, T.H., Caton, D., Thatcher, W.W., Barron, D.H. and Fields, M.J. (1982). Ovarian function during the estrous cycle of the cow: ovarian blood flow and progesterone release rate. J. Anim. Sci. *55*, 627–637.

II. physiology of reproduction

3
Hormones, Growth Factors, and Reproduction

E.S.E. Hafez

ENDOCRINOLOGY OF REPRODUCTION

Endocrinology of reproduction deals with biochemistry, physiology, pharmacology, and molecular biology of hormones and their receptors. Hormones synthesized and secreted by endocrine glands are transported into the blood circulatory system to stimulate, inhibit, or interact with the functional activity or specific target organ producing a wide range of physiologic responses. Extensive investigations have been conducted to study the function, structure, and biochemical composition of actin and transmission as well as clinical application of the endocrine glands of farm animals (Dickson, 1984; Genuth, 1988; Griffin and Ojeda, 1988). These aspects are summarized in Tables 3–1 to 3–5.

Primary and Secondary Hormones of Reproduction

Reproductive hormones are derived primarily from four major systems (Tables 3–6 and 3–7):
1. Varous areas of the hypothalamus
2. Anterior and posterior lobes of the pituitary gland
3. Gonads: testis and ovary including their interstitial tissues and corpus luteum
4. Uterus and placenta

The hormones of reproduction are also classified into two groups, according to their mode of action.
1. Primary hormones regulate the various reproductive processes
2. Metabolic hormones, which indirectly influence reproduction.

TABLE 3–1. **Techniques Used in Reproductive Endocrinology**

Procedure	Protocol and Application
Ablation gland	Surgical removal of endocrine gland leads to a deficiency of hormone produced by that gland
	Castration of males removes androgen, resulting in a change in physical characteristics
Replacement therapy	Deficiency caused by ablation may be overcome by implantation of the gland back into the animal or by injection of crude extracts from removed gland
Isolation of hormone	Isolation or separation of hormone from other substances in the crude extract of endocrine gland involves intensive chemical separation procedures coupled with sensitive assays to measure the hormone
	Once hormone is isolated, it is chemically identified and synthesized if possible
Regulation of endocrine gland	Changes in synthesis and release rate of hormone from endocrine gland studied under endocrine physiological conditions by assay techniques

TABLE 3–2. Classes of Hormones Based on Structure

Biochemical Structure	Hormones

Peptides and proteins	Glycoproteins
	    Follicle-stimulating hormone (FSH)
	    Human chorionic gonadotropin (hCG)
	    Luteinizing hormone (LH)
	    Thyroid-stimulating hormone (TSH)
	Polypeptides
	    Adrenocorticotropic hormone (ACTH)
	    Glucagon
	    Growth hormone
	    Insulin
	    Insulin-like growth
	    Peptides (somatomedins)
	    Oxytocin
	    Proclatin
	    Relaxin
	    Somatostatin
	    Vasopressin (antidiuretic hormone—ADH)

Steroids	Aldosterone Cortisol Estradiol Progesterone Vitamin D
Amines	Epinephrine Norepinephrine Thyroxine (T4) Triiodothyronine (T3)

Several techniques have been conducted on the physiology/biochemistry of primary/secondary hormones of reproduction (Table 3–1). The primary hormones are involved in various aspects of reproduction, spermatogenesis, ovulation, sexual behavior, fertilization, implantation, maintenance of gestation, parturition, lactation, and maternal behavior. Metabolic hormones—necessary for the general well-being, metabolic state, and growth of the animal—permit the full effect of the primary hormones of reproduction.

The primary hormones of reproduction, based on their chemical structure, are divided into three groups:

1. Proteins: These are polypeptide hormones ranging in size from a molecular weight of 300 up to 70,000 daltons. Because they are easily digested by enzymes, they cannot be given orally, but must be administered by injection.

2. Steroids: These have a molecular weight of approximately 300 to 400 daltons. Natural steroids are not effective by oral administration, but

TABLE 3–3. Chemical Composition of Hormones of Reproduction

Hormones	Molecular Weight (Daltons)	Characteristics
Steroids	300–400	Natural steroids are not effective by oral administration Synthetic and plant steroids can be administered orally or by injection
Proteins	300–70,000	Easily broken down by enzymes Cannot be given orally; must be administered by injection
Fatty acids	400	Can be administered only by injection

TABLE 3–4. Mode of Action of Hormones of Reproduction

Hormones	Mechanism of Action
Proteins and polypeptide	Regulate cell function by binding to a cell-membrane-specific receptor; controls the activity of the enzyme, adenylate cyclase, which catalyzes the conversion of adenosine triphosphate (ATP) to cyclic adenosine monophosphate (cAMP) and pyrophosphate
	cAMP acts on an enzyme cAMP-dependent protein kinase
	Synthesis of new mRNA returns to the cytoplasm to produce the new protein that may be an important enzyme in steroid biosynthesis
Steroids	Steroidal hormones are transported through both cell membrane and cell cytoplasm by simple diffusion
	Binding of steroidal hormone to its receptor starts the synthesis of specific mRNA, which is translocated to the cytoplasm, where it directs synthesis of specific proteins

synthetic or plant steroids can be administered orally and by injection.

3. Fatty acids: These have a molecular weight of 400 daltons and can be administered only by injection.

Secondary hormones indirectly related to reproduction are secreted by the pituitary, thyroid, parathyroid, adrenal cortex, uterus, and pancreas (Table 3–7 and Figs. 3–1 and 3–2).

Endocrinology of Puberty

The onset of puberty is regulated by the maturity of the hypothalmic adenohypophysial axis rather than by inability of the pituitary to produce gonadotropins or by an ovarian insensitivity to their effects. With the approach of puberty, the frequency of LH peaks increases, followed by a transient rise in the preovulatory surge of LH, which is associated with behavioral estrus during this pubertal period.

Prepubertal males show an increase in the amplitude of LH peaks up to about 3 months of age, when the amplitude of these LH peaks begins to decline. The frequency of LH pulses increases until 4 months of age, the plasma levels of LH increase in a linear fashion. Initially, the Leydig cells require a high level of LH for testosterone secretion. This threshold begins to decline at about 6 months of age.

Endocrinology of Lactation

Lactating animals have a longer anestrous period; unless milking or suckling ceases, either through machine milking or the suckling of the calf, there is a negative influence on the release of gonadotropic hormones. The negative effect is related

TABLE 3–5. Modes of Transmission of Hormones of Reproduction (Compiled from Reece, 1991)

Mode of Transmission	Physiologic Mechanisms
Epicrine	Hormones pass through gap junctions of adjacent cells without entering extracellular fluid
Neurocrine	Neurocrine transmission
	Hormones diffuse through synaptics clefts between neurons as neutrotransmitters
	Hormones are synthesized in the neuron's cell body, stored in axons (like neurotransmitters), but secreted into blood
Paracrine	Paracrine transmission
	Hormones diffuse through interstitial fluid, e.g., prostaglandins
Endocrine	Endocrine transmission
	Hormones transported through blood circulation, typical of most hormones.
Exocrine	Hormone secreted to exterior of body
	Hormones affect cell activity more distal to point of secretion
	Hormones, such as somatostatin, exocrine transmission (secretion to intestinal lumen), act as inhibitors of many functions, including intestinal motility and intestinal absorption

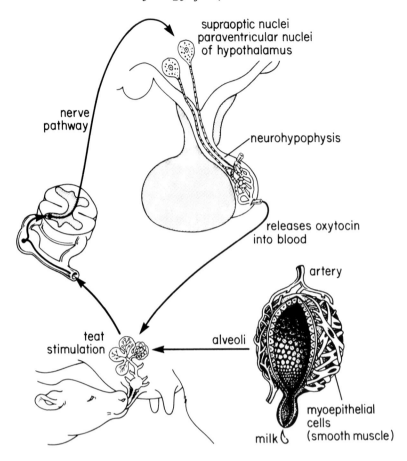

FIG. 3–1. Milk letdown may be considered a neuroendocrine reflex. The stimulation of the teat induces a neural signal to the hypothalamus to release oxytocin from the neurohypophysis, which stimulates the myoepithelial cells to constrict the alveoli, resulting in milk secretion.

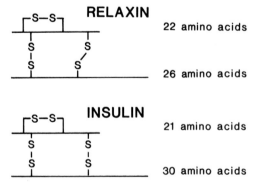

FIG. 3–2. The chemical structures of relaxin and insulin are similar, but their biologic actions are different.

to the amount of milk produced and is related directly to a lower pulsatile release of LH (see Fig. 3–1).

Feedback Mechanisms

The synthesis, storage, and release of hypothalamic hormones are regulated by both pituitary and steroid hormones through two feedback mechanisms: a long and a short loop. Long feedback involves interaction among the gonad, pituitary, and hypothalamus. In the short feedback system, the levels of pituitary gonadotropins can influence the secretory activity of the releasing hormones without mediation of the gonads. Depending on their concentration in the blood, steroid hormones may exert a stimulatory (positive) or an inhibi-

TABLE 3–6. Major Hormones of Reproduction

Source or Gland	Releasing Hormones	Physiologic Functions
Hypothalamus	Luteinizing hormone-releasing hormone (LH-RH)	Stimulates release of FSH and LH
	Growth hormone-releasing hormone (GH-RH)	Stimulates release of growth hormone
	Growth hormone-inhibiting hormone (GH-LH) (Somatostatin)	Inhibits release of growth hormone
	Thyrotropin-releasing hormone (TRH)	Stimulates release of thyroid-stimulating hormone (TSH) and prolactin
	Prolactin-inhibiting factor (PIF)	Inhibits release of prolactin
	Corticotropin-releasing hormone (CRH)	Stimulates release of ACTH
Anterior pituitary	Follicle-stimulating hormone (FSH)	Stimulates follicular growth, spermatogenesis, estrogen secretion
	Luteinizing hormone (LH)	Stimulates ovulation, corpus luteum function: stimulates secretion of progesterone, estrogen, and androgen
	Prolactin (PRL)	Promotes lactation, stimulates corpus luteum function and progesterone secretion in some species, promotes maternal behavior
		*Promotes tissue and bone growth
Posterior pituitary	Oxytocin (stored in posterior pituitary; also produced in ovary)	Stimulates uterine contractions, parturition, and sperm and egg transport
		Facilitates milk ejection
		Possible luteolytic function
Placenta	Human chorionic gonadotrophin (primates only) (hCG)	LH activity
	Maintains corpus luteum of pregnancy in primates	
	Pregnant mare serum gonadotropin (PMSG)	FSH activity
		Stimulates formation of accessory corpora lutea in the mare
	Placental lactogen	Regulates transport of nutrients from dam to fetus not fully elucidated
	Pregnancy protein B	
Ovary	Estrogens (E)	Promotes sexual behavior; stimulates secondary sex characteristics, growth of reproductive tract, uterine contractions, and mammary duct growth
		Controls gonadotropin release, stimulates calcium uptake in bones, has anabolic effects
	Progestins (progesterones) (P)	Acts synergistically with estrogen in promoting estrous behavior and preparing reproductive tract for implantation
Testis	Androgens	Develops and maintains accessory sex glands; stimulates secondary sexual characteristics, sexual behavior, and spermatogenesis; has anabolic effects
	Inhibin and activin	Inhibits and stimulates FSH
Uterus	Relaxin	Dilates cervix
	Prostaglandins	Causes uterine contractions and is luteolytic

TABLE 3–7.   **Secondary Hormones of Reproduction**

Source	Hormone	Some Functions
Placenta	Human chorionic go-nadotropin (hCG)	LH-like
	Estradiol	See Ovary (Table 3–6)
	Progesterone	See Ovary (Table 3–6)
Anterior Pituitary	Somatotropin hor-mone (STH)	Body growth; protein synthesis
	Thyroid-stimulating hormone (TSH)	Stimulates thyroid gland Thyroxine release and iodine up-take by thyroid
	Adrenocorticotropic hormone (ACTH)	Stimulates adrenal cortex Release of adrenal corticoids
Posterior Pituitary	Antidiuretic hor-mone (ADH; Vaso-pressin)	Water balance
Thyroid	Thyroxine	Body growth; development and maturation; oxidation of feeds
Parathyroid	Parathormone	Calcium and phosphorus metab-olism
Adrenal Cortex	Aldosterone	Electrolyte and water metabolism
	17-OH corticoids (cor-tisone; cortisol)	Carbohydrate, protein, and fat metabolism
Pancreas	Insulin	Carbohydrate, fat, and protein metabolism

tory (negative) feedback. Positive feedback results when an estrogen or a progestin stimulates the release of a gonadotropin, such as LH. Negative feedback results when large levels of progesterone prevent the release of a gonadotropin.

Stimulatory Feedback (A Positive Feedback)

In this system, an increasing level of hormones causes subsequent increase of another hormone. For example, increasing levels of estrogen during the preovulatory phase trigger an abrupt release of pituitary LH. These two events are precisely synchronized, because an LH surge is necessary for the rupture of ovarian follicle.

Inhibitory Mechanism (A Negative Feedback)

This system involves reciprocal interrelationships with two or more glands and target organs. For example, as the ovary is stimulated, estrogen secretion increases, and FSH levels decline. Also, when pituitary hormones reach a certain level, some hypothalamic nuclei respond by decreasing the production of their particular releasing hormone. The decreased levels of releasing hormones causes a decline in secretion of pituitary tropic hormone and, subsequently, a lower level of target gland function.

Immunoendocrine Aspects

The endocrine and immune systems interact extensively to regulate each other. Several endocrine organs are involved in some aspect of this regulatory process: hypothalamus, pituitary, gonads, adrenals, pineal, thyroid, and thymus. Many of these organs are themselves affected by immune function. The autonomic nervous system is also involved in this regulation; it affects the hypothalamus, pituitary, adrenal, thymus, gut-associated lymphatic tissue, lymph nodes, and bone marrow.

Hormone Receptors

Each hormone has a selective effect on one or more target organs. This phenomenon is achieved through two mechanisms:

1. Each target organ has a specific method of binding that hormone not found in other tissue.
2. The target organs have certain metabolic pathways capable of responding to the hormone-metabolic pathways not shared by nontarget tissue.

Specific binding is the usual mechanism. For example, all target tissues that respond to steroid hormones contain a receptor protein within the cell, which specifically binds the activating hormone. Within the target cell, the steroid hormone is found in the cytoplasm, bound to a relatively large protein (molecular weight, 200,000 daltons). This steroid protein complex migrates across the process, and the protein changes in shape and size. The newly transformed complex enters the nucleus and causes a sequence of physiologic responses specific for that cell.

The target cells of the anterior pituitary possess cell membrane receptors that recognize and selectively bind the protein hormones, including gonadotropins (Figs. 3–3, 3–4). The binding phenomenon triggers the synthesis and secretion of the pituitary hormone via the cyclic AMP–protein kinase system of the cell. Gonadotropin receptors, in turn, are influenced by estrogen levels (McDonald and Capen, 1989).

Hormone Assays

Several techniques are used to study endocrinology: ablation of a gland, organ replacement therapy, and isolation of hormones (Table 3–1). Quantitive measurements of hormones are based on bioassays, immunologic assays, and radioreceptor assays (RIAs).

Bioassays. Biologic assays have been used to measure activity of all hormones. The hormone is administered to the animal to induce a measurable biologic response.

Radioimmunoassays. RIA, one of the major advances in analytic endocrinology, allows rapid measurement of large numbers of samples containing low concentrations of hormones. The principle of the RIA is based on the theory that in the absence of unlabeled antigen or hormone (H), the labeled radioactive hormone (H*) has maximal opportunity to react with a limited number of antibody-binding sites (Ab).

PITUITARY GLAND (HYPOPHYSIS)

The pituitary gland is located in the sella turcica, a bony depression at the base of the brain. The gland is subdivided into two distinct anatomic parts: an anterior lobe and posterior lobe. There are remarkable species variations in the anatomy of the pituitary gland. For example, the pars intermedia is well developed in the hypophysis of cattle and horses.

The anterior pituitary has five different cell types that secrete the seven hormones of the anterior pituitary:

1. Somatotrope cells, which secrete growth hormone
2. Corticotrope cells, which secrete adrenocorticotropic hormone (ACTH)
3. Mammotrope cells, which secrete prolactin
4. Thyrotrope cells, which secrete thyroid-stimulating hormone (TSH)
5. Gonadotrope cells, which secrete FSH and LH (Fig. 3–5)

The release of pituitary hormones in blood serum is cyclic. FSH and LH are not released in the blood at a constant rate but rather by a sequence of small dosages.

Pharmaceutical companies obtain animal pituitary glands from slaughter houses and extract several hormones for commercial and experimental uses.

Vascular Supply

The vascular connection between the hypothalamus and the anterior pituitary is unique. Arterial blood enters the pituitary by way of the superior hypophyseal artery and inferior hypophyseal artery. The superior hypophyseal artery forms capillary

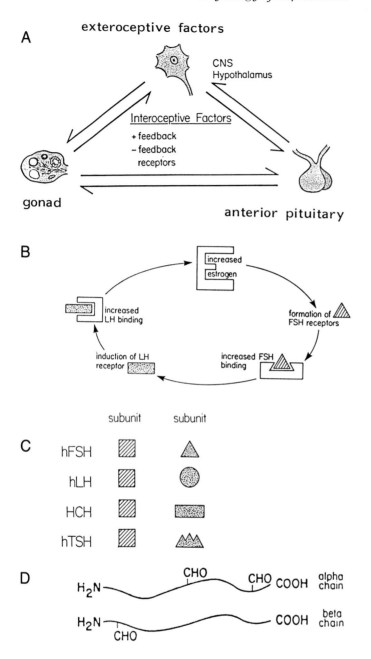

FIG. 3–3. *A*, The endocrine relationships of exteroceptive and interoceptive factors as they affect the functions of the hypothalamus, pituitary gland, and gonads. *B*, Diagram showing the formation of gonadotropin receptors as affected by estrogen level. *C*, Subunits of pituitary protein hormones. Note that the biologic activity is determined by β-subunits, whereas α-subunits are similar in structure. *D*, The α- and β-subunits of LH (a glycoprotein). Shown is the approximate position of the polysaccharide units (CHO). The peptide bonds linking the amino acid chains are not shown.

loops at the medial eminence and pars nervosa. From these capillaries, the blood flows into the hypothalamohypophyseal protal vessels, which pass down the pituitary stalk to terminate in capillaries in the anterior pituitary. The hypothalamohypophyseal portal system is the vascular pathway that transports hypothalamic hormones to the anterior pituitary (see Fig. 3–4). The inferior hypophyseal artery transports blood to the anterior and posterior pituitary. The interruption of these blood vessels in the stalk of the pituitary gland leads to gonadal atrophy. If, however, the stalk of the pituitary is allowed to revascularize, gonadal functions can re-

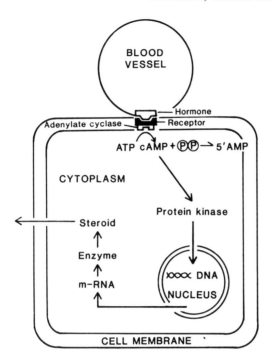

BLOOD VESSEL

Adenylate cyclase — Hormone — Receptor

ATP cAMP + ℗℗ → 5'AMP

CYTOPLASM

Protein kinase

Steroid
↑
Enzyme
↑
m-RNA
↑

xxxx DNA
NUCLEUS

CELL MEMBRANE

FIG. 3–4. Schematic mechanism of action of protein hormones. The sequence of cellular events that occur following binding of a protein hormone to a receptor in the membrane of a target cell is shown.

sume. On the other hand, electrical or hormonal stimulation of specific nuclei of the hypothalamus can regulate gonadal function.

PITUITARY GONADOTROPINS

The anterior pituitary gland secretes four major gonadotropic hormones: FSH, LH, prolactin and TSH. Prolactin and proprionic acid can dissociate FSH, LH, and TSH into two nonidentical subunits termed α- and β-subunits. The α-subunit is identical within species for FSH, LH, and TSH. The molecular weight of each of the glycoprotein hormones is approximately 32,000 daltons, with each subunit having a molecular weight of 16,000 daltons. The α- and β-subunits of any of these hormones by themselves have no biologic activity. If the α-subunit of one hormone (LHα) is recombined with the β-subunit

of another hormone (FSHβ), the molecule regains FSH biologic activity or the activity of the β-subunit. If two α-subunits or two β-subunits are combined, no biologic activity is noted. These hormones have primary action on the gonads.

Follicle-Stimulating Hormone. FSH stimulates the growth and maturation of the ovarian follicle. FSH does not cause secretion of estrogen from the ovary by itself, but in the presence of LH, it stimulates estrogen production from either the ovary or testis. In the male, FSH acts on the germinal cells in the seminiferous tubule of the testis. FSH is also responsible for spermatogenesis up to the secondary spermatocytes, after which androgens are responsible for final stages of spermatogenesis.

In women, after menopause the pituitary output of FSH increases tremendously, which is due to the lack of steroids. This increase in FSH output is at such high concentrations that it passes through the kidney and goes directly to the urine and is called *human menopausal gonadotropin* (hMG). The biologic activity of hMG is increased over FSH from women with active ovaries and is available commercially as a fertility hormone for women (Pergonal). FSH is primarily used in the stimulation of follicular development to induce multiple ovulations for embryo transfer.

Luteinizing Hormone LH is a glycoprotein composed of an α- and a β-subunit with a molecular weight of 30,000 daltons and a half-life of 30 minutes. Tonic or basal levels of LH act in conjunction with FSH to induce estrogen secretion from the large ovarian follicle. The preovulatory surge of LH is responsible for rupture of the follicle wall and ovulation. The interstitial cells of both the ovary and testis are stimulated by LH. In the male, the interstitial cells (Leydig cells) produce androgens after LH stimulation.

Tonic LH and FSH Release. Serum LH and FSH are released in a tonic or basal fashion in both sexes. Tonic levels of LH and FSH are controlled by negative

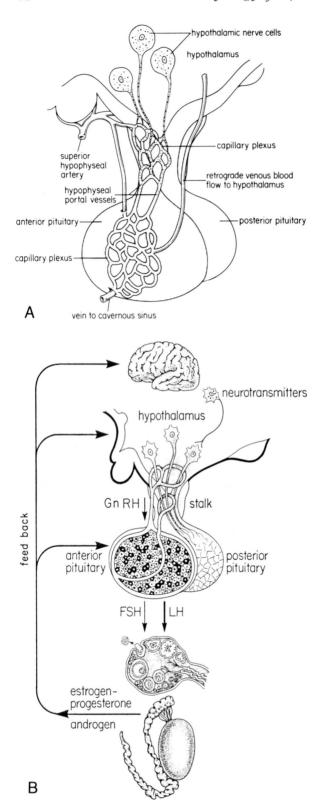

hypothalamic nerve cells

hypothalamus

capillary plexus

superior
hypophyseal
artery

retrograde venous blood
flow to hypothalamus

hypophyseal
portal vessels

anterior pituitary

posterior pituitary

capillary plexus

A   vein to cavernous sinus

neurotransmitters

hypothalamus

Gn RH   stalk

anterior
pituitary

posterior
pituitary

feed back

FSH   LH

estrogen-
progesterone

androgen

B

FIG.   3–5. Hypothalamus–pituitary–gonadal complex. *A,* Hypothalamic nerve cells releasing neurohormones into the portal vessels for transport to the anterior pituitary via the hypothalamohypophyseal portal vessels. Solid particles in nerve cells represent neurohormones. Blood is also transported by the retrograde venous system back to the hypothalamus. *B,* Endocrine–neuroendocrine relationship among hypothalamus, pituitary gland, and gonad (ovary–testis). Hypothalamic neurosecretory materials (GnRH) are transported by the portal blood capillaries to the cells of the anterior pituitary. FSH and LH stimulate the gonads. Estrogens and androgens secreted by gonads exert a feedback.

feedback from the gonads. The tonic level of LH is not stationary but shows oscillations about every hour. Tonic serum LH levels are elevated after castration in both males and females. The increased levels of LH and FSH after gonadectomy is due to the lack of a negative feedback from the gonadal steroids on the tonic LH control center in the hypothalamus.

The LH and FSH surges also induce the final stages of oocyte maturation, just before ovulation, to metaphase II. The levels of estradiol fall after the LH and FSH surge, and the psychic manifestations of estrus abate. Ovulation occurs 24 to 30 hours after the initial maximal gonadotropin surge. At the time of ovulation, the levels of estradiol, progesterone, and LH are low.

Preovulatory LH and FSH Release. A second type of LH and FSH release, called the *preovulatory surge of LH and FSH,* is evident in the female before ovulation. The preovulatory surges of LH and FSH are responsible for ovulation, and they last from 6 to 12 hours. The preovulatory surge of LH is initiated by an increase in the circulating estrogen concentration, which has a positive effect on the hypothalamus, inducing release of LH-RH (LH releasing hormone) which results in the preovulatory surge of LH and FSH. Anestrous ewes treated with estradiol-17β exhibit a surge of LH and FSH within 15 or 16 hours after treatment. The site of estrogen action is the anterior hypothalamus. Because of the cost of purification of LH from pituitaries, the less costly, but equally effective, human chorionic gonadotropin (hCG) is used in place of pituitary LH. The uses of this LH-like molecule are induced ovulation, primarily in cows with cystic ovaries, or to aid in superovulation of embryo-transfer cows.

Coitus may prolong the LH surge. Mating can modulate the preovulatory surge of LH by prolonging the duration of LH release rather than by increasing plasma concentrations. Mating affects the time of ovulation in species that ovulate spontane-

ously, such as rats and sheep. In beef cattle, clitoral stimulation hastens the onset of ovulation, and cervical stimulation reduces the time from the beginning of estrus to the occurrence of LH surge. Various neural pathways exist between the reproductive system and hypothalamic–pituitary axis. In sows, natural mating affects ovulation by shortening the interval from onset of estrus to ovulation and by reducing the interval from the first to last ovulation. Naturally mated sows have higher concentrations of plasma LH immediately after mating. Coitus or mechanical stimulation of the vagina and cervix stimulated LH release in spontaneously ovulating rats. FSH, LH, and prolactin levels increase 20 minutes after mating in both intact and pelvically neuroectomized female rats.

Gonadotropins and Ovulation Induction. Various preparations of gonadotropic hormones are used to induce ovulation and pregnancy in anovulatory women. Excessive dosages of FSH, a higher concentration of LH than FSH in the preparation, or prolonged treatment with hCG, may cause multiple ovulation and multiple pregnancies. To avoid multiple ovulation, the patients are carefully selected, and their endocrine profiles are monitored throughout treatment.

Effect of Hormones in Vitro FSH and LH promote physiologic maturation in vitro. Cumulus cell-enclosed germinal vesicle stage mouse oocytes were matured in medium containing FSH or LH with or without FSH antiserum. The physiologic maturity of the oocytes can be evaluated in vitro by examining their potential for fertilization and development to blastocysts. FSH and LH significantly increase the rate of blastocyst development from oocytes. The beneficial effects of FSH and LH on oocyte maturation were abolished when added simultaneously. In whole-follicle cultures, when combined with LH, FSH inhibits the maturation-inducing effect of LH alone (Jinno et al., 1990). FSH initially increases the cyclic adenosine monophosphate (cAMP) level in cumulus–oocyte complexes and in suppression of meiotic resumption.

FSH may stimulate the production of a positive maturation signal by the cumulus cells through a cAMP-dependent process. Stimulation of maturation by LH may occur via a reduction in the level of a maturation inhibitor in the cumulus cells. Estrogens do not enhance the rate of blastocyst development, but blastocyst hatching may be enhanced. The results of the oocytes maturation in whole-follicle culture also suggest that precise balance and sequence of steroids is necessary for the full maturation of oocytes.

Prolactin

Ovine prolactin is a 198 amino acid protein with a molecular weight of 24,000 daltons. Prolactin molecules are similar in structure to growth hormones, and in some species, these hormones have similar biologic properties. Prolactin is termed a *gonadotropic hormone* because of its luteotropic properties (maintenance of corpus luteum) in rodents. In domestic animals, LH is the main luteotropic hormone, with prolactin being of less importance in the luteotropic complex. Prolactin acts on the central nervous system (CNS) to induce maternal behavior. In women, high levels of prolactin suppress menses (galactorrhea–amenorrhea syndrome); however, prolactin levels have not been associated with lack of breeding in cows or sheep.

Growth Hormone

Growth hormone (GH) is also known as *somatropic hormone (STH)* because of its stimulating effect of the somatic cells (body cells). STH is needed throughout life as well as during the growth phase. These metabolic effects include the following:

1. Increases rate of protein synthesis in all body cells.
2. Increases mobilization of fatty acids from fat and increases the use of fatty acids for energy.
3. Decreases rate of glucose uptake throughout the body.

Growth hormone has no specific target gland but acts on several tissues in the body. Secretion of GH is controlled mainly, but not exclusively, by the hypothalamus.

Posterior Pituitary Hormones

The hormones of the posterior pituitary, peptides formed by nerve cell bodies within hypothalamic nuclei, are transported by axons to terminal positions in the neurohypophysis (posterior pituitary) for storage. The posterior pituitary hormones, antidiuretic hormone (ADH) and oxytocin, are neurosecretions.

Oxytocin

Oxytocin and vasopressin are synthesized in the hypothalamus and stored in the neurohypophysis (posterior pituitary). They were the first hormonal peptides to be synthesized. Arginine vasopressin, also called *ADH*, is identified. Lysine vasopressin is identified in domestic pigs.

Oxytocin and ADH are synthesized in the supraoptic and paraventricular nuclei of the hypothalamus and are only stored and released from the neurohypophysis. These hypothalamic hormones (neurohypophyseal hormones) are synthesized together with the carrier proteins called *neurophysins*. As with other neurosecretions, oxytocin and vasopressin are transported in small vesicles enclosed by a membrane. These secretory vesicles flow down the hypothalamic–hypophyseal nerve axons by axoplasmic streaming. They are stored at the nerve endings next to the capillary beds in the neurohypophysis until their release into the circulation (see Fig. 3–5). Oxytocin is also produced in the corpus luteum. Thus, oxytocin has two sites of origin, the ovary and the hypothalamus.

Function. Oxytocin has several functions: contraction of uterine muscle, increased contraction frequency in the oviduct, the transport of both female and male gametes in the oviduct, and milk letdown. Estrogen enhances responsiveness of smooth muscle to oxytocin. The lactating female becomes conditioned to visual and tactile stimuli associated with suckling or milking. This conditioning induces the release of oxytocin into the circulation, to act on the myoepithelial cells (smooth muscle cells) that surround the alveoli in the mammary gland, resulting in milk letdown (see Fig. 3–1). Ovarian oxytocin is involved in luteal function by acting on endometrium to induce prostaglandin $F_{2\alpha}$ ($PGF_{2\alpha}$) release, which has a luteolytic action (regression of the corpus luteum).

Oxytocin has several applications: It induces female animals to let down milk after parturition, it induces expulsion of retained placentas, and it aids delivery in young animals when the period of labor is extended.

HYPOTHALAMUS

The hypothalamus, which occupies only a very small portion of the brain, consists of the region of the third ventricle, extending from the optic chiasma to the mammillary bodies (Fig. 3–6) The hypothalamus, an important neuroendocrine center, releases several hormones. Naturally occurring releasing hormones, extracted from thousands of ovine and procine hypothalami have been used to determine the biochemical structure of these hormones. For example, the hypothalamic gonadotropin-releasing hormone (GnRH) is a decapeptide composed of 10 amino acids. Several of the hypothalamic hormones have been synthesized and marketed for clinical use.

Function

The hypothalamus regulates various vital automatic processes, such as appetite, heart rate, temperature control, sexual behavior, and neuroendocrine activity. Various centers in the hypothalamus integrate physiologic signals in the body, such as the CNS, metabolic status, functional activity

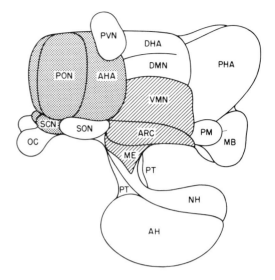

▦ control centers of preovulatory LH and FSH

▨ control centers of tonic LH and FSH secretion

FIG. 3–6. Schematic drawing of hypothalamic nuclei and pituitary. *AH*, adenohypophysis; *ARC*, arcuate nucleus; *AHA*, anterior hypothalamic area; *DHA*, dorsal hypothalamic area; *DMN*, dorsal medial nucleus; *ME*, median eminence; *NH*, neurohypophysis; *MB*, mammillary body; *PM*, premammillary nucleus; *OC*, optic chiasm; *PVN*, paraventricular nuclei; *PON*, preoptic nuclei; *PHA*, posterior hypothalamic area; *PT*, pars tuberalis; *SCN*, suprachiasmatic nucleus; *SON*, supraoptic nuclei; *VMN*, ventromedial nucleus. The diagonal lines show nuclei that control tonic LH and FSH release from the pituitary. The dotted areas are nuclei that control the preovulatory surge of LH and FSH from the pituitary.

of target glands, and the internal environment. The hypothalamus then responds by elaboration of specific releasing hormones. Thus, the hypothalamus acts as a processing and integrating center for received information and translates it into a neurohormonal signal that evokes physiologic responses (Tables 3–8, 3–9, Figs. 3–6 to 3–8).

The main hormones released by the hypothalamus that regulate reproduction include the gonadotropin-releasing hormone (GnRH or LH-RH), ACTH, and prolactin-inhibiting factor (PIF). The hypothalamus is also the source of oxytocin

TABLE 3–8. Nomenclature of LH- and FSH-Releasing Hormones

Name*	Abbreviation
Luteinizing hormone-releasing hormone	LH-RH or LRH
Luteinizing hormone-releasing hormone/follicle-stimulating hormone-releasing hormone	LH-RH/FSH-RH
Gonadotropin-releasing hormone	Gn-RH
Luteinizing hormone-releasing factor	LH-RF or LRF
Luliberin	LH-RH
Gonadoliberin	Gn-RH
Cystorelin	Gn-RH
Factrel	Gn-RH

* All hormone names conform with those listed in *The Merck Index,* 10th-Ed. Rahway, NJ, Merck, 1983.

TABLE 3–9. Hypothalamic Hormones that Regulate Anterior Pituitary Hormones

Name of Hormone	Abbreviation	Number of Amino Acids	Function
Luteinizing hormone-releasing hormone	LH-RH	10	Releases LH and FSH
Growth hormone-releasing hormone	GH-RH	44	Releases GH
Growth hormone-inhibiting hormone (Somatostatin)	GH-IH	14	Inhibits GH release
Thyrotropin-releasing hormone	TRH	3	Releases TSH and prolactin
Corticotropin-releasing hormone	CRH	41	Releases ACTH

and vasopressin, the hormones stored in the posterior lobe of the pituitary gland.

Mode of Action

Specific hypothalamic neurons synthesize several peptide hormones, which controls the release and synthesis of hormones of the anterior lobe of the pituitary gland. The role of the hypothalamus in reproduction involves both the triggering effect of steroid hormones on sexual behavior and simultaneously the control of the secretion of pituitary gonadotropins. The local action of steroids administered by intrahypothalamic implant or injection induces the development of sexual behavior in the gonadectomized animal. The hypothalamus plays a critical role in initiating the mechanisms of sexual behavior as a response to hormones. The hypothalamic centers controlling tonic LH secretion in anestrous ewes respond more rapidly to the stimulatory effects of the introduction of rams in the morning than in the evening.

The neurons involved in such a "sex center" do not form an anatomically individualized nucleus but appear to be scattered in an area extending from slightly posterior to the optic chiasm to the anterior preoptic area. The neural pathways involved in sexual behavior seem to be located in more anterior and superior parts of the hypothalamus. The activation of copulatory patterns seems to be under varying degrees of inhibitory control by the CNS. Lesions in the junction of diencephalon and mesencephalon cause an increase in the copulatory performance of male rats. The hypothalamus may control sexual behavior in several ways: (a) fixation of sexual steroids and slow-acting elaboration of sexual motivation, (b) direct control of sexual activity, and (c) sexual satisfaction.

Hypothalamic Hormones

Several hypothalamic hormones have been isolated and structurally identified:

Follicle-stimulating releasing hormone (FSH-RH)

Luteinizing hormone-releasing hormone (LH-RH)

Gonadotropic releasing hormone (GnRH)

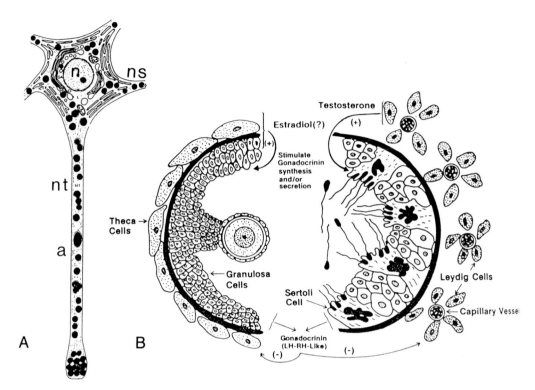

FIG. 3–7. *A,* Structural characteristics of a neurosecretory neuron in the hypothalamus. The nerve cell body (n, nucleus) has dendritic and axonal (a) processes with arrays of rough endoplasmic reticulum, a prominent Golgi apparatus, and neurotubule (nt). Hormone-containing, membrane-limited neurosecretory granules (ns) are formed in the Golgi apparatus and transported along the axon to the site of release at the termination on capillaries. Neurosecretory neurons synthesize the releasing and release-inhibiting hormones of the adenohypophysis and the hormones of the neurohypophysis (oxytocin, antidiuretic hormone). The feedback to the theca cells and Leydig cells may inhibit steroidogenesis by decreasing the number of receptors; it also would interfere with the activation of the cAMP system (From Capen, C.C. and Martin, S.L.: The pituitary gland. *In* Veterinary Endocrinology and Reproduction. L.E. McDonald and M.H. Pineda (eds.). Philadelphia, Lea & Febiger, 1989). *B,* Postulated physiologic function of gonadotropins on the Sertoli and granulosa cells. (Adapted from different sources, including R.N. Sharp (1982). J. Reprod. Fertil. *64,* 517.)

Thyrotropin-releasing hormone (TRH)

Somatostatin or growth hormone-inhibiting hormone (GH-Ih)

Growth hormone-releasing hormone (GH-RH)

Corticotropin-releasing hormone (CRH)

The amino acid numbers and function of hypothalamic hormones is shown in Figure 3–9.

In 1977, two American scientists, Schally and Guillemin, shared the Nobel prize for their independent research on determining the chemical structures of hormones of the hypothalamus that control pituitary function. LH-RH is a decapeptide (10 amino acids) with a molecular weight of 1183 daltons. This hormone induces release of both LH and FSH from the pituitary. Stimulatory analogs have been synthesized that induce release of more LH and FSH than natural LH-RH. The release of FSH and LH is controlled by LH-RH (see Tables 3–4, 3–5). The half-life of LH-RH is 7 minutes in the ewe. The

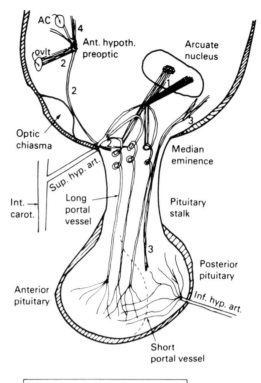

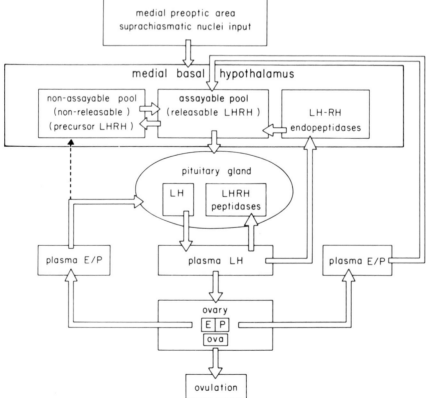

FIG. 3–8.   *(Top)* Schematic representation of LH-RH: 1. The main LH-RH pathway originates in the arcuate nucleus and terminates in the median eminence at the origin site of the long portal vessels. 2. Tracts from the anterior hypothalamic-preoptic area to the organum vasulosum laninae terminalis (ovlt.) and to the median eminence. 3. Tracts from the hypothalamus to the posterior pituitary. 4. Tracts from the anterior commissure (AC) into the limbic system. (Ferin, M. (1982). Neuroendocrine control of ovarian function in the primate. J. Reprod. Fert. *69*, 369–381.)

(Bottom) Some of the control systems that regulate the preovulatory surge of LH.

(a). Prior to the initiation of the preovulatory LH surge, estrogen rises in circulation and increases the pituitary gland's responsiveness to LH-RH. This steroid also may alter thresholds of excitability within the preoptico-tuberal unit and may be responsible, in part, for the initial release of the LH-RH, which primes the pituitary gland (f).

(b). On presentation of an intrinsic stimulus (unknown), LH-RH is released into portal plasma and activates the discharge of LH.

(c). The release of self-priming amounts of LH-RH also may be manifested by a decrease in the releasable (assayable) pool of MBH-LH-RH. Further, a decline in this releasable pool of LH-RH is detected by an intrinsic short-loop feedback system, and it is replenished. This may be accomplished by an increase in synthesis of new LH-RH and suggested rhythmic pulsatile release of LH-RH into the portal circulation. During this interval of LH-RH release, the presensitized pituitary gland responds by the discharge of markedly increased amounts of LH into plasma.

(d). When ovarian LH threshold concentrations are reached, follicular rupture and ovulation occur. Also, while LH is rising, estrogen declines and progesterone increases in plasma.

(e). The cessation of pituitary LH release may be the consequence of an LH feedback system that activates endopeptidases located both within the pituitary gland and the hypothalamus whose function is to degrade LH-RH.

(f). The changing plasma steroid levels (during the LH surge) may also alter the release of MBH-LH-RH such that it declines in portal plasma. With the cessation of LH-RH release, this hormone then remains in steady-state concentrations within the MBH throughout the remainder of the cycle until the time of the next preovulatory LH surge.

Progesterone also serves to facilitate the release of LH-RH, perhaps by augmenting the LH release response following prior estrogen exposure. (Barraclough, C.A. (1979). Central nervous regulation of the preovulatory release of FSH and LH from the pituitary gland. *In* Human Ovulation Mechanisms, Prediction, Detection and Induction. E.S.E. Hafez (ed.). Amsterdam, North Holland.)

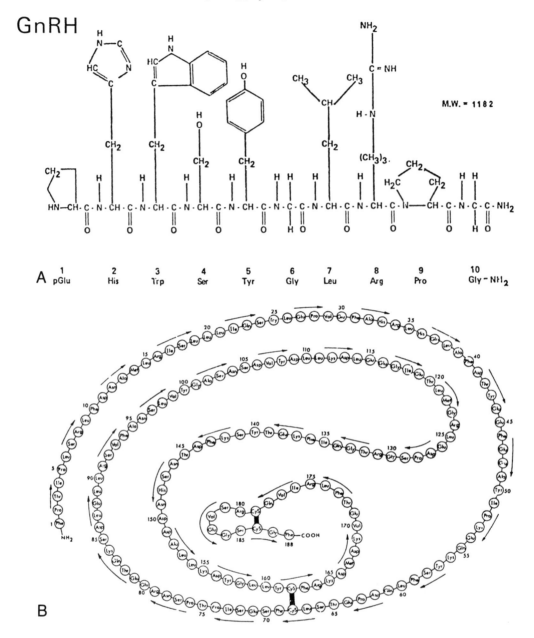

FIG. 3–9. *A*, Amino acid sequence of gonadotropin-releasing hormone (GnRH). (From Capen, C.C., and Martin, S.L. (1989). The pituitary gland. *In* Veterinary Endocrinology and Reproduction. L.E. McDonald and M.H. Pineda (eds.). Philadelphia, Lea & Febiger.) *B*, Amino acid sequence of the human somatotropin hormone (STH) molecule (Adapted from Lich, 1969).

short half-life LH-RH has made its application to the livestock industry difficult. LH-RH is effective in overcoming cystic follicles in cows. In this instance, 100 μg of LH-RH induces the release of substantial amounts of endogenous LH to induce luteinization or rupture of the cystic follicle. Cows with a treated cystic ovary exhibit estrus 19 to 23 days later and can then be bred. TSH stimulates the synthesis of colloid by thyroid gland cells and stimulates the release of thyroid hormone. Associated with these functions are the accumulation of iodine, organic binding of iodine, and formation of thyroxine within the thyroid gland.

Clinical Uses of Hypothalamic-Releasing Hormones

GnRH has been used for the treatment of delayed puberty and various infertility problems in both men and women. GnRH and TRH injected intravenously in microgram quantities provide a valuable diagnostic tool to distinguish between hypothalamic and pituitary defects. TRH is used to increase milk production by nursing mothers.

PLACENTAL HORMONES

The placenta secretes several hormones either identical to, or with biologic activity similar to, hormones of mammalian reproduction: Pregnant mare serum gonadotropin (PMSG), hCG, placental lactogen (PL), and protein B (Tables 3–10, 3–11).

Pregnant Mare Serum Gonadotropin

PMSG was discovered when blood from pregnant mares produced sexual maturity in immature rats (Cole and Hart, 1930). PMSG is a glycoprotein with α- and β-subunits similar to LH and FSH but with a higher carbohydrate content, especially sialic acid. The higher sialic acid content appears to account for the long half-life of several days for PMSG. Thus, a single injection of PMSG has biologic effects on the target gland for more than a week.

This placental gonadotropin is secreted by the equine uterus. The endometrial cups are formed at about day 40 of pregnancy and persist until day 85 of pregnancy. The secretion of PMSG stimulates development of ovarian follicles. Some of these follicles ovulate, but most form a luteinized follicle, which is due to the LH-like action of the PMSG. These accessory corpora lutea produce progestogens important to the maintenance of pregnancy in the mare. PMSG has both FSH and LH biologic actions, with the FSH actions be-

TABLE 3–10. Placental Hormones and Their Biologic Actions

Hormone	Species	Body Fluids Present in	Biologic Actions
Pregnant mare serum gonadotrophin (PMSG)	Horse	Blood	Primary FSH action, some LH activity
Human chorionic gonadotrophin (hCG)	Monkey	Blood and urine	Primary LH action, some FSH activity
Placental lactogen (PL)	Cow Sheep Rodent	Blood	Growth hormone and prolactin
Protein B	Sheep Cow	Blood	Unknown

TABLE 3–11. Gonadotropic Hormones Clinically Used to Stimulate the Ovaries and to Induce Ovulation and Corpus Luteum Formation in Anovulatory Females

Hormone	Preparation	Source of Extraction
hCG	Human chorionic gonadotropin	Urine of pregnant women
FSH	Follicle-stimulating hormone	Postmortem human pituitary gland
LH	Luteinizing hormone	
hMG	Human menopausal gonadotropin	Urine of postmenopausal women
PMSG	Pregnant mare serum gonadotropin	Serum of pregnant mares
Various preparations	Animal pituitary gonadotropin	Pituitary glands of animals

ing dominant. PMSG is isolated from the blood of pregnant mares and is not found in urine. PMSG was one of the first commercially available gonadotropins and is used to induce superovulation.

Human Chorionic Gonadotropin

The glycoprotein hCG consists of α- and β-subunits with a molecular weight of 40,000 daltons. The α-subunit has 92 amino acids and two carbohydrate chains. The α-subunit of hCG is similar to the α-subunits of human, porcine, ovine, and bovine LH. The β-subunit has 145 amino acids and five carbohydrate chains. Human chorionic gonadotropin, synthesized by the syncytiotrophoblastic cells of the placenta of primates, is found in both the blood and urine. It is detected in the urine 8 days after conception by sensitive radioimmunoassays.

Because hCG appears early in human pregnancy, detection of hCG in the urine is the basis of immunologic human pregnancy tests. In addition, the LH-like action of hCG has made it the first hormone available for treatment of cystic ovaries in cattle. The hCG treatment of a cow with cystic ovaries usually requires 5,000 to 10,000 IU of hCG, after which the follicle either ovulates and forms a corpus luteum or more often, luteinizes. In either case, the luteal structure produces progesterone and the corpus luteum is functional for 20 days and regresses normally, allowing the cow to cycle 21 days after treatment. At that time she is expected to breed almost as successfully as a noncystic cow. Certain malignancies, such as chorioepithelioma and hydatiform moles in women are associated with high levels of urinary gonadotropins.

Placental Lactogen

Placental lactogen is a protein with chemical properties similar to prolactin and growth hormone. Its molecular weight is 22,000 to 23,000 daltons in the ovine with 192 amino acids. Placental lactogen is isolated from placental tissue but cannot be detected in the serum of the pregnant animal until the last trimester of pregnancy. Placental lactogen is more important for its growth hormone properties than its prolactin properties. It is important in regulating maternal nutrients to the fetus and possibly is important for fetal growth. Placental lactogen may play a role in milk production because the level is higher in dairy cows (high milk producers) than in beef cows (low milk producers).

Protein B

Protein B has a long circulating half-life of 7 days. It has been isolated (Butler et al., 1982) from bovine placental, and an assay has been developed (Sasser et al., 1986), which can detect it in the blood of pregnant cows as early as 22 days after conception. It is not found in the milk or urine of cows. A radioimmunoassay for protein B in cattle detects the substance in sheep but not in pigs or horses. The physiologic action of protein B may be involved in sending a message from the placenta to the cow or ewe, preventing destruction of the corpus luteum spurium. This placental hormone has the potential to be the first reliable hormonal pregnancy test for cattle.

GONADAL STEROID HORMONES

Steroid hormones secreted by the ovary, testes, placenta, and adrenal cortex have a basic or common nucleus called the *cyclopentanoperhydrophenanthrene nucleus*, consisting of three, six-membered fully hydrogenated (perhydro) phenanthrene rings designated *A, B and C,* and one five-membered cyclopentane ring designed *D* (Fig. 3–10). In 1967, the International Union of Pure and Applied Chemistry (IUPAC) established rules from the number of carbons in a steroid; its biologic action can usually be predicted. An 18-carbon steroid has estrogen activity, a 19-carbon steroid has androgen activity, and a 21-carbon steroid has progestogen properties. Cholesterol, a 27-carbon steroid,

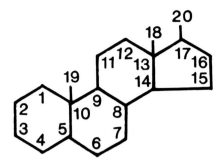

FIG. 3–10. International Union of Pure and Applied Chemistry (IUPAC) nomenclature of steroid nucleus. Letters designate ring and numbers designate carbon.

becomes pregnenolone (20-carbon) when its side chain is cleaved. Pregnenolone is subsequently converted to progesterone, which is in turn converted to an androgen and on to estrogens (Fig. 3–11).

Several enzymes regulate the biosynthesis of steroid hormones from cholesterol in several endocrine glands, for example, the ovary, testis, adrenal glands, and placenta. The testis primarily synthesizes androgens, whereas the ovaries synthesize two major types of steroids: 18-carbon estrogens and the 21-carbon progestins.

In the blood plasma, a large portion of each steroid hormone is bound to albumin, a plasma protein with low affinity and high capacity for steroids. Another portion of the steroid hormone is bound to one or more specific proteins with high affinity. The half-life of naturally occurring steroids in the body is very short. Therefore, several steroids with modified biochemical structure have been synthesized for clinical use.

Steroid hormones cause a variety of physiologic responses in target tissues, such as cell division, tissue differentiation, growth, synthesis of specific proteins, and contraction of smooth muscle. These responses are responsible for various reproductive processes, including sexual behavior, sexual receptivity, priming the uterus for implantation of the blastocyst, prepara-

CHOLESTEROL

PREGNENOLONE

PROGESTERONE

TESTOSTERONE

ESTRADIOL

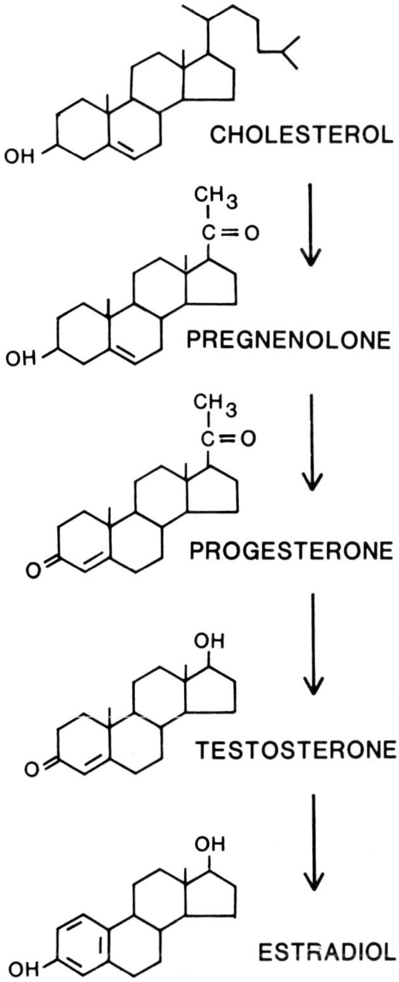

FIG. 3–11. The biosynthesis of steroid hormones from cholesterol. This scheme provides a simplistic view of a highly organized and complicated process that requires multiple enzyme systems.

tion of mammary development for milk production, and regulation of uterine contractions during parturition. Sex steroids also play a major role in the phenotypic expression of sex. The differentiation of male or female fetus depends on the ratios of testosterone to estrogen production during prenatal development.

The secretory activity of steroid hormones by the gonads is under endocrine control of the anterior pituitary. Hypophysectomy before or after puberty causes the gonads to atrophy. The secretory activity of the gonad is restored by injection of pituitary preparation or implantation of pituitary tissue.

Estrogens

Estradiol is the primary estrogen, with estrone and estriol representing other metabolically active estrogens. Androgens are 19-carbon steroids with a hydroxyl or oxygen at positions 3 and 17 and a double-bond at position 4. The androgens are called 17-ketosteroids when oxygen is found at position 17. Several substances of estrogenic activity are found in both the animal and plant kingdom. At least eight estrogens are secreted by the ovary.

Estradiol is the biologically active estrogen produced by the ovary, with smaller quantities of estrone. Except for the possible secretion of small amounts of estriol in the luteal phase of the cycle, most estriol and related urinary estrogens are metabolic breakdown products of secreted estradiol/estrone. All estrogens secreted by the ovary are produced from androgenic precursors.

Function. Estrogens, like androgens, are carried by binding proteins in the circulation. Of all the steroids, estrogens have the widest range of physiologic functions. Estrogen acts on the CNS to induce behavioral estrus in the female; however, small amounts of progestrogen with estrogen are needed in some species such as the ewe and cow to induce estrus. The first ovulation in the ewe at puberty or the start of a breeding season is without estrus because only estrogen is present in circulation. At the second ovulation, however, the estrogen from the follicle will cause ovulation, and the progesterone from the waning corpus luteum together induce behavioral estrus in the ewe. Estrogens act on the uterus to increase the mass of both the endometrium and myometrium. The increased growth is due to both cell hyperplasia and hypertrophy. It also acts on the uterus to increase both amplitude and frequency of contraction by potentiating the effects of oxytocin and PG $F_{2\alpha}$.

Physical development of female secondary sex characteristics are attributed to estrogen. Estrogen stimulates duct growth and causes the development of the mammary gland. Estrogens have both a negative and positive feedback control through the hypothalamus on LH and FSH release: The negative effect is on the tonic center in the hypothalamus, and the positive effect is on the preovulatory center.

Clinical Applications. Nonreproductive effects of estrogens include stimulation of calcium uptake and ossification of bones. Estrogens cause maturation of epiphyseal cartilage of the long bone and inhibit further long bone growth. In contrast, in ruminants, estrogens also have a protein anabolic effect to increase in weight gain and growth. The possible mechanism for increased growth appears to be that estrogen stimulates the pituitary to release more growth hormone.

Plant estrogens (isoflavons) are found primarily in legumes such as subterranian clover and alfalfa. Two of these compounds, genistein and coumestrol, cause infertility problems primarily in females and less frequently in males. Zeronal (Ralgro), a compound with estrogen activity produced by a mold, is an ear implant and promotes growth of feedlot animals. These compounds act like estrogens but do not have the 18-carbon steroid nucleus (Fig. 3–12). They should therefore be called *nonsteroidal plant estrogens.*

Synthetic nonsteroidal estrogens are used in livestock industry, primarily as growth promotants in ruminants. Diethylstibesterol (DES), a synthetic nonsteroidal estrogen, was used for growth promotion in cattle and sheep (Fig. 3–13). DES binds to estrogen receptor, and acts with the same potency as 17β-estradiol. It has been removed from the market for use in feedlot cattle to be replaced by other estrogenic implants.

Estrogens have been used to abort cows and sheep because they have a luteolytic

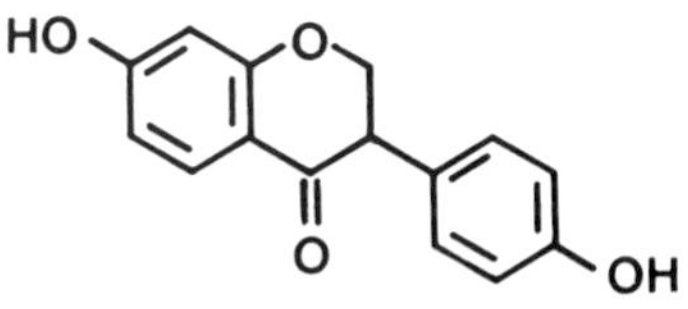

GENISTEIN

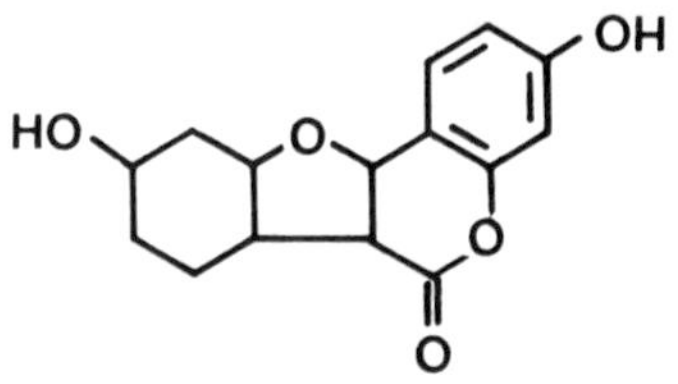

COUMESTROL

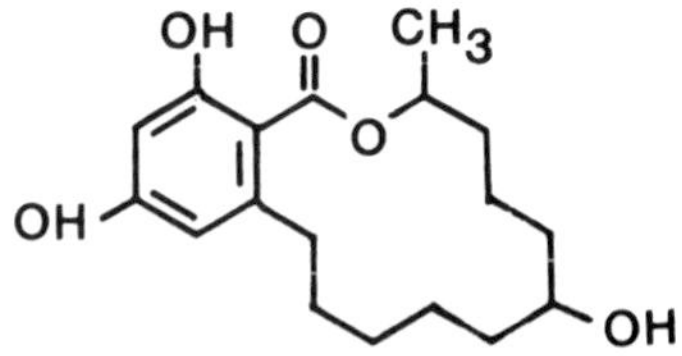

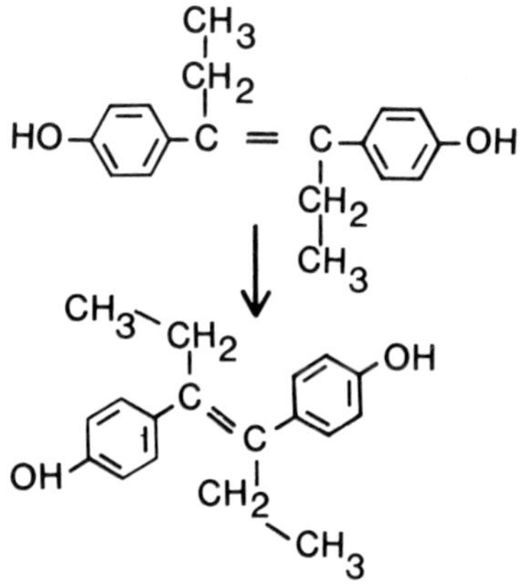

DES

FIG. 3–13. The structure of DES does not resemble estrogen unless it is drawn three-dimensionally.

ZERANOL

FIG. 3–12. The chemical structure of common plant estrogens lacks a steroid nucleus but contains biologic actions similar to estrogen.

action (regression of CL), probably caused by $PGF_{2\alpha}$. In the sow, estrogens have a luteotrophic action (helps to maintain CL). Thus, estrogens are used to synchronize estrus to hold sows in luteal phase until estrogen treatment is withdrawn and followed by a $PGF_{2\alpha}$ injection, which causes regression of the corpus luteum.

Progestogens

Progesterone is secreted by luteal cells of the corpus luteum, by the placenta and adrenal gland. Progesterone is transported in blood by a binding globulin as androgens and strogens. Progesterone secretion is primarily stimulated by LH.

Function. Progesterone prepares the endometrium for implantation and maintenance of pregnancy by increasing secretory glands in the endometrium and by inhibiting the motility of the myometrium. Progesterone acts synergistically with estrogens to induce behavioral estrus. It develops the secretory tissue (alveoli) of the mammary glands. High levels of progesterone inhibit estrus and the ovulatory surge of LH. Thus, progesterone is important in the hormonal regulation of the estrous cycle. Uterine motility under the influence of progesterone is characterized by spontaneous contractions of low frequency and high amplitude. Progesterone has little effect on the genital tract if administered alone but has striking effects of given after estrogen.

Clinical Applications. Progestogens are given to prevent abortion in females prone to abortion as a result of insufficient secretion of endogenous progesterone. The most common use is in birth control pills for women to prevent LH surge and subsequent ovulation. Synthetic progestogens are commercially available to synchronize the estrous cycle of cows. Melengesterol acetate (MGA), a synthetic progestogen, is used to increase gains in feedlot heifers. MGA is effective only in heifers with intact ovaries. Continuous administration of MGA inhibits LH surge, which prevents ovulation but allows development of ovarian follicles.

Androgens

Testosterone is one of the steroids known as *androgens.* In the male, androgens are produced by the interstitial cells (Leydig cells) of the testes, with a limited amount produced by the adrenal cortex. The horse is a unique species because the seminiferous tubules and epididymis also produce testosterone in high levels. Horsemen have known for centuries that if part of the epididymis is left attached to the vas deferens when a horse is castrated, the gelding will look and behave like a stallion, as a result of the androgens produced by the remaining epididymis. Allowing part of the epididymis to remain is termed "cutting a horse proud." This high level of androgen prolongs the life of epididymal sperm in the stallion rather than acting on the secondary male sex characteristics.

Testosterone (Fig. 3–14) is transported in the blood by an α-globulin designated *steroid-binding globulin.* Some 98% of circulating testosterone is bound. The remaining testosterone is free to enter the target cell, where an enzyme in the cytoplasm converts testosterone to dihydrotestosterone, which can act on the nuclear receptor (Fig. 3–15). Androgens stimulate late stages of spermatogenesis and prolong the life span of epididymal sperm. They promote growth, development, and secretory activity of the accessory sex organs of the male such as the prostate, vesicular glands, bulbourethral gland, vas deferens, and the external genitalia (penis and scrotum). The maintenance of secondary sex characteristics and sexual behavior or libido of the male is controlled by androgens. The synthetic androgen, testosterone proprionate, is administered to cows or steers used as teaser animals for detection of estrus. These androgenized cows are more popular in the industry than sterilized bulls for teaser animals.

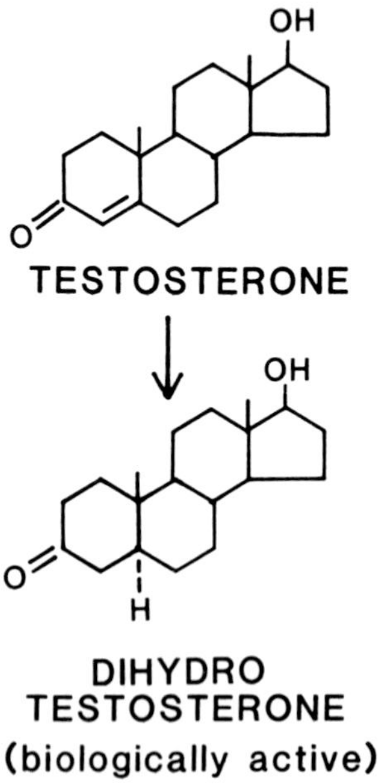

Relaxin

Relaxin is a polypeptide hormone consisting of α- and β-subunits connected by

OH

TESTOSTERONE

↓

OH

DIHYDRO TESTOSTERONE (biologically active)

FIG. 3–14. Testosterone is not the biologically active form, but it is converted to dihydrotestosterone, which binds to the nuclear receptor.

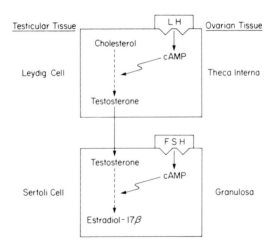

FIG. 3–15. Model of the two-cell two-gonadotropin hypothesis. (Modified from Dorrington et al., 1978.)

two disulfide bonds. It has a molecular weight of 5700 daltons and has structural similarity to insulin. Although relaxin and insulin have a similar structure, they have different biologic actions. Relaxin is secreted primarily by the corpus luteum during pregnancy. In addition, the placenta and uterus secrete relaxin in some species. The main biologic action of relaxin is dilation of the cervix and vagina before parturition. It also inhibits uterine contractions and causes increased growth of the mammary gland if given in conjunction with estradiol. In the guinea pig, relaxin causes separation of the pubic symphysis bone within 6 hours after injection. Separation of the pubic symphysis normally occurs during parturition in this species.

Inhibin

Inhibin, a protein hormone, is produced by the Sertoli cells in the male and the granulosa cells in the female. Inhibin can inhibit FSH release from the pituitary without altering LH release and is partially responsible for the differential release of LH and FSH from the pituitary.

ENDOCRINE MECHANISMS OF SEXUAL BEHAVIOR

The steroid hormones in the male and the female have close biochemical similarities, but the rhythm of their release into the bloodstream is totally different. The secretion of androgens is not permanent. In the male, it takes place in the form of several peaks within 24 hours, reflecting the pulsatile release of pituitary gonadotropins. However, the total amount secreted is practically constant from day to day. Any seasonal fluctuations are progressive and slow. Stallions produce and excrete large quantities of estrogens compared to those produced by males of most other mammalian species. The estrogens are produced by the testes. Concentrations of estradiol-17 (estradiol) are seasonal in stallions and are parallel to the concentrations of LH and testosterone. In the fe-

male, however, estrogen levels are high during a few days of the estrous cycle. The effects of the deprivation of the gonadal hormones and therapy in males are completely different from those in females.

Hormonal Mechanisms of Male Sexual Behavior

Castration of males is routinely used in animal husbandry. The depressing action of castration varies with the species, the individual, and the physiologic and behavioral status of the animal at the time of operation.

Some mounting activity is retained after prepubertal castration in bulls and rams, but the underdevelopment of the genital tract resulting from the lack of androgen during ontogeny, drastically inhibits mating. There seems to be wide species variation in the effect of castration. There is variable activity in rams castrated before puberty. In contrast, male rodents and cats rarely mount if castrated prepubertally. Following postpubertal castration, erection, intromission, and even ejaculation may persist for a long time, but with a decreased frequency. Among eight tropical male goats, only one had lost the ejaculatory response 1 year after castration. Normal sexual behavior is dramatically altered by castration. Two parameters of normal sexual behavior seem to be somewhat independent: the animal's desire to mount and thrust and the ability to ejaculate. After castration, the desire to mount is retained for a longer period than the ability to ejaculate. The attainment of an erection is the last aspect of normal sexual behavior to disappear after castration. This behavioral pattern is noted in impotent stallions and in those with other forms of abnormal sexual behavior (Pickett et al, 1975; Pickett and Voss, 1975).

The loss of ejaculation potency may be due to modifications of androgen-dependent structures of the copulatory organs. The persistence of the other behavioral patterns cannot be attributed to the presence of androgen from adrenal origin; for example, adrenalectomy does not change the sexual behavior of castrated dogs.

Precastration sexual experience influences the persistence of libido. The patterns of sexual behavior gradually reappear under daily androgen treatment in an order inverse to their disappearance. Their frequency reaches a plateau similar to the precastration level of activity. The only effect of increasing the daily dose of hormone is to accelerate the recovery of the precastration activity. The hormonal therapy allows the male to recover the preoperative level of copulatory activity, but the pre-existing differences cannot be overcome by an extra dosage of hormone. The endocrine balance appears only to reveal the potential intensity of reaction without modifying it. Libido and the ability to ejaculate are gradually lost after castration. Testosterone can restore both aspects of sexual behavior within 2 weeks. Estradiol effectively restores libido at the higher dosage but is less effective in restoring the ability to ejaculate. The pH of the gel-free semen increases after castration and is subsequently decreased by treatment with testosterone or the combination of both steroids. Weights of the seminal vesicles, ampullae, and prostate are greater in geldings treated with testosterone or with both steroids than in estradiol-treated or control geldings.

Hormonal Mechanisms of Female Sexual Behavior

Female sexual behavior depends on an appropriate endocrine balance resulting in the development of the ovarian follicles. Ovariectomy inhibits sexual behavior, but in the cow and sow, sexual behavior is restored in ovariectomized females after the injection of a minimal dose of estrogen following 8 to 12 days of progesterone pretreatment. In the sow and ewe, there is a linear dose–response relationship between the duration of estrus and the logarithm of the dose of estrogen. There is also a relationship between duration of natural

estrus and the number of the ovulations in the sow and ewe.

Progesterone inhibits the female's sexual reaction when it is injected after the appropriate hormonal sequence during the long-lasting period of latency.

The action of exogenous hormones in the intact female depends on her physiologic state at injection. When estrogens are injected during proestrus, sexual receptivity is hastened. During the luteal phase of the cycle, the inhibitory action of progesterone prevents an estrous response. The effects of hormonal treatment during anestrus are similar to those observed in spayed females.

Sex Specificity of Endocrine Control of Behavior

The sex specificity of steroid hormones—androgens for males, estrogens and progestogens for females—raises the question of a direct influence of the hormone on the behavioral response. The rhythm of secretion, however, differs between males and females, and a possible sexualization of the brain may influence the reaction. The treatment of gonadectomized animals with the hormone of the other sex shows that the sex specificity of the hormone is limited as far as the behavioral responses are concerned. Daily injections of estrogen allow a complete recovery of male activity in castrated rams, whereas a single treatment with testosterone induces a normal female receptivity in the ovariectomized female.

Neural Mechanisms of Sexual Behavior

The physiologic signal that initiates sexual motivation is the secretion of steroid hormones. Once released in the bloodstream, hormones are rapidly bound to receptor sites in the CNS. Maximal estrogen levels in the blood of the ewe and sow occur about 24 hours before onset of estrus. When the animal is sexually motivated, behavioral events are initiated. Specific or unspecific sensory stimuli acting on the sense organs, through innate or acquired mechanisms, are integrated in the brain to elicit appropriate motor reactions. The nervous organization of the sexual behavior, integrating humoral and physiologic signals as well as elaborated sensory information, involves the participation of the various levels.

PROSTAGLANDINS

The prostaglandins, first isolated from accessory sex gland fluids, were termed *prostaglandins* because of their association with the prostate gland. They are secreted by almost all body tissues. The prostaglandins, derived from arachidonic acid, are short-acting. Some forms never appear in the blood, whereas others are degraded after they circulate throughout the liver and lungs. $PGF_{2\alpha}$ is the natural luteolytic agent that terminates the luteal phase (corpus luteum) of the estrous cycle and allows for the initiation of a new estrous cycle in the absence of fertilization. $PGF_{2\alpha}$ is particularly potent in terminating early pregnancy (Table 3–12).

Unlike other humoral agents, prostaglandins are not localized in any particular tissue. Most prostaglandins act locally at the site of their production on a cell-to-cell interaction and therefore do not conform exactly to the classic definition of a hormone. They are transported in the blood to act on a target tissue away from the site of production. All prostaglandins are 20-carbon unsaturated hydroxy fatty acids with a cyclopentene ring (reviewed by Reeves, 1987). Prostaglandins in at least six parent compounds and numerous metabolites exhibit a wide variety of pharmacologic effects. Prostaglandins are involved in control of blood pressure, lipolysis, gastric secretion, blood clotting, and other related physiologic processes including renal and respiratory function. Blood levels of prostaglandins are generally low but are elevated under certain conditions such as parturition.

Prostaglandins are rapidly degraded in the blood, and it is only after injection with pharmacologic or high levels of prosta-glandin that a sustained physiologic effect is noted. Archiodonic acid, an essential fatty acid, is the precursor for prostaglandins most closely associated with reproduction, mainly $PGF_{2\alpha}$ and prostaglandin E_2 (PGE_2) (Fig. 3–16).

Functions

Prostaglandins may be considered hormones, which regulate several physiologic and pharmacologic phenomena, such as contraction of smooth muscles in the reproductive and gastrointestinal tracts, erection, ejaculation, sperm transport, ovulation, formation of the corpus luteum, parturition, and milk ejection. Prostaglandins are involved in ovulation (DeSilva and Reeves, 1985; Murdock and Dunn, 1983). For example, in the ewe and cow, ovulation is blocked by the administration of indomethacin, an inhibitor of prostaglandin synthesis. LH release is not affected in these animals, so the action and synthesis of prostaglandin is probably at the level of the ovarian follicle involving either or both $PGF_{2\alpha}$ and PGE_2 (Fig. 3–17).

An increase in estrogen, which increases myometrium growth in the uterus, stimulates $PGF_{2\alpha}$ synthesis and release. In pregnant animals, some unknown signal is sent from the embryo to the uterus, preventing $PGF_{2\alpha}$ release, thus allowing the corpus luteum of the cycle to become the corpus luteum of pregnancy. In the cow and ewe, $PGF_{2\alpha}$ does not cause regression or prevent formation of the corpus luteum during its first 5 days of life. In the sow, it does not cause regression until day 12 of the estrous cycle.

Human semen contains high concentrations of prostaglandins. Low levels of prostaglandins in semen may be related to male infertility because the concentration of PGE in the seminal plasma is about 18 μg/ml in infertile men and 55 μ/ml in fertile men.

TABLE 3–12.   Chemistry, Functions, and Applications of Prostaglandins (PGs) in Farm Animals

Chemistry	Function	Applications to Animals
PGs are found in the form of at least six parent compounds that induce various pharmacologic responses.	PGs are involved in ovulation in the ewe and cow when ovulation is blocked by the administration of indomethacin, an inhibitor of prostaglandin synthesis.	Various treatments with PG are used to synchronize estrus for artificial insemination. Cows are treated twice at 10-day intervals, after which they will all theoretically exhibit estrus 3 days after second injection.
PGs are 20-carbon unsaturated hydroxy fatty acids with a cyclopentane ring.	LH release is not affected, so the action and synthesis of PG is at level of ovarian follicle involving $PGF_{2\alpha}$ and/or PGE_2.	PG used in timed breeding in mares and abortion in cattle.
Arachidonic acid, an essential fatty acid, is the precursor for the PG most closely associated with reproduction, mainly prostaglandin $F_{2\alpha}$ ($PGF_{2\alpha}$) and prostaglandin E_2 (PGE_2).	PGE_2 stimulates contraction of the uterus, dilates blood vessels, and has no luteolytic action. $PGF_{2\alpha}$ stimulates contraction of uterus, aids in sperm transport in the male and female, causes constriction of blood vessels, and has luteolytic properties.	Trade names of these compounds are Lutalyse and Estrumate for the cow and Prostin for the mare.
PGs are involved in control of blood pressure, lipolysis, gastric secretion, blood clotting, and other general physiologic processes including renal and respiratory function.	Venoconstrictive effects of $PGE_{2\alpha}$ induce hypoxia, which in turn leads to luteolysis.	$PGF_{2\alpha}$ aids in treating infected uterus of dairy cows. Mechanism of action is twofold: (a) Regression of CL, if present, induction of follicle growth and estrogen production, and (b) contraction of uterus, under the action of estrogen.
Blood levels of PGs are generally low but are elevated in certain conditions such as parturition.	If the uterus is removed, the corpus luteum (CL) will not regress for at least the length of the respective gestation.	
	Mechanism by which $PGF_{2\alpha}$ transports from uterus to the ovary: $PGF_{2\alpha}$ passes directly through walls of utero-ovarian vein into ovarian artery and directly to CL.	
	An increase in estrogen, which increases myometrium growth in the uterus, stimulates $PGF_{2\alpha}$ synthesis and release.	
	If the female animal becomes pregnant, some signal is sent from embryo to uterus preventing $PGF_{2\alpha}$ release, thus allowing CL of cycle to become CL of pregnancy. In the cow and ewe, $PGF_{2\alpha}$ will not cause regression or prevent formation of CL during its first 5 days of life. In the sow, it will not cause regression until day 12 of cycle.	

Clinical Application

PGE_2 stimulates contraction of the uterus, dilates blood vessels, and has no luteolytic action. $PGF_{2\alpha}$ stimulates contractions of the uterus, aids in sperm transport in the male and female, causes constriction of blood vessels, and has luteolytic properties in domestic animals. The prostaglandins are responsible in part for regression of corpora lutea. Venoconstric-

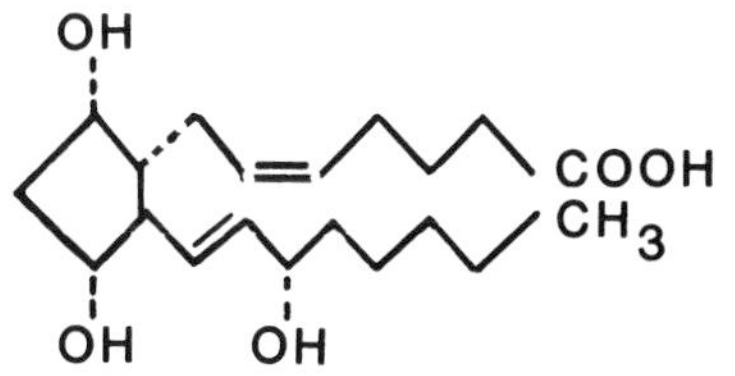

OH

COOH
CH₃

OH   OH

PGF₂α

O

COOH
CH₃

OH   OH

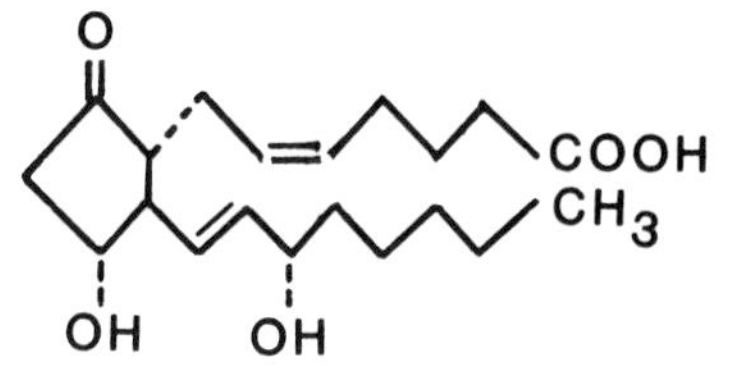

PGE₂

FIG. 3–16. Chemical structure of PGF$_{2\alpha}$ and PGE$_2$.

tive effects of PGF$_{2\alpha}$ may induce hypoxia, which in turn leads to luteolysis. If the uterus is removed from farm animals, the corpus luteum does not regress for at least the length of the respective gestation. This is not the case in primates, because the mechanism controlling luteolysis is not in the uterus; hysterectomy does not alter cyclic function. The mechanism by which PGF$_{2\alpha}$ travels from the endometrium to the ovary is unique in that PGF$_{2\alpha}$ passes directly through the walls of the utero-ovarian vein into the ovarian artery and directly to the corpus luteum (McCracken, 1980).

Prostaglandins are used to regulate breeding in cows and mares and in abortion of cattle. The trade names of these compounds are Lutalyse and Estrumate for the cow and Prostin for the mare. PGF$_{2\alpha}$ is used in treating the infected uterus of dairy cows. Its mechanism of action is twofold: (a) regression of the CL, if present, and thus, induction of follicle growth and estrogen production, and (b) contraction of the uterus, both from its action and from the action of estrogen.

ANDROLOGY AND HORMONES

Male reproductive processes are regulated by short loop, long loop and ultra-short loop. The long loop involves FSH–inhibin and LH–tesosterone interactions. The short loop between the interstitial and seminiferous epithelium involves growth factors and hormones. The ultrashort loop regulates Sertoli cell–germ cell–myoid cell interactions. Several circulating proteins are internalized through the basal compartment into Sertoli cells by endocrine mechanisms: transferrin, androgen bound protein (ABP), insulin growth factor (IGF), and related growth factors. Proteins secreted by Sertoli cells in the adluminal compartment are internalized by a paracrine mechanism in germ cells. Spermatocytes and early spermatids are preferential targets of Sertoli cell proteins in the testis.

Sertoli Cells and Leydig Cells

Sertoli cells and germ cells reciprocally regulate each other's cyclic secretion of proteins along the length of the seminiferous tubule, and myoid cells amplify this process through transforming growth fac-

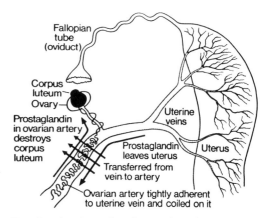

FIG. 3–17. Postulated route by which prostaglandin manufactured by the progesterone-primed uterus is able to enter the ovarian artery and destroy the corpus luteum in sheep. (From Short, (1972). *In:* Reproduction in Mammals, Book 3. Austin and Short (eds.). Cambridge, Cambridge University Press.)

tors, humoral modulators, and extracellular matrix. Sertoli cells are provided with low-resistance pathways for intercellular transport of cell metabolites, which coordinates the activity of the seminiferous epithelium.

Activin and Inhibin

This family of gonadal glycoproteins possesses remarkable mechanisms to generate signal diversity: Differential subunit association can result in the generation of dimers with opposing biologic actions in multiple tissues. These heterodimeric hormones are composed of an α-subunit and one of two β-subunits (βA or βB) that suppress FSH secretion by the anterior pituitary. Activins are potent FSH-releasing dimers (dimers of inhibin β-subunits) and are purified from gonadal fluids. Activin and inhibin also act within the gonads and placenta as autocrine and paracrine modulators of the production of steroids and other hormones and growth factors. Inhibin is a glycoprotein hormone produced by the gonad to regulate FSH secretion with minimal effect on LH secretion by the pituitary. The name *inhibin* was coined in 1932 for a water-soluble substance from the testis.

Transferrin β_2 Microglobulin, and Albumin in Seminal Plasma

The levels of transferrin, β-microglobulin, and albumin in seminal plasma are related to sperm count. There is a general relationship between seminal plasma proteins and sperm numbers; some products of the sperm themselves regulate the transport of plasma proteins into the seminal plasma (Chard et al, 1991). Seminal plasma transferrin can be used as a clinical index of Sertoli cell function. The levels of unrelated plasma proteins, albumin β-microglobulin, and transferrin all increase on the transfer from circulation in the lower genital tract.

SECONDARY HORMONES OF REPRODUCTION

Thyroid Gland

The thyroid gland is located on the trachea, just caudal to the larynx. In cattle, it consists of two laterally placed, flattened lobes joined by an isthmus. The thyroid gland comprises numerous follicles lined by simple epithelial cells and filled with a colloid fluid. The surface area of the lining epithelium is increased by villi that project into the follicle. The thyroid hormones, derived from the amino acid tyrosine, contain iodine that is bound organically in the thyroid gland. Thyroid hormones are combined with plasma proteins for transport in the blood. The major plasma protein is termed *thyroxine-binding globulin (TBG)*. This protein has a high affinity for the thyroid hormones. Calcitonin is a hormone of the thyroid gland secreted by parafollicular or C cells in the walls of thyroid gland follicles. Calcitonin is a polypeptide of 32 amino acids.

The parathyroid glands, located near or embedded within the thyroid gland, are sometimes so close to the thyroid gland that differentiation is difficult.

Adrenal Glands

The two adrenal glands immediately cranial to the kidney have an outer cortex and an inner medulla. The adrenal cortex has three distinct cell types arranged in zones from the outside to the inside: the zona glomerulosa, zona fasciculata, and zona ritcularis. The adrenal medulla is homogenous and contains secretory granules. Seven adrenocortical steroids (corticosteroids) are formed mainly from cholesterol, as follows:

Corticosteroids: corticosterone, cortisol, cortisone, and 11-dehydrocorticosterone

Mineralocorticoids: 11-deoxycorticosterone, 17-hydroxy-11-deoxycorticosterone, and aldosterone

Mineralocorticoids promote membrane transport between intracellular and extracellular fluid compartments. The glucocorticoids are secreted by the zona fasciculata of the adrenal cortex. Their secretion is regulated by ACTH of the anterior pituitary. Stimuli such as stress cause ACTH secretion, which increases glucocorticoid concentrations above normal levels, as noted with the overcrowding of domestic chickens. Excess ACTH secretion causes adrenal hypertrophy because of glucocorticoids. The hormones of the adrenal medulla, known as "catecholamines," belong to the amine chemical class and are referred to as epinephrine (adrenalin) and norepinephrine (noradrenalin). The actions of epinephrine and norepinephrine are similar, and differences are expressed according to the receptors, which have a preference for epinephrine or norepinephrine. The two adrenergic receptors are α- and β-receptors.

GROWTH FACTORS

During the last few years, remarkable investigations have been conducted on growth factors related to hormone receptors, peptides and intratesticular regulators, molecular cloning of reproductive proteins and peptides, ovarian proteins and peptides, early pregnancy factors, endometrial placental proteins, and peptide hormone-binding proteins. Growth factors elicit cellular responses by binding to specific cell surface receptors in their target tissues. Polypeptide growth factors regulate the proliferation on many cell types and regulate growth of the reproductive tract (Tables 3–13, 3–14). These factors have a wide range of cell types that express the appropriate growth factor receptors (Earp, 1991).

Endogenous opioid peptides (EOP) seem to have an autocrine and paracrine regulation on Leydig cell steroidogenesis and participate in the intratesticular hormonal control of vascular permeability. β-Endorphin is present in the testicular interstitial fluid (TIF), in a concentration manyfold higher than that found in plasma. Two families of compounds regu-

TABLE 3–13. Growth Factors and Animal Reproduction

Acronym	Term
bFGF	Basic fibroblast growth factor
CSF	Colony-stimulating factor
EGF	Epidermal growth factor
FGF	Fibroblast growth factor
FRP	Follicular regulating protein
FSHBI	FSH binding inhibitor
G-CSF	Granulocyte colony-stimulating factor
GM-CSF	Granulocyte–macrophage colony-stimulating factor
HFGRP	Human follicular gonadotropin-releasing peptide
IF	Inhibin F (folliculostatin or follicular fluid inhibin)
IGFS	Insulin-like growth
LF	Lactoferrin
LI	Luteinization inhibitor
LS	Luteinization stimulator
MIS	Müllerian inhibiting substance
NGF	Nerve growth factor
NP-Gα	Neuropeptides GnRHα
NP-Gβ	Neuropeptides GnRHβ
OMI	Oocyte maturation inhibitor of meiotic division
OFFP	Ovarian follicular fluid peptide
PDGF	Platelet-derived growth factor
TGF	Transforming growth factor
VIP	Vasoactive intestinal peptide

late the hypothalamo–pituitary–gonadal complex. Plasminogen activators are found in three major categories:

1. Urokinase type of plasminogen activator (u-PA)
2. Tissue type of plasminogen activator (t-PA)
3. Other types of plasminogen activator

u-PA has a molecular weight of 50,000, and its active form is a two-chain glycoprotein.

Uterine cell membranes contain specific, and high-affinity receptors. The molecular weight of uterine epidermal growth factor (EGF) receptor is 170,000 daltons. These growth factors stimulate myometrial contractibility. The effect of EGF is due to the release of arachidonic acid and subsequent conversion to prostaglandins. Thymosine (thymus hormone) is found in lower concentration in seminal plasma of infertile men. Some thymus fractions exert an effect on sperm motility

TABLE 3–14. Growth Factors and Reproductive Function in Domestic Animals (Compiled from the Literature)

Growth Factors	Function
CLE (corpus luteum extract)	Stimulate luteal growth and proliferation; activate intraovarian mitogen (OSEO plays a major role in postovulovarian morphogenesis)
CSF (colony-stimulating factor)	Mononuclear phagocytic growth factor increases dramatically during gestation in trophoblast, decidua, amniotic fluid
EGF (epidermal growth factor)	May stimulate regrowth of epithelium following disruption of ovarian surface at ovulation
	Human myometrial cells respond to this factor by stimulation of their proliferation; their activities are additive when used in combination and synergistically enhanced by progesterone
EGF-like (EGF-like peptides)	Growth and development of neonatal uterus; relation of these peptides with estrogen action unknown?
FGF (fibroblast growth factor)	18,000-Dalton protein stimulates proliferation of various cell types required with blastocyst implantation and embryonic development
GHRH (Growth Hormone Releasing Hormone)	Modulatory action of GHRH on gonadal function is FSH dependent
	Locally formed GFR exerts synergistic action during ovarian follicle maturation
GM-CSF (granulocyte-macrophage colony-stimulating factor)	Secreted by placental cells, autocrine within certain cells of fetal placenta
	One of the major cytokines that serve as a basis for interaction between maternal immune system reproductive tissues during mammalian pregnancy
	Maternal decidual tissue produces CSF, which may regulate adjacent fetal trophoblastic cells in placenta (rat)
IGF (intrafollicular growth factor)	Regulates steriodogenesis in granulosa cells in large ovarian follicles via aromatase activity
	Estrogens initiate granulosa cells' responsiveness to IGF-I during follicular development (marmoset)
IFN (Interferon)	Cytokines with complex effects on cells of immune system in ovine and bovine conceptus produce IFN as their major secretory before implantation
IGF (insulin growth factor)	Plays a role in early pregnancy in ruminants
	Endometrium synthesizes and secretes four IGF regulated by progesterone
	Progesterone indirectly affects IGF action in endometrium by regulating specific IGF-binding protein synthesis
	Putative intraovarian regulators involve receptors and binding
	Granulosa cells regulate its own destiny by enhancing ovarian androgen provision to suit its aromatizing capability and the estrogen requirements of the developing follicle
	Testicular EGF plays a role in regulation of spermatogonial division and testicular IGF-I production stimulated by retinol without cyclic changes in testicular IGF-I concentrations
IGF-I (insulin growth factor-*r*)	Removal of fetus decreases serum E_2 and growth hormone and elevates serum levels of IGF-I; these effects reversed by A and E_2 Fetus, via secretion of estrogen precursors, regulates placental and maternal IGF-I production and maternal serum concentrations for IGF-I during pregnancy
LF (lactoferrin)	Constitutes 20% of total uterine proteins secreted under influence of estrogen
	Iron-building glycoprotein in secretions of many types of glandular epithelium expressed in two stages: (a) mammary gland undergoing rapid growth and morphogenesis and (b) differentiated, nongrowing lactating mammary glands where LF is actively secreted into milk
	Regulates mammary gland growth and differentiation
PDGF (platelet-derived growth factor)	Promotes hatching and blastocyst outgrowth after in vitro microinjection of anti-PDGF antibodies into uterine lumen
PAF (platelet-activating factor)	Phospholipid (l-o-alkyl-acetyl-sn-gylceryl-3-phosphocholine) secreted by human blastocyst, an autocrine growth factor, needed for implantation
	PAF antagonists prevent implantation
	PAF forms antiluteolytic and luteotropic function during pregnancy
Relaxin	Polypeptide, closely related structure to insulin and insulin-like growth factors, synthesized and secreted by corpus luteum
TNF (tumor necrosis factor)	Immunohistochemically localized in ovary: granulosa cells of antral follicle
	Increases thecal progesterone production and inhibits basal and FSH-stimulated progesterone in granulosa cells
	TNF and hCG increase progesterone secretion above maximal dose of hCG
	Synergism between TNF and hCG is due to increase in hCG binding to granulosal and luteal cells by TNF

in vitro. EDF, platelet-derived growth factor (PDGF), and insulin receptors have profound effects on endometrial and myometrial cells by stimulation of their proliferation.

Intraovarian Regulators and Intraovarian Growth Factor

Intraovarian growth factor (IGF) plays three main functions in the ovary: (a) Amplification of gonodotropin action required for the exponential nature of follicular development; (b) integration of follicular development; and (c) selection of dominant follicles, assuming timely and selective activation of the IGF–I system "chosen" follicles (Adashi et al., 1991). Little is known about the role of growth hormones in the breeding season and anestrous season in farm animals (Fig. 3–18).

Implantation and Gestation

Several growth factors are involved in implantation of the blastocyst. PDGF, a glycoprotein (molecular weight, 30,000 daltons) supports the growth of serum-dependent cells. PDGF is normally confined to paracrine and autocrine actions. PDGF secreted by some human blastocysts is present in human uterine secretions. Growth factors mediate cell proliferation, differentiation, migration, and invasion during preimplantation development, implantation, and subsequent stages of gestation. Growth factors in the zygote, morula and blastocysts include the following:

Transforming growth factor _____ (TGFB1)
Transforming growth factor _____ α (TGFF-α)
IGF _____ (IGFII)
PDGF
_____ (KFGF)
Interleukin-6 (IL-6)

Other growth factors and related isoforms are not transcribed by the morula and blastocyst:

IGF-I
_____ (bFGF)
Epidermal growth factor (EGF)
Nerve growth factor (NGF)
_____ (G-CSF)

Platelet-Activating Factor

Platelet-activating factor (PAF) [1-0-alkyl-2-acetyl-sn-glycero-3-phosphocholine (AGEPC)] is a potent phospholipid mediator produced by several cell types: neutrophils, macrophages, endothelial cells, and preimplantation embryos. PAF induces a wide range of physiologic and pharmacologic responses involving reproductive processes (Harper, 1989), platelet aggregation, anaphylaxis, and vascular permeability. PAF is produced by sperm and enhances sperm motility and in vitro fertilization during coincubation of sperm and egg.

Müllerian-Inhibiting Substance

Müllerian-inhibiting substance (MIS) is a 140-kDa glycoprotein synthesized and secreted by the gonads, with a sexually dimorphic pattern of expression. In the male, MIS is produced initially by the fetal gonad. Maximal blood levels of MIS are reached after birth and fall to basal levels at puberty. This Sertoli cell product is responsible for the regression of the Müllerian duct, the early precursors of the uterus, oviduct, cervix, and upper vagina. In the female, MIS is secreted by the ovarian granulosa cells only at puberty, when MIS levels in the blood reach that of the adult male. In the female, MIS inhibits meiosis and blocks spontaneous breakdown of the germinal vesicle ovarian oocytes.

Abbreviations Used in this Chapter

ACTH	Adrenocorticotropic hormone
CBG	Corticosteroid-binding globulin
DHEA	Dehydroepiandrosterone
EGF	Epidermal growth factor

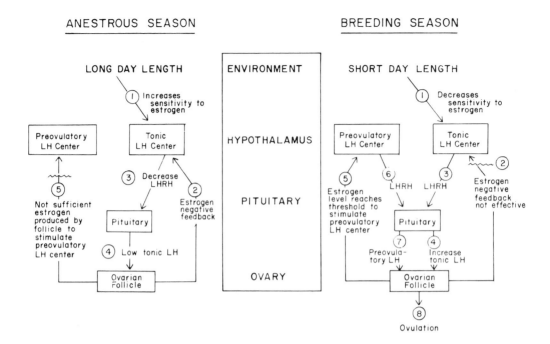

FIG. 3–18.   The four major components to consider in the model for hypothalamic control of the anestrous season in the ewe are external environment (day length), hypothalamus, pituitary and ovary. During the anestrous season or long days, the ewe does not show reproductive cyclic activity. The length of daylight by some mechanism, probably through the optic nerve, sensitizes the tonic LH center in the hypothalamus to become sensitive to circulating estrogen concentrations (1). Estrogen (2) then negatively feeds back on the tonic LH control center and less LH-RH is released (3). Less tonic LH is released into circulation (4), resulting in lower estrogen production (5) from the ovarian follicle. The circulating estrogen concentrations cannot reach a threshold concentration to stimulate the preovulatory LH center in the hypothalamus, resulting in the lack of ovulation during the anestrous season. During the breeding season of the ewe, the day length decreases (1) and the tonic LH control center in the hypothalamus becomes refractory to circulating estrogen (2). Increasing levels of estrogen do not negatively affect the tonic LH control center at this time, resulting in increased LH-RH release (3), which induces increased tonic LH release from the pituitary (4). The increased tonic LH release induces sufficient estrogen levels (5) in circulation to stimulate the preovulatory LH center of the hypothalamus, resulting in increased LH-RH release (6). The resulting preovulatory surge of LH (7) induces ovulation (8) (Reeves, 1987.)

Abbreviations Used in this Chapter (*continued*)

FGF	Fibroblast growth factor	**hGH**	Human growth hormone
FSH	Follicle-stimulating hormone	**hPL**	Human placental lactogen
		IGFs	Insulin-like growth factors
GnRH	Gonadotropin-releasing hormone	**LH**	Luteinizing hormone
		PDGF	Platelet-derived growth factor
hCG	Human chorionic gonadotropin		
hCGnRH	Human chorionic gonadotropin-releasing hormone	**TRH**	Thyrotropin-releasing hormone
hCS	Human chorionic somatomammotropin	**TSH**	Thyroid-stimulating hormone (thyrotropin)

REFERENCES

Adashi, E.Y., Resnick, C.E., Hernandez, E.R., Hurwitz, A., Roberts, C.T., Leroith, D. and Rosenfeld, R. (1991). The intraovarian IGF-I system. *In* Serono Symposium. D.W. Schomberg (ed.). New York, Springer Verlag.

Butler, J.E., Hamilton, W.C., Sasser, R.G., Ruder, C.A., Hass, G.N. and Williams, R.J. (1982). Detection and partial characterization of two bovine pregnancy-specific proteins. Biol. Reprod. *26*, 916–925.

Capen, C.C. and Martin, S.L. (1989). The pituitary gland. *In* Veterinary Endocrinology and Reproduction. L.E. McDonald and M.H. Pineda (eds.). Philadelphia, Lea & Febiger.

Chard, T., Parslow, J., Rehmann, T. and Dawnay, A. (1991). The concentrations of transferrin microglobulin, and albumin in seminal plasma in relation to sperm count. Fertil. Steril. *55*, 211–213.

Cole, H.H. and Hart, G.H. (1930). Potency of blood serum of mares in progressive stages of pregnancy in affecting sexual maturity of immature rats. Am. J. Physiol. *93*, 57.

DeSilva, M. and Reeves, J.J. (1985). Ovulation blockage by intrafollicular injection of indomethacin in the cow. J. Anim. Sci. *75*, 547.

Dickson, W.M. (1984). Endocrine glands. *In* Dukes' Physiology of Domestic Animals. 10th Ed. M.J. Swenson (ed.). Ithaca, NY, Cornell University Press.

Dorrington, J.H., Fritz, I.B., and Armstrong, D.J. (1978). Control of testicular estrogen synthesis. Biol. Reprod. *18*, 55.

Earp, S. (1991). The epidermal growth factor receptor: control of synthesis and signaling function. *In* Serono Symposium. D.E. Schomberg (ed.). New York, Springer-Verlag.

Fortune, J.E. and Armstrong, D.T. (1978). Hormonal control of 17-estradiol biosynthesis in proestrous rat follicles: estradiol production by isolated theca versus granulosa. Endocrinology *102*, 227.

Genuth, S.M. (1988). The hypothalamus and the pituitary gland. *In* Physiology. 2nd Ed. R.M. Berne and M.N. Levy (eds.). St. Louis: C.V. Mosby.

Griffin, J.E. and Ojeda, S.R. (eds.) (1988). Textbook of Endocrine Physiology. New York, Oxford University Press.

Harper, M.J.K. (1989). Platelet-activating factor: a paracrine factor in preimplantation stages of reproduction. Biol. Reprod. *40*, 907–913.

Jinno, M., Iizuka, R., Sandow, B.A. and Hodgen, G.D. (1990). In vitro maturation of oocytes. Assisted Reprod. Tech. Andr. *I*, 54–68.

Li, C.H. (1969). Recent studies on the chemistry of human growth hormone. *In* La Specificite Zoologique des Hormones Hypophysaires et de Leurs Activites. M. Fontaine (ed.). Paris, Centre National de la Recherche Scientifique.

Murdock, W.J. and Dunn, T.G. (1983). Luteal function after ovulation blockage by intra-follicular injections of indomethacin in the ewe. J. Reprod. Fert. *69*, 671.

McCracken, J.A. (1980). Hormone receptor control of prostaglandin F secretion by the ovine uterus. Adv. Prostaglandin Thromboxane Leukotriene Res. *8*, 1329.

McDonald, L.E. and Capen, C.C. (1989). Introduction. Veterinary Endocrinology and Reproduction. L.E. McDonald and M.H. Pineda (eds.). Philadelphia, Lea & Febiger.

Niswender, G.D., Reimers, T.J., Diekman, M.A. and Nett, T.M. (1976). Blood flow: a mediator of ovarian function. Biol. Reprod. *14*, 64.

Pickett, B.W. and Voss, J.L. (1975). Abnormalities of mating behavior in domestic stallions. *In* Equine Reproduction. I.W. Rowlands, W.R. Allen and P.D. Rossdale (eds.). Oxford, England, Blackwell Scientific Publications.

Pickett, B.W., Faulkner, L.C. and Voss, J.L. (1975). Effect of season on some characteristics of stallion semen. *In* Equine Reproduction. I.W. Rowlands, W.R. Allen and P.D. Rossdale (eds.). Oxford, England, Blackwell Scientific Publications.

Reece, W.O. (1991). Physiology of Domestic Animals. Philadelphia, Lea & Febiger.

Reeves, J.J. (1986). Endocrinology of reproduction. *In* Reproduction in Farm Animals. 5th Ed. E.S.E. Hafez (ed.). Philadelphia, Lea & Febiger.

Schomberg, D.W. (ed.) (1990). Growth Factors in Reproduction. New York, Springer-Verlag.

Sasser, R.G., Ruder, C.A., Ivani, K.A., Butler, J.E. and Hamilton, W.C. (1986). Detection of pregnancy by radioimmunoassay of a novel pregnancy-specific protein in serum of cows and a profile of serum concentrations during gestation. Biol. Reprod. (in press).

Trautmann, A. and Febiger, J. (1952). Fundamentals of the Histology of Domestic Animals. Ithaca, NY, Comstock Publishing.

4
Reproductive Cycles

E.S.E. HAFEZ

The reproductive cycle relates to various phenomena: puberty and sexual maturity, the breeding season, the estrous cycle, postpartum sexual activity, and aging. These components are regulated by environmental, genetic, physiologic, hormonal, behavioral, and psychosocial factors. The level of fertility initiated at the time of puberty is maintained for a few years before it begins to gradually decline due to aging. Farm animals, however, are slaughtered well before the decrease in fertility levels (Fig. 4–1).

PRENATAL AND NEONATAL PHYSIOLOGY

Gonadotropins

Secretion of the gonadotropins FSH and LH and their hypothalamic-releasing factor, hormone LH-RH, always begins during fetal life. In the ewe and cow it starts early, shortly after sex differentiation (month 1 or 2 of pregnancy) and in the sow only toward the end of fetal life (about 1.5 months after gonadal sex differentiation).

This secretion temporarily regresses; it is slightly reduced 2 months before birth in cattle, near term in sheep, and 1 month after birth in pigs. The damping of gonadotropin secretion must be related to the maturation of the central nervous system. It occurs when superior brain structures take charge of hypothalamic activity. Gonadotropin levels remain low up to the onset of puberty. The duration of this "infancy" is highly variable. It lasts a few days

in the rat, 1 month in sheep and pig, 3 months in cattle, and 6 to 7 years in humans.

At the onset of the pubertal period, gonadotropin secretion rises. This process occurs in normal animals as well as in animals that had been castrated early in which the process is clearer, owing to the absence of negative feedback from the gonadal steroid (Fig. 4–2). Gonadotropin rise results in the removal of the inhibitory control of the central nervous system when the body's development progressively attains a level compatible with reproduction.

The Gonads

During prenatal and neonatal life, gametogenesis and steroidogenesis seem independent, while at the onset of puberty they become closely related.

The Testis. The basic structure of the testis (seminiferous cords and interstitial tissue) remains unchanged from gonadal sex differentiation at the beginning of fetal life to the onset of puberty. The seminiferous cords are lined with supporting cells, whereas undifferentiated germ cells or gonocytes occupy the central part. The only modification during this period is a slow increase in the relative number of gonocytes.

Interstitial tissue that fills the space between the sex cords is composed of elongated conjunctive-type cells and steroidogenic cells. The Leydig cells secrete androgens as soon as the testis differentiates and before the gonadotropic function

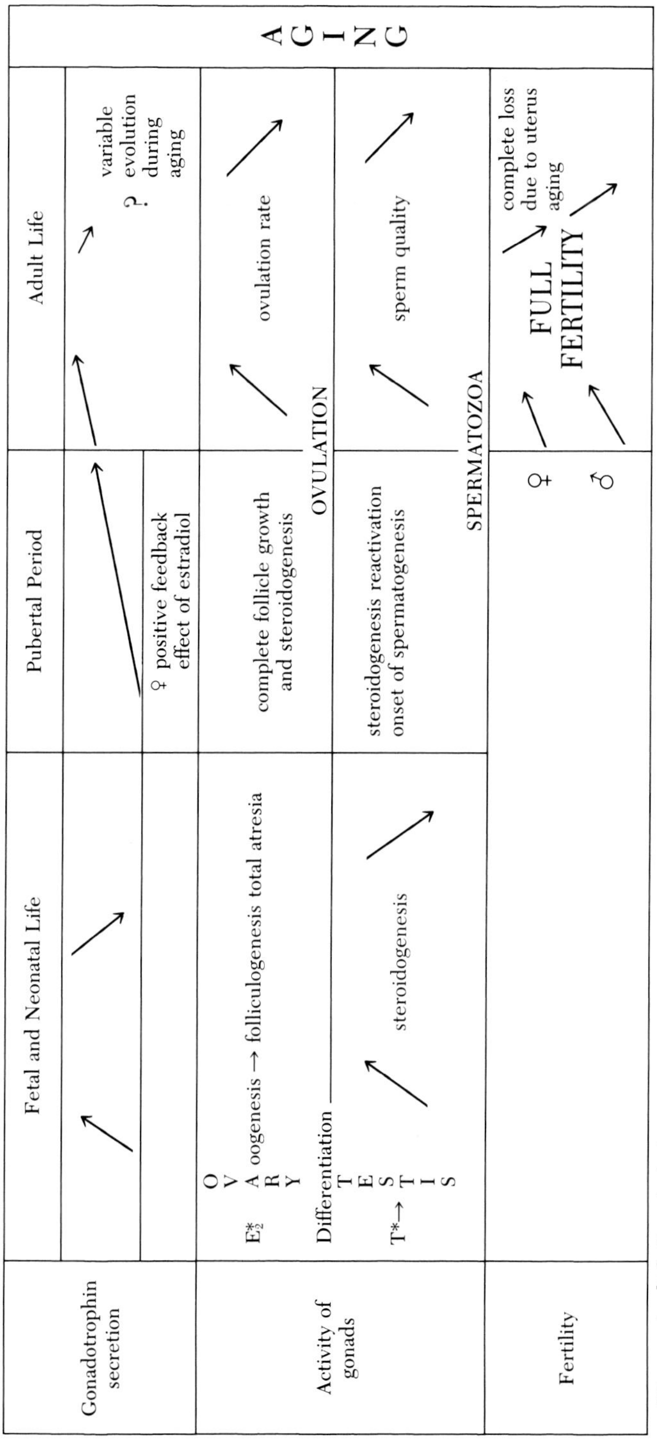

	Fetal and Neonatal Life	Pubertal Period	Adult Life
Gonadotrophin secretion			variable evolution during aging ?
Activity of gonads	OVARY E₂* A oogenesis → folliculogenesis total atresia	♀ positive feedback effect of estradiol	
		complete follicle growth and steroidogenesis	ovulation rate
		OVULATION	
	Differentiation TESTIS T*→ steroidogenesis	steroidogenesis reactivation onset of spermatogenesis	sperm quality
		SPERMATOZOA	
Fertility		♀ ♂	FULL FERTILITY complete loss due to uterus aging

AGING

FIG. 4–1. Neonatal, pubertal, and maturity stages.

*E₂ = estradiol, T = testosterone

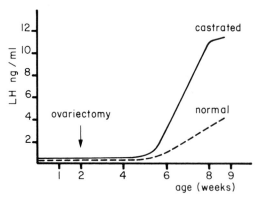

FIG. 4–2. Comparative evolution of plasma LH levels in normal and castrated ewe lambs. The pubertal rise occurs at the same age in both animals, but the increase is more pronounced in the castrated. (From Foster et al., (1975) Endocrinology, *96*, 15.

is triggered. However, the Leydig cells are gonadotropin sensitive and their continued steroidogenic activity closely depends on gonadotropic secretion. In swine, a transitory testosterone secretion occurs about day 55 when the Leydig cells differentiate; this secretion then drops until the fetus begins to secrete LH shortly before birth. The further decrease of gonadotropins 1 month after birth causes testosterone secretion to regress again during the short period of "infancy." In cattle and sheep, gonadotropin secretion begins earlier; the fetal Leydig cells are quickly stimulated by LH and testosterone is secreted until gonadotropic function regresses (Fig. 4–2).

At the onset of puberty, gonadotropin secretion resumes and Leydig cells are reactivated. In swine the Leydig cells, which were active during fetal and neonatal life, occupy large areas between the tubules, while after puberty the peritubular cells are more active.

The Ovary. Initial ovarian structure is not fundamentally different from that of the testis. Sex cords, formed by somatic and germ cells, are present at the beginning of ovarian and testicular differentiation. While these structures remain basically unchanged in the testis as seminiferous cords or tubules, in the ovary germ cells actively divide, sex cords vanish, and finally each oocyte is wrapped by a few somatic cells to form the primordial follicle. At the end of oogenesis, the ovary encloses millions of primordial follicles within a framework of interstitial tissue and is lined with ovarian epithelium erroneously called *germinal epithelium.* Oogonia and oocytes are formed during the first half of fetal life in the ewe and the cow. Oocyte formation also begins early during fetal life in the sow; however, oogenesis is completed only during the first weeks after birth (Fig. 4–3).

The appearance of meiotic prophase early in life is one of the main differences between ovarian and testicular germ cell evolution (Fig. 4–4). Moreover, as oogonia completely disappear, the oocytes formed during the fetal and neonatal period are the only source of oocytes available during the entire sexual life. As soon as the primordial follicle reserve is constituted, it rapidly diminishes by atresia. A cow fetus that has 2,700,000 oocytes at day 110 of gestation has only 70,000 oocytes at birth. From the end of the period of oogenesis, some primordial follicles continuously begin growth, but up to puberty all disappear owning to atresia (Fig. 4–4).

PUBERTY

From a practical point of view, a male or female animal has reached puberty when it is able to release gametes and to manifest complete sexual behavior sequences. Puberty is basically the result of a gradual adjustment between increasing gonadotropic activity and the ability of the gonads to simultaneously assume steroidogenesis and gametogenesis.

Endocrine Mechanisms of Puberty

At the onset of puberty, the circulating concentrations of gonadotropins increase, which is due to the rise of both the amplitude and the frequency of the periodic impulses of gonadotropins. This results

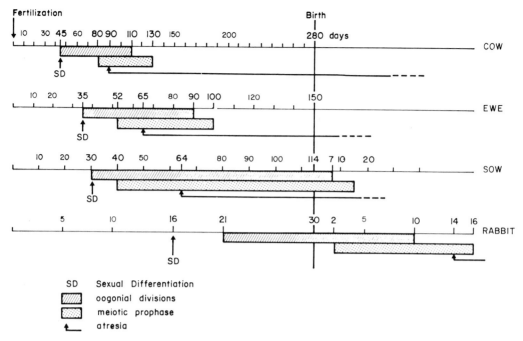

FIG. 4–3.   Species differences in patterns of oogenesis in some mammals.

from sex steroids and possibly from an increase in responsiveness of the hormone LH-RH, secreted from the hypothalamus to regulate gonadotropins. In 2- to 8-week old lambs, pulse frequencies increase from 1 to 5 in a 6-hour period; the magnitude of the surge is augmented threefold during that time.

In the male in response to gonadotropin secretion, testosterone progressively rises from very low to adult levels. Every LH pulse is followed at a 1-hour interval by a transitory rise of testosterone secretion. The extent of the testosterone secretion increases as puberty advances, and finally the average testosterone level remains definitively high. The increase of blood testosterone level eventually causes a decrease in gonadotropin secretion by a negative feedback effect. In the female, estrogen secretion gradually increases in response to the pubertal gonadotropin rise as long as antral follicle formation has begun. This is the case in the ewe and the cow. On the other hand, estrogen level only rises in the gilt toward week 11 after

birth, when the first antral follicles appear, while pubertal gonadotropic secretion begins 3 weeks earlier at 8 weeks of age.

Gametogenesis

Spermatogenesis.   At the onset of puberty in male swine, cattle and sheep, the gonocytes migrate to the periphery of the tubules and differentiate into spermatogonia, whereas supporting cells produce Sertoli cells. These changes occur when prepubertal gonadotropin elevation is already evident. The Sertoli cells remain present during the whole sexual life, and their number is the limiting factor in sperm production.

Manipulation of certain factors during the prepubertal period may reduce the onset of puberty further or increase testicular growth rate. Gonocytes develop at random through the testis into definitive A-spermatogonia. This, together with the formation of Sertoli cells, marks the end of the prepubertal period and the onset of spermatogenesis (Curtis and Amman, 1981).

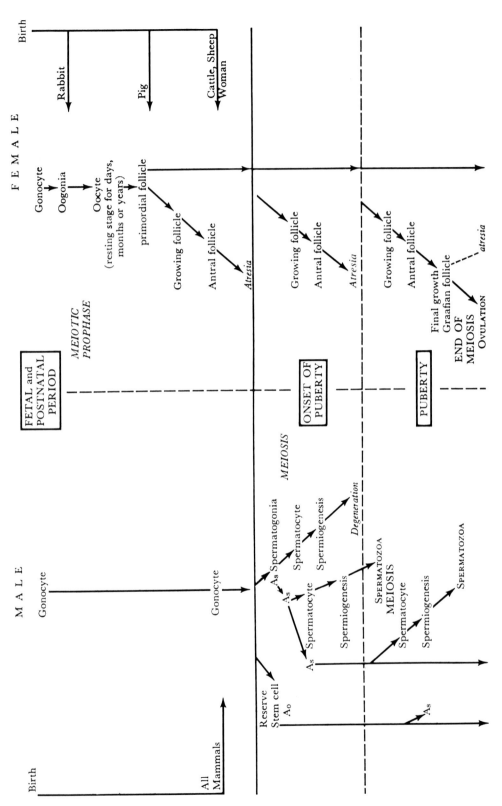

Fig. 4-4. Comparison of gametogenesis in male and female mammals from fetal life to active sexual life. A_o = reserve stem cells, A_s = stem cell spermatogonia.

During the fetal and neonatal period, the testis grows slowly, mainly through the lengthening of the seminiferous cords. Spermatogonial differential and formation of the first spermatogenetic lines mark the beginning of rapid testicular growth. After the attainment of full spermatogenetic activity, a slow growth rate is maintained during some months (ram) or years (bull) in response to the continuous increase of the stem cell population.

The concentration of the spermatozoa's progressive motility, the seminal protein concentration, and the percentage of spermatozoa with a normal head, tail, and acrosomal morphology increases from puberty through 16 weeks after puberty; rapid increases in the percentage of spermatozoa exhibiting normal head morphology (excluding acrosomes) and progressive motility are associated with rapid decreases in the percentage of spermatozoa with proximal cytoplasmic droplets (Lunstra and Echternkam, 1982).

Follicular Development. The first antral follicles appear during the prepubertal period (sow, rabbit) or even earlier (cow, ewe). However, complete follicular development, resumption of oocyte meiosis, and ovulation are observed only when FSH and LH have reached adult profiles.

Age at Puberty

In normal breeding conditions puberty occurs at about 3 to 4 months of age in rabbits; 6 to 7 months in sheep, goats, and swine; 12 months in cattle, and 15 to 18 months in horses.

The age of puberty is influenced by physical environment, photoperiod, age and breed of dam, breed of sire, and sires within breed, heterosis, environmental temperature, body weight as affected by nutrition, and growth rates before and after weaning. The onset of puberty is more closely related to body weight than to age. Dairy cattle reach puberty when the body weight is 30 to 40% that of the adult weight, whereas in beef cattle this percentage is higher (45 to 55% that of

adult body weight) (Roy et al., 1975). The same difference occurs in sheep (Romney ewes: 40%; Suffolk: 50%; Scottish Blackface: 63% of adult body weight) (Hafez, 1952). Nutritional levels modulate age at puberty. If growth is accelerated by overfeeding, the animal reaches puberty at a younger age. On the other hand, if growth is slowed down by underfeeding, puberty is delayed.

Puberty and regularity of estrous cycles in gilts is affected by the breed, type of housing, and season of the year during sexual maturation. Both gilts reared in confinement and gilts not reared in confinement that were exposed to a boar reached puberty at an earlier age than gilts reared without exposure.

In seasonal breeders, the age of puberty depends on the birth season. Ewes born in January attain puberty 8 months later, whereas those born in April become pubertal when 6 months old (during full adult breeding season in both cases). Puberty occurs earlier in gilts bred in a group than those bred alone. The presence of an adult boar hastens puberty in both situations (Mavrogenis and Robinson, 1976).

Full reproductive efficiency is not attained in any species at the first appearance of estrus or ejaculation. There is a period of "adolescent sterility." This period is remarkably short (some weeks) in domestic animals as compared with humans (1 year or more).

Practical Applications for Age of Puberty. The age of sexual maturity in ewes is related to adequate energy intake and the attainment of sufficient body weight. Early onset of sexual maturity provides economic advantages through increased lifetime reproductive rate. Thus, it is advantageous to maximize growth rates in ewe lambs being added to the breeding flock. The application of multiple lambing systems permits the rearing of lambs throughout various seasons of the year. Growth and maturation are, therefore, subject to a variety of seasonal influences.

The genetic improvement achieved by artificial insemination of dairy cattle has resulted from the use of proven-tested sires. Obtaining semen at the earliest possible age from bulls being proven-tested is desirable to hasten identification of superior sires. Ultimately, the genetic impact of a superior sire is limited by the number of sperm produced, which is a direct function of testicular size.

ESTROUS CYCLES

Mating is limited during estrus, coinciding with the time of ovulation. In humans and other primates, mating is not restricted at any time of the menstrual cycle, and ovulation occurs during midcycle (Fig. 4–5). The length of the estrous cycle is 16 to 24 days: ewe: 16 to 17 days; cow, sow, goat: 20 to 21 days; mare: 20 to 24 days. The duration of estrus is species dependent and varies slightly from one female to another within the same species. This is also true in respect to the time of ovulation, which occurs 24 to 30 hours after the onset of estrus in most ewes and cows, 35 to 45 hours in sows, and 4 to 6 days in mares (Table 4–1).

The length of estrus and the time of ovulation also vary in relation to internal and external factors. In ewes the interval between the onset of estrus and LH ovulatory surge (and therefore the interval between estrus and ovulation) lengthens as the number of ovulations increases (Fig. 4–6).

Endocrine Regulation of Estrous Cycles

The estrous cycle is regulated by endocrine and neuroendocrine mechanisms, namely the hypothalamic hormones, the gonadotropins, and the steroids secreted by the testis and ovary.

Regulation of gonadotropin secretion during the estrous cycle requires a delicate balance between complex hormonal interactions. One component known to be an important influence is luteinizing hormone-releasing hormone (LH-RH). Changes in the rates of LH-RH synthesis and release, as well as the rate of degradation of this hormone, are additional factors

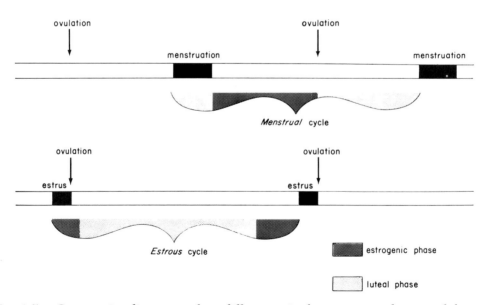

FIG. 4–5. Comparative diagram to show differences in the patterns and stages of the estrous cycle in farm animals as compared to the menstrual cycle in women. Note the incidence of ovulation in relation to estrus and menstruation. (Adapted from an illustration by Professor C. Thibault.)

TABLE 4–1.   Estrous Cycle, Estrus, and Ovulation in Farm Animals

	Length of Estrous Cycle (Days)	Duration of Estrus (Hours)	Time of Ovulation
Ewe	16–17	24–36	
		32–40	30–36 hours from beginning of estrus
Goat	21 (Also short cycles)		
Sow	19–20	48–72	35–45 hours from beginning of estrus
Cow	21–22	18–19	10–11 hours after end of estrus
Mare	19–25	4–8 days	1–2 days before end of estrus

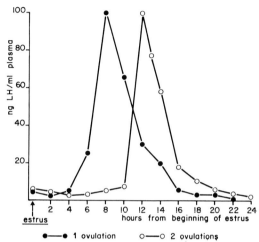

FIG. 4–6. Timing of LH surge in ewe according to number of ovulations (Ile-de-France breed). (From Thimonier and Pelletier, (1971) Ann. Biol. Anim. Biochim. Biophys. *11*, 559.

that modify its role in influencing gonadotropin release (O'Conner et al., 1984).

At the ovarian level, the estrous period is characterized by high estrogen secretion from preovulatory graafian follicles. Estrogens stimulate uterine growth by a mechanism that involves interaction of the hormone with receptors and the increase in synthetic processes within cells. Estrogens also stimulate the production of prostaglandins by the uterus. On the other hand, indomethacin has an inhibitory action on the production of prostaglandins by the uterus and other tissues. Indomethacin prevents the production of products of the enzyme, which influences various reproductive processes.

At the end of estrus, ovulation occurs followed by corpus luteum formation resulting in progesterone secretion. The corpus luteum is made of two distinct steroidogenic cell types, both of which contribute significantly to the total progesterone secreted during the luteal phase of the estrous cycle. The small luteal cells secrete little progesterone unless stimulated by LH, while large luteal cells spontaneously secrete progesterone at a high rate. The corpus luteum of pregnancy is resistant to the luteolytic effect of $PGF_{2\alpha}$.

The corpus luteum is the main source of progesterone and relaxin in pregnant swine where relaxin may play a role in parturition and the onset of lactation. The ovary is the primary source of relaxin in several species that require this organ throughout gestation, that is, pigs and rodents. Relaxin is distributed uniformly throughout ovarian tissue and is not confined to corpora lutea.

Prostaglandin $F_{2\alpha}$ ($PGF_{2\alpha}$) is the uterine luteolytic hormone in several mammalian species. Uterine $PGF_{2\alpha}$ controls the life span of the corpus luteum, which in turn regulates the length of the cycle. If pregnancy occurs, the luteolytic influence of the uterus has to be negated since progesterone secreted by the corpus luteum is necessary for the maintenance of pregnancy.

The period of corpus luteum activity is called the *luteal phase;* it lasts 14 to 15 days in ewes and 16 to 17 days in cows and sows. The follicular phase, from the regression of the corpus luteum to ovulation, is relatively short: 2 to 3 days in ewes and goats and 3 to 6 days in cows and sows. This short follicular phase does not reflect the true duration of graafian follicle growth (Fig. 4–7). Thus, estrous cycle length is closely related to the duration of the luteal phase. Corpus luteum regression is not caused by a decreased secretion of pituitary luteotrophic hormones (LH and prolactin) but by the action of a luteolytic factor, $PGF_{2\alpha}$.

Postpartum Estrus and Ovulation

The duration of postpartum anestrus is affected by several environmental, genetic, physiologic, and metabolic factors including breed, strain, nutritional level, suckling, milk production, frequency of milking, and level of and genetic potential for milk yield. The duration of postpartum anestrus is also affected by the rate of uterine involution, the rate of development of

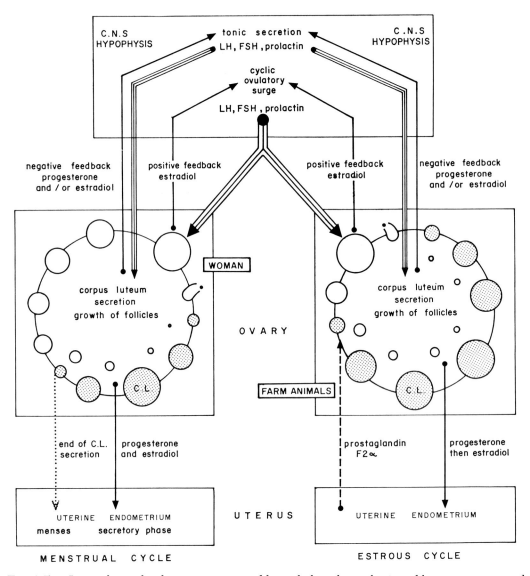

FIG. 4–7. Interrelationship between ovary and hypothalamohypophysis and between ovary and uterus.

ovarian follicles, pituitary and peripheral concentrations of gonadotropins, peripheral levels of estrogens and progesterone, onset of episodic secretion, and changes in body weight and energy intake (Stevenson and Britt, 1980). In cattle energy balance during the first 20 days of lactation is important in determining the onset of postpartum ovarian activity (Butler et al., 1981). The time required for postpartum uterine involution varies from 4 to 6 weeks (Table 4–2).

In modern swine production systems, it is important that sows return to estrus rapidly following weaning. Several factors influence the weaning to estrus interval such as type of feed and feed intake during gestation, lysine intake during lactation, protein intake during gestation and lactation, postweaning feed intake, lactation length, and altered suckling stimulus (Reese et al., 1982).

Altering the nursing pattern of pigs may be effective in either inducing estrus in the dam before weaning or decreasing the interval to remating after weaning. In general sows exhibiting prolonged weaning to estrus intervals are thin. Energy intake during lactation is inversely related to sow weight loss during lactation, thus low energy intake during the lactation may cause delayed estrus following weaning.

Endocrine Factors. A relatively high level of progesterone is absolutely necessary throughout gestation. Progesterone is secreted by the corpus luteum and in some species (cow, ewe) mainly by the placenta. The continuous progesterone secretion suppresses estrus and, in most mammals, ovulation.

Following parturition, progesterone drops to undetectable levels and estrus and ovulation can resume. The sow exhibits estrus within 48 hours after parturition, but there is no ovulation. The high plasma estrogen rise after farrowing (Shearer et al., 1972) may explain the estrous behavior (Fig. 4–8). In mares there is a fertile estrus 1 to 3 weeks after parturition. In cows, ewes, and goats silent ovulations can occur 2 to 3 weeks following parturition; however, fertile estrous cycles return later (Casida, 1968; Hunter, 1968). Postpartum anestrous females have short estrous cycles in response to weaning. Approximately 80% of the postpartum anestrous cows that exhibited estrus within 10 days after weaning their calves have estrous cycles of 7 to 12 days in length with a short serum progesterone rise after the first estrus. The early decline of progesterone after the first estrus is not due to lack of LH in serum. However, lower levels of FSH before this first ovulation may be due to the reduced life span of the subsequent corpus luteum (Ramirez-Godinez et al., 1982).

It would appear that the corpora lutea associated with the short cycles in cattle

TABLE 4–2. The Expected Time Course of Postpartum Uterine Involution in Farm Animals *(Hunter, 1982)*

Species	Involution Characteristics	Time Required (Days)
Cow	Initial shrinkage of uterus within 7–10 days of birth. Sloughing and discharging of caruncles completed by 10–12 days. New epithelium formed by 25–30 days. Uterus fully restored by 40–45 days.	35–40
Sheep	Necrosis and sloughing of caruncles completed within 7–8 days. Regeneration of epithelium within 25–30 days. Uterus restored to cyclic dimensions in 30–35 days; this may be delayed due to seasonal anestrus.	25–30
Pig	Some discharge for up to 1 week postpartum. No sloughing of endometrial tissue as in ruminants. Normal columnar epithelium formed by 21 days. Uterus fully restored in size by 21–28 days.	25–28

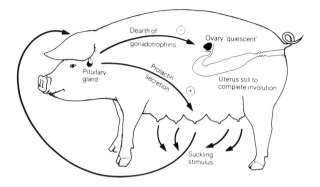

FIG. 4–8. Endocrine relationships in the post-partum sow showing the active secretion of prolactin early in the suckling period and the relative dearth of gonadotrophin secretion associated with lactational anestrus and incomplete involution anestrus and incomplete involution of the uterus. A change in the relative secretion of gonadotropins and prolactin occurs as the incidence of suckling decreases with the interval after birth. (Hunter, R.H.F. (1982). Reproduction of Farm Animals. New York, Longman.)

have a short life span as a result of (a) lack of luteotrophic support; (b) failure of the luteal tissue to recognize a luteotropin; or (c) enhanced secretion of a luteolytic agent.

Suckling and Lactation. The extent of postpartum anestrus depends on the degree of mammary stimulation the dam receives and on the nutritional status of the dam during late gestation and early lactation. During this period of frequent nursing, serum concentrations of prolactin are elevated and are inversely related to the concentrations of circulating FSH and LH (Moss et al., 1980). In dairy cattle the interval from parturition to first ovulation is related to the level of milk production and is longer in cows with a higher genetic potential for milk yield. Because high-producing cows cannot maintain a positive energy balance during the early lactation and must mobilize body reserves, the postpartum ovarian activity is more closely associated with milk production than with total digestible nutrient intake (Butler et al., 1981).

The inhibitory relationship between the mammary gland and reproductive function may be due to neural stimulation, secretion of an inhibitory substance, or the hormonal milieu. The level of nutrition also influences postpartum reproduction, although the effect of suckling is not related to the nutritional effect. The interval from parturition to uterine involution may be shortened by suckling. Suckling cows

exhibit shorter intervals to uterine involution.

The interval from parturition to first ovulation is shortened in unilateral ovariectomized cattle when surgery is performed 5 days postpartum. There is also a significant interaction between the effect of suckling and unilateral ovariectomy. Unilateral ovariectomy shortens the interval to the first postpartum estrus, and compensatory ovarian hypertrophy occurs in suckled animals, while, in nonsuckled animals, unilateral ovariectomy does not further shorten the already short interval (Grass and Hauser, 1981).

In nursing beef cattle, the interval from parturition to first estrus varies from 60 to 100 days. Several attempts were made to initiate ovarian cycles in anestrous-suckled beef cows through early weaning, limited nursing, gonadotropin-releasing hormone treatment, and treatment with a combination of sex steroids. Early weaning, limited nursing, LH-RH, and steroids all induce ovulation in anestrous beef cows. However, the luteal phase of the first postpartum estrous cycle and the first estrous cycle following early weaning limited nursing, and LH-RH treatment is shorter than in normal estrous cycles.

The importance of suckling on the duration of postpartum anestrus is demonstrated in sheep by experimentally induced pregnancy during seasonal anestrus so that lambing occurs during the breeding season. Dried off ewes usually return to estrus after about 1 month, while suckling ewes present the first estrus some weeks later. In sheep and cattle, the duration of postpartum anestrus varies with the breed and seems to be constant for the same female during successive pregnancies.

Fertility is low during the first estrus, particularly when the female suckles. Maximal fertility in the cow occurs 60 to 90 days after calving (Fig. 4–9). In sows fertility is nil during weaning; a highly fertile estrus occurs a few days after weaning.

BREEDING SEASON

In wild animals, there is a well-defined breeding season when both sexes have sexual activity. The Barbary sheep, a wild breed, exhibit two sexual seasons, one in October through January and the other in April through June. In domestic mammals, the nature and extent of the breeding season is variable. Cattle and swine exhibit no seasonality of breeding, whereas sheep, goats, and horses have a breeding season that also varies in duration.

Nature of Breeding Season. In sheep and goats there are important breed dif-

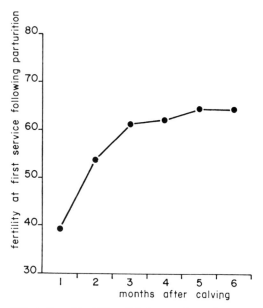

FIG. 4–9. Fertility of dairy cattle at first service following parturition. (From Casida, (1968) Wise, Expt. Sta. Research Bull. No. 270.)

ferences in the duration of the sexual season. Préalpes and Mérino sheep are long-season breeders, whereas Blackface and Southdown are short-season breeders. The length of the sexual season in these breeds is 260, 200, 139, and 120 days, respectively. A long sexual season is a dominant genetic character. All Mérino crosses exhibit a long sexual season like the Mérino. A cross of Dorset Horn and Persian ewe has produced a breed—the Dorper—which has only a 1-month anestrus (Fig. 4–10).

Silent ovulatory cycles always occur at the beginning and end of the sexual season. These ovarian cycles continue during the anestrous period in a variable number of ewes. In Ile-de-France Préalpes ewes, the frequency of silent cycles rises temporarily in spring. If a ram is present, behavioral estrus appears, thus permitting a second annual sexual season in these breeds.

In goats the sexual season is well defined in temperate climates. The ovaries in the Alpine goat are slightly active from February to March and quiescent from April to July; activity is abruptly resumed in all goats in September. Quiet ovulations are less frequent than in ewes. As in sheep in tropical climates, Creole goats exhibit continuous sexual activity.

Although rams can mate throughout the year, testis weight, testosterone, and gonadotropin levels are minimal from January to May during female anestrus (Fig. 4–11). Similarly, in the billy-goat the plasma testosterone level remains low from January to August, when it rises suddenly at the beginning of the breeding season.

An annual reproductive cycle in horses is well documented from both hemispheres. In northern temperate countries, ovarian silence in mares and low plasma testosterone and LH levels in stallions are observed from October to February.

In cattle and pigs estrus occurs regularly throughout the year, and seasonality is discrete. Local breeding conditions often mask its expression. In cattle a seasonal variation of fertility in temperate climates

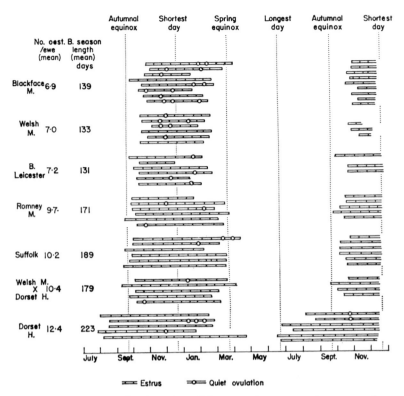

FIG. 4–10.   Breed differences in the duration of the sexual season and nonsexual season in adult ewes in Great Britain. Some breeds such as the Dorset Horn had a prolonged sexual season, whereas those such as the Welsh Mountain had a restricted sexual season. In nearly all cases, the sexual season was within the period from the autumnal equinox and the spring equinox, and the middle of the season corresponded rather closely to the shortest day of the year, or December 21. This illustrates the close relationship between the sexual season and length of day. Note that some estrous cycles double or triple the usual length occurred, which is due to quiet ovulations or to the failure to detect heat in the nonpregnant females observed. (After E.S.E. Hafez, (1952). J. Agric. Sci. *42*, 305.)

only becomes evident after studying a large number of herds over a period of several years (Fig. 4–12). Minimal fertility occurs in June and maximal fertility in November. This variation may be related to photoperiodism rather than to temperature and breeding, which can fluctuate from year to year. Cows are mainly responsible for the seasonal variation of fertility, as shown by nonreturn rates after insemination in spring and fall with frozen semen collected in fall or spring. Fertility in the sow is lower in the summer than in other seasons, and the litter size is also smaller then (Fig. 4–13).

Role of Photoperiodism and Temperature.   Photoperiods and environmental

temperature affect the annual sexual cycles; the former is the most efficient factor.

The most conclusive experience showing the control of reproduction by photoperiodism has been conducted in sheep. Using two photoperiodic cycles per year, ewes experience two annual breeding seasons. (Fig. 4–14). When the ewe is allowed to mate regularly, lambing occurs every 6½ months, since the 5-month gestation is followed by a lactational anestrus of 1½ months. The mare is a long-day seasonal breeder with reproductive cyclicity occurring from early May to October in northern latitudes. The arbitrary assignment of January 1st as the birth date for all foals born in a given year has created

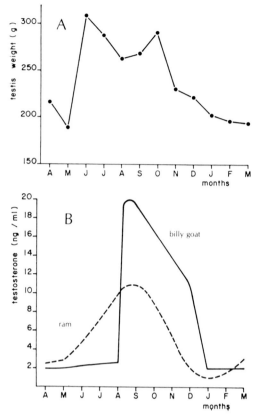

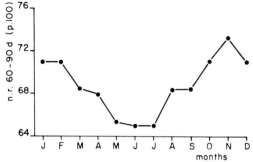

FIG. 4–12. Seasonal variation of fertility in cattle from 320,000 artificial inseminations over seven years (Montbéliard breed in French Jura, 47° N). The nonreturn rate is lower in spring and higher in autumn. (From Courot et al. (1968). Ann. Biol. Anim. Biochim. Biophys. *8,* 209.)

FIG. 4–11. *A,* Seasonal variation of testis weight in Ile-de-France ram (testis weight is adjusted to body weight) (47° N). (From Pelletier (1971). Ph.D. Thesis, University of Paris.) *B,* Seasonal variations of testosterone plasma levels in Ile-de-France ram and Alpine billy goat. (Ram: from Attal, (1970) Ph.D. Thesis, University of Paris; billy goat: from Saumande and Rouger (1972). C.R. Acad. Sci. Paris D, 274, 89.)

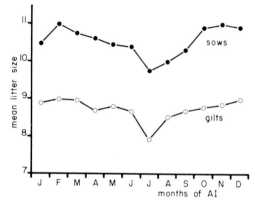

FIG. 4–13. Evolution of litter size in artificially inseminated sows and gilts in the west of France (46° N). This study includes 4,510 gilts and 13,324 sows and covers three consecutive years. (From Courot and Bariteau (1978). Personal communication.) Pig fertility is minimal under conditions of long days and high temperatures, as evidenced in sows and gilts by the smaller litter size in July. Note that adult sows have 1.5 piglets more per litter than gilts all the year round.

a demand in the equine industry for the administration of hormones to advance the onset of the natural breeding season in mares by 3 to 4 months. Thus foals would be born nearer to the first of the year.

In the northern hemisphere, increasing the daylight ratio up to 16 hours in November and December advances the beginning of the sexual season in the mare; first ovulation occurs up to 3 months earlier than under natural photoperiod. Induced cycles are endocrinologically nor-

mal and fertile (Oxender et al., 1977). Several hormonal treatments were used with varying success, such as pregnant mare serum gonadotropin (PMSG), human chorionic gonadotropin (hCG), gonadotropin-releasing hormone (GnRH), progesterone, and equine pituitary extracts (Hart et al., 1984).

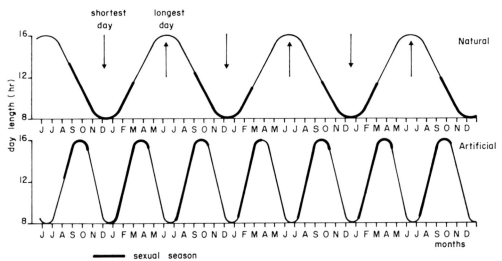

FIG. 4–14.   Periods of sexual activity in Limousine ewes. *Top:* Under natural photoperiodicity, estrus normally occurs during decreasing daylight period. *Bottom:* Under 6-month photoperiodic cycles, estrus occurs during the increasing daylight period. (From Mauleon and Rougeot (1962). Ann. Anim. Biochim. Biophys. *2*, 209.)

Similar manipulations are also effective with rams. Using two photoperiodic cycles per year, the ram exhibits two periods of decreasing spermatogenetic activity coinciding with the two periods of increasing day length (Ortavant and Thibault, 1956). Photoperiodism is basically a synchronizer of sexual activity. When ewes are placed under 12 hours of daylight every day or under constant illumination for many years, a breeding season is maintained for 1 or 2 years, then estrus becomes more random throughout the year.

Seasonal variation of temperature plays a major role in the regulation of sexual function in lower vertebrates, particularly in reptiles. In mammals, when environmental temperatures remain within the limit compatible with thermoregulatory mechanisms, seasonal temperature variation effect on fertility is rarely reported (Hafez, 1968). Nevertheless, the postfertilization period appears to be a critical one in domestic females. Cow, ewe, and sow embryos are susceptible to damage during the first 10 days of development (Ortavant and Loir, 1978).

In swine, photoperiodism and temperature interact unfavorably on fertility.

Sperm output, sperm motility, and farrowing rate are severely lowered when boars are submitted to summer temperatures (35°C) under long days (16 hours).

Breeding Season in Males

The duration of the breeding season of males is longer than in the females of the species. Although rams can mate throughout the year, testis weight, testosterone, and gonadotropin levels are minimal from January to May during female anestrus (Fig. 4–11). Similarly, in the billy-goat, the plasma testosterone level remains low from January to August, when it rises suddenly at the beginning of the breeding season. An annual reproductive cycle in stallions is also well documented from both hemispheres. In northern temperate countries, low plasma testosterone and LH levels in stallions are observed from October to February.

Breed differences exist in mature rams with regard to secretory patterns of hormones. Breed differences in serum gonadotropin and testosterone are apparent only during the short days of the year when the hypothalamo–pituitary–testicular axis is considered most active. Likewise, breed differences in prolactin are noted only during the long days, when secretion of this hormone is enhanced. Breed differences in LH, FSH, and testosterone secretion in rams during short days might be related to seasonality of mating and/or fecundity or breed types (D'Occhio et al., 1984).

There are distinct breed differences in hormone secretion in rams. These differences seem to be related to both seasonality of mating and fecundity of breed types and thus may provide important insight into the neuroendocrine mechanisms underlying seasonal variations in reproduction of this species. The between animal variability in gonadotropin secretion, noticeable particularly in Dorsets and Rambouillets, may similarly prove useful in identifying the most prolific individuals within a breed (D'Occhio et al., 1984).

Factors Regulating Breeding Season. Environmental, physiologic, and social factors regulate the onset and maintenance of the breeding season. The patterns of photoperiod, rainfall, and temperature are considered environmental cues that either entrain an endogenous rhythm or directly trigger the physiologic changes of the breeding season (Ruiz de Elvira et al., 1982). These are mediated by endocrine and neuroendocrine mechanisms.

In several mammalian species photoperiodic variation is a major environmental cue synchronizing reproductive function with season. Among the domesticated bovine species, the Zebu cattle exhibits the most distinct seasonality in reproductive efficiency. For example, the frequency of estrus and ovulation, as well as conception rate in Zebu cattle is higher during the summer than during the winter in Kenya (Rhodes III et al., 1982). Temperature may modify the seasonal effect of photoperiod on reproductive function. However, the length of daylight seems to be the primary stimulus for seasonality in reproductive parameters.

Endocrine and Neuroendocrine Mechanisms

Photoperiodism effect involves at least two separate mechanisms. First, there is a direct action on the hypothalamic pituitary axis. In the castrated ram and spayed mare, in which negative feedback from sexual steroids does not occur, gonadotropin levels reach a maximum during the normal breeding season and decrease during the nonbreeding season. Secondly, there is a simultaneous change in the sensitivity of the central nervous system to negative feedback from steroids.

The injection of testosterone or estradiol into castrated sheep causes two responses: (a) reduced gonadotropins to undetectable levels during the nonbreeding season and (b) slight depression of gonadotropins during the normal sexual season or under short days. The interactions among photoperiod, steroid hormones, gonadotropins and LH-RH are shown in Fig. 4-15. Similarly, estrus in spayed ewes is more regularly induced by progesterone/estrogen treatment during the normal breeding season than during anestrus (Reardon and Robinson, 1961).

Neural impulses are generated as a result of light incident on photoreceptors in the eye. The impulses are transmitted to the pineal gland, where they regulate the synthesis and secretion of melatonin. The pineal gland, and possibly melatonin, seem to mediate changes in neuroendocrine-gonadal activity in response to a changing photoperiod. In the mare, both superior cervical ganglionectomy and pinealectomy have altered the ability to respond to a stimulatory photoperiod (Hart et al., 1984). The hypothalamic content of LH-RH along with anterior pituitary concentrations of LH, but not the number of LH-RH receptors or concentration of FSH in the anterior pituitary, may be one of the hypothalamic-hypophyseal factors responsible for seasonal anestrus in the mare. It is possible that the low concentration of LH in the pituitary available for release

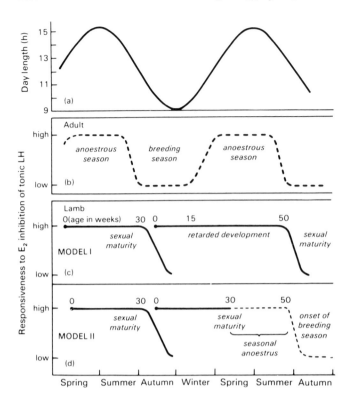

Fig. 4–15. Alternative models for the influence of photoperiod on the decrease in responsiveness to estradiol inhibition of tonic LH secretion in the lamb. Models I and II are based on the age and season of the decrease in responsiveness to estradiol feedback and initiation of ovulation in lambs born in the spring and autumn in relation to (a) natural photoperiod and (b) annual changes in responsiveness and ovarian cyclicity in the adult. Responsiveness is schematically illustrated as the inverse of circulating LH concentrations in chronically estradiol-treated ovariectomized females. Responsiveness is considered to be high when LH secretion is suppressed and is low when LH secretion is not suppressed; intact females are acyclic during periods of high responsiveness and are cyclic during periods of low responsiveness. (Foster, D.L. (1981). Mechanism for delay of first ovulation in lambs born in the wrong season. Biol. Reprod. *25*, 85–92.)

delays ovulation during the period of transition into the breeding season.

How is change in daylight ratio perceived by the central nervous system as a stimulus to gonadotropic function? There is no evidence in mammals, as in birds, of direct light perception by hypothalamic photosensitive neurons; the retinal pathway seems the more probable route. The length of the daylight period necessary for sexual stimulation does not mean that light must stimulate the nervous system during the whole light period. Light is efficient only during a precise period of the 24-hour dark–light cycle. According to species, this sensitive period occurs 10 to 20 hours after light on (dawn). The photosensitive period is short in birds (about 1 hour) and remarkably broad in the ram (7 hours). In rams submitted to 8 hours of light per day given in two parts (7 hours plus 1 hour given at various intervals in the night), LH level

was higher when the one-hour flash was given 11 to 20 hours after the beginning of the 7-hour light period (Fig. 4–15). Under natural condition, LH levels are higher in the summer than in the winter months.

These results are apparently in opposition to those that show an increase of FSH, LH, testosterone, and spermatogenesis in rams when they are under short days (8L/16D) after being under long days (16L/8D) (Lincoln et al., 1977). However, a correct understanding of the mechanism involved in natural seasonality must include varying levels of other hormones, such as prolactin and thyroxine, which interfere with the gonadotropic function or with gonad responsiveness. Prolactin and thyroxine secretion are also modulated photoperiodically. Under the same photoperiod of 8 hours of light given in a 7-hour period plus a 1-hour period, maximal prolactin secretion was obtained in the ram when the 1-hour flash was given 17 hours after light on. Moreover, a photoperiod enhancing either gonadotropin and prolactin secretion or maximal testis enlargement is never followed by sustained pituitary and gonadal responses. A fatigue or refractory period generally ensues. The frequency of LH and FSH pulsatile discharges changes at critical periods of sexual activity. For instance, five peaks of LH per 24 hours have been observed during the summer months in rams as compared to three peaks per 24 hours in the winter.

AGING AND FERTILITY

Herd fertility is evaluated by the percentage of pregnant females and the litter size. These parameters increase for a few years after puberty, reach a maximum, and then decrease slowly. The maximal pregnancy rate is reached around 3 to 4 years in sows, 4 to 6 years in ewes, and 5 to 7 years in cows. Maximal litter size occurs in third, fourth and fifth pregnancies in the sow. Maximal frequency of two pregnancies appears from the fifth pregnancy onward in cows (Table 4–3). In ewes the rate of twins increases up to 6 to 7 years and then decreases slowly (Fig. 4–16).

As in other mammals, ovulation and fertilization rates decrease only slightly in aged domestic females, but embryonic mortality, stillbirth, and postpartum losses

TABLE 4–3. Twinning Frequencies in the Cow According to Age (Gestation Number)

Gestation No.	Twin Pregnancies (%)	
	Monozygotic	Dizygotic
1	0.15	0.33
2	0.17	1.36
3	0.14	1.96
4	0.24	2.30
5	0.17	2.54

(Swedish breed, from Johansson I., Lindhé B. and Pirchner F. (1974) Hereditas *78*, 201.

increase. Early embryonic mortality may result from poor egg quality in aging female, as shown in the rabbit by the relatively unsuccessful development of blastocysts transferred from old donors to young foster mothers (Adams, 1970). However, high rates of embryonic and perinatal loss mainly result from the fact that the aging uterus reacts too slowly to the demands of the rapidly growing fetus and to the stimulus initiating parturition. Increased sperm production continues during aging, but at a slower rate. Apart from pathologic disturbances, male fertility, sperm production, and semen quality decrease slowly during aging. In bulls, the daily sperm output falls from 6×10^9 at 3 to 4 years to 4×10^9 between 6 and 13 years. Fertility decreases in the same proportion from 65% of nonreturn at 3 to 4 years to 54% at 12 years (Bishop, 1970). The re-

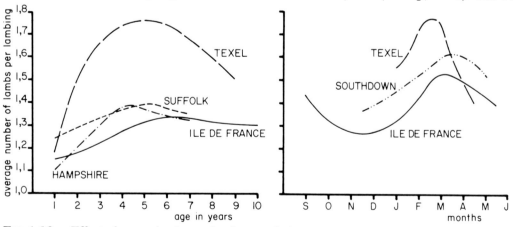

FIG. 4–16. Effect of age on lambs per lambing and of season on lambing rate. (Institut technique de l'Elevage ovin et caprin. Paris, France, 1972.)

markable decline in the reproductive parameters may be due to endocrine factors that affect body growth, sexual development, metabolism, and homeostasis. Endocrine failure may represent either a reduction in hormone secretion or a reduction in the response of target cells to hormonal stimulation (Morrison et al., 1981). Reduction may be associated with the compensatory increase in the secretion of prolactin or growth hormone.

REFERENCES

Adams, C.E. (1970). Ageing and reproduction in the female mammal with particular reference to the rabbit. J. Reprod. Fertil. Suppl. *12*, 1.

Bishop, M.W.H. (1970). Ageing and reproduction in the male. J. Reprod. Fertil. Suppl. *12*, 65.

Butler, W.R., Everett, R.W. and Coppick, C.E. (1981). The relationships between energy balance, milk production and ovulation in postpartum Holstein cows. J. Anim. Sci. *53*, 742–749.

Casida, L.E. (1968). Studies on the postpartum cow. Wisc. Exp. Station Res. Bull. No. 270.

Curtis, S.K. and Amann, R.P. (1981). Testicular development and establishment of spermatogenesis in Holstein bulls. J. Anim. Sci. *53*, 1645–1659.

D'Occhio, M.J., Schanbacher, B.D. and Kinder, J.E. (1984). Profiles of luteinizing hormone, follicle-stimulation hormone, testosterone and prolactin in rams of diverse breeds: effects of contrasting short (8L:16D) and long (16L:8D) photoperiods. Biol. Reprod. *30*, 1039–1054.

Foster, D.L., Lemons, J.A., Jaffe, R.B. and Niswender, G.D. (1975). Sequential patterns of circulating luteinizing hormone and follicle-stimulating hormone in female sheep from early postnatal life through the first estrous cycles. Endocrinology *97*, 985.

Grass, J. and Hauser, E.R. (1981). The influence of early age mastectomy and unilateral ovariectomy on reproductive performance of the bovine. J. Anim. Sci. *53*, 171–176.

Hafez, E.S.E. (1952). Studies on the breeding season and reproduction of the ewe. J. Agric. Sci. *42*, 189.

Hafez, E.S.E. (1968). Environmental Effect on Animal Productivity. *In* Adaptation of Domestic Animals, E.S.E. Hafez (ed.), Philadelphia, Lea & Febiger.

Hart, P.J., Squires, E.L., Imel, K.H. and Nett, T.M. (1984). Seasonal variation in hypothalamic content of gonadotropin-releasing hormone (GnRH), pituitary receptors for GnRH, and pituitary content of luteinizing hormone and follicle-stimulating hormone in the mare. Biol. Reprod. *30*, 1055–1062.

Hunter, G.L. (1968). Increasing frequency of pregnancy in sheep. Anim. Breed. Abstr. *36*, 347, 533.

Hunter, R.H.F. (1982). Reproduction of Farm Animals. London, Longman.

Lincoln, G.A., Peet, M.J. and Cunningham, R.A. (1977). Seasonal and circadian changes in the episodic release of follicle-stimulating hormone, luteinizing hormone and testosterone in rams exposed to artificial photoperiods. J. Endocrinol. *72*, 337.

Lunstra, D.D. and Echternkamp, S.E. (1982). Puberty in beef bulls: acrosome morphology and semen quality in bulls of different breeds. J. Anim. Sci. *55*, 638–648.

Mavrogenis, A.P. and Robinson, O.W. (1976). Factors affecting puberty in swine. J. Anim. Sci. *42*, 1251.

Morrison, M.W., Davis, S.L. and Spicer, L.J. (1981). Age-associated changes in secretory patterns of growth hormone, prolactin, and thyrotropin and the hormonal responses to thyrotropin-releasing hormone in rams. J. Anim. Sci. *53*, 160–170.

Moss, G.E., Adams. T.E., Niswender, G.D. and Nett, T.M. (1980). Effects of parturition and suckling on concentrations of pituitary gonadotropins, hypothalamic GnRH and pituitary responsiveness to GnRH in ewes. J. Anim. Sci. *50*, 496.

O'Conner, J.L., Lapp, C.A. and Mahesh, V.B. (1984). Peptidase activity in the hypothalamus and pituitary of the rat: fluctuations and possible regulatory role of luteinizing hormone releasing hormone-degrading activity during the estrous cycle. Biol. Reprod. *36*, 855–862.

Ortavant, R. and Loir, M. (1978). The environment as a factor in reproduction in farm animals. World Congr. Anim. Prod., Buenos Aires.

Ortavant, R. and Thibault, C. (1956). Influence de la durée d'éclairement sur les productions spermatiques du Bélier. C.R. Soc. Biol. *150*, 358.

Oxender, W.D., Noden, P.A. and Hafs, H.D. (1977). Estrus, ovulation and serum progesterone, estradiol and LH concentrations in mares after an increased photoperiod during winter. Am. J. Vet. Res. *38*, 203.

Ramirez-Godinez, J.A., Kiracofe, G.H., Schalles, R.R. and Niswender, G.D. (1982). Endocrine patterns in the postpartum beef cow associated with weaning: a comparison of the short and subsequent normal cycles. J. Anim. Sci. *55*, 153–158.

Reardon, T.F. and Robinson, T.J. (1961). Seasonal variation in the reactivity to oestrogen of the ovariectomized ewe. Aust. J. Agric. Res. *12*, 320.

Reese, D.E., Moser, B.D., Peo, E.R., Jr., Lewis, A.J., Zimmerman, D.R., Kinder, J.E. and Stroup, W.W. (1982). Influence of energy intake during lactation on the interval from weaning to first estrus in sows. J. Anim. Sci. *55*, 590–598.

Rhodes, R.C., III, Randel, R.D. and Long, C.R. (1982). Corpus luteum function in the bovine: in vivo and in vitro evidence for both a seasonal and breed type effect. J. Anim. Sci. *55*, 159–168.

Roy, J.H.B., Gillies, C.M. and Shotton, S.M. (1975). Factors affecting first oestrus in cattle and their effects on early breeding. *In* The Early Calving of Heifers and its Impact on Beef Production. J.C. Taylor (ed.). Brussels, European Economic Communities.

Ruiz de Elvira, M.C., Herndon, J.G. and Wilson, M.E. (1982). Influence of estrogen-treated females on sexual behavior and male testosterone levels of a social group of Rhesus monkeys during the nonbreeding season. Biol. Reprod. *26*, 825–834.

Shearer, I.J., Purvis, K., Jenkin, G. and Haynes, N.B (1972). Peripheral plasma progesterone and oestradiol 17β levels before and after puberty in gilts. J. Reprod. Fertil. *30*, 347.

Stevenson, J.S. and Britt, J.H. (1980). Models for prediction of days to first ovulation based on changes in endocrine. J. Anim. Sci. *50*, 103–112.

5

Folliculogenesis, Egg Maturation, and Ovulation

E.S.E. HAFEZ

The ovary performs two major functions: (a) the cyclic production of fertilizable ova and (b) the production of a balanced ratio of steroid hormones that maintain the development of the genital tract, facilitate the migration of the early embryo, and secure its successful implantation and development in the uterus. The follicle is the ovarian compartment that enables the ovary to fulfill its dual function of gametogenesis and steroidogenesis.

FOLLICULOGENESIS

In the primordial follicle reserve, formed during fetal life or soon after birth, some primordial follicles begin to grow continuously throughout life or at least until the reserve is exhausted. The role of the oocyte in the initiation of follicular growth was stressed initially from measurements of oocyte and follicle diameters. Enlargement of the oocyte, however, follows changes in the shape of the follicular cell from flat to cuboid. When any follicle is released from this reserve, it continues to grow until ovulation or until the follicle degenerates, which is the case with the majority of follicles (Tables 5–1 and 5–2). The largest follicle is responsible for most estrogen secretion by the ovary at estrus. Estrogen secretion by the largest follicle decreases rapidly at the time of the LH peak.

Cattle ovulate a single follicle that can be identified by its size about 3 days before the onset of estrus, when there are one or two large follicles on ovaries. In sheep, one or two large follicles secrete more estrogens and bind more gonadotropins to granulosa cells than smaller follicles. In sows, recruitment of the ovulatory follicles into the ovulatory population continues during the follicular phase. Thus, the development of smaller follicles may be promoted rather than inhibited by larger "dominant" follicles. Androgen availability, rather than low granulosa cells or aromatase activity may limit estrogen production, which itself may be functionally related to LH binding to granulosa cells.

The final growth in ewes, cows, and sows ranges between 12 and 34 days; the total duration of follicular growth is longer than 20 days and presumably about 6 months. The growth of the follicle up to the stage of antrum formation is not strictly gonadotropin dependent. In hypophysectomized females, the formation of preantral follicles continues at a more or less normal rate. On the other hand, antrum formation and final growth are entirely FSH and LH dependent (Figs. 5–1 and 5–2).

Follicle Growth

Follicular growth and maturation represent a series of sequential subcellular and molecular transformations of various components of the follicle such as the oocyte, granulosa, and theca (Testart et al., 1982).

TABLE 5–1. Some Morphologic, Physiologic and Biochemical Aspects of Ovarian Follicles

Components	Morphologic and Physiologic Characteristics
Thecal cells	Produce androgens in response to increasing basal LH. Have LH receptors from early stage of follicular growth. After ovulation, theca develop in theca lutein cells.
Follicular wall	Made of granulosa and theca, separated by basement lamina, undergo developmental changes related to organogenesis of an endocrine/exocrine gland that synthesizes steroid hormones.
Granulosa cells	In antral follicles, microfibrils link granulosa cells to basal lamina and thecal cells to reticular lamina. In preovulatory follicles, granulosa cell projections connect through the ruptured basal lamina. After ovulation, granulosa layer is invaded by vessels and connective material. Granulosa cells of goat follicles acquire the ability to secrete oxytocin before ovulation, probably as a response to the preovulatory LH surge.
Corona radiata	Before ovulation the egg lies at one side of the ovarian follicle, embedded in a solid mass of follicular cells, cumulus oophorus
Primordial follicle	Follicles with centrally located oocytes and a single layer of granulosa cells. Follicles are separated from one another by stroma made of fibroblasts, bundles of collagen, and reticular fibers. Differentiate from primordial germ cells (oogonia) and remain in an arrested meiotic prophase until they resume maturation, preliminary to either ovulation or atresia. Made of basement membrane and/or two layers of granulosa cells and a dictyate oocyte. Early follicle formation regulated by tubular rete ovarii. Follicle growth, proliferation of granulosa cells, zona pellucida formation, theca cell differentiation. A constant percentage of follicles grow in unit time irrespective to endocrine profile of female. Follicle growth monitored precisely and sequentially at similar rates.
Secondary follicle	With increase in number of granulosa cells by mitosis, the cells become cuboidal.
Vesicular follicle	Follicles with accumulation of follicular fluid in antrum within epithelial cells.
Follicular fluid (in antrum)	Antrum separated from vascular theca by basement membrane of selective permeability. Contains steroids, glycosaminoglycans, and many metabolites; K^+ and Na^+ in similar concentrations as in serum. Some components are physiologically active: oocyte maturation inhibitor, LH-binding inhibitor, inhibin, and various enzymes and chondroitin sulphuric acid. Contains, only in large follicles, high percentage of estradiol-17 in follicular phase and progesterone at ovulation. High concentration of progesterone after LH surge inhibits aromatoze activity locally in ovary.
Follicular fluid (between granulosa cells)	Fluid within granulosa cells and especially in the cumulus complex is viscous and rich in hyaluronic acid. Fluid accumulates as ovulation approaches. Many old oocytes remain on the follicular surface after ovulation until removed by fimbria. Proliferation is stimulated by estrogen. Fluid contains FSH receptors exclusively. Fluid contains estradiol receptors. FSH stimulates accumulation of cAMP. Increased responsiveness of granulosa cells to FSH occurs without change in number of FSH receptors, but this requires estradiol. LH receptors and LH-responsive adenylate cyclase are acquired only at late follicle development. Androgens are aromatized to estrogen. Estradiol-17 enhances ability of FSH to induce LH receptors. Separation of granulosa and theca is broken as basement membrane dissolves. Lutein cells develop after ovulation and are major source of progesterone in corpus luteum.

TABLE 5–2.   **Regulatory and Physiologic Parameters of Some Components of the Follicle**

Component	Morphologic Characteristics	Physiologic and Regulatory Mechanisms
I. Granulosa cells	A. Granulosa cells increase in number during follicle growth by mitosis, possibly in response to estrogen or intraovarian factors, thus forming unilaminar, bilaminar, trilaminar and multilaminar follicles. B. With an accumulation of follicular fluid in the antrum, granulosa cells are separated into a membrane granulosa lying adjacent to the basement lamina and into several to many concentric layers, forming cumulus oophorus around the oocyte. C. Cells ionically coupled to one another and to the ovum become uncoupled when the follicle ruptures at ovulation.	A. Granulosa cells control follicular development. B. Meiosis is arrested and oocytes enter dictyotene stage in the fetal or neonatal ovary as they are enclosed by granulosa cells during the formation of primordial follicle; oocytes that evade granulosa cells continue meiosis to metaphase-II and become atretic. C. Several mechanisms stimulate the replication of granulosa cells: low molecular weight peptides, epidermal growth factor, fibroblast growth factor, insulin, transferrin, steroids, thyroxine, and follicular fluid. FSH stimulates the differentiation of granulosa cells and promotes antrum formation.
II. Cumulus cells	A. Cumulus corona cells interdigitate with the oocyte through cytoplasmic processes, which cross the zona pellucida and make contact with adjacent cumulus cells through gap junctions. B. Cells undergo remarkable morphologic transformation—from a compact cell mass into an expanded and mucinous structure. C. Cells become progressively separated from each other; cumulus cells anchored to zona pellucida remain surrounding the oocyte, forming corona radiata.	A. Cells use glucose to supply pyruvate for metabolic exchange with egg; with the separation of cumulus cells, metabolic exchange occurs only through follicular fluid. B. Resumption of meiosis and oocyte maturation is triggered by preovulatory gonadotrophin surges; the degree of cumulus mucification and corona dispersal is correlated with the stage of oocyte meiotic maturation; oocyte maturation occurs in a medium that is biochemically similar to blood serum, although more dilute. C. Investments of the oocyte protect the egg from polyspermic fertilization by providing a physical barrier to the sperm. This can improve the chance for fertilization by increasing the target size for the sperm. Due to the radial arrangement of the corona radiata, the cells can help to guide the sperm toward the egg. D. While the presence of an intact cumulus oophorus may facilitate penetration of spermatozoa into the dissolution of these cells by mechanical or enzymatic treatment, it does not seem to impair in vitro fertilization.
III. Oocyte growth	A. Enlargement of cytoplasm of deutoplasm (yolk) B. Development of an egg zona pellucida and the mitotic proliferation of follicular epithelium and adjacent tissue. C. Growth of oocyte in two phases: (1) rapid growth of oocyte and development of ovarian follicle and antrum formation, (2) the oocyte does not grow in size while the ovarian follicle is responding to pituitary hormones and increases rapidly in diameter. Growth is confined to follicles in which the egg has attained full dimensions. Oocyte matures. Nucleus enters into prophase of meiotic division.	A. Primary oocyte undergoes two meiotic divisions; in the first division two daughter cells arise, each containing one-half of the chromosome complement (2n); in the second division the egg acquires almost all cytoplasm. This cell is known as the secondary oocyte. B. In a second maturation division, the secondary oocyte divides into ootid (n) and a second polar body (n). C. Oocyte continues maturation until fertilization.

TABLE 5–2. **Continued**

Component	Morphologic Characteristics	Physiologic and Regulatory Mechanisms
IV. Zona pellucida	A. A thick acellular, gelatinous, glycoprotein layer between the surface of the growing oocyte and granulosa cells. B. Made of polysaccharides, mucopolysaccharides, proteins, and glycoprotein. C. In some species, the zona pellucida consists of more than one layer and has a variable chemical composition. D. Microvilli and follicle cell processes embedded in the zona pellucida greatly increase in number as the oocyte and granulosa cells differentiate, increasing the surface area during oocyte growth. E. A fibrous network-like structure interspersed with numerous pores; the canaliculi, bounded by the fibers, provides viaducts by which processes of granulosa cells may traverse the zona pellucida and interact with vitelline surface.	A. Has important functions in the initial stages of fertilization, as the sperm must recognize, develop contact, and traverse it before establishing contact with the plasma membrane of the egg. B. Has physiochemical properties and antigenicity.

These are governed by several intraovarian factors, intrafollicular factors, and hormonal signals, which lead to the secretion of androgens and estrogens (mainly estradiol).

Follicle growth involves hormonally induced proliferation and differentiation of both theca and granulosa cells, leading ultimately to the increased ability of follicles to produce estradiol and to respond to gonadotropins. Production of estradiol determines which follicle will gain the LH receptors necessary for ovulation and luteinization. Disturbances in the responsiveness of the granulosa and theca to the gonadotropin signals, which stimulate and maintain maximal rates of estrogen and androgen biosynthesis, lead to cessation of follicle growth and initiation of atresia.

Recruitment and Selection of Ovarian Follicles

The ovarian follicle is a balanced physiologic unit whose structure and function depend not only on extracellular factors such as gonadotropins but also on a complex system of intrafollicular relationships. In sheep, all healthy follicles 2 mm in size are recruited, and once selection has occurred, recruitment is blocked. Booroolas sheep differ from Merinos because of the extended time during which recruitment takes place, the low incidence of selection, and the ability of fully grown follicles to wait for the LH peak. In contrast, Romanov sheep differ from Ile-de-France ewes because of a higher number of follicles recruited between days 13 and 15. Thus, it is likely that different control systems operate to generate a high ovulation rate in prolific breeds (Draincourt and Cahill, 1984).

Follicular Fluid

Follicular fluid originates mainly from the peripheral plasma by transudation across the follicle basement lamina and accumulates in the antrum formed by the coalescence of small pockets of fluid.

Biochemical Composition of Follicular Fluid. Follicular fluid, a serum transudate modified by follicular metabolic activities, contains specific constituents such as steroids and glycoproteins synthesized by the cells of the follicle wall. During follicular growth, an equilibrium is established

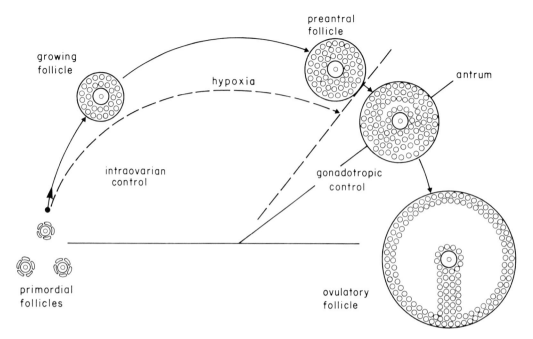

FIG. 5–1. Some follicles begin to grow every day. The growth of the primordial follicle up to the preantral stage occurs in the hypophysectomized female but at a lower rate. The number of primordial follicles beginning growth every day is controlled by an unknown intraovarian factor. Antrum formation and final follicle growth up to the ovulatory size is gonadotropin dependent. This second phase of follicle growth is shorter than the first one. Meiosis only resumes when the oocyte is released from the granulosa cells. *In vivo,* this occurs after the gonadotropin ovulatory surge, which causes loosening of granulosa cell junctions and the release of the oocyte into the follicular fluid. *In vitro,* meiosis resumes when oocytes are cultured, isolated or "grafted" on theca cells. Complete oocyte maturation (resumption of meiosis and cytoplasmic maturation) only occurs in the follicle after gonadotropin ovulatory surge. (Thibault and Levasseur (1978). La fonction ovarienne chez les Mammiferes. Masson, Paris.)

between serum and follicular fluid. The metabolite concentrations in the two compartments are similar. These concentrations are similar to those in oviductal secretions. The fluid contains several compounds of major physiologic significance, and most of them are concentrations similar to blood serum (Tables 5–3 to 5–5).

In large antral follicles (but not in small follicles), the follicular fluid contains remarkably high levels of estradiol-17β in the follicular phase and progesterone as ovulation approaches. Polycystic ovaries, however, have high levels of androstenedione. In porcine follicles, lipids are less concentrated in follicular fluid than in serum but more concentrated in the oviduc-

tal secretions. This is associated with a decline in follicular lipid levels at the end of follicular growth.

Viable ovarian follicles accumulate and secrete steroid hormones, primarily estradiol, progesterone, and 4-androstenedione; several physiologically active nonsteroids such as an oocyte maturation inhibitor (OMI), a polypeptide weighing about 1,500 daltons; luteinization inhibitor, a complex protein; inhibitory protein, a protein of about 1,400 daltons; relaxin, polypeptide of about 9,000 daltons; and inhibin activity protein (FSH-suppressing activity), a protein of high molecular weight (Tables 5–3 and 5–4).

Functions of Follicular Fluid. The fol-

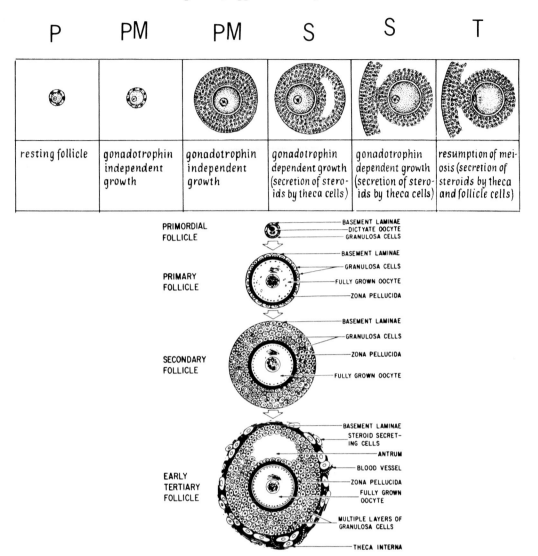

P	PM	PM	S	S	T
resting follicle	gonadotrophin independent growth	gonadotrophin independent growth	gonadotrophin dependent growth (secretion of steroids by theca cells)	gonadotrophin dependent growth (secretion of steroids by theca cells)	resumption of meiosis (secretion of steroids by theca and follicle cells)

FIG. 5–2. Physiologic (top) and morphologic (bottom) classification of ovarian follicles: *P,* primordial follicle; *PM,* primary follicle; *S,* Secondary follicle; and *T,* tertiary follicle. Note the differences in the number of granulosa cells and the degree of expansion of the antrum with accumulation of follicular fluid. (Dvorak, M. and Tesarik, J. (1980). Ultrastructure of human ovarian follicles. *In* Biology of the Ovary. P.P. Motta and E.S.E. Hafez (eds.). London, Martinus Nijhoff.)

licular fluid plays a major role in the physiologic biochemical and metabolic aspects of the nuclear and cytoplasmic maturation of the oocyte, and the release of the egg from the ruptured follicle, and sperm hyperactivation.

The follicular fluid undergoes remarkable changes throughout the estrous cycle and performs several functions including the following:

1. Regulation of the functions of the granulosa cells, initiation of follicular growth and steroidogenesis.
2. Oocyte maturation, ovulation and egg transport to the oviduct.
3. Preparation of the follicle for the for-

TABLE 5–3. Some Components and Metabolites of the Follicular Fluid that Exhibit Physiologic Functions

Biochemical Components	Compounds
Proteins	(e.g., albumins, globulins, IgA, IgM, fibrinogen, lipoproteins, peptides)
Amino acids	ASP, Thr, Glu, Gln, Gly, Ala
Enzymes	Intracellular and extracellular
Carbohydrates	Glucose, fructose, fucose, galactose, mannose
Glycoproteins	Glucosamine, galactosamine, hyaluronic acid, sulfated glycosaminoglycans, heparin and heparin sulfates, plasminogen
Gonadotropins	FSH, LH and their subunits; prolactin
Steroids	Cholesterol, androgens, progestins, estrogens
Prostaglandins	PGE, $PGF_{2\alpha}$
Elements and salts	Sodium, potassium, magnesium, zinc, copper, calcium, sulphur, chloride, inorganic phosphate, phosphorus
Immunoglobulins	IgG is the predominant immunoglobulin. IgA is present in amounts second to IgG. The concentration of IgG in fluid increases as the follicles enlarge to preovulatory size. Follicular fluid of prepubertal gilts contains slightly higher IgA concentration compared to sow follicular fluid, although its IgG content is much less.

TABLE 5–4. Regulatory Function of Follicular Fluid with Stimulatory or Inhibitory Responses

Substance	Physiologic Responses
Inhibitors	
Oocyte maturation inhibitor (OMI)	Inhibits completion of oocyte meiosis
Luteinization inhibitor	Prevents or inhibits luteinization of granulosa cells
FSH receptor-binding inhibitor	Depresses the binding of FSH to granulosa cells
Inhibin (FSH suppressing substance)	Depresses the secretion of FSH
Other factors	Promote capacitation and acrosome reaction of sperm
Stimulator	
Luteinization stimulator	Stimulates luteinization of granulosa cells

Table 5–5. Steroid Concentration in the Follicular Fluid of Ovine Follicles

	Steroid Hormones in Follicular Fluid (Pmol/ml)		
Diameter of Follicles (nm)	Estradiol	Testosterone	Progesterone
3–6 (large, nonatretic follicles)	860	70	150
3–6 (large, atretic follicles)	100	190	120
2–3 (small, nonatretic follicles)	140	280	40

Large healthy follicles are characterized by a high estradiol content and relatively low testosterone value. When large follicles are atretic, estradiol level is lower than that of testosterone. The same low estradiol/testosterone ratio is observed in small healthy follicles; however, their progesterone content is lower than that of large follicles, whether they are atretic or not. Intrafollicular steroid content reflects the steroidogenic potency of these follicles. (From Moor et al. (1978). J. Endocrinol. *77*, 309.)

mation of the subsequent corpus luteum.

4. The stimulatory and inhibitory factors in the fluid regulate the follicular cycle (Table 5–4).

5. The volume of fluid released at ovulation is also important, since it is a significant component, along with the oviductal secretions, of the environment in which sperm metabo-

lism, capacitation, and early embryonic development take place.

ENDOCRINOLOGY OF FOLLICULAR GROWTH AND OVULATION

Growth, maturation, ovulation, and luteinization of the Graafian follicle depend on appropriate patterns of secretion, sufficient concentrations, and adequate ratios of FSH and LH in the serum. These hormones include steroids, prostaglandins, and glycoproteins (combinations of sialic acid and bichained polypeptide), and they are all secreted by the B cells of the anterior pituitary.

FSH plays a major role in the initiation of antrum formation. This gonadotropin stimulates granulosa cell mitosis and follicular fluid formation. Estradiol enhances FSH mitotic effect. FSH stimulates granulosa cells through membrane receptors whose number per cell remains constant during follicular growth. Moreover, FSH induces granulosa cell sensitivity to LH by increasing the number of LH receptors. In sows, LH receptors increase from 300 in small follicles to 10,000 in large preovulatory follicles. The LH-receptor increment prepares the luteinization of granulosa cells in response to LH ovulatory surge (Figs. 5–3 and 5–4).

On the other hand, theca cells are stimulated only by LH, and LH receptors are present from the beginning of theca cell formation. In sows the number of receptors per theca cell only doubles during final follicular growth.

Steroidogenesis

Steroidogenic activity of the follicle also depends on FSH and LH acting on granulosa and theca cells, respectively. The primary steroid secreted is usually estradiol-17β. However, progestins and androgens are also produced (Table 5–1). Follicular androgens are important in the female. In rabbits, androgens can naturally overpass estrogen secretion. The androgen-estrogen ratio in the follicular fluid reflects the physiologic integrity and viability of the follicle. In sheep, a high androgen content is normal in small, healthy follicles, but it signals atresia in large follicles (Table 5–1). Immunization against androstenedione has revealed the unlikely role of ovarian androgens acting at the hypothalamopituitary level, because the ovulation rate doubles in immunized ewes.

During follicular growth, estradiol production results from the coordinated steroidogenic activity of the theca interna and the granulosa cells (Table 5–5). In vitro experiments have shown that theca cells mainly secrete testosterone, while granulosa cells convert testosterone intro estradiol as a result of high aromatase activity (Fig. 5–5). In the ewe, granulosa cells secrete only estradiol when testosterone is present in the culture medium; secretion is higher if FSH is added. On the other hand, theca cells from large follicles of cattle and sheep synthesize testosterone. Because FSH mainly stimulates granulosa cells, testosterone production, the FSH-LH ratio is an important endocrine parameter to evaluate ovarian steroid production (Fig. 5–6).

Follicular Growth During "Follicular" and "Luteal" Phases

Active corpora lutea are present in the ovaries during a large part of the estrous cycle called the *luteal phase*. The *follicular phase*, the period from corpus luteum regression to the following ovulation, is apparently short (2 days in ewes and 4 to 5 days in cows and sows). However, the presence of antral follicles throughout the luteal phase suggests that the real duration of the follicular phase is longer than 2 to 5 days, if "follicular phase" refers to the period from antral follicle formation to ovulation. Therefore, the luteal phase in domestic mammals would partially overlap the true follicular phase, obscuring the relationship between basal plasma FSH and LH levels and follicular growth.

Figure 5–7 illustrates some species differences regarding these phases: (a) animal species with no luteal phase, such as

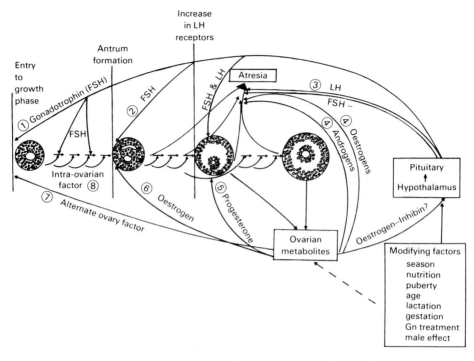

FIG. 5–3.   Some regulating mechanisms controlling preantral and antral follicles.

	Hormone Involved	*Physiologic Mechanism*
1	Gonadotropin (probably FSH)	Initiation of follicle growth
	FSH	Facilitation of growth of pre-antral follicles
2	FSH	Antrum formation
3	LH	Enhancement of atresia of antral follicles
	FSH	Inhibition of atresia of antral follicles
4	Androgens	Enhancement of atresia of antral follicles
	Estrogens	Inhibition of atresia of antral follicles
5	Progesterone	Inhibition of the growth rate of large antral follicles
6	Estrogens	Synergistic effect with FSH on follicles at antrum formation
7	Unknown	Enhancement of follicles to enter growth phase following hemicastration
8	Unknown	Intraovarian regulation resulting in correlations between number and growth rates of follicles

rodents with 4-day estrous cycles; (b) primates with quite distinct follicular and luteal phases; and (c) domestic mammals with overlapping "follicular" and "luteal" phases.

In rodents, plasma FSH profiles differ from those of LH. After the preovulatory discharge of both gonadotropins, FSH surges again after ovulation. Preventing the effect of this FSH surge with FSH anti- bodies shows that the surge is responsible for the formation of the antral follicles destined to ovulate 3.5 days later at the subsequent estrous cycle. In primates, a rise of FSH begins during menstruation at the end of the luteal phase. This elevation presumably initiates antrum formation of the follicle that will ovulate 2 weeks later and also of others that become atretic at the end of the first week of the follicular phase.

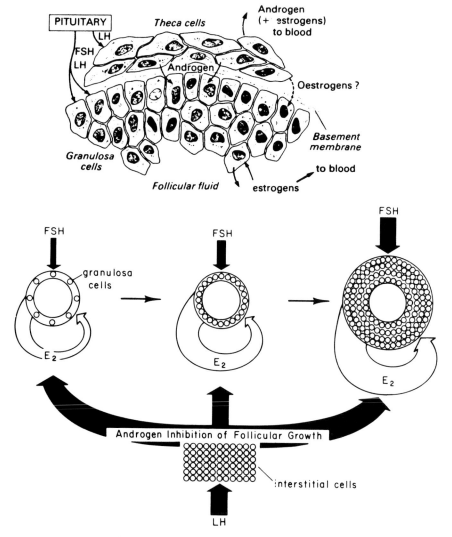

FIG. 5–4. *(Top)* Part of follicle showing sites of action of gonadotropins and production and action of steroids. *(Bottom)* Relationship between pituitary hormones and ovarian steroids in growing preantral follicles. (Peters, H. and McNatty, K.P. (eds.). The development of the ovary in the embryo. *In* The Ovary. Berkeley, University of California Press, 1980.)

In domestic mammals, there is also a second rise of FSH 20 to 30 hours after the preovulatory surge of LH and FSH. This postovulatory FSH rise triggers antrum formation in the follicle population that includes candidates for ovulation 1 or 2 cycles later. In ewes the second peak of FSH is significantly larger in those animals with a higher ovulation rate, and the magnitude of this peak is highly correlated with the number of antral follicles present in the ovary 17 days later. From estimations of the duration of growth of antral follicles, the time lapse from antral formation to ovulation is either 17 or 34 days.

Only a few of these differentiated antral follicles grow to ovulation; the others become atretic and degenerate. FSH levels near the end of the follicular phase in rodents are related to the rate of atresia. The

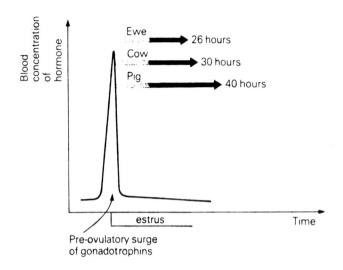

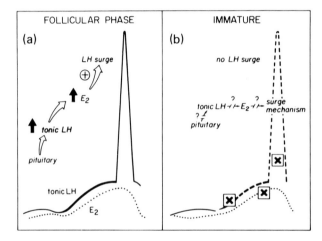

FIG. 5–5. *(Top)* The interval between the surge of gonadotropin secretion found at the onset of estrus and ovulation of the follicle(s) 26 to 40 hours later, according to species. (Hunter, R.H.F. (1982). Reproduction of Farm Animals. New York, Longman.)
(Bottom) Schematic diagram of (a) follicular phase: relationships between LH and estradiol during the follicular phase of the estrous cycle of the adult ewe. (b) Immature: three possible endocrine events that may fail in the immature female and could explain the absence of LH surges and ovulation before puberty. (Foster, D.L. and Ryan, K.D. (1981). Endocrine mechanisms governing transition into adulthood in female sheep. *In* Reproductive Endocrinology of Domestic Ruminants. R.J. Scaramuzzi, D.W. Lincoln and B.J. Weir (eds.). J. Reprod. Fertil. Suppl. *30,* pp. 75–90.

same physiologic regulation is noted in domestic mammals, and superovulation occurs when PMSG (a gonadotropin with high FSH potency) is injected just before atresia begins.

The relatively long duration of the follicular phase in domestic mammals as compared to rodents probably results from the slowing down of follicular growth by progesterone from the corpus luteum. When fully functional corpora lutea are induced in rodents by cervical stimulation, the duration of the estrous cycle and of follicular growth increases several days. On the other hand, reduction of the progesterone level during the luteal phase in cows and ewes by corpus luteum enucleation or prostaglandin luteolysis is followed by shortening of the cycle; ovulation occurs within 3 days, showing an immediate acceleration of follicular growth. This is the physiologic basis of the well-known practice of estrus synchronization in cattle after prostaglandin luteolytic treatment or in sheep after withdrawal of exogenous progestogens (vaginal sponge).

EGG MATURATION

The maturation of mammalian oocytes comprises two stages: (a) a period of growth and (b) a period of final nuclear and cytoplasmic preparation prerequisite

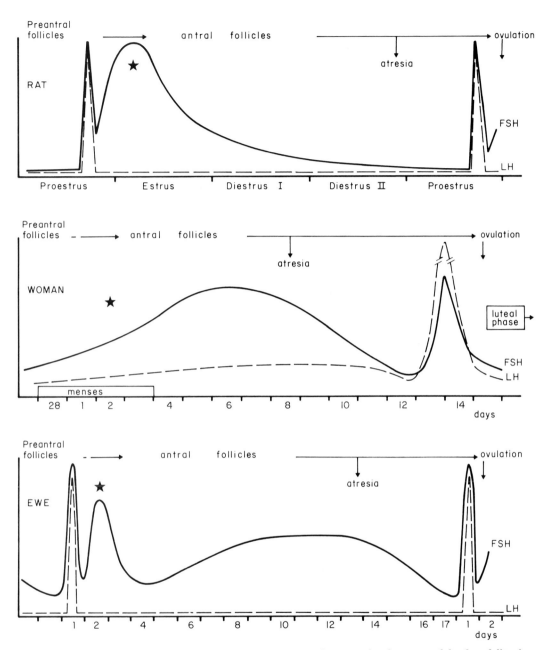

FIG. 5–6. Final growth of follicles destined to ovulate. Whatever the duration of the first follicular growth phase, follicles attain the preantral stage every day. From this follicle population, recruitment of antral follicles destined to ovulate is assumed by FSH postovulatory surge (★), which occurs before the beginning of corpus luteum secretion in the rat and ewe. In primates, this surge is postponed and occurs after corpus luteum regression. Some of these follicles become atretic when FSH returns to low basal levels. PMSG injection at this stage rescues these follicles and permits superovulation. FSH appears as the most important gonadotropin to support follicular growth, whereas LH plays a major role in ovulation. (Hafez et al., 1980.)

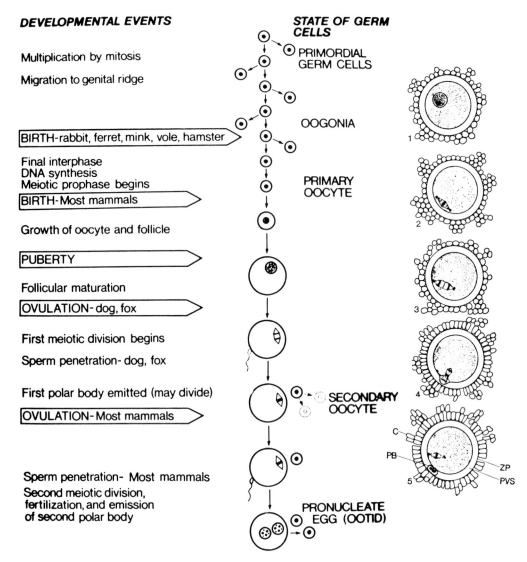

DEVELOPMENTAL EVENTS

Multiplication by mitosis

Migration to genital ridge

BIRTH-rabbit, ferret, mink, vole, hamster

Final interphase
DNA synthesis
Meiotic prophase begins
BIRTH-Most mammals

Growth of oocyte and follicle

PUBERTY

Follicular maturation

OVULATION-dog, fox

First meiotic division begins

Sperm penetration- dog, fox

First polar body emitted (may divide)

OVULATION-Most mammals

Sperm penetration- Most mammals
Second meiotic division,
fertilization, and emission
of second polar body

STATE OF GERM CELLS

PRIMORDIAL GERM CELLS

OOGONIA

PRIMARY OOCYTE

SECONDARY OOCYTE

PRONUCLEATE EGG (OOTID)

C
PB
ZP
PVS

FIG. 5–7. Developmental events. (From Baker, T.G. Oogenesis and ovulation. *In* Reproduction in Mammals. C.R. Austin and R.W. Short (eds.). Cambridge, University Press.)

to fertilization and normal development (Figs. 5–7 and 5–8).

Oocyte Growth

When a primordial follicle is released from the reserve, the oocyte and its follicle begin to grow. Oocyte growth is almost complete at the time of antrum formation. Through cellular processes, the inner cumulus cells actively cooperate to achieve oocyte growth, as they establish close contact with the oocyte cell membrane. During the formation of the external membrane of the oocyte (the zona pellucida), the cumulus cell processes are strengthened and the membrane junctions are retained. The cytologic, morphologic, metabolic, chromosomal, physiologic, biochemical, and hormonal aspects of oocyte growth are summarized in Table 5–6.

The maturation of oocytes is independent of (a) the nature of follicular stimulation, (b) the diameter of the follicle from

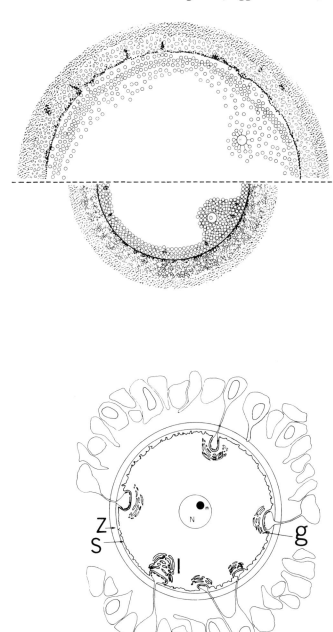

FIG. 5–8. *(Top)* Bovine ovarian follicle before (left) and 24 hours after (right) shows ovulation edema of the theca with dissociation of the round cells of the theca interna. *(Bottom)* Anatomic and physiologic relationships between the egg and the surrounding follicular cells: *g,* Golgi body; *S,* perivitelline space; *Z,* zona pellucida. (Thibault, C. and Levasseur, M.C. (1979). La Fonction Ovarienne chez les Mammiferes. Masson, Paris.) The vitellus composes most of volume with the zona pellucida at time of ovulation. After fertilization, it shrinks, and a perivitelline space is formed between the zona pellucida and the vitelline membrane in which the polar bodies are situated.

which the oocytes have been removed, and (c) the source of the follicular fluid or its filtrate from diverse follicles and different females. Maturation is inhibited when a protease inhibitor is added to fluids; this inhibitor may preserve the potential of the maturation inhibitor in follicular fluid.

In gilts, the removal of one ovary results in compensatory growth of the other ovary as measured by the increased number or growth of follicles in an increased volume of follicular fluid (Redmer et al., 1984). Thus, the removal of one ovary from a sow results in nearly the same litter

TABLE 5–6.   Major Physiologic, Biochemical, Biophysical, and Neuroendocrine Characteristics of Follicular Growth and Maturation

Parameters	Mechanisms
I. Recruitment and selection of follicles to ovulate	Throughout the estrous cycle, each ovary has numerous antral follicles on its surface. Two processes lead to the development of these preovulatory follicles. A. First, the recruitment process establishes a group of follicles capable of ovulating. B. Second, the individual follicles are selected to continue development to ovulation from a cohort of grossly similar follicles that degenerate. This selection occurs in the absence of detectable changes in hormone receptor concentrations, hormone levels in serum, or local blood.
II. Development of follicles	Development of ovarian follicles is classified according to the following A. Size of follicle. B. Number of layers of granulosa cells. C. Development of theca layers. D. Position of the oocyte within its surrounding cumulus oophorus. E. Presence of an antrum (fluid-filled space).
III. Number of follicles that develop	A. Number of follicles that develop per estrous cycle depends on hereditary and environmental factors. B. In cattle and horses, one follicle usually develops more rapidly than others, so that at each estrus only one egg is released; remaining follicles regress and become atrophied. C. In swine, 10–25 follicles ripen at each estrus. D. In sheep, one to three follicles may reach maturity depending on breed, age, and stage of sexual season.
IV. Nuclear maturation	A. Meiosis starts in the fetal ovary but stops before birth at the prophase of the first reduction division; oocytes then enter the dictyate state, which is a state of nuclear rest. Such nuclear rest may last until the first oocyte is ovulated at puberty. B. Resting or immature oocytes have a large nucleus known as the *germinal vesicle.* C. Meiosis progresses from the germinal vesicle (prophase of the first reduction division) to metaphase of the second reduction division, where it stops once again. D. The first polar body is extruded into the perivitelline space. E. Chromosomes in the first polar body, as well as those of the metaphase plate of second maturation spindle, are double-stranded.
V. Cytoplasmic maturation	A. Resumption of meiosis results from the release of an inhibitory effect exerted by follicular cells on the oocyte. B. This inhibition release coincides with loosening of granulosa and other cells around the oocyte as a result of gonadotrophin stimulation.
VI. Ovum maturation	Upon appropriate stimulation from circulating FSH and LH, or in some species, after removal from graafian follicles and culture in vitro, the dictyate-stage oocytes resume meiosis (reductional cell division), resulting in the final maturation of the oocyte within the mature, preovulatory follicle(s).
VII. Stigma formation	A. With formation of stigma, a thin circumscribed area of follicular apex, the whole apical wall becomes thin; prior to ovulation, inner layers of the follicular wall protrude through a gap to form a papilla of thin translucent stigma. B. Stigma thins out, bulges on the surface of the ovary and becomes completely avascular. C. At ovulation the bulging stigma ruptures at the apex, releasing some of the follicular fluid.

TABLE 5–6. Continued

Parameters	Mechanisms
VIII. Release of eggs	A. Cumulus-oocyte complex oozes out in visous follicular fluid. Granulosa cells, theca interna, and surrounding stoma, including surface epithelium, undergo cellular, subcellular and molecular changes in response to a preovulatory LH surge, which brings about ovulation. B. Theca and granulosa cells are no longer separated as the basement lamina is dissolved. C. Cumulus oophorus is made of several layers of cells randomly dispersed in a gelatinous matrix containing the egg surrounded with a layer of corona radiata cells. D. Gelatinous mass comprising contents of the follicle is gradually extruded until it is released to be picked up by cilia heat of fimbria. E. Ovulation point appears as a centrally located crater-like region containing follicular cells, erythrocytes, and a mucin-like substance.
IX. Steroidogenesis	A. All cell types of the ovary, particularly granulosa cells and theca cells, have the capacity to make steroids. B. Steroid hormones secreted by a particular cell type are determined by the stage of the estrous cycle. Ovaries of farm animals lack the relatively large amounts of steroid secreting interstitial tissue that is so prominent in the ovaries of rodents and rabbits. C. Theca cells of farm animals appear to differentiate almost completely during the atretric process; thus, these animals lack an important source of certain steroids present in those animals that have large amounts of interstitial tissue. D. Some progesterone produced by the granulosa cells may be used by the theca cells for synthesis of androgens and estrogens. Following ovulation, the luteinized granulosa cells become vascularized and secrete increased amounts of progesterone in the ovarian vein.
X. Anomalies of follicular growth and ovulation	A. Various anomalies occur in follicular growth, ovulation, and luteinization of the ruptured follicle. Growth can be arrested at specific stages, leading to conditions in which the follicles release androgens and other steroids, as in the development of cystic ovaries. B. Follicles are similar to nonovulatory follicles and may have accumulated through absence of feedback effects from larger follicles within the ovary. C. Abnormal follicle growth may arise through deficiencies in the hypothalamic-pituitary axis. D. *Luteinized unruptured follicle.* The luteinization of a follicle without the release of the egg; luteinization of follicles proceeds normally in the absence of follicle rupture. This condition is due to subtle defects in the endocrine profile or in follicular maturation that may accelerate, delay or even prevent the rupture of the follicle and release of the ova.
XI. Association of follicle and corpus luteum	A. Physiologic association between follicles and functional corpora lutea exists because follicular development is enhanced in the ovary containing a corpus luteum. B. Follicular fluid weight and the number of large follicles are greater in the ovary bearing a corpus luteum. In ewes follicles in ovaries that contain corpora lutea grow faster than follicles on the opposite ovaries without corpora lutea. Such an effect may be mediated through differences in local concentrations of progesterone in the two ovaries. C. Progesterone may act both systemically and locally to alter time-dependent changes in follicle size, thus making it possible for some follicles to grow while others undergo atresia. D. Effect of progesterone on follicular growth rates does not appear to be mediated through induction or alteration of ovarian estradiol-17β content. E. Estrogens affect follicles directly, both preventing atresia and stimulating growth.

(di Zerega and Hodgen, 1981; Draincourt and Cahill, 1984; Sluss and Reichert Jr., 1984; Hafez et al., unpublished data.)

size per farrowing as in an intact sow; however, the lifetime production of piglets by a sow with a unilateral ovariectomy appears to be reduced.

Oocyte Preparation for Fertilization

From oogenesis onward, the diplotene nucleus of the oocyte remains in the resting stage called the *dictyate nucleus.* Meiosis never resumes normally before gonadotropin ovulatory surge (Figs. 5–9 and 5–10). When the oocyte is removed from the antral follicle and cultured in a gonadotropin-free medium, it spontaneously resumes meiosis up to metaphase I or metaphase II, the stage normally reached at the time of ovulation. Co-culture of oocyte and granulosa or theca cells, as well as culture of the follicle cell-free oocyte in a medium with follicular fluid regulates the maintenance of the oocyte nucleus in a dictyate state, which results from the re-

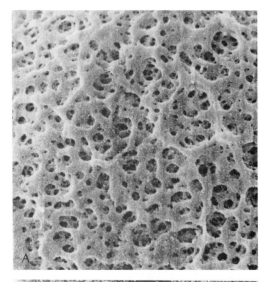

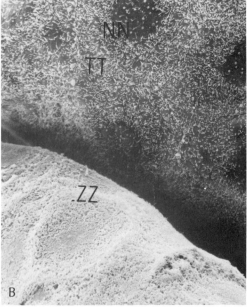

FIG. 5–9.   Scanning electron micrographs of the zona pellucida as shown from the outside surface (A) and inside surface (B). *A,* Note the characteristic mesh of the zona through which the sperm will penetrate. *B,* The spongy appearance of the inner surface of the zona (ZZ) as it is peeled off the trophoblastic layer of the blastocyst. Trophoblastic cells (TT) are characterized by microvilli. The nucleus (NN) is bulging from the cellular membrane. Species differences are noted in thickness of zona pellucide.

Species	Z.P. Thickness (μm)
opossum	1
mouse	5
hamster	8
human	13
sheep	15
pig	16
cow	27

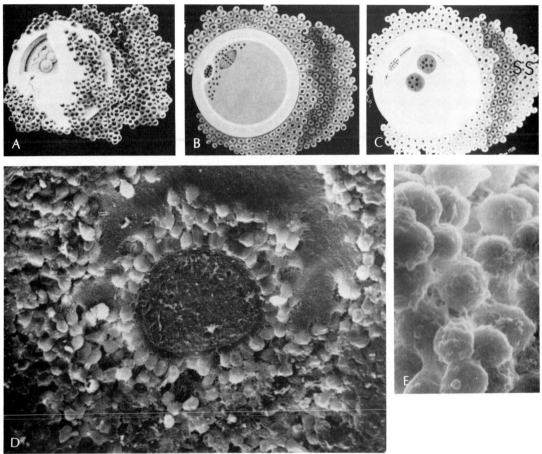

FIG. 5–10. The major cytologic changes in the ovarian cycle. *A, B, C,* Arrangements and cytologic connections between granulosa and the zona pellucida of the oocyte. Note some cytologic differences in distinct layers (SS) of the granulosa cells. *D, E,* scanning electron micrographs of the ovarian follicles (*d*) and higher magnifications of granulosa cells (*e*) showing differences in the surface of the cells probably indicating different degrees of cellular maturity or a cell cycle.

gressive effect of the granulosa on the oocyte.

The gonadotropin ovulatory discharge suppresses production of the granulosa cell meiotic-inhibiting factor. The gonadotropin surge is followed by metabolic modification of that follicular layer.

Meiotic resumption (nuclear maturation) is only one aspect of egg maturation; cytoplasmic maturation must also occur. In cows and ewes embryonic development never progresses normally when extrafollicular oocytes, which have reached the second meiotic division *in vitro,* are transferred into recipient females (Fig. 5–

11). The nucleus of the fertilizing sperm transforms into an abnormal pronucleus, although all other aspects of fertilization (second polar body formation, appearance of female pronucleus, timing of the first cleavage) proceed normally in these eggs.

OVULATION

Preovulatory follicles undergo three major changes during the ovulatory process: (a) cytoplasmic and nuclear maturation of the oocyte, (b) disruption of cumulus cell cohesiveness among the cells of the granulosa layer and (c) thinning and

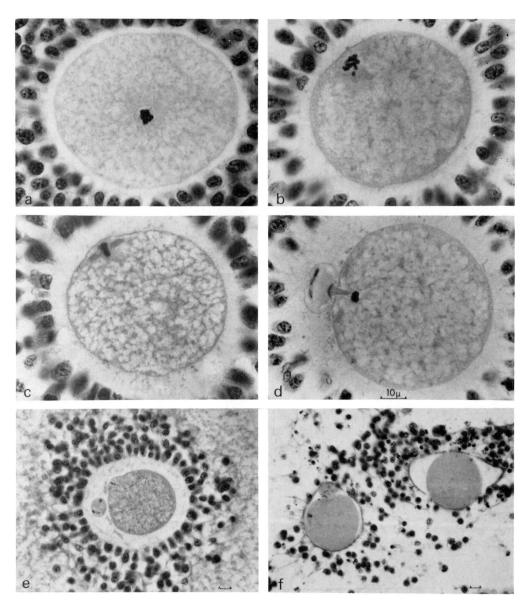

FIG. 5–11.   Mammalian oocytes showing typical maturation changes. (a) Dense chromatin mass in late germinal vesicle; cells of cumulus surround oocyte. (b) Diakinesis: nucleus has migrated to the periphery, and its envelope is about to break down; corona radiata forms around oocyte. (c) First metaphase; spindle axis is parallel to surface of oocyte. (d) Late first telophase; spindle is perpendicular to oocyte surface, and polar body is almost separated. A crescentic "midbody" persists where polar body is still attached. (e) Second metaphase; small second spindle formed in oocyte. Chromatin is now separated, first polar body is also in abortive mitosis. Cumulus oophorus has become detached from follicle wall. (f) Ovulated secondary oocytes in oviduct (rodent). Second metaphase spindle and first polar body visible at left. Zona pellucida of both eggs is intact, but cumulus cells are dispersing. (All markers are 10 μ; a to d at same magnification.) (Courtesy of Drs. Hill, R., Franchi, L.L. and Baker, T.G. (1980). Oogenesis and follicular growth. *In* Human Reproduction: Conception and Contraception. 2nd Ed. E.S.E. Hafez and T.N. Evans (eds.). Hagerstown, MD, Harper & Row.)

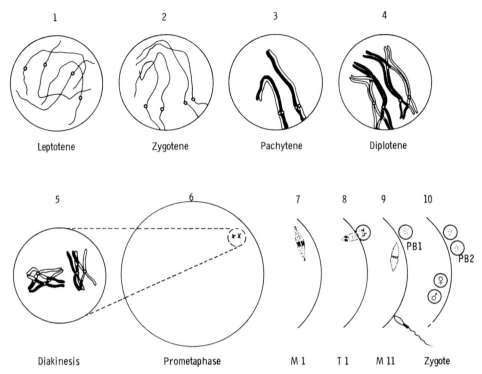

FIG. 5–11. Continued.   Cytogenetic changes in mammalian oocytes showing typical chromosomal events during meiosis. For simplicity, only two pairs of homologues are shown. (From Franchi, L.L. and T.G. Baker, (1973). Oogenesis and follicular growth. *In* Human Reproduction: Conception and Contraception. E.S.E. Hafez and T.N. Evans (eds.). Hagerstown, MD, Harper & Row.)

rupture of the external follicular wall (Fig. 5–12).

The distribution of capillary flow to follicles of different sizes was measured; the relative blood flow seemed to be inversely related to the mass of follicular tissue. After the ovulatory surge of gonadotropins, blood flow increases to all classes of follicles. The follicle destined to ovulate, however, not only receives the largest volume of blood in absolute terms (ml/min) but also has capillaries that are more permeable than those in other follicles.

Follicular Atresia

The ovarian follicles undergo degenerative changes during which the follicles lose their integrity. Most oocytes are lost at variable stages of their growth, as well as during all stages of the ovarian cycle. This loss occurs more frequently in the advanced stages of follicular growth. Figure 5–13 illustrates the distribution of proliferating and pyknotic granulosa cells during anovulatory cycles.

Atresia is associated with several morphologic, biochemical, and histologic changes that vary greatly with the stage of follicle growth, as well as with the animal species. They may be related to an altered role of granulosa cells and also to an altered passage of nutritive substances from the plasma into the follicles. Degeneration is accompanied by loss of the oocyte, granulosa cells, and receptors for various hormones, leaving behind the thecal cells, which form ovarian interstitial gland cells possessing the features of steroidogenic tissues.

Factors Affecting Atresia.   Several factors regulate follicular atresia: age, the stage of the reproductive cycle, pregnancy, lactation, the balance between estrogen and androgen of extraovarian or

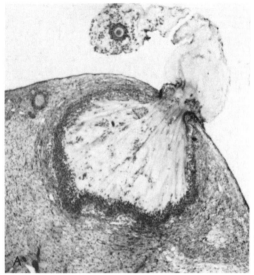

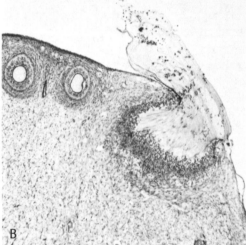

FIG. 5–12.   *A,* A section through a follicle of the rabbit in which ovulation has been completed. Note the protrusion of the cumulus and matrix through the stigma and its adherence to the surface (54×).

B, Section through an ovulated follicle in the rabbit ½ hr after ovulation. The egg has been pulled away from the protruding matrix. The material remaining will be removed from the surface in approximately 1 hour by the ciliary activity of the fimbriae (54×). (From Blandau, R.J. (1969). Gamete transport; comparative aspects. *In* The Mammalian Oviduct. E.S.E. Hafez and R.J. Blandau (eds.). Chicago, University of Chicago Press).

C, Oocyte as it appears in (A). Note the corona radiata cells around the oocyte and the follicular fluid (f) accumulating in the follicular antrum.

Term	Definition
Corona cells	Radiant, slightly expanded, compact or absent, even or clumped
Expanded cumulus mass	Present in thin matrix of acid mucopolysaccharide, dense matrix or absent, even distribution or clumped
Follicular membrana granulosa cells	Amount of cytoplasm, loose aggregation or compact appearance, pale color, or dark and clumped

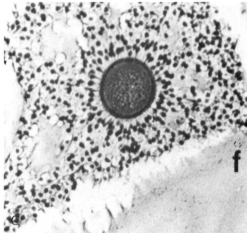

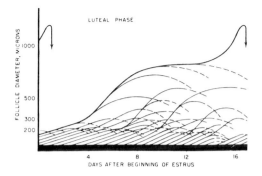

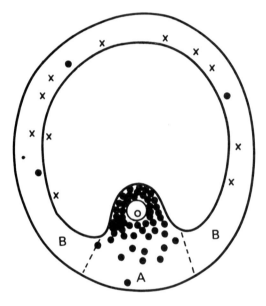

FIG. 5–13. Follicular cycle in the guinea pig. The heavy solid line indicates the average diameter of the largest follicles. Ovulation occurs at the arrow. The other solid and broken lines represent the concomitant growth and atresia, respectively, of other groups of follicles that do not normally ovulate.

intraovarian sources, a genetic "program," nutrition, and ischemia. There may be several processes and mechanisms of atresia depending on the stage of follicular growth; different hormonal treatments influence the rate at which the follicles become atretic. The ability of a developing follicle to release high concentrations of estrogens, which stimulate growth and cell differentiation of granulosa, is central

to selection of a given follicle for maturation and ovulation. Interruption of estrogen production at any step results in atresia of follicles.

The effect of the corpus luteum on the ovarian follicle is determined by the type of follicle and the stage of pregnancy. The reduction in the diameter of the largest follicle and the accumulation of the medium-sized follicles is due to the effect of the corpus luteum on reducing the rate of growth and atresia of the follicle.

Site of Ovulation

The mammalian ovary is normally arranged so that ovulation can occur at any point on its surface, except at the hilus. However, ovulation in mares always occurs in a limited ovarian area called the *ovulation fossa*. The ovary of horses begins its development in the usual way, and germinal epithelium covers the whole ovary, but during the neonatal period, this epithelium becomes concentrated in one area, the ovulatory fossa.

In cattle, sheep, and horses, ovulation occurs at random with respect to which ovary contains the previous corpus luteum. However, in some mammals ovulation consistently alternates between the ovaries. In the ewe, the side of ovulation is independent of the location of the corpus luteum of the previous ovarian cycle, and the duration of the estrous cycle is unaffected by the relative locations of the corpus luteum. There is no difference between left and right ovaries in size or occurrence of ovulation in horses. The frequency of multiple ovulations for ponies is about 10%. The ovulatory season appears to be shorter, with fewer ponies ovulating through the year. The percentage of mares ovulating during the fall in the younger age groups (under 5 years) is less than in the older groups, indicating a shorter breeding season for young mares. Ovarian activity appears to decrease after 15 years. The onset of puberty occurs at 12 to 15 months of age (Wesson and Ginther, 1981). In ponies there is a decrease in the number of large follicles during late estrus. There are two waves of follicular growth during the ovulatory cycle, and there are also differences in follicular end points in relation to the time of the year attributed to monthly differences in cycle gonadotropin patterns.

Cellular Events

Several tissue layers separate the oocyte from the outside of the follicle. These are the surface epithelium, the collagen-rich tunica albuginea, the theca externa, the thin basement lamina separating the capillary network from the membrana granulosa, and the membrana granulosa itself. Before ovulation, all tissue layers are broken down. Moreover, the necessary increase in follicular elasticity during preovulatory growth is associated with changes in granulosa and theca cell relationships. Such changes are also prerequisite to further corpus luteum organization.

As the enlarging follicle begins to protrude from the surface of the ovary, the vascularity of the follicular surface increases except at its center, which seems devoid of blood vessels. This avascular area is the future point of rupture.

The same processes occur in all mammalian species (Fig. 5–14).

Oocyte. The cumulus cells of growing graafian follicles are cytologically indistinguishable from the granulosa cells. In rabbits, cavities appear 1 to 2 hours after coitus within the cumulus mass, and the cells progressively separate from each other. Only the cumulus cells anchored in the zona pellucida remain, surrounding the oocyte and forming the corona radiata (Fig. 5–15). Cumulus cell dissociation frees the oocyte from the granulosa layer, and meiosis resumes about 3 hours after the gonadotropin surge. This process, called *nuclear maturation,* ends 1 hour before ovulation when the first polar body has been extruded.

Cumulus cells actively secrete glycoproteins, which form a viscous mass enclosing the oocyte and its corona. After follicular

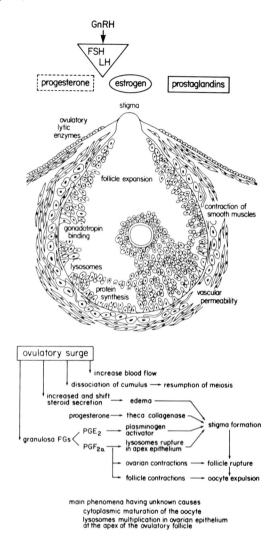

FIG. 5–14. *(Top)* Diagram of some of the morphologic, physiologic, cytologic and biochemical mechanisms involved in ovulation. *(Bottom)* Tentative synthesis of biochemical processes in ovulation.

rupture, the viscous mass spreads at the ovarian surface to facilitate the "pick up" of the oocytes by the fimbriae. Ultrasonography is used extensively to recover preovulatory eggs from the ovarian follicle to be used for *in vitro* fertilization (IVF) (Fig. 5–16).

Granulosa Cells. The granulosa layer is completely dissociated only at the follicular apex and finally disappears. This pro-

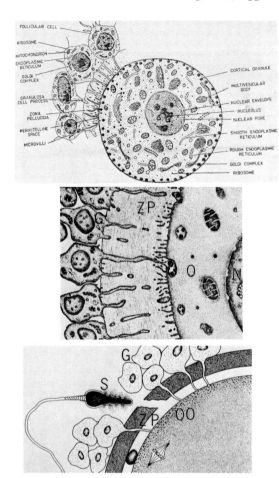

FIG. 5–15. *(Top)* Diagram of ultrastructure of various components of growing oocyte and of a portion of its zona pellucida associated with follicular cells that show various organelles. Granulosa (or follicle) cell processes. Microvilli are also seen in the zona pellucida. (From Guraya, S.S. (1984). Recent advances in the cellular and molecular biology of ovarian follicles. *In* Human Fertility, Health and Food: Impact of Molecular Biology and Biotechnology. D. Pruett (ed.). New York, United Nations Fund for Population Activities.) *(Middle).* Structure of fully formed zona pellucida (ZP) around an oocyte in Graafian follicle. Microvilli arising from oocyte interdigitate with processes from granulosa cells (G). These processes penetrate into cytoplasm of oocyte (O) and may provide nutrients and maternal protein. (N), oocyte nucleus. (From Baker (1972). *In:* Reproduction in Mammals. C.R. Austin and R.V. Short (eds.). Cambridge University Press.). *(Bottom)* Penetration of the spermatozoon through the granulosa cells (G), Zona pellucida (ZP) and oocyte (O). Note acrosomal enzymes released from the sperm (S) during vesiculation.

cess begins 6 hours after coitus and terminates before ovulation 4 hours later. About 2 hours before ovulation, granulosa cell growth processes penetrate through the lamina basalis, preparing the invasion of theca cells and blood vessels into the granulosa after ovulation in the developing corpus luteum. This process is associated with the production of the early pregnancy factor (EPF) (Fig. 5–17 and 5–18).

Theca Cells. The follicular volume rapidly increases in the few hours preceding ovulation without any increment of follicular fluid pressure, owing to the increased elasticity of the follicle. This results from a looser cohesion of the theca externa cells owing to the invasive edema of this layer and to collagen fiber dissociation, which begins 4 hours after coitus. Dissociation of bundles of collagen fibers also results from proteolytic enzyme activity on the proteinaceous matrix of the fibers. Plasmin activity increases after the gonadotropin surge, and this proteolytic enzyme causes an increase in follicular wall elasticity.

Apex Changes. The rupture of the follicle outside the ovary involves interaction between the ovarian epithelium and the underlying follicular wall. The wall of the follicular apex becomes exceedingly thin in a circumscribed area called the "stigma." The stigma thins out, bulges on the surface of the ovary, and becomes completely avascular. At ovulation the bulging stigma ruptures at the apex, releasing some of the follicular fluid and the viscous glycoprotein mass embedding the oocyte.

Mechanisms of Ovulation

Ovulation occurs in response to a combination of physiologic, biochemical, and biophysical mechanisms including: (a) neuroendocrine and endocrine mechanisms, LH-RH, steroids, and prostaglandins; (b) neurobiochemical and pharmacologic mechanisms; (c) neuromuscular and neurovascular mechanisms, and enzymatic interactions.

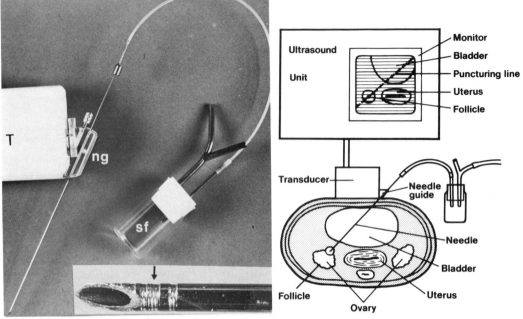

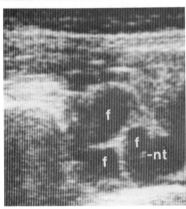

FIG. 5–16.   1. Aspiration equipment for ultrasonically guided percutaneous follicle puncture: *T*, transducer; *ng*, needle guide; *sf*, sampling flask. 2. Needle tip with the shallow tracks (arrow) in the needle tip. 3. Schematic illustration of the ultrasonically guided puncture technique. 4. Illustration of ultrasonically guided puncture of a human follicle. The white echo inside the follicle (f) represents the needle tip (nt). (Wikland et al., 1983.)

The relative importance of any of these factors is still controversial (Tables 5–7 and 5–8). A gonadotropin-induced preovulatory increase in follicular prostaglandin, produced by granulosa cells, is needed for ovulation. Prostaglandins may stimulate ovarian contractions and activate thecal fibroblasts to proliferate and release proteolytic enzymes that digest the follicle wall and basement lamina. Steroids, especially progesterone, may also be involved. Prior to ovulation, a progressive dissociation and decomposition of various cellular layers surrounding the apex of the preovulatory follicle occurs as a result of activities of proteolytic enzymes, produced by the granulosa cells and/or by surrounding fibroblasts in response to LH, progesterone, and prostaglandins. The contractions of smooth muscle cells during ovulation appear to influence the detachment of the cumulus oophorus, the expulsion of the follicular contents after the opening of the apical wall and related vascular phenomena, and the collapse of the follicle and its transformation into a corpus luteum.

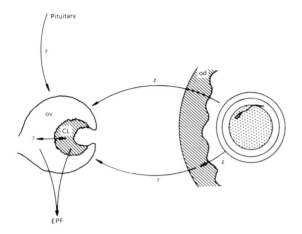

Fig. 5–17.   Schematic representation of the production of early pregnancy factor (EPF). *CL*, corpus luteum; *od*, oviduct; *ov*, ovary; *z*, zygotin. (Nancarrow et al. (1982). The early pregnancy factor of sheep and cattle. *In* Reproductive Endocrinology of Domestic Ruminants. R.J. Scaramuzzi, D.W. Lincoln and B.J. Weir (eds.). J. Reprod. Fertil. Suppl., 30.)

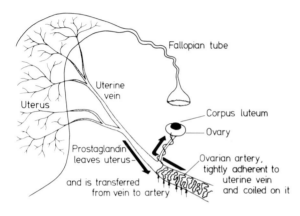

Fig. 5–18.   Diagram of the utero-ovarian vasculature in the sheep and of the route that PGF$_{2\alpha}$ travels from the uterus to the ovary. (Peters, H. and McNatty, K.P. (eds.) (1980). The development of the ovary in the embryo. *In* The Ovary. Berkeley, University of California Press.)

The ovarian follicle undergoes two major changes: (a) the stimulation of steroid synthesis by LH, and (b) activation of an ovulatory enzyme by the steroid released. The sequence of events leading to steroidogenesis involves the activation of adenyl cyclase by an LH-receptor complex, perhaps through the local action of a prostaglandin, which results in increased tissue levels of cAMP.

Biochemical Mechanisms of Ovulation

The gonadotropin preovulatory surge first induces an immediate and temporary rise in steroid levels due to an increased secretion of progesterone and related progestins. Later, estradiol and PGF$_2$ secretion are also augmented. Inhibition of either prostaglandin or steroid secretion prevents ovulation. Thus, the gonadotropin surge induces ovulation by a cascade of biochemical changes.

Changes in Steroid Secretion.   The enhancement of steroid secretion and the switch of the estradiol-progesterone ratio that follow the gonadotropin surge are easily detectable in the follicular fluid. In sow follicles, the estradiol-progesterone ratio decreases from 2.0 to 0.15. These changes are slightly noticeable in the ovarian venous blood and are undetectable in the peripheral blood. Inhibition of progesterone synthesis prevents ovulation. The role of progesterone is to stimulate collagenase activity in the follicular wall. Moreover, the thecal edema may result from the transitory but important rise of steroid levels.

TABLE 5–7.   Some Neuroendocrine and Endocrine Mechanisms of Ovulation

Parameters	Physiologic and Biochemic Mechanisms
I. Neuroendocrine	A. Structures within the preoptic and suprachiasmatic hypothalamus regulate ovulatory discharge of gonadotropins, which exert cyclic control of ovulation. The tonic center is under the negative feedback control of estrogen. B. Gonadotropins are secreted in a pulsatile fashion in response to the similar pulsatile release of LH-RH from neurosecretory neurons centered in the hypothalamus. C. Gonadal steroids exert their feedback effects both directly on the pituitary and through modulation of the pulsatile pattern of LH-RH secretion. They may also influence subsequent biologic activity of gonadotropins. D. LH-RH release is under the control of catecholaminergic neurotransmitters. Norepinephrine acts as an excitatory agent, whereas dopamine inhibits LH-RH secretion. E. Dopamine inhibits prolactin release and may be the prolactin-inhibiting factor. F. The endorphins are endogenous apiate peptides, and through modulation of neurotransmitter mechanisms, the endorphins may affect both prolactin and gonadotropin secretion.
II. Endocrine	A. LH is at a steady level during early follicular phase and rises slightly before ovulation. B. A remarkable surge of LH occurs prior to ovulation; LH levels return to low level during the luteal phase. C. Number of ovarian follicles that develop and the proportion that subsequently degenerate are regulated by relative ratio of FSH and LH. D. Cyclic changes in estradiol and FSH levels stimulate one or two waves of follicular growth and regulate ovulation rates (1) during the transition from preantral to antral stage and (2) some days before ovulation when atresia reduces the number of preovulatory follicles. E. Granulosa cells secrete progesterone into follicular fluid and act as precursor for estrogen synthesis in surrounding theca interna cells. F. 17-β-Estradiol and 17-α-hydroxyprogesterone produced by partially luteinized cells of theca interna, causing gradual rise in estrogen production. G. Follicular development under influence of high LH levels, estradiol level increase, and pituitary gland become increasingly responsive to LH-RH; pituitary LH reserves may increase to provide future hormone pools. H. At preovulatory LH surge, LH-RH is released in pulsatile bursts to activate the pituitary discharge of LH and FSH. I. As LH reaches critical concentrations in plasma, it exerts a negative feedback within the CNS. J. Rate of follicular development and the number that fully mature per estrus depend on pituitary gonadotropins. In adult females, a limited number of hormones are available to the ovary. During each estrous cycle, as a result of the release of sufficient FSH by pituitary gland, a crop of "growing" follicles is stimulated to undergo further growth and maturation. K. Several follicles grow during first stages of the estrous cycle, but few reach preovulatory maturity. L. Less FSH may be required to initiate the growth of small follicles than to maintain larger follicles and bring them to ovulatory size since the number of follicles that mature can be greatly increased (superovulation) by injecting animals with pharmacologic doses of gonadotrophins.
III. Prostaglandins	A. Theca is the predominant site of prostaglandin production, and the capacity of both granulosa and theca cells increases with the stage of follicular development; the rupture of follicles is associated with follicular synthesis of prostaglandin. B. Porcine granulosa cells and thecal tissue isolated from follicles 1 to 3 days after PMSG treatment produce prostaglandin E_2 (PGE), prostaglandin $F_{2\alpha}$ (PGF) and 6-keto-prostaglandin-$F_{1\alpha}$ in tissue culture. C. Concentration of prostaglandins E and F in follicular fluid of preovulatory follicles increases markedly as time of ovulation approaches; indomethacin blocks follicular rupture by inhibiting prostaglandin production. D. Exogenous LH increases prostaglandin E and prostaglandin F within the whole ovaries, graafian follicles and follicular fluid.

Hafez et al., 1980.

TABLE 5–8. Biophysical, Biochemical, Muscular, Neuromuscular, and Neurovascular Mechanisms of Ovulation

Parameters	Mechanisms and Some Functions
Biophysical	A. Remarkable and sudden changes in ovarian arterial and venous blood flow and lymph flow as judged by distribution of capillary flow to follicles of different sizes. B. Relative blood flow is inversely related to the mass of follicular tissue. An increase in follicular flow near ovulation occurs in all classes of follicles. C. The follicle destined to ovulate receives the largest volume of blood in absolute terms (ml/min) and has capillaries more permeable than those in other follicles. D. Rapid response of ovarian microcirculation to LH and increased metabolism of follicles after gonadotropin stimulation suggest that enhanced vascularity may be an inherent effect of LH on follicles. E. Increase in intrafollicular pressure does not seem to affect mechanical rupture of follicle.
Biochemical	A. Granulosa cells elaborate plasminogen activator in response to increases in LH and intracellular cAMP; plasminogen activator converts plasminogen into plasmin to weaken the follicle wall. B. Tensile strength of follicle wall decreases at time of rupture; numerous proteolytic agents can reduce the strength. C. Enzymes involved in breakdown are detected in follicular fluid. This is enhanced by ischemia developing in follicular apex. D. Synthesis of collagenase-like enzymes, under progesterone influence, causes distention of follicular wall and rupture of apex.
Muscular	A. Ovarian musculature is not indispensable for follicular rupture. Even if ovarian contractions do facilitate rupture, the latter may still occur in the absence of any such contractility. B. Contraction of ovarian musculature during ovulation may influence the detachment of the cumulus oophorus, the expulsion of the follicular contents after opening of the apical wall, and related vascular phenomena, as well as collapse of the follicle and its transformation into a corpus luteum.
Neuromuscular and neurovascular mechanisms	A. Concentric layers of theca externa of follicles contain smooth muscle cells richly innervated by autonomic nerve terminals. B. Mechanical process of ovulation is influenced by intraovarian autonomic nerves and/or receptors mediating their actions on follicular musculature. C. Prostaglandins are involved in neuronal functions and other local processes within the follicle. This does not necessarily imply that musculature acts by simply increasing the follicular pressure to rupture follicular wall. D. Follicle wall tension may increase during follicular development with no increase in intrafollicular pressure. E. Ovarian musculature provides a mechanical basis for maintenance of constant intrafollicular pressure prior to follicular rupture.

Prostaglandins. The increase of $PGF_{2\alpha}$ and PGE_2 levels in follicular fluid does not immediately follow the gonadotropin surge, as the steroid elevations do. In sows an increase of prostaglandins begins only 30 hours after ovulatory discharge, and the maximal level occurs about 40 hours later as ovulation approaches. Prostaglandins play a basic role in follicular rupture; inhibition of their synthesis always prevents ovulation, and their action is exerted at the level of the albuginea and follicular epithelium. When prostaglandin synthesis is inhibited, the oocyte remains inside the luteinizing follicle or may be "ovulated" inside the ovary. $PGF_{2\alpha}$ is involved in follicular rupture; and PGE_2, in the remodeling of the follicular layers, terminating in corpus luteum formation.

$PGF_{2\alpha}$ contributes to the rupture of epithelial cell lysosomes at the follicular apex, as suggested both by the relation between the elevation of the $PGF_{2\alpha}$ level and lysosomal rupture and by the well-known detrimental effect of $PGF_{2\alpha}$ on lysosomal membrane. Increases of $PGF_{2\alpha}$ must also be related to preovulatory enhancement of ovarian contractions. $PGF_{2\alpha}$ stimulates the production of plasminogen activator, thus increasing plasmin activity. Plasmin is generally involved in tissue cell migration and presumably plays a role in the mixing of theca and granulosa cells during corpus luteum formation.

Gonadotropins. The freeing of the oocyte inside the follicle is the only direct gonadotropic action known; *in vitro* cumulus cell dissociation is exclusively obtained by FSH and LH.

Neuromuscular Mechanisms

The ovarian stroma and the concentric layers of the theca externa of preovulatory follicles contain smooth muscle cells that are richly innervated by autonomic nerve terminals. Drug inhibition of β-adrenergic receptors delays ovulation and reduces ovulation rate, demonstrating a role of neuromuscular systems in follicular rupture. The frequency of spontaneous ovarian contractions begins to increase 2 to 3 hours before ovulation, reaching a maximum around ovulation time. The role of $PGF_{2\alpha}$ is evidenced both by *in vitro* stimulation of ovarian contractions by $PGF_{2\alpha}$ and by the *in vivo* relationship between increasing contraction frequencies and increasing $PGF_{2\alpha}$ levels in follicular fluid. Thus, ovarian contractions facilitate follicular rupture after the follicular apex has been thinned.

Before rupture, the follicle itself does not contract spontaneously, as shown *in vivo* by stable intrafollicular pressure and *in vitro* by the absence of contractions in the isolated follicle. However, strips of follicular wall contract spontaneously and respond to drugs and $PGF_{2\alpha}$ as the entire ovary does. Thus, after follicular rupture, the thecal neuromuscular system, stimulated by $PGF_{2\alpha}$, contributes to the extrusion of the oocyte.

Neuroendocrine Control of the Ovulatory Gonadotropic Discharge

A preovulatory gonadotropin surge occurs at the beginning of estrus when progesterone has fallen to its minimal blood levels and when estradiol reaches its highest cyclic values.

A typical preovulatory LH surge is obtained only when the duration of estradiol treatment and blood estradiol levels narrowly mimic the natural estradiol increase before the cyclic LH surge. Simultaneous administration of progesterone always suppresses estradiol positive feedback.

Estradiol acts at two levels: the pituitary and the hypothalamus. Estradiol increases the sensitivity of pituitary gonadotropin-producing cells to the competent hypothalamic hormone LH-RH. During postpartum anestrus in lactating females, estradiol positive feedback may be prevented by high prolactin levels related to the suckling stimulus.

Egg "Pick-Up"

The ovary, attached to the back of the broad ligament, lies free in the peritoneal cavity. The oviduct curls over the ovary to facilitate egg "pick-up" by the mucosal folds of the fimbriae. At the time of ovulation, the ovum, together with the surrounding cells in a gelatinous mass, protrudes at the ovarian surface and is swept into the ostium of the oviduct by the action of the motile kinocilia of the fimbriae.

In Vitro Ovulation

Several culture media are used to induce ovulation *in vitro* with or without ovarian perfusion. The selection of quality follicles is favored by the choice of season for the experiments and also by the absence of any ovarian stimulation when the follicle ovulates; thus, the granulosa cell mass will be well preserved. The same culture system is used for *in vivo* fertilization of oocytes matured in their follicles in vitro. The proportion of follicles ovulating, particularly after addition of progesterone to the medium, is appreciably higher than that previously obtained after the culture of whole ovaries.

Collection of Preovulatory Eggs. Follicle-guided ultrasonography has been extensively used to recover preovulatory eggs from the ovarian follicles of women, monkeys, and farm animals.

Anomalies of Ovulation and Reproductive Failure

The absence of ovulation and the subsequent formation of follicular cysts are the main causes of reproductive failure in cows and aged sows. An efficient treatment for preventing cyst formation, which reduces fertility in cystic cows, is the stimulation of gonadotropin release by LH-RH or the direct stimulation of the ovary with *h*CG. It is probable that the presence of cystic follicles reflects a disorder in gonadotrophic function at the hypothalamic level.

REFERENCES

Blandau, R.J. (1969). Gamete transport: comparative aspects. *In* The Mammalian Oviduct. E.S.E. Hafez and R.J. Blandau (eds.). Chicago, University of Chicago Press.

diZerega, G.S. and Hodgen, G.D. (1981). Folliculogenesis in the primate ovarian cycle. Endocr. Rev. *2,* 27–49.

Draincourt, M.A. and Cahill, L.P. (1984). Preovulatory follicular events in sheep. J. Reprod. Fertil. *71,* 205–211.

Dvorak, M. and Tesarik, J. (1980). Ultrastructure of human ovarian follicles. *In* Biology of the Ovary. P.P. Motta and E.S.E. Hafez (eds.). London, Martinus Nijhoff.

Foster, D.L. and Ryan, K.D. (1981). Endocrine mechanisms governing transition into adulthood in female sheep. *In* Reproductive Endocrinology of Domestic Ruminants. R.J. Scaramuzzi, D.W.

Lincoln and B.J. Weir (eds.). J. Reprod. Fertil. Suppl. *30,* 75–90.

Franchi, L.L. and Baker T.G. (1973). Oogenesis and follicular growth. *In* Human Reproduction: Conception and Contraception. E.S.E. Hafez and T.N. Evans (eds.). Hagerstown, MD, Harper & Row.

Guraya, S.S. (1984). Recent advances in the cellular and molecular biology of ovarian follicles. *In* Human Fertility, Health and Food: Impact of Molecular Biology and Biotechnology. D. Puett (ed.). New York, United Nations Fund for Population Activities.

Hafez, E.S.E., Levasseur, M.C. and Thibault, C. (1980). Folliculogenesis, egg maturation and ovulation. *In* Reproduction in Farm Animals. 4th Ed. E.S.E. Hafez (ed.). Philadelphia, Lea & Febiger.

Hunter, R.H.F. (1982). Reproduction of Farm Animals. London, Longman's.

Peters, H. and McNatty, K.P. (1980a). Morphology of the ovary. *In* The Ovary. H. Peters and K.P. McNatty (eds.). Berkeley, University of California Press.

Peters, H. and McNatty, K.P. (1980b). Corpus luteum function, *In* The Ovary. H. Peters and K.P. McNatty (eds.). Berkeley, University of California Press.

Redmer, D.A., Christenson, R.K., Ford, J.S. and Day, B.N. (1984). Effect of unilateral ovariectomy on compensatory ovarian hypertrophy, peripheral concentrations of follicle-stimulating hormone and luteinizing hormone, and ovarian venous concentrations of estradiol-17β in pre-puberal gilts. Biol. Reprod. *31,* 59–66.

Sluss, P.M. and Reichert, Jr. L.E. (1984). Porcine follicular fluid contains several low molecular weight inhibitors of follicle-stimulating hormone binding to receptor. Biol. Reprod. *30,* 1091.

Testart, J., Thebault, A., Frydman, R. and Papiernik, E. (1982). Oocyte and cumulus oophorus changes inside the human follicle cultured with gonadotrophins. *In* In-vitro Fertilization and Embryo Transfer. E.S.E. Hafez and K. Semm (eds.). Lancaster, England, MTP.

Thibault, C. and Levasseur, M.C. (1979). La Fonction Ovarienne chez les Mammiferes. Paris, Masson.

Wesson, J.A. and Ginther, O.J. (1981). Influence of season and age on reproductive activity in pony mares on the basis of a slaughterhouse survey. J. Anim. Sci. *52,* 119–129.

Wikland, M., Nilsson, L., Hansson, R., Hamberger, M.L. and Janson, P. (1983). Collection of human oocytes by the use of sonography. Fertil. Steril. *39,* 603.

6
Transport and Survival of Gametes

E.S.E. HAFEZ

The mammalian sperm–egg complex undergoes various maturational changes in preparation for fertilization (Table 6–1). While the female sheds 1 or 2 ova (or 10 to 15 ova in the case of swine), each estrous cycle, the male discharges massive numbers of spermatozoa at copulation. Since the survival time of ova and spermatozoa is relatively short (20 to 48 hours), fertiliza-tion depends primarily on the synchro-nous transport of the gametes in the female reproductive tract. Gamete transport is the result of the inherent con-tractility of the female tract as modified by central nervous system reflexes and hormonal activity. Pharmacologically ac-tive substances in the semen stimulate and modulate the contractility of the female

TABLE 6–1. Sperm and Egg Physiology Related to Fertilization

Parameters	Oogenesis and Characteristics of Ova	Spermatogenesis and Characteristics of Sperm
Mitosis in the gonad	Ceases during fetal life; no new eggs are formed after birth	Continues throughout reproduc-tive life of the male
Meiosis in the gonad	Begins during fetal life	Begins at puberty and continues throughout reproductive life
First maturational division in gamete	First maturational division is completed in preovulatory follicle	First meiotic division results in two cells of equal size
Second maturational division	Second maturational division is completed only when egg is penetrated by sperm	Not comparable
Number of gametes produced during reproductive life	Thousands of oogonia are found in neonate ovary	Millions of sperm are produced in each ejaculate from puberty, with reduced numbers during senility
Sex chromosome in gamete	X	X or Y
Amount of cytoplasm in gamete	As oocyte matures, the amount of its cytoplasm increases	As spermatid develops into sperm, the amount of cytoplasm decreases, acrosome and tail develop in late spermatid
Motility of gamete	Oocytes, surrounded by follicular cells, are immotile	Sperm motility develops gradually in various parts of epididymis and increases at ejaculation
Plasma membrane at fertilization	Egg acquires plasma membranes from sperm	Sperm loses its plasma membranes to egg
Survival in female reproductive tract	12 to 24 hours after ovulation	Ferilizability is maintained 24 hours after ejaculation

reproductive tract. The oviductal cilia and fluids, cervix, uterotubal junction and ampullary–isthmic junction play roles in gamete transport.

SPERM TRANSPORT IN THE FEMALE TRACT

Species differences exist in the sites at which the ejaculate is deposited in the female reproductive tract during copulation (Table 6–2). In cattle and sheep, the small volume of semen is ejaculated into the cranial end of the vagina and onto the cervix (Fig. 6–1). In horses and swine, the voluminous ejaculate is deposited through the relaxed cervical canal into the uterus. The spermatozoa are unique because they are transported through various luminal fluids of completely different physiologic and biochemical characteristics, such as testicular fluid, epididymal fluid, seminal plasma, vaginal fluid, cervical mucus, uterine fluid, oviductal fluid, and peritoneal fluid (Fig. 6–1).

Physicochemical and immunologic factors in the vagina and cervix at the time of insemination play an important role in sperm survival and transport into the uterus and oviduct (Table 6–2 and Figs. 6–2 to 6–4). The vaginal secretions immobilize spermatozoa within 1 to 2 hours of insemination. The rapid elimination and immobilization of spermatozoa in the vagina make the rapid transport of sperm to a more favorable environment essential.

Seminal plasma plays a major role in the transport and physiology of spermatozoa. However, spermatozoa removed from the vas deferens and epididymis are successfully used in artificial insemination, and the removal of various accessory organs of the male tract rarely decreases fertility so long as ejaculation still results in the release of a few million spermatozoa.

Unlike the vagina, the epithelial lining of the cervix, uterus, and oviduct is composed of nonciliated secretory cells and kinociliated cells. In general, secretory cells have a dome-shaped surface covered with numerous microvilli, and their cytoplasm contains numerous secretory granules. The percentage of kinociliated cells in the epithelium, which varies in different parts of the reproductive tract, is maximal in the fimbriae and oviductal ampulla and minimal in the uterus and uterine cervix. The ciliated cells are covered with kinocilia that beat rhythmically toward the vagina (Figs. 6–3 and 6–4).

Sperm Distribution in the Female Reproductive Tract

Three stages are recognized in sperm transport in the female reproductive tract: short, rapid sperm transport; colonization of reservoirs; and slow, prolonged release.

TABLE 6–2.   Species Differences in the Site of Ejaculation and Semen Characteristics in Several Mammals

Site of Ejaculation		Semen Characteristics	Species
Vagina	Incipient plug	Slight coagulation of ejaculate	Man Rabbit
	Incipient plug	Instant coagulation of ejaculate	Monkey
	Little accessory fluid	Semen with high sperm concentration	Cattle Sheep
	Voluminous	Distention of cervix	Horse
Uterus	Voluminous	Retention of penis during copulation	Dog Pig
	Vaginal plug	Spasmodic contraction of vagina	Rodents

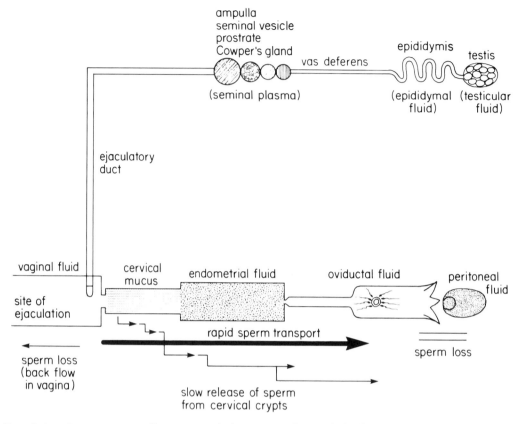

FIG. 6–1.   Diagrammatic illustration of the various luminal fluids in which spermatozoa are suspended from the time of sperm production in the seminiferous tubules to the time of fertilization in the oviduct.

Rapid Transport. Immediately after insemination, spermatozoa penetrate the micelles of the cervical mucus where some are quickly transported through the cervical canal. This phase takes 2 to 10 minutes and may be facilitated by sperm motility (Fig. 6–5) as well as increased contractile activity of the myometrium and mesosalpinx during courtship and coitus. Some spermatozoa reach the internal os of the cervix within 1.5 to 3 minutes after insemination. Thus, some sperm can reach the site of fertilization rapidly. Whether the first spermatozoa entering the oviduct participate in fertilization of the ovum is not known; it has been proposed that fertilization occurs only when a minimal number of spermatozoa reach the site of fertilization.

Colonization of Sperm Reservoirs. Massive numbers of spermatozoa are trapped in the complex mucosal folds of the cervical crypts. This process is facilitated by the fact that the micelles of the cervical mucus direct spermatozoa to the cervical crypts where the reservoir is formed. Fewer leukocytes are found in the cervical secretions compared with those of the vagina or uterus; this suggests that less phagocytosis of spermatozoa takes place in the cervix. Concentration gradients of spermatozoa in different segments of the reproductive tract are important for fertility. The more spermatozoa that enter the cervical reservoir, the more that will reach the oviduct, thus increasing the chance of fertilization. In addition, the larger the reservoir, the longer an ade-

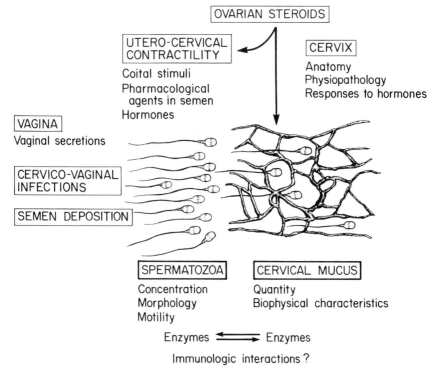

FIG. 6–2. The biophysical, physiologic, biochemical, and immunologic interaction among spermatozoa, cervical mucus, and various segments of the female reproductive tract.

quate population of spermatozoa will be maintained in the oviduct. Spermatozoa may leave the cervix by means of their own motility or be passively transported by cervical and uterine contractions.

In species in which ejaculation occurs in the uterine horns, sperm reservoirs are localized in the uterotubal junction, as in the pig, or in the endometrial glands, as in the dog. No evidence indicates that spermatozoa are released after their entry into the endometrial glands of any species (Fig. 6–6). Sperm transport is affected by prostaglandins (Fig. 6–7) in the semen of some species.

Slow Release and Transport. After adequate sperm reservoirs have been established within the reproductive tract, the spermatozoa are released sequentially for a prolonged period. This slow release, which involves the innate motility of spermatozoa and the contractile activity of the myometrium and mesosalpinx, ensures

the continued availability of spermatozoa for entry to the oviduct to effect fertilization of the egg. However, various anatomic and physiologic barriers prevent massive numbers of spermatozoa in the ejaculate from reaching the site of fertilization (Fig. 6–8), presumably to avoid polyspermy, which is lethal to the fertilized egg.

Sperm Transport in the Cervix

The endocervical mucosa is an intricate system of clefts, grooves, and crypts grouped together. Several functions have been ascribed to the cervix and its secretion: (a) it is receptive to sperm penetration at or near ovulation and inhibits migration at other phases of the cycle; (b) it acts as a sperm reservoir; (c) it protects spermatozoa from the hostile environment of the vagina and from phagocytosis; (d) it provides spermatozoa with energy requirements; (e) it filters defective and

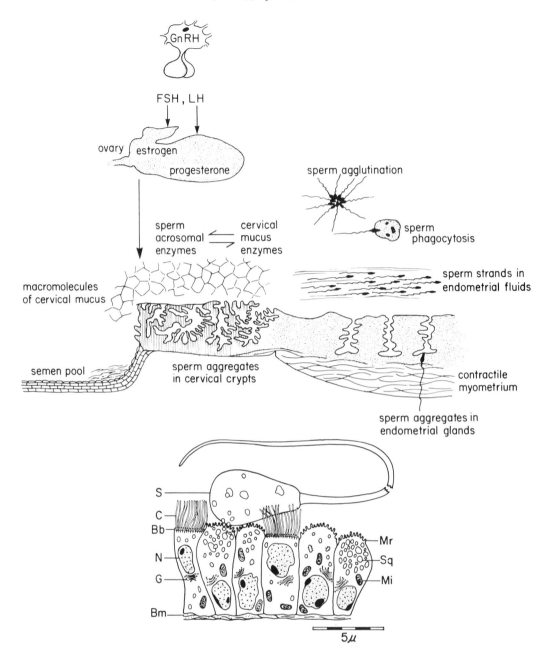

FIG. 6–3. Sperm transport through the cervix to the uterus. *Top,* Sperm transport through the cervix to the uterine lumen involves biochemical mechanisms as well as biophysical and physiologic changes in cervical mucus, which in turn are controlled by endocrine factors. *Bottom,* The size of spermatozoa (S) in relation to the nonciliated secretory cells and ciliated cells of the cervical epithelium. *Bb,* Basal bodies of cilia; *Bm,* basal membrane of epithelium; *C,* cilia; *G,* Golgi apparatus; *Mi,* mitochondria; *Mr,* Microvilli of nonciliated cells; *N,* nucleus; *Sg,* Secretory granules.

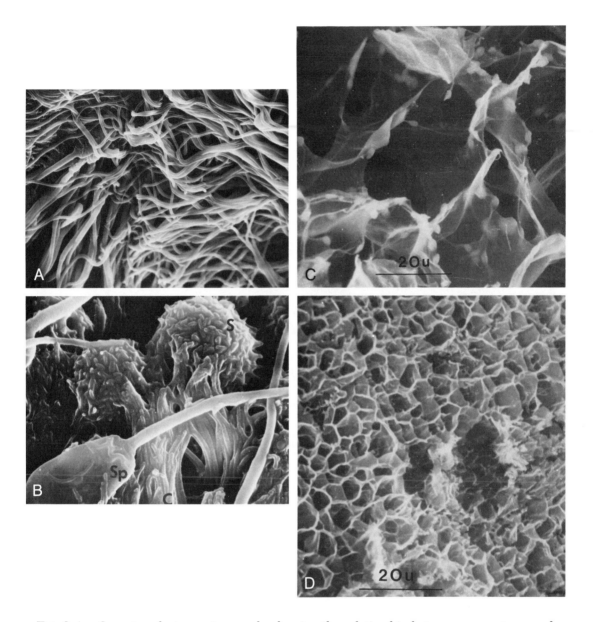

FIG. 6–4. Scanning electron micrographs showing the relationship between spermatozoa and ultrastructure of cervical mucus. *A,* Spermatozoa on the cervical epithelium 1 hour postcoitum. Note the arrangement of sperm tail in a parallel formation. (Hafez, E.S.E. (1973). J. Reprod. Med. Vol. 73, 217.), *B,* Cervical epithelium showing nonciliated secretory cells (S) with microvilli, ciliated cells (C) with kinocilia. Note the relative size of the spermatozoa (Sp) and kinocilia. *C,* Cervical mucus (human) during the ovulatory phase of the cycle. Note the wide spacing of the honeycomb-like meshwork that allows the transport of spermatozoa. Note the relative size of sperm (arrow) and the mesh. *D,* Cervical mucus (human) during the luteal phase of the cycle. Note the narrow meshwork of mucus that inhibits sperm transport to the uterine cavity. (*C, D,* from Daunter, B. and Lutjen, P.L. (1982). Cervical mucus. *In* Atlas of Human Reproduction by Scanning Electron Microscopy. E.S.E. Hafez and P. Kenemans (eds.). Lancaster, England, MTP Press.)

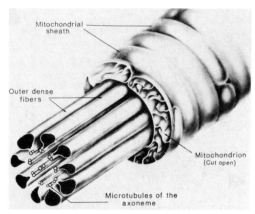

FIG. 6–5. Organization of the principal piece of the sperm tail showing some of the ultrastructural characteristics involved in sperm motility. (From Pedersen, H. and Fawcett, D.W. (1976) Functional anatomy of the human spermatozoon. *In* Human Semen and Fertility Regulation in Men. E.S.E. Hafez (ed.). St. Louis, C.V. Mosby.)

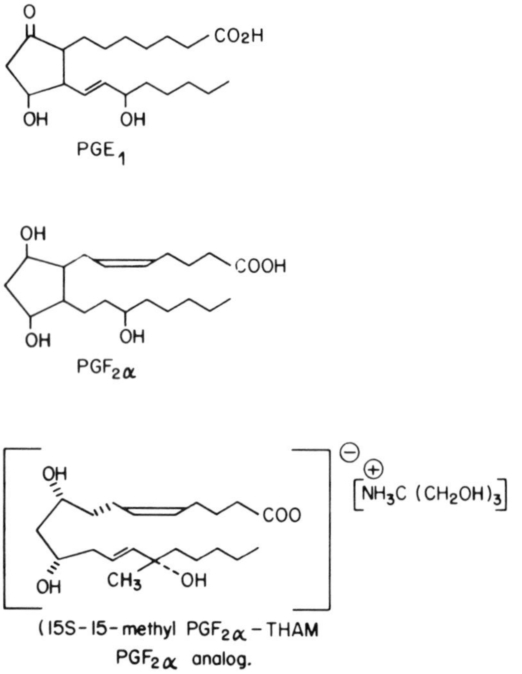

PGE_1

$PGF_{2\alpha}$

(15S–15-methyl $PGF_{2\alpha}$–THAM $PGF_{2\alpha}$ analog.

FIG. 6–7. Chemical formula of various types of prostaglandins found in the semen. On ejaculation in the vagina, some of these prostaglandins cause an increase in the tone and patterns of contractility of the musculature of the uterus and/or the oviduct. These responses affect the quantitative and qualitative components of sperm transport.

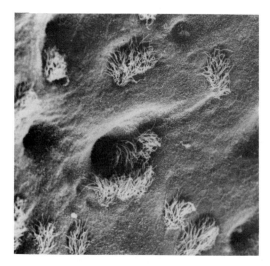

FIG. 6–6. (*Top*) Scanning electron micrograph of the endometrium showing the openings of the uterine gland and the presence of ciliated cells near these openings. (Courtesy of Professor P. Motta.) (*Bottom*) Diagram showing the action of the cilia in the gel and sol portion of the cervical mucus. The kinocilia beat with a wavelike motion within the sol layer of mucosa. Tips of cilia strike the inner surface of gel.

immotile spermatozoa, and (f) it possibly participates in the capacitation of spermatozoa.

Cervical Mucus. Cervical mucus that accumulates in the vaginal pool may contain endometrial, oviductal, follicular, and peritoneal fluids as well as leukocytes and cellular debris from uterine, cervical, and vaginal epithelia. The cervical mucus is a hydrogel, which consists of water and a solid component composed of three or more units forming a three-dimensional network. The secretions are heterogeneous in composition, due to the presence of two types of low- and high-viscosity components. Cervical mucus has rheologic properties such as viscosity, flow elasticity, spinnbarkeit, thixotropy, and tack (stickiness). Low-molecular-weight organic components include free simple sug-

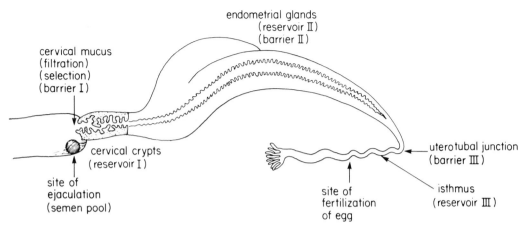

FIG. 6–8.   Various anatomic and physiologic barriers prevent massive numbers of spermatozoa in the ejaculate from reaching the site of fertilization, presumably to avoid polyspermy.

ars (glucose, maltose, and mannose) and amino acids. The mucus also contains proteins, trace elements, and enzymes.

A physiologic balance of ovarian steroids is necessary for the initiation and maintenance of a cervical population of spermatozoa following artificial insemination, particularly after estrus synchronization.

Sperm Penetration in Cervical Mucus. Ejaculated spermatozoa rapidly penetrate watery cervical mucus during midcycle, aided principally by sperm motility as well as the micro- and macrorheologic properties of mucus. The rate of sperm penetration in the mucus varies throughout the estrous cycle.

Spermatozoa are mechanically oriented toward the cervical internal os. As the flagellum beats and vibrates, the sperm head is propelled forward in the channels of least resistance. The tail frequency sets up a mechanical resonance between itself and the oscillation frequency of the molecular lattice. Hydrodynamic principles seem to apply to sperm motility; thus, motile spermatozoa are in dynamic equilibrium with the viscous force of the medium rather than being affected by the inertial force that influences large moving objects.

Dead pig spermatozoa inseminated in pigs were transported to the oviduct less efficiently than live spermatozoa; it appears that sperm mobility facilitates penetrability but is not absolutely necessary.

Although spermatozoa appear to move at random in the cervical secretion, they probably follow the path of least resistance along strands of cervical mucus. When migration of a spermatozoon in mucus is impeded, the sperm usually resumes its forward course with a sudden deflection into an adjacent parallel path. When semen is mixed with cervical mucus *in vitro,* a sharp boundary occurs between the two fluids and the cervical mucus is penetrated by fingerlike phalanges. Phalanx formation may function to increase the surface area between semen and cervical mucus, provide pockets of semen within the mucus to protect spermatozoa from the hostile vaginal environment, or facilitate sperm migration into the uterine cavity.

Sperm Transport in the Uterus

The contractile activity of the vagina and myometrium plays a major role in the transport of spermatozoa into and through the uterus. Massive numbers of spermatozoa invade the endometrial glands. It is believed that the presence of spermatozoa in the uterus induces endometrial leukocytic response, which enhances phagocytosis of excessive numbers of living and probably dead spermatozoa.

Spermophagy.   The uptake of spermatozoa by phagocytes is of special physiologic significance because infiltration of leukocytes into the uterine lumen, and their activation to ingest sperm following mating seems to be a major mechanism for the removal of these cells from the female reproductive tract (Koehler et al., 1982). Spermatozoa in the uterus are taken into phagocytic vacuoles and digested by the macrophages (Fig. 6–9). Phagocytotic sperm may not have been initially damaged or necrotic.

Transport in the Oviduct

The oviduct has the unique function of conveying spermatozoa and eggs in opposite directions almost simultaneously. The pattern and rate of sperm transport through the oviduct are controlled by several mechanisms, such as peristalsis and antiperistalsis of oviductal musculature, complex contractions of the oviductal mucosal folds and the mesosalpinx, fluid currents and countercurrents created by ciliary action, and possibly the opening and closing of the intramural portion. The relative importance of these mechanisms in sperm transport through the oviduct is unknown. Oviductal contractions alter the configuration of the oviductal compartments momentarily, so that fluids and suspending spermatozoa may be transported toward the fimbriae from one compartment to the next. In the oviducts of the pigeon and the tortoise, there are two systems of kinocilia: One beats toward the ovary and the other toward the cloaca. These two ciliary systems are capable of moving particles in opposite directions.

The rate and pattern of sperm transport through the oviduct are attributed to peristalsis and antiperistalsis of musculature and contractions of the mucosal folds and mesosalpinx. The frequency and amplitude of contractions of oviductal circular and longitudinal musculature, mesosalpinx and mesotubarium are controlled by ovarian hormones, adrenergic and nonadrenergic activity, and such components of seminal plasma as prostaglandin.

The pattern and amplitude of contractions vary in different segments of the oviduct. In the isthmus, peristaltic and anti-

peristaltic contractions are segmental, vigorous, and almost continuous. In the ampulla, strong peristaltic waves move in a segmental fashion toward the midportion of the oviduct.

Endocrine Control of Sperm Transport

More is known about the endocrine control of ovulation and spermatogenesis than about the endocrinology of sperm transport in the female tract. Ovarian hormones affect (a) the structure, ultrastructure, and secretory activity of the cervical, uterine, and oviductal epithelia; (b) the contractile activity of the uterotubal musculature; and (c) the quantitative and qualitative characteristics of cervical mucus and uterine and oviductal secretions. Changes are noted in the protein content, enzyme activity, electrolyte composition, surface tension, and conductivity of these fluids. Increasing the amount of endogenous estrogen during the preovulatory phase of the cycle or administering synthetic estrogens produces copious amounts of thin, watery, cervical secretions. Endogenous progesterone during the luteal phase of the cycle or in pregnancy produces scanty, viscous, cellular cervical mucus with low spinnbarkeit and ferning properties. The penetrability of spermatozoa is inhibited greatly in progestational cervical mucus. It is possible that the cyclic changes that occur in cervical mucus are mechanisms to protect the female from unnecessary exposure to the foreign proteins of semen.

Hyperactivation of Sperm

Cumulus cells, by using substances in the culture medium, can provide the ovum with intermediary metabolites for maturation and/or zygote cleavage. Cumulus cells also act as a sperm "reservoir," maintaining many spermatozoa within a close cellular matrix immediately apposing the zona pellucida.

The velocity of spermatozoa and the pattern of sperm motility are altered as the sperm are transported through differ-

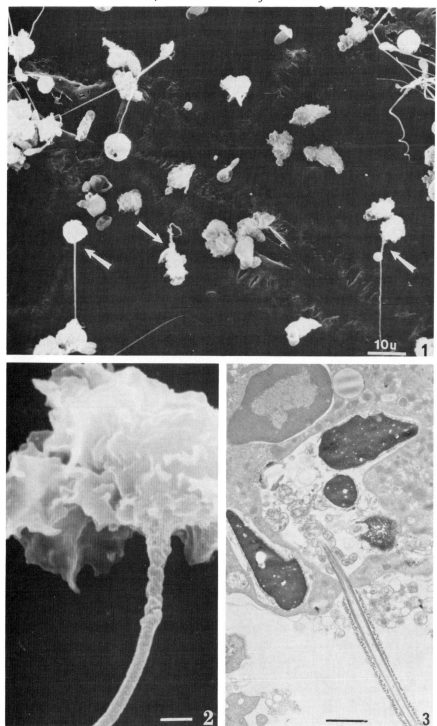

FIG. 6–9. *1,* Scanning electron micrograph of an ejaculate from a patient with idiopathic infertility showing massive infiltration of leukocytes. Few "free" spermatozoa are present; most are associated with the ruffled white cells. The smooth contoured cells may be immature forms of early spermatid ($13,000\times$). *2,* Scanning electron micrograph of ruffled leukocyte with a sperm during spermophagy. *3,* Transmission electron micrograph portions of four sperm nuclei in phagocytic vacuoles in addition to the flagellum extending from the cell. This cell is most likely a neutrophil. (From Koehler, J.K. et al. (1982) Spermophagy. *In* Atlas of Human Reproduction by Scanning Electron Microscopy. E.S.E. Hafez and P. Kenemans (eds.). Lancaster, England, MTP Press.)

ent segments of the female reproductive tract. Sperm hyperactivation occurs primarily in the oviduct near the time of ovulation and may be instrumental in the final sperm transport, the completion of sperm capacitation, and the acrosome reaction. Sperm are normally retained in the isthmus portion of the oviduct. Biophysical and biochemical properties of the isthmus may impede the upward migration of spermatozoa and facilitate sperm storage. Physical characteristics of the isthmus include narrow isthmic lumen, a viscous isthmic mucus, reduced local temperatures, prouterine ciliary beat, and oviductal muscular contractions, which are directed primarily towards the uterus. Physiologic interaction between the spermatozoa and the isthmic environment involves the modulation of sperm motility.

Active swimming of spermatozoa is readily induced by dilution of the isthmic contents with ampullary fluid or an artificial media. When pyruvate is present in the medium, hyperactivated flagellar bending is stimulated, whereas these movements are virtually absent when glucose alone is present. Alterations in the concentrations of both K^+ and pyruvate may have a role in regulating the motility of spermatozoa in the oviductal isthmus, K^+ being inhibitory and pyruvate stimulatory (Burkman et al., 1984). When in vitro fertilization media are used, immediate vigorous sperm motility is noted and many of the isthmic sperm display hyperactivation. The depression of isthmic sperm motility may be accomplished by the presence of one or more motility inhibitors in the isthmic environment. A similar suppression of sperm movement occurs in the epididymal lumen (Burkman et al., 1984).

The pH of the female reproductive tract fluids varies considerably. The vagina is acidic, around pH 4.0; cervical mucus is basic, pH 8.4, and the uterus is intermediate, pH 7.8. The pH of oviductal fluid is around 7.1 to 7.3 in the follicular phase and 7.5 to 7.8 in the luteal phase. Thus it is important that sperm maintain good motility over a relatively wide range of extracellular pH values.

Sperm Transport and Fertility

The continuous flow of spermatozoa from the cervix is associated with phagocytosis of spermatozoa within the uterus and sperm loss into the peritoneal cavity. Thus, a population of fertile spermatozoa is maintained at the site of fertilization near the ampullary–isthmic junction of the oviduct. The percentage of morphologically normal spermatozoa is higher in the oviducts and uterus than in the ejaculate. Some morphologically abnormal spermatozoa may reach the oviduct, although to a lesser extent than normal spermatozoa. The filtering of dead, abnormal, and incompetent sperm during their passage through the reproductive tract ensures the greatest viability of the zygote.

Head-to-head and tail-to-tail sperm agglutination may occur, causing inhibition in sperm transport (Fig. 6–10). The immunologic significance of sperm agglutination in relation to infertility is not known.

Effect of Estrous Synchronization on Sperm Transport. The survival and transport of spermatozoa in the female reproductive tract generally decrease after any alteration of the estrous cycle. The

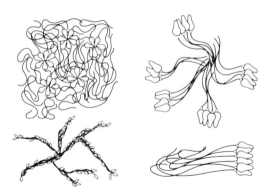

FIG. 6–10. Different patterns of head-to-head and tail-to-tail sperm agglutination, a phenomenon that interferes with sperm transport. Little is known about the immunologic significance of sperm agglutination in relation to infertility.

number of sperm in the oviduct is reduced after regulation of estrus by the administration of progestogen and prostaglandin F_2 (Fig. 6–7), which cause regression of the corpora lutea. Regulation of estrus with progestogen or prostaglandin allows only limited numbers of sperm to reach the oviducts, thus causing lowered ovum fertilization rates and low fertility.

Uterine contractions, observed *in vivo* or measured *in vitro,* differ between control ewes and ewes in regulated estrus. Three compounds, when added to semen used for insemination or injected into females near the time of insemination, increase the number of sperm in the oviducts. These compounds include a combination of prostaglandin E_1 and F_2 for sheep and estradiol-17β for rabbits and sheep (Hawk et al., 1982).

A positive relationship exists between the number of sperm in the oviduct around the time of ovulation and the number of accessory sperm per ovum and the resulting percentage of ova fertilized. The increased fertilization rate is associated with increased numbers of accessory sperm per ovum. Moreover, the number of sperm in the oviduct around the time of ovulation is reduced in hormone-treated ewes when compared with untreated ewes.

Survival of Spermatozoa

Once ejaculation has occurred, spermatozoa have a finite life span. Certain components of the seminal plasma stimulate sperm motility, whereas others inhibit motility. Much information is known about the duration of spermatozoal motility, but little is known about the duration of fertilizing capacity, which is lost long before motility. A relationship exists between the pH of the intravaginal seminal pool and the motility of the spermatozoa.

When migrating in the genital tract, sperm are separated rapidly from the seminal plasma and resuspended in the female genital fluid. In the oviduct, spermatozoa are greatly diluted. Since only a few sper-

matozoa appear in the oviduct, their survival time is difficult to estimate, and if they remain motile, they migrate into the peritoneal cavity.

During transport to the site of fertilization, spermatozoa are significantly diluted with luminal secretions from the female reproductive tract and are susceptible to changes in the pH of luminal fluids. Acidity or excessive alkalinity of the mucus immobilizes spermatozoa, whereas moderately alkaline mucus enhances their motility.

The cervical mucus secreted at the time of ovulation provides an environment suited to the maintenance of metabolic activity of spermatozoa. This mucus undergoes biochemical changes, such as a decrease in albumin, alkaline phosphatase, peptidase, antitrypsin, esterase and sialic acid, as well as an increase in mucins and sodium chloride.

Transport of spermatozoa into the uterus may influence capacitation because the sperm are separated from an excess of "decapacitation factor" and from other enzyme inhibitors in the seminal plasma.

Loss of Spermatozoa

Although millions of spermatozoa are deposited into the reproductive tract of the female, few ever reach the egg at the site of fertilization. Most spermatozoa perish at the selective barriers: uterine cervix, uterotubal junction, and oviductal isthmus. Little is known about the fate of those that invade the endometrial glands in large numbers. In the uterine cavity, spermatozoa undergo phagocytosis by leukocytes (Fig. 6–9). A continual loss of sperm also occurs in the vaginal and peritoneal cavities.

The introduction of semen into the uterine cavity initiates the leukocytic response: the appearance of polymorphonuclear leukocytes. The biologic relationship between leukocytes and spermatozoa with respect to capacitation and/or sperm survival is not known. In the bovine cervix, the majority of leukocytes occur in the central mass of the mucin, a fact indicating that most of them have invaded the cervix from the uterus. Most viable spermatozoa, lodging in the cervical crypts, escape the leukocytes, so an adequate population of sperm would survive.

Damaged spermatozoa are carried passively back through the ectocervix with the help of ciliated cells beating toward the vagina. Such spermatozoa, advancing only a short distance into the cervical mucus core, do not reach the cervical crypts and greatly decrease in number within a few hours after coitus. Since spermatozoa that become immotile elsewhere are not rapidly eliminated, the ratio of immotile spermatozoa that are being eliminated is higher in the cervix than in other segments of the female reproductive tract. Large amounts of cervical mucus are produced, and numerous spermatozoa are expelled with the mucus through the vulva in cattle. Spermatozoa that reach the fimbriae may be released into the peritoneal cavity.

RECEPTION OF EGGS (OVA PICKUP)

The viscid mass of cumulus oophorus that contains oocyte and corona cells adheres to the stigma and remains attached to it unless it is removed by the action of the kinocilia of the fimbriae. Ovum transport through the ostium itself and the first few millimeters of the ampulla is effected by the action of the cilia.

The physiologic mechanism by which freshly ovulated eggs are picked up into the oviducts depends on four main factors:

1. The structural characteristics of the fimbriae of the infundibulum and its relationship to the surface of the ovary at the time of ovulation
2. The pattern of release of the cumulus oophorus and its contained egg from the follicle at the time of ovulation
3. The biophysical properties of the follicular fluids and the fluids that comprise the matrix of the cumulus oophorus

4. The coordinated contraction of the fimbriae and the utero-ovarian ligaments

At the time of ovulation, the fimbriae are engorged with blood and are brought into close contact with the surface of the ovary by the muscular activity of the mesotubarium. The ovary is moved slowly to and from and around its longitudinal axis by contractions of the ligamentum ovarii proprium. This chain of reactions is controlled by anatomic and hormonal mechanisms.

The ovary is located inside the ovarian bursa to which the ampulla of the oviduct and part of the fimbriae are attached. The ovary can move readily from this location to the surface of the fimbriae, which is positioned at the open portion of the ovarian bursa. This movement is controlled by both the *ligamentum ovarii proprium* and the mesovarium, which hold the ovary and oviduct in position.

The fimbriae and the infundibulum are basically composed of an erectile structure that is rich in vascular and muscular tissues. During estrus, the fimbriae distend from the increased blood flow; furthermore, the margins of the fimbriae become edematous and translucent.

The contractile activities of the fimbriae, oviduct and ligaments are partly coordinated by hormonal mechanisms involving the estrogen/progesterone ratio. Egg reception is most efficient about the time of estrus, but it occurs to some degree throughout the cycle. In some species neurohormonal mechanisms also stimulate the contractile activity of the fimbriae at the time of copulation.

EGG TRANSPORT IN THE OVIDUCT

The transport time of ova in the oviduct varies with the species (Tables 6–3 and 6–4). In cattle, sheep and swine, the transport time ranges from 72 to 90 hours (Figs. 6–11 and 6–12). Unfertilized ova are retained in the oviduct of the mare for several months. It is critical that fertilized

TABLE 6–3. Sequence of Major Physiologic Phenomena Associated with Sperm Transport in the Male and Female Reproductive Tract

Site	Physiologic Phenomena	Mechanisms Involved
Male reproductive tract	Sperm stored in cauda epididymidis undergo maturation.	Neuromuscular
	At ejaculation, sperm released from epididymis are mixed with male accessory secretions.	Metabolic
Vagina	Semen deposited in several ejaculatory pulsations.	Copulatory motor activities
	Semen mixed with vaginal and cervical secretions.	
Cervix	Sperm migrate through micelles of cervical mucus.	Biophysical
	Abnormal sperm filtered (gross selection of sperm) through cervical canal.	Biochemical
	Cervical crypts establish "sperm reservoir" or rid excessive sperm causing massive reduction in sperm number.	Mechanical (kinocilia of epithelium)
Uterus	Sperm separated from seminal plasma and transported to oviduct.	Myometrial contraction
	Surface plasma of sperm removed.	Agglutination of sperm
	Metabolic changes and capacitation of sperm.	Phagocytosis of sperm by leukocytes
	Acrosomal proteinase (trypsin-enzyme) inactivated by trypsin inhibitors from seminal plasma.	Enzymatic
Uterotubal junction	Quantitative selection of sperm.	Mechanical
Isthmus	Sperm numbers reduced.	
Ampullary–isthmic junction	Control of egg transport in oviduct.	Neural
	Sperm plasma membrane changes (acrosome reaction), sperm capacitation.	Biochemical
Ampulla	Sperm motility increases in oviductal fluid to be able to penetrate corona radiata and zona pellucida.	Mechanical
	Reduction division of gametes completed.	Metabolic
	Acrosomal proteinases released.	Enzymatic
	Selection at egg surface (receptors?) by sperm.	Biophysical
Fimbriae	Excessive sperm lost into peritoneal cavity.	Sperm motility

TABLE 6–4. Transport Time of Ova in the Oviduct of Farm Animals Compared with Some Other Mammals

Species	Time in Oviduct (hours)
Cattle	90
Sheep	72
Horse	98
Pig	50
Cat	148
Dog	168
Monkey, rhesus	96
Opossum	24
Woman	48–72

eggs reach the uterus at an appropriate progestational stage of the estrous cycle.

The rate of egg transport is faster from the infundibulum to the ampullary–isthmic junction than through the isthmic portion. This delay in ovum transport appears to be required for subsequent implantation of the embryo. The time of entry of the ovum into the uterus is relatively precise compared with the movement of the ovum past the ampullary–isthmic junction into the isthmus.

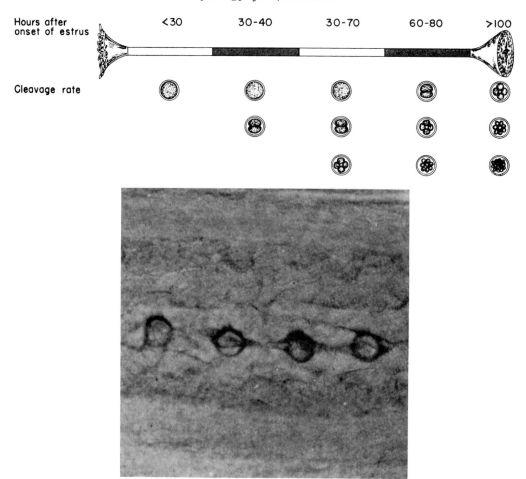

FIG. 6–11.   (*Top*) Rate of transport and cleavage of eggs in swine. Eggs pass through the first half of the oviduct rapidly, and they remain in the third quarter, which contains the ampullary–isthmic junction, until 60–75 hours after onset of estrus. The eggs enter the uterus between 66 and 90 hours after onset of estrus. (Data from Oxenreider and Day, J. (1965) Anim. Sci., *24,* 413.) (*Bottom*) The isthmus of the oviduct is shown after using the clearing technique showing the transport of the ova.

The transport of the egg through the oviduct is regulated by four primary forces:

1. The frequency, force, and programming of contraction of oviductal musculature and related ligaments, as influenced by endocrine, pharmacologic, and neural mechanisms
2. The direction and rate of currents and countercurrents of luminal fluids as affected by the rate and direction of the beat of kinocilia lining the mucosal folds
3. The secretory activity of nonciliated cells in the oviductal epithelium as influenced by the estrogen progesterone ratio
4. The hydrodynamics and rheologic properties of luminal fluids at the critical times that ova are being transported (Figs. 6–13, 6–14).

Oviductal Contraction

The various patterns of oviductal contraction regulate to some extent the rate of egg transport (Table 6–5). However,

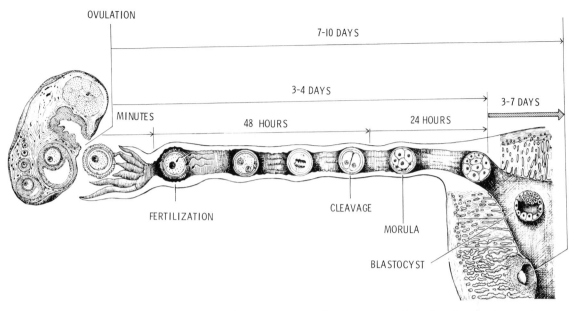

OVULATION

7-10 DAYS

3-4 DAYS

3-7 DAYS

MINUTES

48 HOURS

24 HOURS

FERTILIZATION

CLEAVAGE

MORULA

BLASTOCYST

FIG. 6–12. Temporal relationships of the major reproductive events that take place in the oviduct such as ova pick-up by the fimbriae and fertilization, cleavage, and formation of the blastocyst in the uterus.

there is little evidence that ova are transported primarily by muscle contractions. The mesovarium, mesosalpinx, mesotubarium, and utero-ovarian ligaments also undergo rigorous contractile activity. These contractions continuously change the position of the ovaries relative to the fimbriae as well as the relation of the various subdivisions of the oviduct to one another. The patterns of contraction vary significantly at various times in the estrous cycle.

After follicular rupture, the ovum is picked up by the oviductal fimbriated end, which is brought in contact with the ovary by means of myometrium contraction, the smooth muscle of the mesosalpinx, as well as the tubo-ovarian ligaments. After a fast passage of the ovum through the distal ampulla, which takes place in a pattern of to-and-fro movements, the ovum is retained in the proximal part of the ampullary region, near the ampullary–isthmic junction, allowing fertilization to take place. About 80 hours after ovulation, the blastocyst reaches the uterine cavity. The transient arrest of the ovum at the ampullary–isth-

mic junction, which seems to be crucial for successful conception to take place, may be an effect of a sphincter-like function.

Neural Mechanisms and Pharmacologic Response

The abundant adrenergic innervation of the oviductal musculature in conjunction with its response to adrenergic drugs has suggested that the sympathetic nervous system is involved in egg transport. Myosalpingeal contraction mediated by adrenergic innervation to the circular muscle of the oviductal isthmus may be involved in delaying ovum transport at the isthmus. In the rabbit, such outbursts occur 36 hours postcoitum, when the majority of ova are in the oviduct. A drop in oviductal motility occurs at 72 hours postcoitum, when most ova are in the uterus (Aref and Hafez, 1973). The α-adrenoceptors (stimulatory) mediate oviductal contraction, whereas the β-adrenoceptors (inhibitory) mediate oviductal relaxation. Nerve stimulation and various autonomic drugs cause variable responses of the oviduct (see Table 6–

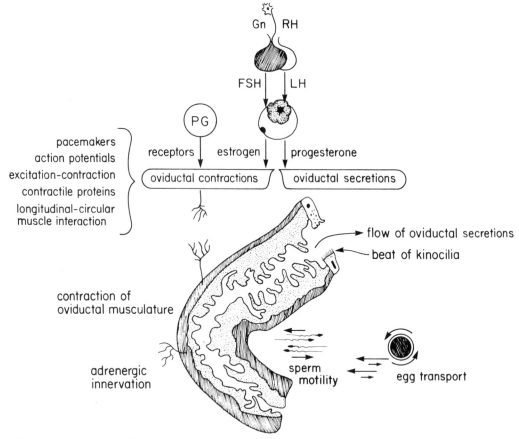

Fig. 6–13. Anatomic and physiologic mechanisms that regulate egg and sperm transport in the oviduct.

5). These responses are highly related to life time of gametes (Table 6–6).

When the muscular activity of the oviduct is pharmacologically blocked with isoproterenol, ampullary egg transport changes its typical discrete "to-and-fro" character and becomes continuous and unidirectional. This implies that the driving forces provided by the ciliary action are indeed asymmetric. Prostaglandins have a remarkable effect on the smooth musculature of the oviducts and the uterus. The formation and release of prostaglandins is brought about by nerve activity.

"Locking" and "Unlocking" of Ova in Oviduct

Various mechanisms cause the slow transport of the ova through the isthmus:

tubal peristalsis, ciliary activity, and fluid currents and countercurrents within the lumen. The physiologic and pharmacologic mechanisms that regulate oviductal locking/unlocking of ova follow:

1. Mechanical blocking (e.g., edema).
2. Myogenic blocking from
   a. sustained contraction of circular musculature of the isthmus;
   b. contractions regulated by myogenic pacemakers, which are somehow coupled in time and space so that they do not force ova transport prematurely to the uterus;
   c. local or general relaxation of muscle.
3. Neurogenic blocking controls one of the myogenic mechanisms.

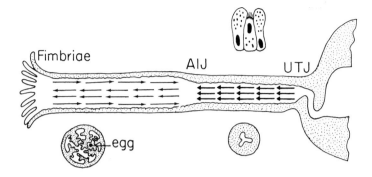

Day I (estrogen)	Cilia beat moves egg to AIJ against flow of secretion	Counter-current of secretion more effective than cilia
	Weak flow of secretion	Less ciliated cells
Day 3 (progesterone)	More cilia beat (+20%)	Less secretion in isthmus

FIG. 6–14.   Diagram to show the rate of estrogen and progesterone on the flow of oviductal secretions in the ampulla and isthmus (shown by arrows toward the fimbriae), the flow of oviductal cilia (shown by arrows toward the uterotubal junction [UTJ]), and egg transport in the oviduct. *AIJ*, ampullary–isthmic junction.

TABLE 6–5.   **Patterns of Egg Transport in the Oviduct as Affected by Type of Oviductal Contractility**

Type of Oviductal Contractility	Pattern of Egg Transport
Peristaltic contractions from ampulla to ampullary–isthmic junction	Fast progress of egg
Peristaltic contraction from uterotubal junction to ampullary–isthmic junction	Obstruction of egg transport
Segmental contraction	Foward and backward shuttling of egg
Outbursts of spastic contraction of circular musculature	Complete obstruction of egg transport at a sphincter
Contraction of related ligaments causing bending of the oviduct	Regulation of rate of egg transport

Gamete Transport and Conception Rate

The rapid transport of live or dead spermatozoa to the upper oviduct within a matter of minutes infers the importance of smooth muscle contractions in this situation. In natural breeding, spermatozoa are deposited during estrus at least 10 to 12 hours before ovulation, and the rate of sperm transport is unlikely to become a critical factor determining conception. In the case of artificial insemination, particularly when this forms part of an estrous synchronization and/or gonadotropin treatment program, the rate and efficiency of sperm transport to the site of fertilization are of fundamental importance.

In cattle, the semen is ejaculated in the anterior vagina near the external cervical os. Penetration of spermatozoa into the cervical canal may depend on muscular activity in the female reproductive tract, which is enhanced by oxytocin released at coitus, but entry into the canal also depends on sperm motility. The condition of the cervical mucus is critical for successful colonization of the cervix, the latter region providing the principal postcoital reser-

TABLE 6–6. Estimates of the Fertile Life of Sperm and Ova, and the Tempo of Embryonic Development

Species	Sperm	Ovum	2-Cell	8-Cell	Into Uterus	Blastocyst	Birth
Cattle	30–48	20–24	1	3	3–3½	7–8	278–290
Horse	72–120	6–8	1	3	4–5	6	335–345
Human	28–48	6–24	1½	2½	2–3	4	252–274
Rabbit	30–36	6–8	1	2½	3	4	30–32
Sheep	30–48	16–24	1	2½	3	6–7	145–155
Swine	24–72	8–10	16–20 hours	2½	2	5–6	112–115

Table header spans: Fertile Life* (hours): Sperm, Ovum. Days after Ovulation†: 2-Cell, 8-Cell, Into Uterus, Blastocyst, Birth.

* *Fertile life* is a relative concept since fertility declines progressively over a period of hours. For sperm, only the period in the female genital tract is included. The life of ova is timed from ovulation. For both, longevity probably depends on a variety of factors, including the hormonal state of the female. It is therefore impossible to give precise figures.

† *These estimates are only approximate since developmental rate is subject to considerable variation both among individuals and among breeds.* In addition, accurate information on the time of ovulation is lacking in several species.

voir of spermatozoa in ruminants, at least during the first 24 hours. Spermatozoa are stored for 2 to 3 days in the endometrial glands and in the folds of the lower isthmus and region of the uterotubal junction. Thus, spermatozoa may be protected from phagocytosis.

Significant numbers of spermatozoa enter the oviducts of estrous cows within 2 hours of mating, although they are found in the ampulla by 8 hours.

Only a small fraction of the ejaculate reaches the upper tube. This phenomenon is important to avoid the pathologic condition of polyspermic fertilization.

Thus, the probability of postovulatory aging of the egg before sperm penetration is extremely low under conditions of natural mating. However, if artificial insemination is employed or under systems of controlled breeding, the eggs may deteriorate before spermatozoa reach the ampulla, even though the fertilizable life of the egg is 20 to 24 hours.

An accelerated descent of eggs through the oviduct occurs after superovulation treatment in cattle, although experiments with pregnant mare serum gonadotropin (PMSG) have not produced this particular response. The disturbance of egg transport is in laboratory animals under steroid hormone treatment well-known, so exces-

sive progesterone production or progestogenic treatments shortly after ovulation may produce a similar result in farm animals, leading to temporary infertility.

FERTILIZABLE LIFE AND AGING OF EGGS

The fertilizable life of the egg is the maximal period during which it remains capable of fertilization and normal development. In most species, the egg is capable of being fertilized for some 12 to 24 hours (Table 6–6). It rapidly loses its fertilizability upon reaching the isthmus and is completely nonfertilizable after reaching the uterus.

The egg may be fertilized near the end of its fertilizable life as a result of delayed breeding. Such eggs may or may not implant and, if so, they produce mostly nonviable embryos. Guinea pigs show a high percentage of abnormal pregnancies and decrease in litter size as the age of the egg increases prior to fertilization (Fig. 6–15). Fertilization of aged eggs in swine is associated with polyspermy and hence abnormal embryonic development. In single-bearing animals, aging of the egg may cause abortion, embryonic resorption, or abnormal development of the embryo. Similar abnormalities may result from aged sperm.

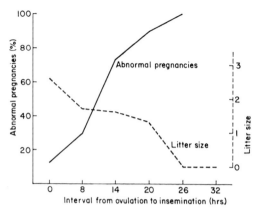

FIG. 6–15. The effect of aging on ova (delayed insemination) on percentage of abnormal pregnancies and litter size in guinea pigs. Note that the ova were fertilized and implanted when the animals were inseminated at 26 hours after ovulation, yet the embryos did not continue development. (Data from Blandau and Young, (1939) Am. J. Anat. *64*, 303.)

In general, fertilization of aged gametes involves one of the following possibilities:

Aged egg and aged sperm
Aged egg and freshly ejaculated sperm
Freshly ovulated egg and aged sperm

Nonviable embryos resulting from any of the foregoing combinations may cause low conception rates in certain herds and flocks. Fertilization with aged sperm increases subsequent embryonic mortality in swine and poultry. At present there is insufficient evidence in farm mammals concerning the relative deleterious effects of gamete aging on fertilization, implantation, and prenatal development. It is possible that some of the congenital abnormalities in postnatal life are a consequence of aged gametes.

If the egg is not fertilized, it fragments into several cytoplasmic segments of unequal size, and in some cases it may even resemble a fertilized egg. All unfertilized eggs eventually disappear through complete disintegration or phagocytosis in the uterus.

TRANSUTERINE MIGRATION AND LOSS OF EGGS

Transuterine migration of the egg through the common body of the uterus is common in ungulates. For example, when one of the ovaries is removed from a sow, approximately half of the embryos develop in each uterine horn, irrespective of which ovary was removed. There is also a tendency in the normal sow for the number of embryos to be equalized between the two horns. Transuterine migration is more common in swine and horses than in cattle and sheep. Nonetheless, cattle and sheep that have double ovulations from one ovary usually have one embryo in each uterine horn. The physiologic mechanisms that govern the movement of eggs, both within individual horns and between horns, is unknown.

Transperitoneal migration of eggs can be accomplished by experimental conditions, for example, removal of one ovary leaving the fimbriae and oviduct intact and ligation of the other oviduct. In this case, the remaining oviduct has the ability to pick up the ovum released by the contralateral ovary and a normal pregnancy may follow. Transperitoneal migration may be avoided by currents and surface tension of the peritoneal fluid.

The egg may never reach the infundibulum as a result of many causes. For example, eggs entrapped in the ruptured follicles can be found in the developing corpora lutea. The egg may also be lost into the peritoneal cavity; such an egg usually degenerates but in rare cases may result in ectopic pregnancy (pregnancy located outside the uterus). Egg loss in the peritoneal cavity may be caused by the immobilization of the oviduct as a result of faulty rectal palpation of the ovaries, postpartum or postabortum infections, endometritis, or nonspecific abdominal infections.

EMBRYONIC DEVELOPMENT IN OVIDUCT

The oviduct takes an active part in maintaining and preparing the eggs for fertilization and subsequent cleavage. The oviductal fluid is rich is substrates and co-factors involved in ovum development, such as pyruvate and bicarbonate, free amino acids, oxygen, CO_2, and carbohydrates, perhaps lipids, nucleosides, steroids, and other compounds. Apparently, these substances are contributed by the cells of the oviductal mucosa to the luminal fluid milieu.

Endocrine factors are important in the early development of embryos in the oviduct. The biochemical composition of the uterine fluid is different from that of the oviduct fluid. Eggs at early cleavage stages require specific substances provided by the oviduct for their development. Thus, premature entry of morulae into the uterus will cause their degeneration. After a certain time, the blastocysts need to enter the uterus for final development and implantation.

REFERENCES

Aref, I. and Hafez, E.S.E. (1973). Oviductal contractility in relation to egg transport in the rabbit. Obstet. Gynecol. *42*, 165.

Blandau, R.J. and Verdugo, P. (1976): An overview of gamete transport-comparative aspects. *In* Ovum Transport and Fertility Regulation. M.J.K. Harper, C.J. Pauerstein, C.E. Adams, E.M. Coutinho, H.B. Croxatto and D.M. Paton (eds.). Copenhagen, Scriptor.

Burkman, L.J., Overstreet, J.W. and Katz D.F. (1984). A possible role for potassium and pyruvate in the modulation of sperm motility in the rabbit oviductal isthmus. J. Reprod. Fertil. *71*, 367–376.

Daunter, B. and Lutjen, P. (1982). Cervical mucus. *In* Atlas of Human Reproduction by Scanning Electron Microscopy. E.S.E. Hafez and P. Kenemans (eds.). Lancaster, England, MTP Press.

Hawk, H.W. and Cooper B.S. (1977). Sperm transport the cervix of the ewe after regulation of estrous prostaglandin or progestogen. J. Anim. Sci. *44*, 63.

Hawk, H.W., Cooper, B.S. and Conley, H.H. (1982). Increased numbers of sperm in the oviducts and improved fertilization rates in rabbits after administration of phenylephrine or ergonovine near the time of insemination. J. Anim. Sci. *55*, 878–890.

Koehler, J.K., Berger, R.E., Smith, D. and Karp L. (1982). Spermophagy. *In* Atlas of Human Reproduction Scanning Electron Microscopy. E.S.E. Hafez and Kenemans (eds.), Lancaster, England, MTP Press.

McLaren, A. 1980. Fertilization and Implantation. *In* Reproduction of Farm Animals. Ed. E.S.E. Hafez, 4th ed., Lea & Febiger. Philadelphia.

Pedersen, H. and Fawcett, D.W. (1976). Functional anatomy of the human spermatozoon. *In* Human Semen and Fertility Regulation in Men. E.S.E. Hafez (ed.). St. Louis, MO, C.V. Mosby.

7

Spermatozoa and Seminal Plasma

D.L. Garner and E.S.E. Hafez

SEMEN

Semen is the liquid or semigelatinous cellular suspension containing the male gametes or spermatozoa and secretions from the accessory organs of the male reproductive tract. The fluid portion of this suspension, which is formed at ejaculation, is known as seminal plasma. A comparison of the seminal characteristics of some farm animals appears in Table 7–1.

SPERM CELLS

Spermatozoa are formed within the seminiferous tubules of the testes. These tubules contain a complex series of developing germ cells that ultimately form the highly specialized male gametes. The fully formed spermatozoa are elongated cells consisting of a flattened head containing the nucleus and a tail containing the apparatus necessary for cell motility (Fig. 7–1). The entire sperm cell is covered by the plasmalemma, or plasma membrane. The acrosome, or acrosomal cap, is a double-walled structure situated between the plasma membrane and the anterior portion of the nucleus. A neck connects the sperm head with its tail (flagellum), which is subdivided into the middle, principal, and end pieces (Fig. 7–1).

Sperm Morphology

Sperm Head. The major feature of the head is the oval, flattened nucleus containing highly compact chromatin (Fig. 7–2). The condensed chromatin comprises

TABLE 7–1. Characteristics and Chemical Components of Semen from Farm Animals*

Characteristic on component	Bull	Ram	Boar	Stallion	Cock
Ejaculate volume (ml)	5–8	0.8–1.2	150–200	60–100	0.2–0.5
Sperm concentration (million/ml)	800–2000	2000–3000	200–300	150–300	3000–7000
Sperm/ejaculate (billion)	5–15	1.6–3.6	30–60	5–15	0.6–3.5
Motile sperm (%)	40–75	60–80	50–80	40–75	60–80
Morphologically normal sperm (%)	65–95	80–95	70–90	60–90	85–90
Protein (g/100 ml)	6.8	5.0	3.7	1.0	1.8–2.8
pH	6.4–7.8	5.9–7.3	7.3–7.8	7.2–7.8	7.2–7.6
Fructose	460–600	250	9	2	4
Sorbitol	10–140	26–170	6–18	20–60	0–10
Citric acid	620–806	110–260	173	8–53	Nil
Inositol	25–46	7–14	380–630	20–47	16–20
Glyceryl phosphoryl choline (GPC)	100–500	1100–2100	110–240	40–100	0–40
Ergothioneine	0	0	17	40–110	0–2
Sodium	225 ± 13	178 ± 11	587	257	352
Potassium	155 ± 6	89 ± 4	197	103	61
Calcium	40 ± 2	6 ± 2	6	26	10
Magnesium	8 ± .3	6 ± .8	5–14	9	14
Chloride	174–320	86	260–430	448	147

*Adapted from Foote, 1980; Gilbert, 1980; Lake, 1971; White, 1980. Mean values of chemical components (mg/100 ml ± S.E.) unless otherwise indicated. Hyphenated values indicate ranges.

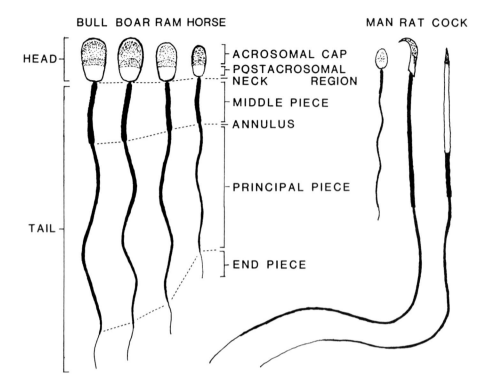

FIG. 7–1. Comparison of the spermatozoa of farm animals and other vertebrates. Note the differences in the relative size and shape.

DNA complexed to a special class of basic proteins known as *sperm protamines.* The chromosome number and hence the DNA content of the sperm nucleus is haploid or half that of somatic cells of the same species. The haploid sperm cell results from the meiotic cell divisions that occur during sperm formation.

Acrosome. The anterior end of the sperm nucleus is covered by the acrosome, a thin, double-layered membranous sac that is closely applied to the nucleus during the last stages of sperm formation (Figs. 7–2 and 7–3). This caplike structure, which contains several hydrolytic enzymes including proacrosin, hyaluronidase, esterases, and acid hydrolases, is involved in the fertilization process (Mann and Lutwak-Mann, 1981). The equatorial segment of the acrosome is important because it is this part of the spermatozoon, along with the anterior portion of the post-

acrosomal region, that initially fuses with the oocyte membrane during fertilization.

Sperm Tail. The tail of the male gamete is composed of the neck, middle, principal and end pieces (Fig. 7–1). The neck or connecting piece forms a basal plate that fits into a depression in the posterior surface of the nucleus. The basal plate of the neck is continuous posteriorly, with nine coarse fibers that project posteriorly throughout most of the tail.

The region of the tail between the neck and the annulus is the middle piece. The central core of the middle piece together with the entire length of the tail make up the axoneme. It is composed of nine pairs of microtubules that are arranged radially around two central filaments. In the middle piece, this 9 + 2 arrangement of microtubules is surrounded by nine coarse or dense fibers that appear to be associated with the nine doublets of the axoneme

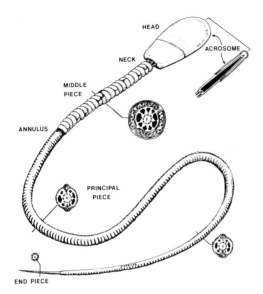

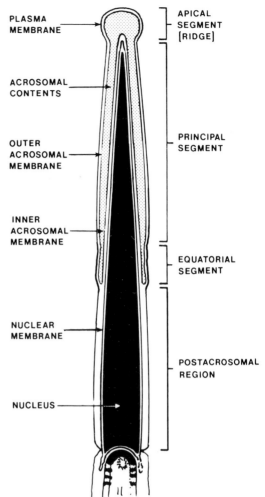

FIG. 7–2. Features of a bovine spermatozoon. The head with its acrosomal cap and the tail with its four anatomic divisions are shown. Cross sections of the middle piece, principal piece (2), and tail piece show the central axonemal core of 9 + 2 microtubules, the nine-coarse outer fibers, the mitochondrial sheath, the dorsal and ventral longitudinal columns, and the circumferential ribs.

(Fig. 7–2). The axoneme and associated dense fibers of the middle piece are covered peripherally by numerous mitochondria (Fig. 7–2). This mitochondrial sheath, which is arranged in a helical pattern around the longitudinal fibers of the tail (Fig. 7–2), generates the energy needed for sperm motility. The mitochondrial sheath terminates at the annulus.

The principal piece, which continues posteriorly from the annulus and extends to near the end of the tail, is composed centrally of the axoneme and its associated coarse fibers. A fibrous sheath is thought to provide stability for the contractile elements of the tail.

The end piece, which is posterior to the termination of the fibrous sheath, contains only the axoneme covered by the plasma membrane.

The axoneme is responsible for sperm motility. The outer pairs of microtubules

FIG. 7–3. A sagittal section of a bovine sperm head showing the various anatomic subdivisions. The acrosome includes the apical (apical ridge), the principal, and the equatorial segments. The outer membranes of the apical and principal segments make up what is called the *acrosomal cap*. The relationship of the acrosome, with its inner and outer membranes, to the nuclear and plasma membranes is also shown.

of the 9 + 2 pattern generate the bending waves of the tail by a sliding movement between adjacent pairs.

The protoplasmic or cytoplasmic droplet, which is usually detached from ejaculated spermatozoa, is composed of residual cytoplasm. Although considered abnormal for ejaculated spermatozoa from most species, the droplet may be retained either in the neck region, where it is known as a proximal droplet, or near the annulus, where it is called a distal droplet.

Chemical Composition of Spermatozoa

The principal chemical components of spermatozoa are nucleic acids, proteins, and lipids. Nearly one third of the dry weight of a single sperm cell is contributed by the nucleus. The nuclear chromatin is composed of approximately half DNA and half protein. The acrosomal cap contains a variety of enzymatic proteins. Many structural, enzymic proteins and lipids are found in the tail.

Inorganic Constituents

Spermatozoa are high in phosphorus, nitrogen, and sulfur. Most of the phosphorus is associated with DNA, whereas the sulfur is derived from both basic nuclear proteins and the keratinoid components of the tail (Mann and Lutwak-Mann, 1981).

Biochemical Components

The spermatozoal nucleus is composed of condensed chromatin in which the DNA is stabilized by conjugation with the sperm-specific proteins collectively known as *sperm histones* (Mann and Lutwak-Mann, 1981). Sperm nuclei from some species contain mostly small sperm histones of low molecular weight known as *protamines,* whereas spermatozoa from other species contain varying amounts of the larger arginine-rich histones. These basic nuclear proteins, which are important for condensation and stabilization of the DNA, are held together by sulfhydryl bonds. The sulfhydryl bonding increases as the cells pass through the epididymis.

During fertilization the spermatozoon undergoes an acrosome reaction in which most of the contents of the acrosome are released or exposed by openings created by fusion of the plasma and outer acrosomal membranes (Fig. 7–3). The released hyaluronidase disperses the cumulus cells that surround the newly ovulated ova. Proacrosin is the precursor for a proteolytic enzyme, acrosin, which is thought to assist in digesting a pathway through the zona pellucida for the penetrating spermatozoon. The specific role of each acrosomal enzyme in fertilization is, however, not completely understood. The equatorial segment differs from the acrosomal cap in that its contents are not released during the initial acrosome reaction but are thought to be exposed when the spermatozoon penetrates the zona pellucida. Biophysical evidence, however, indicates that spermatozoa may be capable of mechanically penetrating the zona pellucida by means of their own motility (Green and Purves, 1984).

The mitochondrial sheath of spermatozoa, which is rich in phospholipid, varies greatly among species in the number of mitochondria and in the chemical makeup. Spermatozoa contain enzymes of the cytochrome-cytochrome oxidase respiratory system and the glycolytic pathway. Other metabolic enzymes, including the sperm-specific lactate dehydrogenase known as LDH-X, are also present. The energy-rich adenine and guanine nucleotides are important components in sperm energetics, as are the axonemal proteins, tubulin and dynein. Sperm dynein, which is the principal protein in the arms of the axonemal microtubules, has been shown to be a divalent cation-activated ATPase.

Sex Chromosomes: X- and Y-Spermatozoa

The process of sperm formation in most mammals results in two types of spermatozoa as far as sex chromatin is concerned. Thus, mammalian males are heterogametic in that approximately one half of the spermatozoa contain an X-chromosome and the other half a Y-chromosome. The males of avian species are, however, homogametic in that they produce spermatozoa with only one kind of sex chromosome. Sex determination in birds therefore occurs with the egg. Of the two types of gametes produced by mammalian males, spermatozoa carrying the X-chromosome produce female embryos on fertilization of an oocyte, whereas spermatozoa carrying the Y-chromosome produce male embryos.

Although the difference in DNA content between X- and Y-chromosome-bearing spermatozoa is only about 4% for domestic livestock, this small difference can be resolved using fluorescent staining and flow cytometry (Garner et al., 1983, 1984). Furthermore, flow cytometers have been modified to sort viable spermatozoa into relatively pure X- and Y-sperm populations (Johnson et al., 1989). When these sorted sperm at near 90% purity were inseminated into females, the sex ratio of the progeny was almost identical to that predicted by the ratio of X- to Y-spermatozoa in the flow-sorted inseminate (Johnson et al., 1989). This accomplishment is a significant step toward development of a practical means of controlling the sex of domestic livestock.

SEMINIFEROUS EPITHELIUM

Spermatogenesis: Spermatogonia, Spermatocytes, and Spermatids

The seminiferous epithelium, lining the seminiferous tubules, is composed of two basic cell types: the Sertoli cells and the developing germ cells. The germ cells undergo a continuous series of cellular divisions and developmental changes, beginning at the periphery and progressing toward the lumen of the tubule (Fig. 7–4). The stem cells, called *spermatogonia*, divide several times before forming spermatocytes. The spermatocytes then undergo meiosis, thereby reducing the DNA content of the cells to one half that of somatic cells. This series of cellular divisions, including the proliferation of the spermatogonia and the meiotic divisions, is known as *spermatocytogenesis*. The haploid cells resulting from this process are called *spermatids*. The spermatids then undergo a progressive series of structural and developmental changes to form sper-

matozoa. These metamorphic changes are known as *spermiogenesis*. The developing germinal cells are closely associated with the large Sertoli or sustentacular cells that surround them during development (Fig. 7–4).

Spermatocytogenesis

During embryonic development, special cells called *primordial germ cells* migrate from the yolk sac region of the embryo into the undifferentiated gonads. After reaching the fetal gonad, the primordial cells divide several times before forming cells called *gonocytes*. In the male, these gonocytes seem to undergo differentiation just before puberty to form the type AO spermatogonia from which the other germ cells originate. The type A1 spermatogonia divide progressively to form type A2, type A3, and type A4 spermatogonia (Fig. 7–5). The type A4 divide again to form intermediate spermatogonia (type In) and then again to form type B spermatogonia. These various types of spermatogonia, which can be identified in histologic sections of the seminiferous epithelium, are the basis for proliferation of the germ cell line.

Some variation exists regarding how spermatogonia are classified, and in certain species, only three rather than four type A spermatogonia are evident. The type A2 cells not only divide to produce the many germinal cells that eventually form sperm, but also a specific division is thought to be used to replace the stem cell population of type A1 spermatogonia. It seems that special reserve stem cells, type AO spermatogonia, replace the stem cell population.

The type B spermatogonia divide at least once and probably twice to form the primary spermatocytes. The primary spermatocytes duplicate their DNA and undergo progressive nuclear changes of meiotic prophase known as *preleptotene, leptotene, zygotene, pachytene,* and *diplotene* before dividing to form secondary spermatocytes. Without further DNA syn-

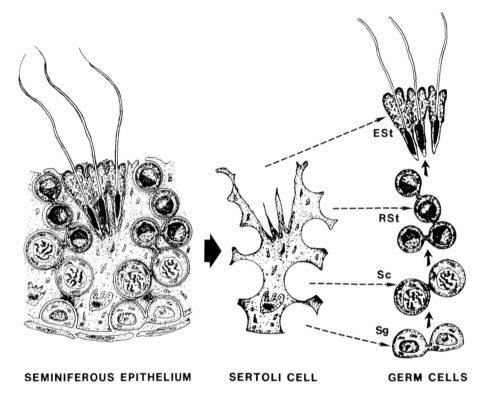

SEMINIFEROUS EPITHELIUM   SERTOLI CELL   GERM CELLS

FIG. 7–4.   The seminiferous epithelium showing the complex nature of the association between Sertoli cells and the developing germ cells along with an illustration depicting dissociation of this cellular complex. The developing germ cells occupy intracellular spaces between adjacent Sertoli cells and move from the basement membrane toward the lumen during spermatogenic process. The germ cells begin their developmental process as spermatogonia (Sg), become spermatocytes (Sc), then round spermatids (RSt), and finally, elongated spermatids (ESt). Schematic dissociation of the seminiferous epithelium shows how the germ cells occupy the expanded intercellular spaces between adjacent Sertoli cells. (Adapted from Fawcett, D.W. (1974) *In* Male Fertility and Sterility, R.E. Mancini and L. Martini (eds.). New York, Academic Press.)

thesis, the resultant secondary spermatocytes divide again to form the haploid cells known as *spermatids.* The entire divisional process of spermatocytogenesis, from spermatogonia to spermatid, takes approximately 45 days in the bull. These divisions are, however, incomplete in that small cytoplasmic or intercellular bridges are retained between most cells of a series or "clone" of developing germ cells (Bloom and Fawcett, 1975). These bridges are thought to be important in coordinating simultaneous development of germ cells as a group.

Spermiogenesis

The round spermatids are transformed into spermatozoa by a series of progressive morphologic changes collectively known as *spermiogenesis.* These changes include condensation of the nuclear chromatin, formation of the sperm tail or flagellar apparatus, and development of the acrosomal cap (Fig. 7–5). The various developmental stages of spermatid transformation are readily classified by using periodic acid-Schiff (PAS) reaction to stain the developing acrosomal components a deep red. Four phases are noted in this develop-

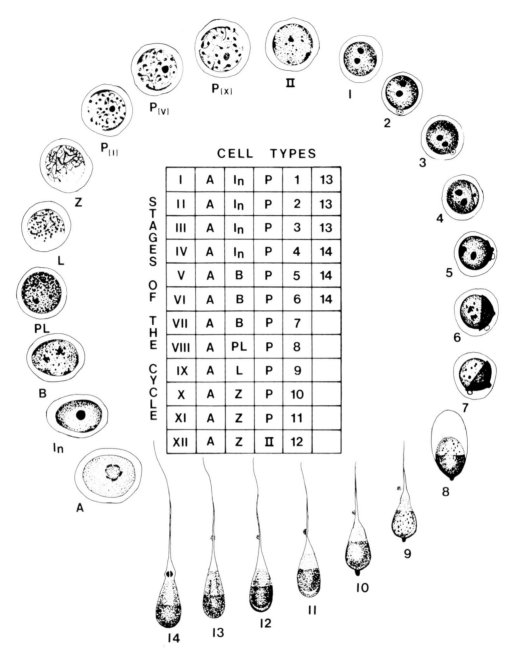

FIG. 7–5. The various steps in spermatogenesis in the bull beginning with a type A spermatogonium. The table in the center indicates the particular cellular association of the 12 stages of the cycle of the seminiferous epithelium. The various cell types are: A, I, B, successive stages of spermatogonia; PL, preleptotene spermatocyte; L, leptotene spermatocyte; Z, zygotene spermatocyte; P, pachytene spermatocytes from stages I, V, and X; II, secondary spermatocyte; 1 through 14 are steps of spermiogenesis showing the Golgi phase (steps 1 to 3), the cap phase (steps 4 to 7), the acrosome phase (steps 8 to 12) and the maturation phase (steps 13 and 14). (Adapted from Berndtson, W.E. and Desjardins, C. (1974) Am. J. Anat., *140*, 167–180.)

mental process: the Golgi, cap, acrosomal, and maturation phases.

Golgi Phase. The Golgi phase of spermiogenesis is characterized by formation of PAS-positive proacrosomal granules within the Golgi apparatus, the coalescence of the granules into a single acrosomal granule, the adherence of the resultant acrosomal granule to the nuclear envelope, and the early stages of tail development at the pole opposite that of the adherence of the acrosomal granule (Fig. 7–5, steps 1–3). The proximal centriole migrates closest to the nucleus, where it is thought to form a basis for attachment of the tail to the head.

Cap Phase. The cap phase is characterized by a spreading of the adherent acrosomal granule over the surface of the spermatid nucleus (Fig. 7–5, steps 4–7). This process continues until nearly two thirds of the anterior portion of each spermatid nucleus is covered by a thin, double-layered membranous sac that closely adheres to the nuclear envelope. During this cap phase, the developing axonemal components of the tail, which are formed from elements of the distal centriole, elongate well beyond the periphery of the cellular cytoplasm. During the early development, the axoneme closely resembles the structure of a cilium in that it consists of two central tubules surrounded peripherally by nine pairs of tubules.

Acrosomal Phase. The acrosomal phase of spermiogenesis is characterized by changes in the nuclei, the acrosomes, and the tails of the developing spermatids. The developmental changes are facilitated by rotation of each spermatid so that the acrosome is directed toward the basement or outer wall of the seminiferous tubule and the tail toward the lumen (Fig. 7–5, steps 8–12). The nuclear changes include condensation of the chromatin into dense granules and reshaping of the spheroidal nucleus into an elongated, flattened structure. The acrosome, which is closely adherent to the nucleus, also condenses and elongates to correspond to the shape of the nucleus. These modifications in nuclear and acrosomal shape appear to be "molded" by the surrounding Sertoli cells. The morphologic changes are slightly different for each species and thus result in elongated spermatids and spermatozoa that are characteristic for each species.

The changes in nuclear morphology are accompanied by displacement of the cytoplasm to the caudal aspect of the nucleus, where it surrounds the proximal portion of the developing tail. Within this cytoplasm, microtubules associate to form a temporary cylindrical sheath called the *manchette*, which projects posteriorly from the caudal border of the acrosome, where it loosely surrounds the axoneme. Within the cylindrical manchette, a specialized cytoplasmic structure called the *chromatoid body* condenses around the axoneme to form the ringlike structure known as the *annulus*. The annulus first forms near the proximal centriole and then during subsequent development migrates posteriorly along the tail. The mitochondria, which were previously distributed throughout the cytoplasm of the spermatid, begin to concentrate close to the axoneme, where they form the sheath that characterizes the middle piece of the tail.

Maturation Phase. The maturation phase of spermiogenesis involves final transformation of the elongated spermatids into cells to be released into the lumen of the seminiferous tubule. The reshaping of the nucleus and acrosome of each spermatid, initiated during the previous phase, produces spermatozoa characteristic for each species. Within the nucleus, the chromatin granules undergo progressive condensation until they form a fine homogeneous material that uniformly fills the entire sperm nucleus (Fig. 7–5, steps 13–14).

During the maturation phase, a fibrous sheath and the underlying nine coarse fibers are formed around the axoneme. The coarse fibers appear to be associated individually with the nine pairs of microtubules of the axoneme and are continuous with columns in the neck of the connecting piece of the spermatid. The fibrous sheath covers the axoneme from the neck to the beginning of the end piece. The annulus migrates distally from its position adjacent to the nucleus along the tail to a point where it will subsequently separate the middle piece from the principal piece of the tail. The mitochondria become tightly packed into a continuous sheath extending from the neck to the annulus.

During the later stages of spermiogenesis, the manchette disappears and the Sertoli cell then forms the cytoplasm remaining after elongation of the spermatid into a spheroidal lobule called *the residual body.* This lobule of cytoplasm, which remains connected to the elongated spermatid by a slender thread of cytoplasm, is also interconnected with other residual bodies by intercellular bridges that resulted from the incomplete division of the germ cells during spermatocytogenesis. Formation of the residual body completes the final maturation, and the elongated spermatids are ready for release as spermatozoa.

Spermiation

The release of formed germ cells into the lumen of the seminiferous tubules is known as *spermiation.* The elongated spermatids, which are oriented perpendicularly to the tubular wall, are gradually extruded into the lumen of the tubule (Fig. 7–5). The lobules of residual cytoplasm through which large syncytial groups of spermatids are connected by intercellular bridges remain embedded in the epithelium. Extrusion of the spermatozoal components continues until only a slender stalk of cytoplasm connects the neck of the spermatid to the residual body (Fig. 7–6) (Fawcett, 1975). Breakage of the stalk results in formation of the cytoplasmic droplet in the neck region of the released spermatozoa (proximal droplet) and retention of the interconnected residual bodies. Following release of the spermatozoa, the residual bodies are rapidly disposed of by the Sertoli cells. Sertoli cells apparently aid in recycling the protoplasmic components. Not only do the Sertoli cells phagocytize the residual bodies remaining from the spermatogenic process, but these cells must also remove considerable numbers of degenerating germ cells. Because the spermatogenic process is relatively inefficient, large numbers of potential sperm cells degenerate before becoming spermatozoa.

Duration of Spermatogenesis

The various cell types within any cross section of the seminiferous epithelium form well-defined cellular associations that undergo cyclic changes. As many as 14 distinct cellular associations or stages are identifiable in some species, whereas only 6 stages are identifiable in man (Clermont, 1963). In the bull, as many as 12 stages of this cycle have been described (Berndtson and Desjardins, 1974) (Fig. 7–5). A complete, time-dependent cycle of the stages known as the *cycle of the seminiferous epithelium* is defined as "a series of changes in a given area of seminiferous epithelium between two appearances of the cellular association or developmental stages" (Clermont, 1963). The steps in spermiogenesis are used to classify the various stages of the cycle. The time necessary to complete a cycle of the seminiferous epithelium varies among domestic species. Duration of the cycle is about 9 days in the boar, 10 days in the ram, 12 days in the horse and 14 days in the bull (Johnson and Everitt, 1984; Swierstra et al., 1968). Depending on the species, four to nearly five epithelial cycles are required before the type A spermatogonia from the first cycle have completed the metamorphosis of spermiogenesis. Each epithelial cycle is analogous to a student attending college (e.g., freshman, sophomore, junior or senior) in that it takes four or more cycles or "years" before a spermatogonial stem cell or "incoming freshman" has completed the process of spermatogenesis or "finished the senior year." Spermiation, which can be thought of as

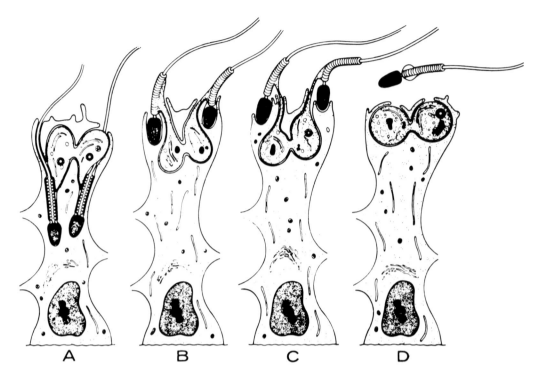

FIG. 7–6. Sperm release in mammals. The successive stages show a gradual extrusion of the elongated spermatid into the lumen with retention of the interconnected residual bodies. Release results from attenuation of the slender stalk of cytoplasm connecting the spermatid to the residual body. Once separated from the residual body, the cell becomes a spermatozoon. (From Fawcett, D.W. (1975) *In* Handbook of Physiology, Vol. V, R.O. Greep and E.B. Astwood (eds.). Bethesda, American Physiological Society.)

"graduation," occurs for the three previous cycles or classes before the stem cell completes the developmental process to become spermatozoa or "the incoming freshman completes the four-year curriculum." Although differences in the rate of spermatogenesis exist among mammalian species, the process is uniform within a species (Setchell, 1978).

Spermatogenic Wave

The stages of the cycle of the seminiferous epithelium change not only with time but also along the length of the tubular loop (Setchell, 1977) (Fig. 7–7). A portion of tubule at one stage is usually adjacent to portions of tubule in stages just preceding or following it in time (Perey et al., 1961) (Fig. 7–8). This sequential change in

stage of cycle along the length of the tubule is known as the *wave of the seminiferous epithelium*. Examination of a loop of seminiferous tubule along its length also reveals that the wave involves a sequence of stages beginning with the less advanced stages in the middle of the loop to progressively more advanced stages nearer the rete testis. Certain irregularities or breaks in the sequential order are noted. Such breaks in sequence, called *modulations*, occur occasionally but involve relatively short lengths of tubule.

Blood–Testis Barrier

Cellular Junctions

The seminiferous tubules are not penetrated by blood or lymph vessels. In addition, the developing germ cells within the

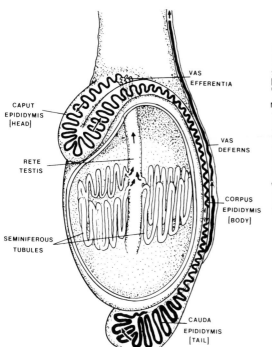

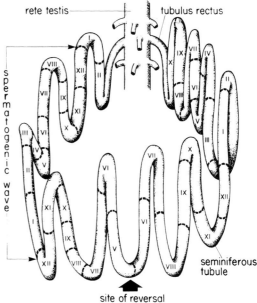

FIG. 7–7.   Loops of the seminiferous tubules, the rete testis and the excurrent duct system of the ram. The pathway by which spermatozoa are transported to the exterior is indicated by arrows. (Modified from Setchell, B.P. (1977) *In* Reproduction in Domestic Animals. H.H. Cole and P.T. Cupps (eds.). New York, Academic Press.)

FIG. 7–8.   A seminiferous tubule in which the wave of the seminiferous epithelium is schematically represented along the length of the tubule. The succession of stages I to XII, the site of reversal in the middle of the tubule and the relationship of the wave to the rete testis are shown. The more advanced stages of each wave are located nearer the rete testis. An actual seminiferous tubule may contain 15 or more complete spermatogenic waves. (Adapted from Perey, B., Clermont, Y. and Leblond, C.P. (1961) Am. J. Anat. The wave of the seminiferous epithelium in the rat. *108*, 47–77.)

tubules are protected from chemical changes in the blood by a specialized permeability barrier. This blood–testis barrier has two principal components: (1) the incomplete or partial barrier of the myoid cells that surround the tubule and (2) the unique junctions between adjacent Sertoli cells (Setchell, 1980).

Myoid Layer.   The basement membrane, or tunica propria, that surrounds the seminiferous tubules contains a layer of contractile myoid cells (Fig. 7–9). In some species a majority of the cell junctions of this layer are sealed by tight apposition of the adjacent cell membranes. This barrier, however, is not well developed in the bull, ram, or boar and may be a relatively unimportant permeability barrier in the testes of farm animals.

Sertoli Cell Junctions.   The principal permeability barrier between the blood and testis is thought to be the complexes at junctions between adjacent Sertoli cells. These Sertoli-Sertoli junctions, which are situated near the cellular base, contain multiple zones of adhesion (tight junctions) where the opposing membranes are fused (Fawcett, 1975). The occluding junctions divide the seminiferous tubules into two distinct compartments: (1) a *basal compartment,* containing spermatogonia and preleptotene spermatocytes, and (2)

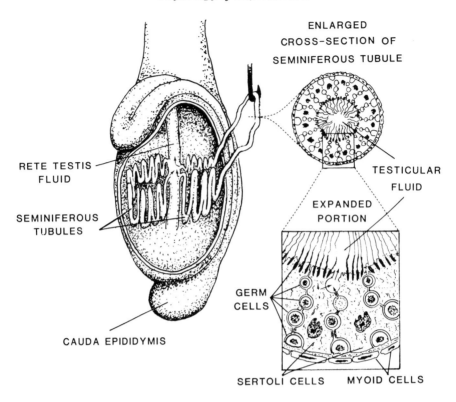

ENLARGED
CROSS-SECTION OF
SEMINIFEROUS TUBULE

RETE TESTIS
FLUID

SEMINIFEROUS
TUBULES

TESTICULAR
FLUID

EXPANDED
PORTION

GERM
CELLS

CAUDA EPIDIDYMIS

SERTOLI CELLS   MYOID CELLS

FIG. 7–9.   Source of testicular and rete testis fluid. These fluids become mixed in the rete testis and are excreted into the excurrent duct system of the male. Testicular fluid is secreted by the Sertoli cells into the lumen of the tubule. One seminiferous tubule has been pulled from the testis and enlarged and expanded in cross section to show the microanatomy of the seminiferous epithelium.

an *adluminal compartment,* containing the more advanced stages of spermatocytes and spermatids, which freely communicates with the lumen of the tubule (Fawcett, 1975).

The basal compartment is freely accessible to components that have previously penetrated the myoid layer. The second barrier, composed of the occluding junctions between Sertoli cells, demonstrates a wide range of permeability from complete exclusion of some substances to nearly free transfer of others. This differential permeability appears to be important in maintaining an environment suitable for the spermatogenic function of the tubules. The blood–testis barrier not only excludes entry of certain substances but also appears to function in retaining specific levels of certain substances, such as androgen-binding protein (ABP), inhibin, and enzyme inhibitors, within the luminal compartments of the tubules.

Fluid Secretions

The spermatids produced during the final phase of spermiogenesis are released during spermiation into the lumen of the seminiferous tubules as immature spermatozoa. These sperm cells, which are immotile, are swept from the tubules by fluid secretions originating from the Sertoli cells. Transit into the epididymis appears to be aided by secretions from the rete testis, by the contractile elements of the testis (e.g., myoid cells and testicular capsule) (Hargrove et al., 1977) and by the cilia lining the efferent ducts.

Testicular fluid is a composite secretion of both the Sertoli cells and the epithelial cells lining the rete testis. The Sertoli cells, however, are thought to be the predominant source of fluid leaving the testis. Fluid secretion from Sertoli cells is thought to occur because active transport processes push solutes into the adluminal compartment, thereby forming an osmotic gradient. This fluid contains several unique proteins including ABP, which is secreted into the lumen of the seminiferous tubule by the Sertoli cells (Hansson et al., 1976). The ABP forms a complex with the androgens produced by the Leydig cells. The resultant complex may assist transit of androgen into the caput epididymis.

Endocrine Control of Spermatogenesis

Normal testicular function requires hormonal stimulation by gonadotropins, which are in turn controlled by pulsatile secretion gonadotropin-releasing hormone (GnRH) from the hypothalamus (Fig. 7–10). Pituitary support is essential because hypophysectomy, surgical removal of the pituitary, results in cessation of spermatogenesis. Restoration of spermatogenesis can be achieved in the hypophysectomized rat by treatment with both FSH and LH or with FSH and testosterone. High doses of testosterone alone will maintain spermatogenesis in hypophysectomized rats, provided treatment begins immediately after removal of the pituitary. Other species, however, require FSH in addition to the steroid for maintenance of spermatogenesis. Other pituitary hormones (e.g., prolactin, growth hormone, and thyroid-stimulating hormone) may have secondary roles in support of testicular function, but confirming evidence is lacking (Schanbacher, 1984).

The major action of androgens appears to be on the Sertoli cells rather than directly on the germ cells. The myoid cells also appear to be androgen dependent. The steroid dependency is met by pulsatile production of androgens by the inter-

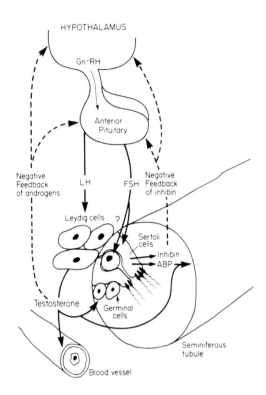

FIG. 7–10. The endocrine control of testicular function in mammals. The hypothalamus secretes gonadotropin, a hormone-releasing hormone (GnRH), that stimulates the secretion of LH and FSH from the anterior pituitary. The LH stimulates the interstitial cells of Leydig to produce androgens, mainly testosterone. The androgens are secreted into the bloodstream, where they cause the development of secondary sex characteristics of the male and development and maintenance of the male reproductive tract. The androgens suppress GnRH, LH, and FSH secretion by negative feedback on the pituitary and hypothalamus. Testosterone is also secreted into the seminiferous tubule, where it is necessary for maintenance of spermatogenesis. The FSH interacts with receptors on the Sertoli cells to cause production of androgen-binding protein (ABP), conversion of testosterone to dihydrotestosterone and estrogen, stimulation of the spermatocytogenesis, completion of sperm release (spermiation), and secretion of inhibin. The inhibin secreted into the bloodstream has a negative feedback effect on FSH but not on LH secretion. (From Kaltenback, C.C. and Dunn, T.G. (1980) Endocrinology of reproduction. *In* Reproduction in Farm Animals, 4th ed., E.S.E. Hafez (ed.). Philadelphia, Lea & Febiger.)

stitial Leydig cells, which are adjacent to the seminiferous tubules (Fig. 7–7). The Leydig cells are stimulated by pulses of pituitary LH to secrete androgens. The androgens produced by the Leydig cells diffuse into the adjacent Sertoli cells and are secreted into the blood, where they feed back both at the hypothalamus and the pituitary to block release of additional LH (Fig. 7–10). The other principal gonadotropin, FSH, stimulates production of ABP and inhibin by the Sertoli cells. ABP forms a complex with androgen and is carried along with the spermatozoa into the epididymis (Ganjam and Amann, 1976). The epithelial cells of the epididymis require relatively high levels of androgen for normal function. Inhibin has a negative feedback effect on FSH secretion but not on LH (Blanc et al., 1981). Although much of the testosterone secreted into the seminiferous tubules is converted into dihydrotestosterone (DHT) by the enzyme 5 α-steroid reductase, some of the testosterone is converted to estrogens by the enzyme aromatase (Dorrington and Armstrong, 1975). A relatively high level of testosterone is required for spermatid maturation (Hafs and McCarthy, 1978).

GROWTH FACTORS

Recent investigations have shown that biologically active growth factors regulate some reproductive processes and are present in seminal plasma. (Adashi et al., 1991; Earp, 1991; Rappolee et al., 1989). Growth factors, which are polypeptides, elicit cellular responses by binding to specific cell surface receptors in target tissues. These growth factors regulate the proliferation of many cell types, thereby influencing growth of the reproductive tract. Cell growth and differentiation are regulated by physiologic interactions among hormones (FSH/LH, estrogen, progestins) and bioactive growth factors. A wide range of cell types expresses the appropriate receptors for these growth factors.

Epidermal Growth Factor (EGF), a 53 amino acid polypeptide, was initially detected in mouse submaxillary gland extracts. This peptide exerts a potent mitogenic action on a variety of epidermal and nonepidermal cells, both *in vivo* and *in vitro*. Specific EFG receptors are found in cultured Leydig cells, testicular membrane extracts, and seminal plasma. Although EGF-like activity is found in testicular tissue and other parts of the male reproductive tract, relatively little is known concerning its physiologic significance in male reproduction.

Some of the growth factors involved with regulation of reproductive processes include the following:

EGF	Epidermal Growth Factor
FGF	Fibroblast Growth Factor
FRP	Follicular Regulating Protein
FSHBI	FSH Binding Inhibitor
G-CSF	Granulocyte-Colony Stimulating Factor
GM-CSF	Granulocyte-Macrophage Colony Stimulating Factor
IF	Inhibin F (Folliculostatin/ Follicular Fluid Inhibin)
IGF	Insulin-like Growth Factor Serum
LI	Luteinization Inhibitor
LS	Luteinization Stimulator
MIS	Müllerian Inhibiting Substance
NP-Gα	Neuropeptides GnRHα
NP-Gβ	Neuropeptides GnRHβ
OFFP	Ovarian Follicular Fluid Peptide
PDGF	Platelet-derived Growth Factor
TGF	Transforming Growth Factor
VIP	Vasoactive Intestinal Peptide

Müllerian Inhibiting Substance (MIS), which is a glycoprotein synthesized and secreted by the gonads, exhibits a sexually dimorphic pattern of expression. In the fetal testis, MIS is produced by the Sertoli cells and causes regression of the Müllerian duct. In the female fetus, MIS inhibits oocyte meiosis and blocks spontaneous breakdown of the germinal vesicle.

Sertoli and germ cells reciprocally regulate each other's cyclic secretion of proteins along the length of the seminiferous tubule. This process is amplified by the myoid cells through transforming growth factors, humoral modulators, and extracellular matrix modification. Activin and inhibin, which are secreted by the Sertoli cells, have remarkable characteristics to generate a diverse series of signals. Activins, potent FSH-releasing dimers (dimers of inhibin β-subunits), have paracrine (inhibiting growth hormone and adrenocorticotropin secretion), and autocrine (stimulating FSH secretion) mechanisms. Activin and inhibin also act within the gonads as autocrine and paracrine modulators of the production of steroids, other hormones, and growth factors. Transforming growth factor (TGF), a multifunctional peptide induced in response to steroids, may be involved in regulation of testicular function. Endogenous opioid peptides (EOPs) seem to have an autocrine and paracrine regulation on Leydig cell steroidogenesis and participate in the intratesticular hormonal control of vascular permeability. Two groups of compounds are involved with regulation of the hypothalamo–pituitary–gonadal axis. These include (a) neurotransmitters, dopamine, serotonin, and norepinephrine and (b) brain opioids and other peptides. Thymosin, a hormone from the thymus, is found in lower concentrations in the seminal plasma of infertile or subfertile males. Other physiologic modulators of cell proliferation such as chalones influence the cell cycle of the seminiferous epithelium.

EPIDIDYMAL TRANSIT, SPERM MATURATION, AND STORAGE

Testicular spermatozoa are transported from the testis through a highly convoluted duct known as the *epididymis* (Fig. 7–7). The epididymis not only transports spermatozoa distally from the testis into the vas deferens but, during this transit,

the spermatozoa also undergo a maturation process in which they gain the potential ability to fertilize ova. This maturation involves several functional changes, including development of the *potential* for sustained motility, progressive loss of water and distal migration, and eventual loss of the cytoplasmic droplet. The functional capabilities of the various epithelial cells lining the epididymis, and hence their influence on the sperm maturation process, are maintained by testicular androgens.

Transport Mechanisms

The passage of spermatozoa through the epididymis depends on localized contractions of the duct wall. These contractions, which have been observed in vitro in rat epididymides, can be stimulated by prostaglandins and progress in one direction at a frequency of about three per minute (Cosentino et al., 1984). Spermatozoa are transported through the epididymis in about 7 days in the bull, 12 days in the boar (Swierstra, 1968), and 16 days in the ram (Amann, 1981). The transit time may be reduced by 10 to 20% by an increased frequency of ejaculation. The contractile elements of the epididymal wall show regional differences in that the content of smooth muscle cells increases progressively from the tail of the epididymis to the vas deferens (Bedford, 1975).

Maturation and Storage of Spermatozoa

The functional changes occurring during epididymal transit of spermatozoa involve maturation of cell organelles. For instance, the development of the capacity for sperm motility reflects both qualitative and quantitative changes in the metabolic patterns of the flagellar apparatus. Although mature epididymal spermatozoa are relatively quiescent within the epididymis, they rapidly demonstrate motility removal and examination. The maturation process in which epididymal spermatozoa attain the capacity for progressive motility involves progressive changes in the flexibility and patterns of movement of their flagella. Rapid forward progression appears first in the middle of the corpus epididymis in a few spermatozoa and becomes the predominating motility pattern in spermatozoa from the cauda and vas deferens (Bedford, 1975).

Secretory components of epithelial cells lining the epididymis, such as "immobilin" in some laboratory animals (Usselman and Cone, 1983) and "quiescence factor" in the bull (Acott and Carr, 1984), probably prolong sperm survival by preventing unnecessary metabolism. Forward motility protein appears to be important to the attainment of progressive motility in bovine epididymal spermatozoa (Acott et al., 1983).

Transit through the epididymis is associated with significant changes within the chromatin of the sperm nucleus. This DNA-protein complex, which was once thought to be relatively inert following its condensation during the latter phases of spermiogenesis, undergoes a qualitative reduction in reactivity to Feulgen staining during epididymal transit (Gledhill, 1971).

During epididymal transit, the droplet migrates from the neck region to a position near the annulus. Presence of the droplet on a significant number of ejaculated spermatozoa is a sign of immaturity.

Changes associated with maturation of the acrosome have been noted in most species during passage through the epididymis. Although marked changes occur in some species, those occurring in farm animals are limited to a rather subtle reduction in acrosome dimensions (Bedford, 1975).

Development of Fertilizing Potential in the Epididymis

Spermatozoa develop their initial ability to fertilize ova during their transport through the epididymis. Their fertilizing capacity is considered potential since they must undergo capacitation before they can penetrate ova. Testicular spermatozoa are infertile even when inseminated in relatively large numbers (Setchell et al.,

1969). The lack of fertility of caput epididymal spermatozoa may be related to motility. Spermatozoa from the caput epididymis possess active circular swimming movement but yet are incapable of the vigorous unindirectional movement of spermatozoa possessing the ability to undergo longitudinal rotation. Changes occurring during epididymal transport such as droplet movement and loss and the increase in specific gravity are difficult to interpret from a functional standpoint. Changes in motility, chromatin structure, acrosome morphology, or plasma membrane change can be interpreted readily as prerequisites to the fertilization process.

The development of fertilizing ability is associated with changes in several aspects of the functional integrity of the spermatozoa: (a) development of the potential for sustained progressive motility, (b) alteration of the metabolic patterns and the structural state of specific tail organelles, (c) changes in nuclear chromatin, (d) changes in nature of the surface of the plasma membrane, (e) movement and loss of the protoplasmic droplet, and (f) modification, at least in some species, of the form of the acrosome (Bedford, 1975).

Sperm Storage

The major site of sperm storage within the male reproductive tract is the caudal portion, or tail, of the epididymis. The tail of the epididymis contains 70% of the total number of spermatozoa in the excurrent ducts, whereas the vas deferens contains only 2% (Amann, 1981). Although the environment is favorable to their survival, spermatozoa are not preserved indefinitely.

Disposal of Unejaculated Spermatozoa

Most unejaculated spermatozoa are gradually eliminated by excretion into the urine. Those spermatozoa that are not eliminated in the urine undergo a gradual senescence. They first lose their fertilizing ability, then their motility, and finally, they disintegrate. Ejaculates collected after prolonged sexual rest usually contain a high percentage of degenerating or "stale" spermatozoa.

Fate of Sperm in the Female Reproductive Tract

Several physiologic mechanisms are involved in removal of spermatozoa in the female reproductive tract. In laboratory animals, the number of intraluminal leukocytes increases abruptly shortly after coitus. The infiltrating leukocytes phagocytize the excess spermatozoa, removing most by 20 hours post coitus. Spermatozoa are more rapidly removed from the uterus if the female had been immunized previously against spermatozoa. Although many sperm are simply eliminated by retrograde flow back out of the vagina, the uptake of spermatozoa by phagocytes, or spermophagy, is of special physiologic significance. The infiltration of leukocytes into the uterine lumen and their activation to ingest sperm following breeding seems to be major mechanism to remove the sperm from the uterine cavity (Koehler et al., 1982). Spermatozoa within the uterus are taken into phagocytic vacuoles and digested by the leukocytes.

SEMINAL PLASMA

The functional significance of seminal plasma is questionable in that pregnancy can be induced in some species by insemination with epididymal spermatozoa. It, however, appears to be an essential component in natural mating because it serves as a carrier and protector of the spermatozoa. The importance of this role varies because spermatozoa are ejaculated directly into the uterus in some species (e.g., sow and mare). Seminal plasma appears to be more important in natural mating of ewe and cow where the ejaculate is deposited in the vagina.

ACCESSORY GLANDS

The source of the constituents of seminal plasma varies with the species as does the number and size of the accessory organs.

The prostate, vesicular and bulbourethral glands pour their secretions into the urethra where, at the time of ejaculation, they are mixed with the fluid suspension of sperm and ampullary secretions from the ductus deferens. All the accessory glands are essentially lobular branched tubular glands with smooth muscle prominent within the interstitial tissue.

Seminal plasma is a composite secretion arising from a number of sources including the testes, epididymides, and accessory glands of the male (Fig. 7–11). The only accessory gland common to all mammals is the prostate. The epididymis or its functional analogue and the vas deferens are the only accessory organs present in male birds and reptiles.

Biochemical Constituents of Seminal Plasma

Seminal plasma contains unusually high levels of citric acid, ergothioneine, fructose, glycerylphosphorylcholine, and sorbitol (Table 7–1). Appreciable quantities of ascorbic acid, amino acids, peptides, proteins, lipids, fatty acids, and numerous enzymes are also present (White, 1980). Antimicrobial constituents including seminalplasmin (Shivaji et al., 1984) and immunoglobulins, mainly of the IgA class (Ablin, 1974), are constituents of seminal plasma. In addition, a variety of hormonal substances including androgens, estrogens, prostaglandins, FSH, LH, chorionic gonadotropin-like material, growth hormone, insulin, glucagon, prolactin, relaxin, thyroid-releasing hormone and enkephalins have been detected in seminal plasma (Mann and Lutwak-Mann, 1981).

Apart from providing a liquid vehicle for sperm transport, the functions of the accessory glands are not fully understood. Spermatozoa from the cauda epididymides can fertilize eggs without the addition of accessory gland secretions. The unique biochemical markers in semen, however,

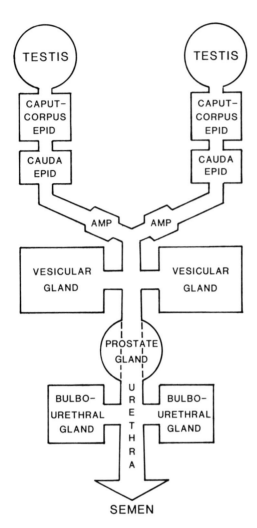

FIG. 7–11.   Ejaculated semen of most farm animals is composed of, in addition to a small amount of testicular fluid, contributions from several accessory organs including the epididymis (CAPUT-CORPUS EPID and CAUDA EPID), ampullary glands (AMP), vesicular glands, prostate gland, and bulbourethral glands. The relative contribution of the glands varies not only among species but also among individuals within a species and among ejaculates from the same animal.

can be used as indicators of specific accessory gland function. Fructose and citric acid are important components of vesicular gland secretions of ruminants. Citric acid alone is found in stallion vesicular glands, whereas the boar vesicular glands

contain little fructose but are characterized by a high content of ergothioneine and inositol. Glycerylphosphorylcholine is a distinctive component of the epididymal secretion. Ergothioneine is a unique characteristic of the ampullary glands of the horse. The gel-like fraction of the boar ejaculate forms a plug in the vagina and uterus of mated sows. This fraction is generally removed from the semen by filtration before use in commercial insemination practices. The stallion also produces a substantial gel fraction during the spring of the year.

The accessory glands of the bull and stallion can be palpated per rectum. In the bull, the seminal vesicles and body of the prostate gland are readily detectable per rectum. The bovine bulbourethral glands, however, are not identifiable because they are covered by muscle. In boars, the size of the bulbourethral glands can be used to differentiate castrate from cryptorchid boars. Prepubertally castrated boars possess small bulbourethral glands, 5 cm long, weighing less than 1 g. Cryptorchid boars, however, have normal-sized glands, each being approximately 10 cm long and weighing 45 grams.

SPERMATOZOAL METABOLISM

The motile character of spermatozoa provides an easily discernible means of assessing their physiologic status. But motility, by itself, is not an accurate predictor of potential fertilizing capacity. The energy required for motility is apparently derived from intracellular stores of ATP. The use of ATP appears to be regulated by the endogenous level of cyclic adenosine monophosphate (cAMP). The cAMP not only regulates ATP breakdown but also has a direct effect on sperm motility. This complex effect of cAMP on sperm motility has been demonstrated *in vitro* by adding to spermatozoa either dibutyryl cAMP or inhibitors such as methyl xanthines that block the normal intracellular degradation of cAMP (Hoskins and Casillas, 1973).

Although spermatozoa lack many of the organelles associated with metabolic processes, they are active metabolically because they possess the enzymes necessary to carry out the biochemical reactions of glycolysis (Embden-Meyerhof pathway), the tricarboxylic acid cycle, fatty acid oxidation, electron transport, and possibly the hexose monophosphate shunt (Mann, 1975).

Glycolysis

Under anaerobic conditions—that is, in the absence of oxygen—spermatozoa break down glucose, fructose, or mannose to lactic acid. This glycolytic activity—or more correctly, fructolytic activity because fructose is the principal seminal sugar—allows spermatozoa to survive under the anaerobic conditions. This characteristic is important during storage of spermatozoa for use in artificial insemination.

Respiration

Spermatozoa use a variety of substrates in the presence of oxygen. Their respiratory activity provides the means of using the lactate or pyruvate resulting from the fructolysis of sugars to yield carbon dioxide and water (Mann, 1975). This oxidative pathway, which is located in the mitochondria, is considerably more efficient in the production of energy than fructolysis. Using these catabolic processes, the spermatozoa convert most of the energy into ATP. Although much of the ATP is used for the energy-consuming process of motility, some is used to maintain the integrity of the active transport processes of spermatozoal membranes. These active transport processes prevent loss of vital ionic components from the sperm cell. In the absence of exogenous substrates, spermatozoa use their intracellular stores of plasmalogen to provide energy on a short-term basis (White, 1980).

IMMUNOLOGIC ASPECTS OF SPERMATOZOA

Antigenicity of Spermatozoa

An important function of the blood–testis barrier is the immunologic isolation of developing gametes. Its importance is that the spermatocytes, spermatids, and spermatozoa are readily recognized as foreign cells by the immune system of the adult male. Thus, sequestering of the developing germ cells behind an immunologic barrier prevents an adult male from developing antibodies against his own sperm cells.

Autoimmunity

Immunization of a male against spermatozoa or isolated spermatozoal antigens results in varying degrees of autoimmune orchitis (inflammation of the testis) and cessation of spermatogenesis (Setchell, 1980). Damage to the blood–testis barrier or the epididymal portion of the excurrent duct system through traumatic injury or

TABLE 7–2. **Age, Weight, and Semen Characteristics at First Breeding**

| Species | Beginning of Breeding Life | | Volume of Ejaculate (ml) | Sperm Concentration (10^8 per ml) |
	Age (Months)	Body Weight	Range	Range
Boar	5–8	250 kg	100–150	0.1–0.2
Bull	12–14	500 kg	3–5	0.8–1.2
Ram	6–8	Varies	0.3–1.0	1.2–2.0
Stallion	20–24	500 kg	50–100	0.1–1.5
Cock	4–6	Varies	0.10–0.3	50–90
Cat	9	3.5 kg	0.01–0.3	1.5–28
Dog	10–12	Varies	2–25	0.6–5.4
Guinea pig	3–5	450 g	0.4–0.8	0.05–0.2
Rabbit	4–12	Varies	0.4–0.6	0.5–3.5

(Adapted from Foote, 1980; Garner and Hafez, 1986; Hamner, 1970).

TABLE 7–3. Semen Evaluation as Related to Unexplained Infertility

Initial evaluation	Motility patterns and concentration Agregation and agglutination Debris and other cellular components	Seminal plasma components Microbiologic contaminants
Sperm motility	Patterns of sperm motility	Duration of motility rating (% motile sperm)
	Computerized evaluation of sperm motility	Progressively motile and vibrating, circular and rolling movement; darting, rotating, asymmetric head and/or flagella Pathologic movement (circular, oscillating, shivering) whiplash motility with small radius Motility within moderate radius of about 20 m Curvilinear Progressiveness ratio 4–6 h after collection; 24 h after collection
Nonsperm cellular components	Leukocytes Erythrocytes Epithelial cells Round cells, medusa formation	
Sperm integrity and fertilizability	Zona-free hamster egg Hemizona assay Penetration in cervical mucus	Bovine, human, *in vivo, in vitro* Immunologic screening

TABLE 7–4. In Vitro Manipulation of Sperm

Technique	Procedure	Rationale
Sperm washing	Modified Ham's F-10 medium, Tyrodes salt solution, or other isotonic media, prewarmed and filtered before use	Retrograde ejaculation Cryopreserved semen and low sperm motility Oligozoospermia Presence of antisperm antibodies
Sperm swim up	Sperm pathologies, increased leukocytes	Decreased motility
Swim down	Reasonable sperm count Increase sperm quality	Oligozoospermia
Semen additive	Arginine, heparin, ionophore	PGE_1 and PGE_2
Mode of action of additives	Stabilize sperm membrane Initiate capacitation	Enhance sperm motility
Semen manipulation for IVF	Swim up and swim down *In vitro* capacitation	Possible separation of X- and Y-sperm Cryopreservation
Micromanipulation of sperm	Microfertilization	Micromanipulators used to introduce one or more sperm in pronuclear vesicle of ova; under the zona pellucida
	Microinsemination	Multiple sperm transfer using drilling of the zona for sperm transfer
	Flow sorting	Live sorting of X- and Y-sperm

IVF = in vitro fertilization.

infection often results in autoimmune orchitis affecting both testes. Vasectomy, the transsectioning and ligation of the vas deferens, also results in varying degrees of autoimmune orchitis. The severity of the orchitis depends on the species and the postoperative time. The autoimmune response of vasectomized males is thought

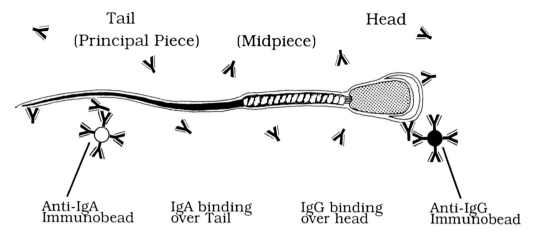

Tail
(Principal Piece)   (Midpiece)   Head

Anti-IgA
Immunobead
IgA binding
over Tail
IgG binding
over head
Anti-IgG
Immunobead

FIG. 7–12. Schematic drawing of the immunobead test for detection of antispermatozoal antibodies. Anti-IgA or anti-IgG covalently linked to polyacrylamide beads binds to IgA or IgG bound to the sperm surface. The amount of antisperm antibody is determined by the number of beads bound to the sperm surface. (Bronson, 1990.)

to occur because intermittent distention and rupture of the ligated duct results in release of spermatozoa into the peritoneal cavity.

As a result of autoimmunity, the seminal fluid concentration of antispermatozoal antibodies can be high. The antibodies are transported into semen from blood plasma in the secretions of the seminal vesicles and prostate. These antibodies, however, cannot enter the seminiferous tubules because of the blood–testis barrier. Thus, males with histologically normal seminiferous tubules can be infertile as a result of impairment by antibodies in the seminal fluid. Sperm cells that bind antibodies over their surface may retain their motility but be unable to penetrate cervical mucus. The antispermatozoal antibodies can result in agglutination of spermatozoa and formation of large clumps. Antibodies directed against spermatozoal antigens obviously can influence male fertility. These antibodies can be detected using immunobead binding with radiolabeled antiglobulins or by using sperm-immobilization and agglutination assays (Fig. 7–12).

Antisperm antibodies can interfere with spermatozoal functions through various pathways (Bronson, 1990):

1. Antibodies may interfere with various cell–cell interactive processes including sperm capacitation and hyperactivation, sperm attachment to cumulus mass, acrosome reaction, and penetration of zona pellucida.
2. Antibodies bound to sperm surface may inhibit survival and penetration of cervical mucus.
3. Autoantibodies to spermatozoa may interfere with spermatogenesis.

The amounts of immunoglobulins bound to ejaculated spermatozoa depend on several mechanisms:

1. The concentration of antispermatozoal antibodies in male accessory gland secretions
2. Local production of antibodies compared with transudation from blood
3. Binding of antibodies to spermatozoa in the epididymis before ejaculation versus that occurring when spermatozoa are mixed with seminal fluid

4. Elapsed time since the last ejaculation
5. Affinity antibody to the sperm surface

IN VITRO EVALUATION OF SEMEN QUALITY

Males should be evaluated for seminal quality before use as breeding animals (Table 7–2). Once semen has been collected from the male, several approaches may be used to assess the quality of the sample. Classic semen evaluation techniques, as well as the new automated semen assessment technologies, yield only estimates of potential fertilizing capacity of spermatozoa. Several *in vitro* methods can be used to assist in determining the specific causes of unexplained cases of male infertility (Table 7–3). Various techniques for micromanipulation of spermatozoa (Table 7–4) can be used to enhance the reproductive potential of genetically superior males.

REFERENCES

Ablin, R.J. (1974). Immunologic properties of sex accessory tissue components. *In* Male Accessory Sex Organs. D. Brandes (ed.). New York, Academic Press.

Acott, T.S. and Carr, D.W. (1984). Inhibition of bovine spermatozoa by caudal epididymal fluid: (II) Interaction of pH and a quiescence factor. Biol. Reprod. *30*, 926–935.

Acott, T.S., Katz, D.F. and Hoskins, D.D. (1983). Movement characteristics of bovine epididymal spermatozoa: effects of forward motility protein and epididymal maturation. Biol. Reprod. *29*, 389–399.

Adashi, E.Y., Resnick, C.E., Hernandez, E.R., Hurwitz, A., Roberts, C.T., Leroith, D. and Rosenfeld, R. (1991). The intraovarian IGF system. *In* Serono Symposium. D.W. Schomberg (ed.). New York, Academic Press.

Amann, R.P. (1981). A critical review of methods for evaluation of spermatogenesis from seminal characteristics. J. Androl. *2*, 37–58.

Bedford, J.M. (1975). Maturation, transport, and fate of spermatozoa in the epididymis. *In* Handbook of Physiology, Section 7, Endocrinology, Vol. V, Male Reproductive System. R.O. Greep and E.B. Astwood (eds.). Washington, D.C., American Physiological Society.

Berndtson, W.E. and Dejardins, C. (1974). The cycle of the seminiferous epithelium and spermatogenesis in the bovine testis. Am. J. Anat. *140*, 167–180.

Blanc, M.R., Hochereau-de Reviers, M.T., Cahoreau, C., Courot, M. and Dacheux, J.C. (1981). Inhibin: effects on gonadotropin secretion and testis function in ram and rat. *In* Intragonadal Regulation of Reproduction. P. Franchimont and C.P. Channing (eds.). New York, Academic Press.

Bloom, D. and Fawcett, D.W. (1975). A Textbook of Histology. Philadelphia, W.B. Saunders.

Bronson, R.A. (1990). Immunology. *In* Infertility: A Comprehensive Text. M.M. Seibel (ed.). Norwalk, CT, Appleton-Lange.

Clermont, Y. (1963). The cycle of the seminiferous epithelium in man. Am. J. Anat. *112*, 35–45.

Cosentino, M.J. and Takihara, H., Burhop, J.W. and Cockett, A.T. (1984). Regulation of rat caput epididymidis contractility by prostaglandins. J. Androl. *5*, 216–222.

Dorrington, J.H. and Armstrong, D.T. (1975). Follicle-stimulating hormone stimulates estradiol-17β synthesis in cultured Sertoli cells. Proc. Natl. Acad. Sci. *72*, 2677–2681.

Earp, S. (1991). The epidermal growth factor receptor: control of synthesis and signaling function. *In* Serono Symposium. D.E. Schomberg (ed.). New York, Academic Press.

Fawcett, D.W. (1974). Interactions between Sertoli cells and germ cells. *In* Male Fertility and Sterility. Proc. of the Serono Symposia, Vol. 5. R.E. Mancini and L. Martini (eds.). New York, Academic Press.

Fawcett, D.W. (1975). Ultrastructure and function of the Sertoli cell. *In* Handbook of Physiology, Sec. 7, Endocrinology, Vol. V, Male Reproductive System, R.O. Greep and E.B. Astwood (eds.), Washington, D.C., American Physiological Society.

Fawcett, D.W. (1979). Contraception: Science, Technology and Application. Proc. of a Symposium Div. of Med. Sci., Assembly of Life Sci., N.R.C., National Academy of Science, Washington, D.C.

Foote, R.H. (1980). Artificial insemination. *In* Reproduction in Farm Animals, 4th ed. E.S.E. Hafez (ed.). Philadelphia, Lea & Febiger.

Friberg, J. (1980). Mycoplasmas and ureaplasmas in infertility and abortions. Fertil. Steril. *33*, 351–359.

Ganjam, V.K. and Amann, R.P. (1976). Steroids in fluids and sperm entering and leaving the bovine epididymis, epididymal tissue and accessory sex gland secretions. Endocrinol. *99*, 1618–1630.

Garner, D.L. (1984). An overview of separation of X- and Y-spermatozoa-sexing. *In* Proceedings of the 10th Technical Conference, National Association of Animal Breeders, Columbia, MO, National Assoc Animal Breeders.

Garner, D.L., Gledhill, B.L., Pinkel, D., Lake, S., Stephenson, D., Van Dilla, M.A. and Johnson, L.A. (1983). Quantification of the X- and Y-chromosome-bearing spermatozoa of domestic animals by flow cytometry. Biol. Reprod. *28:* 312–321.

Garner, D.L. and Hafez, E.S.E. (1986). Spermatozoa and seminal plasma. *In* Reproduction in Farm Animals, 5th ed. E.S.E. Hafez (ed.). Philadelphia, Lea & Febiger.

Gilbert, A.B. (1980). Poultry. *In* Reproduction in Farm Animals, 4th ed. E.S.E. Hafez (ed.). Philadelphia, Lea & Febiger.

Gledhill, B.L. (1971). Changes in deoxyribonucleoprotein in relation to spermateliosis and epididymal maturation of spermatozoa. J. Reprod. Fertil. Suppl. *13,* 77–88.

Green, D.P.L. and Purves, R.D. (1984). Mechanical hypothesis of sperm penetration. Biophysical J. *45,* 659.

Hafs, H.D. and McCarthy, M.S. (1978). Endocrine control of testicular function. *In* Beltsville Symposium in Agricultural Research 3, Animal Reproduction. H.W. Hawk (ed.). New York, Halsted Press, pp. 345–364.

Hamner, C.E., 1970. The semen. *In* Reproduction and Breeding Techniques for Laboratory Animals. E.S.E. Hafez (ed.). Philadelphia, Lea & Febiger.

Hansson, V., Weddinton, S.C., French, F.S., McLean, W., Smith, A., Nayfeh, S.N., Ritzen, E.M. and Hagenas, L. (1976). Secretion and role of androgen-binding proteins in the testis and epididymis. J. Reprod. Fertil. Suppl. *24,* 17–33.

Hargrove, J.L., MacIndoe, J.H. and Ellis, L.C. (1977). Testicular contractile cells and sperm transport. Fertil. Steril. *28,* 1146–1157.

Hoskins, D.D. and Casillas, E.R. (1973). Function of cyclic nucleotides in mammalian spermatozoa. *In* Handbook of Physiology, Section 7, Endocrinology, Vol. V, Male Reproductive System. R.O. Greep and E.B. Astwood (eds.). Washington D.C., American Physiological Society, pp. 453–460.

Johnson, L.A., Flook, J.P. and Hawk, H.W. (1989). Sex preselection in rabbits: live births from X and Y sperm separated by DNA and cell sorting. Biol. Reprod. *41:* 199–203.

Johnson, M. and Everitt, B. (1984). Essential Reproduction, 2nd ed. Blackwell Scientific Publications.

Kaltenback, C.C. and Dunn, T.G. (1980). Endocrinology of reproduction. *In* Reproduction in Farm Animals, 4th ed. E.S.E. Hafez (ed.). Philadelphia, Lea & Febiger.

Koehler, J.K., Berger, R.E., Smith, D. and Karp, L. (1982). Spermophagy. *In* Atlas of Human Reproduction by Scanning Electron Microscopy. E.S.E. Hafez and P. Kenemans (eds.). Lancaster, England, MTP Press.

Lake, P.E. (1971). The male in reproduction. *In* Physiology and Biochemistry of the Domestic Fowl. D.J. Bell and B.M. Freeman (eds.). New York, Academic Press.

Mann, T. (1975). Biochemistry of semen. *In* Handbook of Physiology, Section 7, Endocrinology, Vol. V, Male Reproductive System. R.O. Greep and E.B. Astwood (eds.). Washington, DC, American Physiological Society.

Mann, T. and Lutwak-Mann, C. (1981). Male Reproductive Function and Semen. New York, Springer-Verlag.

Perey, B., Clermont, Y. and Leblond, C.P. (1961). The wave of the seminiferous epithelium in the rat. Am. J. Anat. *108,* 47–77.

Quinn, P.J., White, I.G. and Wirrick, B.R. (1965). Studies of the distribution of the major cations in semen and male accessory secretions. J. Reprod. Fertil. *10,* 379–388.

Rappolee, D.A., Sturm, K.S., Schultz, G.A., Pedersen, R.A. and Werh, Z. (1989). The expression of growth factor ligands and receptors in preimplantation mouse embryos. *In* Early Embryo Development and Paracrine Relationships. S. Heyner and L. Wiley (eds.). New York, Alan R. Liss. pp. 11–26.

Schanbacher, B.D. (1984). Hormonal regulation of the male pituitary. *In* Proc. 10th Int. Congress on Animal Reprod. and Artif. Insem., Urbana-Champaign, Vol. IV, pp. I1–I8.

Setchell, B.P. (1977). Male reproductive organs and semen. *In* Reproduction in Domestic Animals. H.H. Cole and P.T. Cupps (eds.), New York, Academic Press.

Setchell, B.P. (1978). The Mammalian Testis. Ithaca, Cornell University Press.

Setchell, B.P. (1980). The functional significance of the blood-testis barrier. J. Androl. *1,* 3–10.

Setchell, B.P., Scott, T.W., Voglmayr, J.K. and Waites, G.M.H. (1969). Characteristics of testicular spermatozoa and the fluid which transports them into the epididymis. Biol. Reprod. *1,* 40–66.

Shivaji, S., Bharagava, P.M. and Scheit, K.H. (1984). Immunological identification of seminalplasmin in tissue extracts of sex glands of bull. Biol. Reprod. *30,* 1237–1241.

Swierstra, E.E. (1968). Cytology and duration of the cycle of the seminiferous epithelium of the boar; duration of spermatozoan transit through the epididymis. Anat. Rec. *161,* 171–185.

Usselman, M.C. and Cone, R.A. (1983). Rat sperm are mechanically immobilized in caudal epididymis by "immobilin," a high molecular weight glycoprotein. Biol. Reprod. *29,* 1241–1253.

White, I.G. (1980). Secretion of the male reproductive tract and seminal plasma. *In* Reproduction in Farm Animals, 4th ed. E.S.E. Hafez (ed.). Philadelphia, Lea & Febiger.

8
Fertilization, Cleavage, and Implantation

F.W. BAZER, R.D. GEISERT, AND M.T. ZAVY

FERTILIZATION

Ovum Maturation

The ovum resumes the process of meiosis from prophase I of the first meiotic division as it begins to mature during folliculogenesis. In most species the ovum is in metaphase II of the second meiotic division when ovulated; however, ova of the horse, dog, and fox are only in their first meiotic division at the time of ovulation. Ovum maturation and meiosis are not completed until after fertilization, when the ovum becomes a zygote.

Sperm Maturation

Spermatozoa require maturational changes that occur during a 10- to 15-day passage through the epididymis, after which fertilization is possible. Spermatozoa maturational changes depend on epididymal secretions and transport time, which are essential for sperm to fertilize the ovum. Sperm maturation is one of three events that spermatozoa must undergo before fertilization can be accomplished. Although sequential, sperm capacitation and the acrosome reaction are two separate events necessary for sperm–ovum fusion.

Capacitation. Chang (1951) and Austin (1951) first observed that sperm must reside in the female reproductive tract before becoming capable of attaching to and penetrating the ovum. This process was termed *sperm capacitation* and is believed to start in the uterus; however, the major site of capacitation appears to be the oviduct, specifically, the isthmic region. Sperm surface components may be modified or removed by genital tract secretions causing the phospholipid bilayer to become destabilized, permitting acrosomal activation. Such changes may include depletion of sperm cholesterol at the sperm surface, alteration in glycosaminoglycans, and changes in ions as sperm traverse the genital tract (Fig. 8–1). Capacitation leads to acrosomal changes needed for sperm penetration of the ovum investments. Therefore, capacitation functions to prevent premature acrosome activation until the spermatozoa reach the site of fertilization and come in contact with the ovum. The true acrosome reaction involves fusion of the sperm plasma membrane with the outer acrosomal membrane (Fig. 8–2) followed by extensive vesiculation over the anterior segment of the acrosome (Bedford, 1983). This differs from the "false" acrosome reaction that occurs during senescence or degeneration of sperm. Fusion and vesiculation of the acrosome release hydrolytic enzymes, for example, hyaluronidase and acrosin implicated in penetration of the ovum.

Interaction of Sperm and Ovum

The fertile life spans of sperm and ovum (Table 8–1) dictate synchronous insemina-

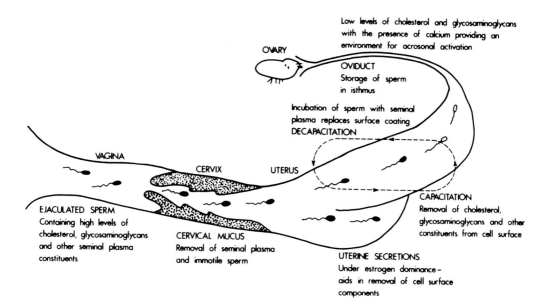

FIG. 8–1. Events in sperm capacitation during transport through the female genital tract. (Drawn by Dr. Geisert.)

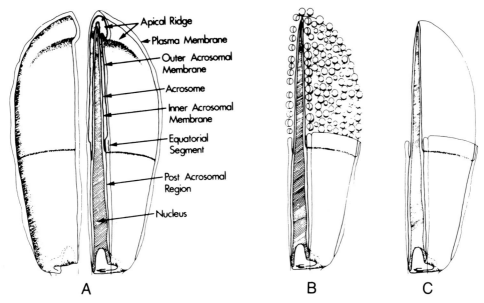

FIG. 8–2. The sequence of events during acrosome reaction in mammalian spermatozoa. *A,* Intact plasma and acrosomal membrane of an unreacted spermatozoon. *B,* Initiation of the acrosome reaction showing multiple fusion points between the plasma membrane and outer acrosomal membrane. Fusion leaves the appearance of numerous vesicles over the cell surface. Note that fusion is absent in the equatorial and postacrosomal regions. Acrosomal enzymes involved with ovum penetration are released and exposed on the inner acrosomal membrane. *C,* The acrosome swells and is eventually lost during penetration of the zona pellucida, leaving only the inner acrosomal membrane exposed on the upper portion of the sperm head. (Adapted from R.G. Saacke and J.M. White, (1972) Proc. 4th Tech. Conf. A.I. and Reprod., Trinto, Italy pp. 22–27.)

TABLE 8–1. Time of Events in Early Embryonic Development

	Species			
Parameter	Cattle	Horse	Sheep	Swine
Gamete Longevity (hours)				
Sperm	30–48	72–120	30–48	34–72
Ovum	20–24	6–8	16–24	8–10
Embryonic Development (days)*				
2-cell	1	1	1	.6–.8
4-cell	1.5	1.5	1.3	1
8-cell	3	3	1.5	2.5
Blastocyst	7–8	6	6–7	5–6
Hatching	9–11	8	7–8	6
Blastocyst transport to uterus				
Hours	72–84	140–144†	66–72	46–48
Cell stage	8–16	Blastocyst	8–16	4
Blastocyst elongation (days)	13–21	NE‡	11–16	11–15
Initial placentation (days)	22	37	15	13
Birth (days)	278–290	335–345	145–155	112–115

*Days after ovulation.
†Unfertilized ova remain in the oviduct.
‡No elongation occurs to form filamentous blastocysts.

tion and ovulation to achieve high conception rates. Females ovulate at various times after onset of estrus. Spermatozoa longevity in the female reproductive tract appears related to the length of estrus. For example, swine and horse sperm have greater longevity than do that of sheep and cattle. Longevity of sperm in the pig and horse increases the probability of viable sperm being present at ovulation when insemination occurs well in advance of ovulation. Regardless of the timing of ovulation, high conception rates result if spermatozoa are present in the oviduct shortly before ovulation. Insemination too early reduces conception rates, which results from loss of sperm viability and the number of sperm at the site of fertilization, whereas loss of ovum viability can result from insemination after ovulation even though fertilization occurs.

Although the male ejaculates billions of sperm into the female reproductive tract, approximately 1,000 to 10,000 spermatozoa are present in the isthmus and only 10 to 100 sperm may be in the ampulla after 4 to 12 hours. Low numbers of sperm in the oviduct do not result from slow sperm transport but rather from their controlled movement into the ampulla by the uterotubal junction and lower isthmus (in the pig) as well as from their movement from the vagina and cervix into the uterus (in ruminants). This relationship regulates the number of spermatozoa at the fertilization site (preventing polyspermy), while providing a sperm reservoir to ensure that capacitated sperm are present until ovulation.

The ability of sperm to adhere and release from the epithelial lining of the ampulla may assist in maintaining adequate numbers of sperm at the site of fertilization (Suarez et al., 1990). When present in the ampulla, spermatozoa become hyperactivated, which increases the probability that they will make contact with the ovum. Although the complete roles of the oviduct and its lumenal contents in ensuring fertilization are not understood, the process is efficient because fertilization rates in all domestic species exceed 90%.

Sperm–Oocyte Encounter. Fertilization in mammals requires three critical events: (a) sperm migration between cumulus cells (if present); (b) sperm attachment and migration through the zona pellucida; and (c) fusion of sperm and ovum plasma membranes.

There is evidence that a substance produced by the cumulus oophorus of rabbit ova may stimulate sperm motility. This factor may play a secondary role in the sperm–ovum encounter since peristaltic contractions of the ampulla increase the chance of ovum–sperm contact (Yanagamachi, 1981). Although necessary in rodents, the role of cumulus cells in sperm attachment has been debated in domestic animals (especially the cow), since they are usually absent 3 to 4 hours after ovulation. Hyaluronidase, present in the bull acrosome, would allow penetration of the cumulus oophorus. Arylsulfatase from boar acrosome also causes cells of the cumulus oophorus to disperse. Therefore, enzymes necessary for cumulus penetration or dispersion are present in these species.

Sperm Attachment. Attachment of the sperm head to the zona pellucida appears to be regulated by receptor sites on the zona surface. Treatment of ova with anti-zona antibodies or the proteolytic enzyme trypsin blocks sperm attachment or binding to the zona pellucida (Fig. 8–3). Binding of sperm to the zona pellucida can also be inhibited by pretreatment of sperm with antisperm antibodies or glycoproteins extracted from the zona pellucida. Antibodies to sperm or zona pellucida, therefore, block or mask sperm receptor sites on sperm and zona surfaces.

The specific sperm receptor in the zona pellucida has been identified as one of the three major glycoproteins that form the extracellular matrix of the zona pellucida. The three glycoproteins, identified as ZP1, ZP2, and ZP3, are synthesized by maturing oocytes, and although variation in these proteins exists, they appear to be present in all mammalian species. The ZP3 functions as the sperm receptor to which only sperm with an intact acrosome can bind. Binding of sperm to the sperm receptors occurs through an interaction with O-linked oligosaccharides on ZP3. The presence of glycosyl transferase, proteinases, and glycosidases on the plasma membrane covering the sperm head could result in binding to ZP3 through a lock and key mechanism such as that for an enzyme and its substrate (Wassarman, 1990).

Sperm Penetration. Penetration of the zona by spermatozoa occurs within 5 to

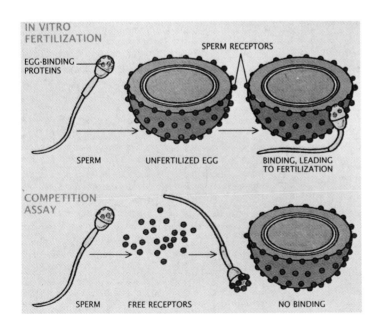

FIG. 8–3. The protein ZP3 in the zona pellucida is the sperm receptor. Exposure of sperm to unfertilized ova results in sperm binding to ZP3 (top). In the competition assay (bottom), sperm are incubated with ZP3 first and then exposed to ova; however, the sperm are unable to bind to the ZP3 proteins on the zona pellucida because their ZP3 binding proteins are already occupied (blocked) by the free ZP3 to which the sperm were introduced before introduction of ova. (Reproduced from Paul M. Wassarman (1988). Scientific American December, p. 83).

IN VITRO FERTILIZATION

SPERM RECEPTORS

EGG-BINDING PROTEINS

SPERM   UNFERTILIZED EGG   BINDING, LEADING TO FERTILIZATION

COMPETITION ASSAY

SPERM   FREE RECEPTORS   NO BINDING

15 minutes after sperm attachment. The acrosome reaction may occur before or after attachment of the sperm head to the glycoprotein receptors on the zona, but an acrosome-intact sperm is essential for attachment. Binding of the sperm head to ZP3 allows interactions with other zona components that stimulate acrosome activation. The acrosome reaction allows release of zona lysin by which spermatozoa digest a path through the zona pellucida to the vitelline membrane. The mammalian acrosome contains enzymes such as hyaluronidase, proacrosin (an inactive form of acrosin), esterases, phospholipase A_2, acid phosphatases, aryl sulphatases, β-N-acetyl glucosaminidase, aryl amidase, and nonspecific acid proteinases; however, quantitative and qualitative differences exist between species.

Acrosin was long considered the essential zona lysin for sperm penetration, but the number of enzymes present in or attached to the acrosomal membrane suggests that a combination of enzymes acts synergistically during penetration. This is consistent with the heterogenous glycoprotein structure of the zona pellucida. Enzymes exposed during the acrosome reaction are needed for the passage of sperm through the zona, but sperm motility is also required (Yanagimachi, 1981). As acrosomal reacted sperm initiate zona pellucida penetration, the glycoprotein ZP2 may serve as a secondary sperm receptor to maintain sperm attachment during passage through the zona.

Gamete Fusion. The vitelline membrane may have less specificity than the zona pellucida in binding foreign spermatozoa; however, some degree of selectivity is apparent since the plasma membrane of the ovum will competitively bind more homologous spermatozoa.

The acrosome reaction is a prerequisite for fusion between ova and spermatozoa plasma membranes, and zona free ova cannot undergo fusion with nonacrosomal activated sperm even though attachment to the membrane surface occurs. Acro-

some activation *in vivo*, however, occurs by the time of sperm attachment and penetration of the zona. Once the sperm has traversed the zona pellucida, the head moves into the vitelline space and contacts the vitelline membrane (Fig. 8–4). Motility

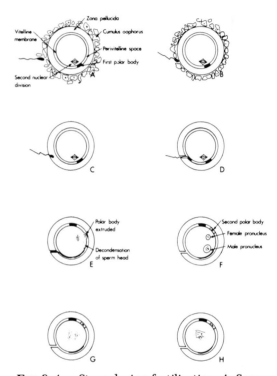

FIG. 8–4.   Steps during fertilization. *A,* Spermatozoon first encounters and penetrates the cumulus oophorus. First polar body is present in the perivitelline space with the metaphase spindle of the secondary oocyte present in the cytoplasm. *B,* The spermatozoon, having undergone acrosomal activation, inner acrosomal membrane contacts the zona pellucida, where enzymes exposed on the membrane surface allow penetration into the perivitelline space (*C* and *D*). *E,* The equatorial region of the sperm head attaches and fuses with the vitelline membrane stimulating completion of the second meiotic division. *F,* The large male pronucleus and smaller female pronucleus form following extrusion of the second polar body. *G,* The pronuclei migrate to the oocyte center, where the nuclear envelopes disperse and prophase of the first mitosis division begins (*F*). (Adapted from McLaren, A. (1980). *In* Reproduction in Farm Animals 4th Ed., E.S.E Hafez (ed.) Philadelphia, Lea & Febiger, p. 229.)

of the spermatozoan tail propels the sperm into the vitelline space, rotating the vitelline membrane within the zona pellucida.

The vitelline membrane is covered by dense microvilli, except for an elevated area adjacent to the surface where the second polar body will be extruded after fertilization. Sperm attachment is seldom observed in this area of the vitelline membrane. Attachment of spermatozoa occurs initially at the equatorial segment of the sperm head with either the microvilli or the intervillous area of the vitelline membrane. Fusion of sperm and egg does not involve the inner acrosomal membrane of the anterior region, but it does involve the plasma membrane over the equatorial segment and postacrosomal region of the sperm head. Subsequently, the surface of the equatorial region of the sperm is incorporated into the plasma membrane of the ovum. The equatorial region of the sperm plasma membrane becomes intermixed with the ovum plasma membrane and can be identified in the egg membrane as late as the eight-cell stage.

Block to Polyspermy. Immediately following fertilization, the ovum surface changes to prevent fusion of additional spermatozoa. When this mechanism fails, polyspermic fertilization can result with formation of polyploid embryos (Hunter, 1976) that undergo embryonic death or abnormal development. The block to polyspermy is at the zona pellucida in most mammals (e.g., sheep, swine) with a secondary physiologic block at the vitelline membrane in some species (e.g., rabbit). Initiation of the block is at sperm penetration of the ovum when cortical granules are released into the perivitelline space. Release of the content of these granules results in extensive reorganization of the zona pellucida and/or vitelline surface referred to as the "cortical reaction." The cortical reaction results in the release of enzymes that cause hardening of the zona pellucida and inactivation of sperm recep-

tors (ZP3). Enzymatic digestion of the O-linked oligosaccharides on ZP3 would remove specific carbohydrates involved in zona binding of sperm. Proteolysis of ZP2 may also alter physical characteristics of the zona to prevent further penetration of accessory sperm.

Although physiologic polyspermy is common in birds and reptiles, the incidence of polyspermy in most mammalian species is only 1 or 2% (McLaren, 1974). The pig appears most susceptible to polyspermy, especially as a result of delayed mating or insemination when up to 15% of the eggs are penetrated by more than one spermatozoan. In sheep, Killeen and Moore (1970) found that late insemination, that is, 36 to 48 hours after onset of estrus was associated with abnormal fertilized eggs in which 39% were polyspermic or contained multinucleated blastomeres.

Development of Pronuclei and Syngamy. On penetration of the vitelline membrane by the spermatozoan, the activated ovum completes meiosis and expels the first and/or second polar body into the perivitelline space (Fig. 8–4). The remaining maternal haploid chromosomes are then enclosed by a pronucleus.

Following fusion with the egg plasma membrane, the spermatozoan nuclear envelope disintegrates and the released chromatin material undergoes decondensation (Fig. 8–4). The sperm nuclear envelope is rapidly replaced by a new envelope within the ovum cytoplasm, forming the male pronucleus. Decondensation of the sperm nuclear envelope appears to require specific components in cytoplasm of the ovum. Immature cow oocytes are unable to decondense the sperm nuclei even when matured *in vitro*. The factor necessary for decondensation has been termed *male pronucleus growth factor* or, in the hamster, *sperm nucleus-decondensing factor*.

Male and female pronuclei migrate to the ovum center, which is probably due to rearrangements in the cytoskeletal framework of the ovum after activation. Once the male and female pronuclei are in close proximity, the nuclear envelopes disperse, allowing intermixing of the chromosomes.

Associated with these events is the initiation of DNA synthesis from cytoplasmic precursors. The chromosomes then aggregate in prophase of the first cleavage division, resulting in formation of a zygote and restoration of the diploid state. Thus, the process of fertilization allows combining of maternal and paternal hereditary elements.

During fusion of sperm and egg, sperm constituents from the cell membranes and sperm head are released into the ooplasm. The importance and fate of these sperm products are not known. The proximal centriole of the sperm tail forms one of the zygote's centrioles. Although possible in theory, attempts to produce homozygous diploid (two male or female pronuclei) mice have failed (Surani and Barton, 1983). Contributions from both the male and female pronuclei appear necessary for normal embryonic development.

Interspecies Fertilization. Interspecies fertilization has been demonstrated only between the snowshoe hare and rabbit, mink and ferret, sheep and goat, and horse and donkey. In addition, *Bos taurus* and *Bos indicus*, European and Asian domestic cattle, will readily produce fertile hybrids that demonstrate a greater disease resistance and heat tolerance than *Bos taurus* cattle. Domestic cattle and American Bison (Bison bison) have also been crossed successfully to produce a hybrid that may have superior cold resistance and forage use capability. Failure in the hybridization process can occur during fertilization and/or cleavage so that successful interspecies fertilization is rare. Development of semen and egg collection methods followed by successful *in vitro* fertilization techniques allow this problem to be addressed. Results using these techniques indicate that from the time of the early cleavage divisions to blastocyst formation the mammalian ovum is tolerant of a foreign environment. After this time,

hybrids succumb, which indicates their dependence on highly specific conditions during the postblastocyst period.

When successful hybridization has been demonstrated, there are marked differences in the success of reciprocal crosses such that a high rate of fertilization is possible in one direction but not in the other; that is, a male snowshoe hare and female rabbit is successful, but a female snowshoe hare and male rabbit is much less so. Fertilization failure between different species is not primarily a result of differences in genetic constitution of sperm or egg but is attributed to genetically determined differences in the physiologic constitution of these gametes in the genital tract.

The importance of the trophoblast in the maintenance of pregnancy has been demonstrated in studies involving interspecies pregnancy, and immunologic involvement has been implicated in the failure of a portion of such pregnancies. This problem has been circumvented using the techniques of embryo micromanipulation. Blastomeres from early (four- to eight-cell) sheep and goat embryos were used to construct chimeric embryos. Blastomeres were positioned so that the outside cells were from the species into which the embryos would be transferred. Trophoblast components, which originate from the outer cell layer, were able to protect cells from the foreign species positioned on the inner cell layer, which gives rise to the embryonic tissues proper. Thus, maternal immune rejection of cells from the "foreign" species could be prevented and the pregnancy maintained.

CLEAVAGE

After the zygote stage, embryos enter into several mitotic divisions. The zygote, or one-cell stage, is quite large, having a low nuclear/cytoplasmic ratio. To attain a ratio similar to somatic cells, cell divisions are without an increase in cell mass. This process is referred to as cleavage. Growth during this period may be considered negative since cellular mass decreases from

20% in the cow to 40% in sheep; however, nuclei do increase in size, and the proper amount of nucleic acid is maintained in the chromosomes (McLaren, 1974). Since cells of mammalian embryos contain little yolk (except for swine and horses), they rely on the mother for much of their metabolic support during early pregnancy. This is provided by oviductal and uterine secretions (histotroph). During early cleavage there is little increase in metabolic rate, but a sharp rise occurs between the morula and blastocyst stage.

Normal Time Course

Cleavage of the zygote is by vertical division through the main axis of the egg from animal (site of polar body extrusion) to vegetal (area of yolk reserve) pole. The cleavage furrow often goes through the area where the pronuclei resided at the initiation of syngamy. The resulting daughter cells are called *blastomeres.* The plane of the second division is also vertical and passes through the main axis but at a right angle to the initial plane of cleavage, producing four blastomeres. The third cleavage division occurs approximately at a right angle to the second, producing eight blastomeres. This doubling sequence is carried on through the remainder of early cleavage. The initial cleavage divisions usually occur simultaneously in all the blastomeres, but the synchronization is inevitably lost and blastomeres start dividing independently of each other.

Cleavage divisions are always mitotic with each daughter cell (blastomere) receiving the full assortment of chromosomes. Mammals and other vertebrates exhibit an indeterminate plan of cleavage in which the developmental ability of the early blastomeres is not as tightly controlled as in the lower animal species. Blastomeres from a two-cell embryo have the developmental latitude to form two healthy offspring; whereas in lower animals with a determinate plan of cleavage, this manipulation would result in an abnormal or partially formed embryo.

Blastomeres from the two- to eight-cell stage in the rabbit are totipotent, that is, fully capable of giving rise to an intact embryo. Totipotency of sheep blastomeres is maintained up to the eight-cell stage (Papaioannou and Ebert, 1986). In four-cell embryos no more than three of four blastomeres are totipotent and in eight-cell embryos no more than one of eight blastomeres is totipotent. After this time, however, the blastomeres appear to differentiate according to their position in the morula.

While blastomeres are encased within the zona pellucida, they must accommodate themselves to this limited area. Once the embryo has formed 8 to 16 blastomeres, but in some cases more, it is referred to as a *morula,* because of its resemblance to a mulberry. Segregation of the inner and outer cells of the 16-cell mouse embryo (or morula) may be initiated by morphogenic changes occurring at the 8-cell stage. At this time, blastomeres flatten on each other to form a rounded embryo and internal cellular components, and surface microvilli become asymmetrically positioned in a process termed *polarization.* The combined processes of flattening of the blastomeres and polarization are referred to as "compaction." Before the 16-cell stage, there is variability in the rate of compaction among embryos as well as in the time of its onset (Sutherland et al., 1990). The compaction process is gradual and may begin as early as the 4-cell stage or as late as the 16-cell stage and is normally completed by the end of the 16-cell stage. The variability in the rate at which compaction occurs is apparently unrelated to viability of the embryo.

The polarization hypothesis states that the asymmetry between the apical and basal aspects of the blastomeres at the 8-cell stage provides the basis for the differences between the inner and outer cells of the morula. The way in which the plane of division occurs during the fourth cleavage division, that is, 8- to 16-cell stage, could segregate the structurally different regions of the 8-cell blastomeres into heterogenous populations. In this situation, division planes that occurred parallel to the blastomere surface or across the axis of polarity would split the blastomere into two daughter cells having different morphologic and behavioral characteristics. In support of this hypothesis, Sutherland et al. (1990) demonstrated that during the fourth cleavage division in mice there were three major division plane orientations; anticlinal (perpendicular to the outer surface of the blastomere); periclinal (parallel to the outer surface of the blastomere); and oblique (at an angle between the other two (Fig. 8–5). The relative number of inner and outer cells in the 16-cell morula would, therefore, depend on the proportion of the types of divisions during the fourth cleavage. By tracing the lineages of four- and eight-cell blastomeres, Sutherland et al. found that the division order of the blastomeres during third or fourth cleavage was associated with the division order of the parent blastomeres during the previous cleavage. Earlier dividing eight-cell blastomeres had a slightly greater tendency to undergo either periclinal or oblique divisions than anticlinal divisions, and this may contribute slightly more descendants overall to the inner cell population in the morula and eventually to the inner cell mass (ICM) of the blastocyst. Similar studies have not been conducted with embryos of domestic species; however, some preimplantation pig embryos have inner cells by the 12- to 16-cell stage (Papaioannou and Ebert, 1988). The proportion of inner cells was low in morula but increased during differentiation of the ICM and trophectoderm in early blastocysts. The proportion of ICM cells then decreased as blastocysts expanded and hatched.

Tight junctions form within the trophoblast layer of 8- to 16-cell mouse embryos (Ducibella, 1977) when the blastomeres are in close apposition during the process of compaction (Fig. 8–6). The formation of tight junctions provides a permeability

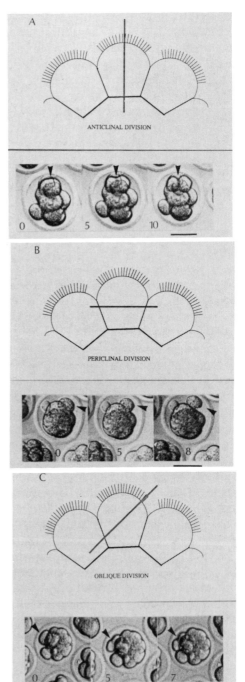

FIG. 8–5. A diagrammatic representation of the "polarization hypothesis," which indicates the lineage of cells contributing to the trophectoderm and inner cell mass during the early cleavage stages of the embryo (From Sutherland, A.E., Speed, T.P. and Calarco, P.G. (1990). Dev. Biol. *137*, 13–25.) Blastomeres may divide in three major division planes, which are called anticlinal (A), periclinal (B) and oblique (C).

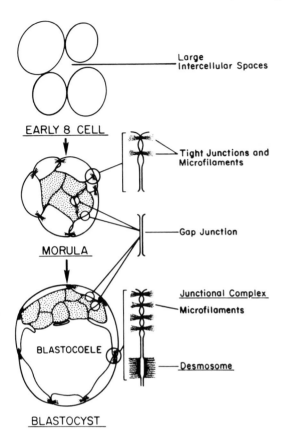

EARLY 8 CELL

Large Intercellular Spaces

Tight Junctions and Microfilaments

MORULA

Gap Junction

BLASTOCOELE

Junctional Complex
Microfilaments

Desmosome

BLASTOCYST

FIG. 8–6. Development of intercellular junctions in preimplantation mouse embryo. Tight junctions act as focal points for membrane fusion, whereas gap junctions allow for intercellular communication. (From T. Ducibella (1977). Development in Mammals. Vol. I. M.H. Johnson (ed.). Amsterdam, North Holland.)

seal that allows fluid to move from the outside to the inside of the blastocyst without substantial leakage and to form the blastocoele. The formation of gap and tight junctions between presumptive trophoblast cells also appears to play an important role in separating cells from contact with the maternal environment, thereby allowing the blastocyst to positionally differentiate into two populations of cells. One population forms the inner cell mass and gives rise to the embryo proper, and the other gives rise to the trophectoderm or trophoblast, which forms the chorion. After this segregation has occurred and the blasto-

cyst has formed, the trophoblast cells become highly attenuated and organized into a simple squamous epithelium, the trophectoderm, and acquire the capacity to translocate organic and inorganic solutes and water from the uterine environment into the blastocoelic cavity.

Cleavage Rates and Variation

The lower region of the ampulla is the site of fertilization in most mammalian species. When the embryo has developed to the 8- to 16-cell stage (4-cell stage in the pig), it is transported into the uterus, where it continues to proliferate. The time embryos spend in the oviduct allows the uterus to prepare for the nutritive role that it must provide once the embryo comes into residence (Table 8–1).

The rate at which the developing embryo moves through the oviduct and into the uterus is thought to be entirely a maternal function controlled by factors that affect the muscular function of the isthmus, such as the local adrenergic system, which can be modified by estrogen and progesterone. Prostaglandins of the F series, acting locally, appear to impede transit of the embryo into the uterus, whereas prostaglandins of the E series appear to accelerate their delivery to the uterus.

Eggs are transported from the oviduct into the uterus whether or not fertilization has taken place, the horse being an exception. In the mare, unfertilized eggs remain within the isthmus and slowly degenerate over several months, while developing embryos pass by them and enter the uterus (Van Niekerk and Gerneke, 1966). The rate at which cleavage divisions progress is impacted by environmental and genetic influences. Warner et al. (1987) described a gene in preimplantation mouse embryos (preimplantation-embryo-development, or Ped gene) which is associated with the murine histocompatibility complex (MHC, or H-2, complex) which influences rate of cleavage of mouse embryos. This gene has two functional alleles, one for fast and one for slow rate of cleavage.

To date, a Ped gene has not been documented for domestic species. However, Bazer et al. (1988) reported that conceptus development in Chinese Meishan gilts, which are known for high prolificacy, was faster and more uniform than in gilts of normal prolificacy. These results suggest that Meishan conceptuses express genes that favor rapid and uniform development that results in higher rates of embryonic survival.

Expression of Genome

Gene expression during early mammalian development has largely been confined to work done with mouse and rabbit embryos in which net RNA content remains constant during early cleavage stages. At ovulation, mouse eggs contain rRNA, mRNA, tRNA, and ribosomes and are fully equipped to synthesize proteins. An ordered set of changes in the synthesis and modification of proteins occurs during oocyte maturation, fertilization, and development until the two-cell stage. Embryos proceed in their development from the first cleavage division—which is largely under the control of informational macromolecules accumulated during oogenesis—to the blastocyst stage, where there is an active transcription and accumulation of new mRNA from the zygote genome (see Schultz, 1986). In mice, the embryo becomes dependent on transcription just after the first cleavage division with a concomitant increase in synthesized protein occurring by the two-cell stage (Bolton et al., 1984). In sheep (Crosby et al., 1988), total protein synthesis is high during the first two cleavage divisions, decreases by 95% by the third cleavage division, remains low in the fourth cleavage division (8 to 16 cells) and increases again in the fifth cleavage division (16 to 32 cells). These results indicate that full activation of transcription in sheep embryos occurs in the fourth cleavage division. Similar findings have been reported for cow embryos (King et al., 1988). Shortly after initiation of embryogenesis, synthesis of all commonly identified classes of RNA is initiated. Ribosomal RNA, 4S-RNA (presumably tRNA) and 5S-RNA are synthesized by the four-cell stage, whereas heterogeneous nuclear RNA (probable precursor of mRNA) and polyadenylated RNA appear to be produced as early as the two-cell stage in mice. In addition, RNA polymerase type II, an enzyme associated with mRNA synthesis, has been identified at the two-cell stage, while polyribosomes containing newly synthesized RNA (presumptive mRNA) have been isolated from blastocyst and morula stages.

Messenger RNA is the template for protein synthesis. The appearance of gene products during embryonic development implies prior synthesis of their corresponding mRNAs and the presence of the translation apparatus. Embryonic gene products such as specific enzymes or antigens can be produced in different ways. For instance, these proteins could be produced at all stages in most, or all, embryonic cells. Proteins in this category include enzymes essential for normal metabolic activity as well as ubiquitous structural proteins such as actin, tubulin, and spectrin. In contrast, other proteins are synthesized at specific periods during development and are referred to as temporal gene products. For example, the serine protease plasminogen activator is present in trophoblast and primitive endoderm cells, absent in primitive ectoderm cells, and is only produced by rodents during the invasive phase of implantation. This protease has also been identified as a temporal product of swine, cow, and sheep (see Menino et al., 1989) embryos during peri-implantation development.

Proteins found in embryos could also represent a translation of transcripts synthesized during oogenesis and not during the early developmental period. Alternatively, genes could have been transcribed during oogenesis, but their mRNAs might not have been translated until after fertilization.

Studies concerning mechanisms for controlling expression of developmental gene products in domestic species are few, but it appears that regulation is at both the transcription and posttranscription levels. Extraembryonic regulatory signals such as hormones, metabolites, and ions may also have roles in the development program of embryonic cells. Preimplantation pig embryos express the proto-oncogene *fos* (*c-fos*) and receptors for insulin-like growth factor I and epidermal growth factor are present on trophectoderm of pig embryos. Simmen and Simmen (1991) suggest that peptide growth factors, their associated proteins (carrier proteins and membrane receptors), and proto-oncogenes (the normal, cellular counterparts of retroviral oncogenes) may play an important role in critical aspects of conceptus growth and uterine–conceptus interactions during the peri-implantation period. However, the exact function of these proteins in early embryonic development is unknown.

Parthenogenesis

Parthenogenesis, development of an egg without intervention of the sperm, occurs in many invertebrate species and in some vertebrate species. Early stages of parthenogenesis can be induced or may occur spontaneously; however, the activated eggs do not usually cleave more than twice before dying.

Mammalian oocytes and eggs do on occasion start developing into embryos in the absence of any detected stimulus. In such cases female germ cells may possess an inherent tendency to divide and differentiate, which is enhanced by fertilization or inducers of the parthenogenic response. Electrical stimulation, temperature shock, and hyaluronidase treatment have resulted in development to the blastocyst stage. Unfertilized eggs from some mammalian species initiate parthenogenesis as they begin to age and will often form a second polar body but are unable to cleave because of the degenerative state of the egg. Available evidence indicates that spontaneous parthenogenesis has never resulted in a successful term pregnancy in any mammalian species.

Studies with mice have shown that successful development of the fetal–placental unit to term requires genetic contributions from the maternal and paternal genomes. For example, activation of oocytes to generate a diploid parthenogenetic embryo having only a maternal genome will, at best, develop to the 25 somite stage and then die. Generation of one-cell embryos using nuclear transfer with two male pronuclei to form "androgenones" or with two female pronuclei to form "gynogenones" can be accomplished experimentally, but both fail to develop to term (Surani et al., 1987). Paternal and maternal contributions to the diploid genome of embryonic cells are necessary because they play complementary roles in the development process. Surani et al. (1987) demonstrated that the parental origin of chromosomes determines their influence during embryogenesis, and therefore contributions from parental genomes are not functionally equivalent during conceptus development. The gynogenones form apparently normal blastocysts more frequently than androgenones. Later in gestation, the gynogenones have poorly developed placentae and reasonably well developed fetuses, whereas androgenones have well-developed placentae but poorly developed fetuses. It should be noted that parthenogenetic and normal embryonic cells can be combined to form "chimeras" that can survive to term. Recently, Renard et al. (1991) used embryo reconstruction techniques with mouse embryos to produce gynogenetic and androgenetic haploid embryos from which blastomeres were obtained at the four-cell stage. Single blastomeres from the androgenones and gynogenones were then fused and allowed to form diploid doublets. Two or three of these doublets were then transferred to a foster mother and some developed to term. These results demonstrate for the first time that the participation of the paternal genome is not required before the eight-cell stage of embryonic development to obtain full-term development of mouse fetuses.

Twinning and Embryo Manipulation

Twinning in monotocous domestic species is most frequently of the dyzygotic type in which more than one egg is ovulated and the eggs are fertilized by different sperm, resulting in offspring no more identical than other full siblings. The twinning rate in domestic animals is affected by factors such as breed, age, and environment.

Among cattle, dairy breeds have twinning rates of about 3.5%, whereas in beef breeds, the average is less than 1.0%. Twin pregnancies, one conceptus per uterine horn, have no detrimental effect on calf viability; therefore, in cattle the major factor limiting increased multiple births appears to be ovulation rate. With twin pregnancy in cattle, fusion of the chorioallantois of adjacent conceptuses results in a common blood circulation. Therefore, 91% of heifers born co-twin with a male are sterile freemartins. Although rare, similar conditions have been reported in sheep, goats, and pigs.

Highly prolific ewes such as Finnsheep and Booroola Merino often produce two or more offspring per lambing. These ewes have a high ovulation rate which, in the Booroola Merino ewe, has been linked to a major F (fecundity) gene (Bindon and Piper, 1984). This gene may be responsible for elevated levels of FSH in both ewe lambs and adult ewes, an observation also reported for other prolific breeds of sheep.

The incidence of dyzygotic twins is 1 to 2% in thoroughbred mares and near 3% in draft-type mares. Double ovulations are fairly common in mares, but one or both embryos usually die early in development, while those that continue to develop are prone to abortion, mummification or, if born alive, neonatal death. Fetal death among twins *in utero* is often attributed to placental insufficiency or inadequate uter-ine capacity since total placental surface area of twins is only slightly greater than that of a single fetus. Twins occurring naturally reflect differences in ovulation rate as well as the ability of the female to maintain a twin pregnancy.

A major factor regulating the number of twin pregnancies is the number of eggs ovulated. Ovulation rate can be increased by exogenous gonadotropin (usually, equine chorionic gonadotropin, ECG) administration in cattle and sheep; however, ovarian response is variable and not conducive to twinning. When two ovulations occur unilaterally, the twin pregnancy rate is low, whereas when a single ovulation occurs on each ovary, the incidence of twinning is higher. This difference has been attributed to competition between embryos since transfer of two embryos to the same uterine horn leads to reduced numbers of cotyledonary attachments compared to results when one embryo was transferred to each uterine horn. A twinning rate of about 60% can be achieved using bilateral embryo transfer.

Immunization against ovarian steroids, particularly androstenedione or estrone, leads to a dramatic increase in the ovulation rate in ewes and to a lesser degree in cows. In ewes, the mean ovulation rate was increased by 0.6 ovulations per ewe, which resulted in an increase in the number of lambs reared. This process, however, results in increased embryonic deaths in sheep (Boland et al., 1986). Immunization against recombinant α-subunit of bovine inhibin results in a three- to four-fold increase in ovulation rate in sheep and a 35% increase in ovulation rate in pigs (see Brown et al., 1990).

Twins can also be monozygotic, in which case a single fertilized egg gives rise to two identical offspring. The incidence of naturally occurring monozygotic twins is rare with only a few species such as humans and cattle having well-documented occurrences. In cattle, monozygotic twins represent 10% or less of twins born. Monozygotic twins usually originate after implantation when the inner cell mass differentiates into two primitive streaks, giving rise to two identical offspring.

Nuclear transplantation involves the transfer of individual nuclei from preimplantation embryos to unfertilized mature oocytes and has been used successfully in the "cloning" of sheep, cow, and rabbit embryos, which has resulted in birth of viable offspring. Offspring produced by nuclear transfer may not be true clones, because most of the mitochondrial genome originates from the cytoplasm of the recipient oocyte. The principle behind this procedure is that nuclei from embryos contain all of the genetic information necessary to give rise to a complete individual having the same genetic makeup. As embryonic development proceeds, the genetic potential of nuclei become increasingly restricted as a result of differentiation, and they are no longer "totipotent" and can give rise only to specific tissues within the embryo. Nuclei can be transplanted to the cytoplasm of a mature oocyte. Factors within the cytoplasm of the mature oocyte "reprogram" the transplanted nucleus to allow it to give rise to a new embryo. Cytoplasm from pronuclear or two-cell embryos is not able to "reprogram" the transplanted nucleus. Initial results of cloning in rabbits and cows indicated that fewer than 4% and 1%, respectively, of the embryos developed to term. More recently, Willadsen et al. (1991), working with cattle, and Collas and Robl (1990), working with rabbits, have increased those percentages to 33% and 21%, respectively.

Production of monzygotic twins can also be achieved by microsurgical separation of blastomeres of two-cell embryos. The technical details of this are discussed in a later chapter.

EARLY EMBRYONIC DEVELOPMENT

Blastocyst Formation

Development of tight intercellular junctions of the morula during compaction is followed by accumulation of fluid within the central cavity forming the blastocoele. Fluid accumulation in the blastocoele results from the solute gradient established by active ion transport (Na^+/K^+ ATPase) and formation of tight junctional complexes between outer cells.

Differentiation of two distinct cell populations occurs after blastocyst formation (Fig. 8–7). The majority of cells form the outside peripheral cuboidal layer, termed *trophoblast* or *trophectoderm*, which is covered by dense microvilli and functions in selective nutrient uptake. Later in development, the trophoblast will form the chorion. A second group of cells residing at one pole beneath the trophoblast form the embryoblast (inner cell mass), which develops into three primary germ layers of the embryo (ectoderm, mesoderm, and endoderm) during the process of gastrula-

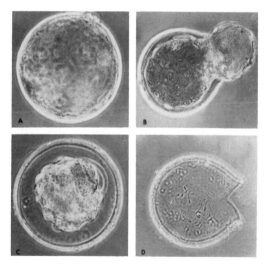

FIG. 8–7. Hatching of blastocyst. *A*, Blastocyst beginning to penetrate zona pellucida. *B*, Blastocyst escaping from zona pellucida. *C*, Blastocyst that collapsed after expanding and did not undergo hatching process. *D*, Empty zona pellucida remains after hatching. (All figures are approximately 240×.) (From D.L. Davis and B.N. Day. (1978) Cleavage and blastocyst formation by pigs in vitro. J. Anim. Sci. *46*, 1043.)

tion. The embryoblast does not remain beneath the trophectoderm in the pig but after hatching moves or digests the overlying trophoblast (Rauber's layer).

Zona Hatching

Release (hatching) of the blastocyst from the zona pellucida (Fig. 8–7) occurs in the uterus 4 to 8 days postovulation (Table 8–1). In the rabbit, zona removal occurs through an enzymatic (termed *blastolemmase*) dissolution of the zona layer by cells of the underlying trophoblast. Zona loss in the mouse may involve rhythmic expansions and contractions of the blastocyst aided by production of a zona lysin from the estrogen-sensitized uterine epithelium. Changes in zona integrity that are due to enzymatic factors produced by the uterus or embryo have been implicated in hatching of pig blastocysts (Linder and Wright, 1978). Exposure to the estrogen-stimulated uterine environment may cause a softening of the zona pellucida and allow the blastocyst to expand and rupture the zona layer. Expansion and contraction of the cow blastocyst appears to play the major role in hatching as the zona becomes torn by distension of the blastocyst, although enzymes involved with zona weakening may also play a role. The zona ruptures on the equatorial plane, allowing the blastocyst to squeeze between the two edges of the opening.

Expansion of the blastocyst involves both cellular hyperplasia and fluid accumulation in the blastocoele. Fluid accumulation within the blastocoele appears to be essential for hatching of mouse blastocysts. Circumstantial evidence suggests that prostaglandins (especially of the E series) are involved with the hatching process since prostaglandin antagonists prevent both blastocyst expansion and hatching (Biggers et al., 1978). Thus expansion of the blastocyst appears to be a vital process for zona hatching with production of uterine or blastocyst enzymatic factors playing a supporting role.

Blastocyst Elongation

Shedding of the zona pellucida is followed by a rapid phase of blastocyst development and growth. During this phase, an inner layer of extraembryonic endodermal cells originating from the embryoblast encloses the blastocoele, forming a bilaminar blastocyst (Fig. 8–8). The extraembryonic endoderm cells develop into a continuous membrane that will become a constituent of the yolk sac.

On day 11 postestrus in the sheep and pig and day 13 in the cow, the blastocyst undergoes a logarithmic elongation phase. The cow blastocyst transforms from a 3-mm spherical shape on approximately day 13 to a 25-cm filamentous threadlike form on day 17. By day 18 of gestation, the blastocyst has extended into the contralateral horn. This rapid lateral conceptus elongation in sheep and cattle occurs through continual hyperplasia of trophectoderm and extraembryonic endoderm. The developing embryoblast, which is still small in comparison to the extraembryonic layers, remains in the horn ipsilateral to the corpus luteum.

Rapid growth of cow and sheep blastocysts occurs over several days, but the rate of elongation of the pig blastocyst is unsurpassed. Pig blastocysts develop from 2-mm spheres on approximately day 10 of pregnancy to 10-mm tubular blastocysts on day 11 to 12 (Fig. 8–9). The tubular blastocysts transform (30 to 40 mm/hour) into a thin filamentous form that measures approximately 20 cm in length. This occurs by cellular reorganization rather than cellular hyperplasia. After this initial elongation phase, the pig blastocyst continues to increase in length and diameter as a result of cellular hyperplasia and reaches lengths of 800 to 1000 mm by day 16. Rapid elongation of the pig blastocyst coincides with blastocyst estrogen production and calcium release from the endometrial epithelium, which may stimulate the elongation process. Blastocyst production of the enzyme plasminogen activator may also reg-

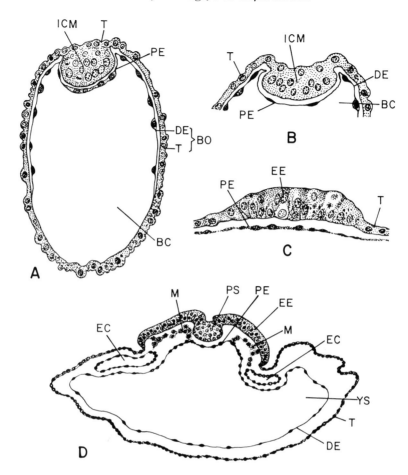

FIG. 8–8. Gastrulation in sheep. *A*, Section of sheep blastocyst 10 days postcoitum. The endoderm can be seen lining the upper half of the blastocyst cavity. *B*, A slightly older blastocyst than A. The inner cell mass is becoming intercalated into the trophoblast. *C*, Section of embryonic disc of a sheep blastocyst 12 days postcoitum. The embryonic ectoderm is now bulging above the level of the adjacent trophoblast. *D*, Section through Hensen's node, 14 days postcoitum. The yolk sac is now completely formed, mesoderm cells are interposed between the embryonic ectoderm and endoderm, and the extra-embryonic coelom can be seen at each side. *BC*, blastocyst cavity; *BO*, bilaminar omphalopleure; *DE*, distal endoderm; *EC*, extra-embryonic coelom; *EE*, embryonic ectoderm; *ICM*, inner cell mass; *M*, mesoderm; *PE*, primary endoderm; *PS*, primitive streak; *T*, trophoblast; *YS*, yolk sac cavity.

ulate cellular movement during elongation.

Rapid blastocyst elongation in pigs is unique to each blastocyst within the litter. Those that reach the tubular stage earliest may have a competitive edge for survival over slower developing blastocysts by obtaining sufficient uterine surface area necessary to support continued development.

Horse blastocysts do not change from a spherical to a filamentous morphology during early development. The embryonic vesicle diameter increases at 2 to 3 mm per day and retains its spherical form until days 17 to 19, when it conforms to the shape of the uterine lumen.

Intrauterine Migration and Spacing

Intrauterine migration and equidistant spacing between embryos is essential to embryonic survival in polytocous species. Pig embryos are found near the tip of the

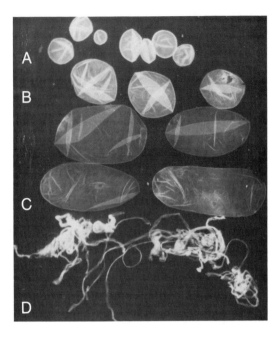

FIG. 8–9.   Collage showing rapid development of pig conceptuses through the early spherical (*A,* Day 10.5), late spherical (*B,* Day 11), tubular (*C,* Day 11.5) and early filamentous (*D,* Day 12) forms. (From Rodney Geisert and Fuller Bazer.)

uterine horn 5 to 6 days after initiation of estrus and then migrate toward the uterine body with embryos entering and mixing with embryos in the opposite uterine horn as early as day 9. Migration and spacing of the embryos is terminated on approximately day 12, when rapid blastocyst elongation occurs. Intrauterine migration and spacing appear to be modulated through peristaltic contractions of the myometrium stimulated by the developing embryo. Estrogens, histamines, and prostaglandins are embryonic products that could stimulate myometrial activity.

Transuterine migration is rare in monovulatory ewes and cows. However, intrauterine migration will occur in sheep but not cows when multiple ovulations occur on the same ovary. Failure of intrauterine migration when both ovulations occur on the same ovary is a major problem when superovulation is used to increase the twinning rate in cattle.

Using ultrasound to monitor embryonic movement in mares, transuterine migrations occurred approximately 13 times per day between days 10 to 16 of gestation (Leith and Ginther, 1984). Fixation of the embryo within the uterine lumen occurs on day 16, although migration is possible as late as days 25 to 30 of gestation. Stabilization of the vesicle within the uterine lumen results from thickening of the uterine wall and increased myometrial tone (estrogen induced) that begins on day 16 and becomes most intense on day 25.

Implantation

Rodents and primates have blastocysts that penetrate the uterine mucosa (Perry, 1981) by penetrating and phagocytizing the uterine luminal epithelium as they migrate into the uterine stroma. This invasive process is accompanied by transformation and proliferation of uterine stromal cells (referred to as *decidualization*) in the vicinity of the developing blastocyst.

In contrast, implantation in domestic animals is superficial and noninvasive (King et al., 1982) and involves phases of trophoblast–uterine epithelial cell apposition and adhesion. The pig trophoblast, however, does exhibit invasive properties when placed in an ectopic site, such as the kidney capsule. This invasive property appears to result from blastocyst production of proteolytic enzymes such as plasminogen activator; but invasive implantation is prevented by uterine epithelial secretion of protease (plasmin/trypsin) inhibitors that coat the blastocyst and protect the uterus from this protease.

Pig blastocysts begin to attach to the uterine surface on day 13, with attachment completed across the trophoblastic surface between days 18 to 24. Attachment is through interdigitation of uterine and trophoblastic microvilli covering the complete interface between the two layers, except where the trophoblast overlies the openings of uterine glands. The trophoblastic surface in these areas becomes modified to form specialized absorptive structures (areolae) that allow nutrient uptake by the developing conceptus.

Placental attachment in ruminants involves both caruncular and intercaruncular areas of the uterine endometrium. A transitory attachment first occurs as cow and ewe trophoblasts develop finger-like villi (papillae) that project into the lumen of the uterine glands (Fig. 8–10). These papillae provide a temporary anchor and absorptive structure for the conceptus as more complete attachment progresses. Loss of trophoblastic surface microvilli permits close surface contact with uterine epithelial microvilli. The uterine epithelium presses into the trophoblastic surface, interlocking with the cytoplasmic projections on the trophoblast surface until the trophoblast microvilli redevelop, forming a more complex attachment.

Attachment is characterized by the appearance of binucleate cells arising from uninucleate cells of the trophoblast. Binucleate cells first appear on day 17 and are present throughout gestation. These cells migrate and fuse with underlying uterine surface epithelial cells to form multinucleate cells or a *syncytium*. The syncytium may be involved in immunologic protection of the conceptus or transfer of placental lactogen synthesized by binucleate cells.

Implantation or attachment does not occur until days 24 to 40 in the mare. Early attachment is through interdigitation between surface epithelium of the embryonic vesicle and uterine lining. Specialized chorionic girdle cells form around the spherical vesicle, detach around day 38, and invade the uterine endometrium to form the endometrial cups that produce equine chorionic gonadotropin. Endometrial cup formation may protect the trophoblast from maternal immune attack. Microvillous attachment becomes more complex as the microvilli branch and coalesce to give rise to thousands of microcotyledonary structures that hold the placenta firmly in place.

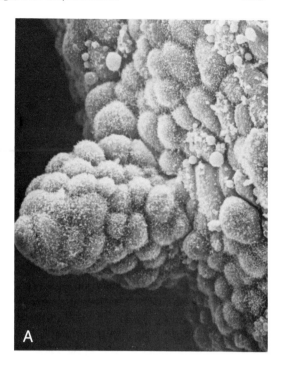

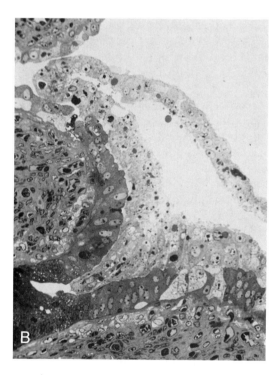

FIG. 8–10.   *A*, Trophectoderm of cow conceptus showing well-developed papillae (870×). *B*, Extension of the trophectodermal papilla into a uterine gland (250×). (From M. Guillomot and P. Quay. (1982) Anat. Rec. *315*, 282.)

During implantation in domestic animals, an outgrowth of extraembryonic mesoderm originates from the embryoblast and migrates between the trophectoderm and endoderm (Fig. 8–8). This mesodermal layer will split and combine with the trophectoderm to form the chorion and endoderm to form the yolk sac. The mesoderm will also contribute to formation of the amnion and allantois. These membranes serve to provide the embryo with a source of attachment and nourishment from the maternal system.

INTERACTION OF CONCEPTUS AND UTERINE ENVIRONMENT

The uterine endometrium of pregnant females is dominated by progesterone, which stimulates development of glandular epithelium. The glandular epithelium becomes highly secretory and produces histotroph, which is believed to be essential for conceptus development (Bazer and First, 1983). Secretory vesicles accumulate in the epithelium of uterine endometrial glands between days 10.5 to 12 of gestation in swine. With the onset of estrogen production by pig blastocysts on days 11 and 12, there is a marked increase in total recoverable calcium, proteins, and prostaglandins in the uterine lumen. The estrogens stimulate calcium release from the plasmalemma and/or mitochondria, which stimulates phospholipase A_2. This results in production of arachidonic acid and lysophospholipids, which may promote fusion of secretory vesicle membranes with the cell membrane and in turn exocytosis.

Proteins released from the secretory vesicles into the uterine lumen serve as transport proteins, enzymes, and regulatory proteins. In the pig, uteroferrin is a purple, progesterone-induced glycoprotein, which transports iron from uterine endometrium to the conceptus during gestation. Retinol and retinoic acid-binding proteins and progesterone-binding proteins have also been demonstrated.

Enzymes identified in pig uterine secretions include acid phosphatase (resulting from uteroferrin), aminopeptidase, glucosephosphate isomerase, lysozyme, and several proteases. These enzymes may be involved in regulating various metabolic activities of the conceptus.

Regulatory proteins secreted by the pig uterine endometrium include a plasmin-trypsin inhibitor, which may prevent invasive implantation. The pig blastocyst is invasive when transferred to an extrauterine site, but *in utero* the protease inhibitor coats the trophectoderm and protects the uterine endometrium from the cascade of proteolytic events that may be initiated by plasminogen activator produced by the trophectoderm. The protease inhibitor may also prevent degradation of proteins in histotroph so that they are available for uptake by the conceptus.

Growth factors known to be present in uterine tissue or uterine fluid include insulin-like growth factor (IGF)-I (pig, sheep, cow); IGF-II (pig, sheep, cow); transforming growth factors-α and -β (TGFα and TGFβ, rat); acidic (α) and basic (β) fibroblast growth factor (pig); epidermal growth factor (EGF, mouse and rat); and uterine luminal fluid mitogen (ULFM, pig), according to Simmen and Simmen (1991). Growth factors are also produced by fetal-placental tissues. The presence of abundant mRNAs for IGF-I and IGF-II in uterine endometrium suggests autocrine and/or paracrine regulation of conceptus development by such factors.

What are the roles of growth factors secreted by the uterus? Are specific growth factors responsible for initiation of morphologic development of conceptuses from spherical to tubular to filamentous forms and initiation of events leading to the secretion of steroids and/or proteins responsible for maternal recognition of pregnancy? Just before initiation of estrogen secretion and morphologic transition from spherical, to tubular to filamentous forms, there is mesodermal outgrowth from the embryonic disc of pig conceptuses. During this period, days 10 to 12 of pregnancy, IGF-I is highest in uterine secretions of both cyclic and pregnant pigs. Furthermore, conceptuses of prolific Chinese Meishan pigs develop more rapidly, secrete more estrogens, and are exposed to higher amounts of IGF-I in uterine secretions than for less prolific Large White pigs. The growth factor associated with inducing mesoderm in amphibians is β-fibroblast growth factor (βFGF), and both αFGF and βFGF stimulate proliferation of mesoderm-derived cells (Kimelman et al., 1988). Fibroblast growth factors are believed to be present in pig endometrium and uterine secretions, but temporal associations between secretion of FGF, morphologic changes in conceptuses, and initiation of secretion of estrogens by pig conceptuses have not been established.

Secretory proteins of the cow, pig, and ewe endometrium are also known to contain immunosuppressive factors (Bazer and First, 1983). In addition, high molecular weight glycoproteins from pig, cow, and ewe conceptuses are immunosuppressive. Immunosuppressive activity is based on evidence that these proteins from the uterine endometrium and conceptus may be responsible for survival of the conceptus allograft within the uterine lumen, which would otherwise be immunologically rejected. Progesterone and its metabolites and prostaglandins E_1, E_2, A, and F_1 may also be involved in suppressing the maternal immune system during pregnancy.

The theory of immunotropism (Wegmann et al., 1989) is contrary to that of immunosuppression during pregnancy. Recent evidence suggests that leukocytes and lymphocytes known to be attracted to the pregnant uterus secrete cytokines and lymphokines that are stimulatory to conceptus development (immunotropic) and beneficial to pregnancy. Cytokines and lymphokines may stimulate development and function of the trophoblast–chorion and, in turn, may benefit fetal development.

MATERNAL RECOGNITION OF PREGNANCY

All Farm Animals

Implantation allows the conceptus and uterine endometrium to achieve intimate contact for nutrient exchange and endocrine communication. At the appropriate time, the conceptus must produce steroid hormones and/or proteins to signal its presence to the maternal system. This "signal" is necessary for corpus luteum maintenance, production of progesterone, and continued endometrial development and secretory activity. This critical period when the conceptus must signal its presence to allow pregnancy to be established is called *maternal recognition of pregnancy*. If the conceptus fails to signal its presence at exactly the correct time, the function of the corpus luteum is terminated by the luteolytic action of prostaglandin $F_{2\alpha}$ ($PGF_{2\alpha}$) from the uterus. This ensures that the female will return to estrus and mate at frequent intervals until a successful pregnancy is established. Uterine $PGF_{2\alpha}$ is produced by endometrium of cows, ewes, mares, and sows (Bazer et al., 1981) and causes morphologic regression of the corpus luteum and cessation of progesterone production. The luteolytic potential of endometrial $PGF_{2\alpha}$ must be blocked if pregnancy is to be established since a functional corpus luteum is essential for the initiation and maintenance of pregnancy in all farm animals. The effect of the conceptus is luteostatic since progesterone production is maintained at a level comparable to that of diestrus during pregnancy. Basal secretion of LH from the anterior pituitary is also essential for corpus luteum maintenance and function during pregnancy.

Pig

Uterine $PGF_{2\alpha}$ is luteolytic, and estrogens produced by conceptuses provide the signal for maternal recognition of pregnancy that occurs between days 11 and 12 of gestation. A second period of estrogen production occurs between days 16 and 30 of pregnancy. Injection of exogenous estrogen (estradiol valerate, 5 mg/day) on days 11 through 15 of the estrous cycle will also allow corpus luteum maintenance for a period equivalent to or slightly longer than during pregnancy. This condition is referred to as *pseudopregnancy.*

Concentrations of $PGF_{2\alpha}$ in utero-ovarian vein plasma are elevated between days 12 and 16 of the cycle and lead to luteolysis. $PGF_{2\alpha}$ in utero-ovarian vein plasma of pregnant and pseudopregnant gilts, however, is significantly lower than for cycling gilts; but greater amounts of $PGF_{2\alpha}$ are recovered in uterine flushings of pregnant and pseudopregnant gilts than cycling gilts. Estrogens do not, therefore, inhibit production of $PGF_{2\alpha}$ by the uterine endometrium but allow $PGF_{2\alpha}$ to be sequestered in the uterine lumen. Secretion of $PGF_{2\alpha}$ in an endocrine direction is blocked, and $PGF_{2\alpha}$ is not available to the corpus luteum to cause luteolysis (Fig. 8–11). Estrogen-induced increases in endometrial receptors for prolactin and prolactin-induced calcium cycling across the endometrial epithelium may be responsible to exocrine secretion of PGF during pregnancy (Young et al., 1989). Pig conceptuses secrete a complex array of proteins during the period of maternal recognition of pregnancy, including Type I conceptus interferons and γ-interferon; however, intrauterine infusion of secretory proteins from day-15 conceptuses does not affect the life span of corpora lutea (Harney and Bazer, 1989).

Conceptuses must be present in both uterine horns of pigs, at least two per uterine horn, for pregnancy to be established. If there are no conceptuses in one uterine horn, the PGF_2 released from the endometrium of the nonpregnant uterine horn will cause luteolysis of the corpora lutea on both ovaries. Failure of pigs to maintain a unilateral pregnancy indicates that conceptuses developing in one uterine horn do not produce a factor that acts systemically to allow bilateral corpora lutea maintenance.

Ewe

In the ewe, uterine PGF is the luteolysin, and protein secreted by the conceptus between days 12 and 21 of gestation inhibit PGF production by uterine endometrium. In cycling ewes, episodes of PGF production between days 14 and 16 increase in frequency to reach five episodes in 25 hours, and corpus luteum regression occurs. Estrogen may stimulate increased oxytocin receptors in sheep endometrium. Oxytocin from the posterior pituitary and/or corpus luteum may then stimulate episodes of PGF (McCracken et al., 1984). An average of 7.6 episodes of PGF occur between days 14 and 15 in nonpregnant ewes versus only 1.3 pulses during that period for pregnant ewes.

Continuous intrauterine infusion of homogenates of day 14 to 15 sheep conceptuses extends corpus luteum life span in ewes; however, infusion of conceptus homogenates into the uterine vein is not effective. The active agent in the homogenate was believed to be a protein. A protein produced by sheep conceptuses between days 12 to 21 of pregnancy was purified and named *ovine trophoblast protein 1* (oTP-1). oTP-1 has high amino acid sequence homology to α- and ω-interferons and is now referred to as a *Type I conceptus interferon.* oTP-1 has antiviral, immunosuppressive, and antiproliferative biologic activities, in addition to antiluteolytic activity described later (Bazer et al., 1991). oTP-1 binds to surface and superficial glandular epithelial cells of the endometrium and selectively enhances secretion of proteins by the uterine endometrium. Total ovine conceptus secretory proteins and highly purified oTP-1 are equally effective in extending corpus luteum life span when introduced into the uterine lumen of cyclic ewes between days 12 and 14.

Introduction of highly purified oTP-1 into the uterine lumen of nonpregnant

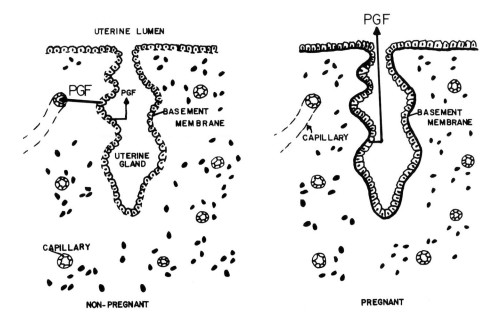

FIG. 8–11. Proposed mechanism for maternal recognition of pregnancy in the pig. $PGF_{2\alpha}$ is released in an endocrine direction during the estrous cycle (nonpregnant) of swine to cause regression of the corpus luteum. Secretion is, however, in an exocrine direction during pregnancy and $PGF_{2\alpha}$ is, therefore, unable to exert its luteolytic effect on the corpus luteum. (From Fuller Bazer.)

ewes inhibits PGF production in response to both estrogen and oxytocin challenges and prevents development of endometrial responsiveness to oxytocin-induced uterine production of PGF. Secretion of significant amounts of oTP-1 begins on day 12, that is, before endometrial receptors for oxytocin are synthesized. Available evidence suggests that oTP-1 inhibits synthesis of endometrial receptors for oxytocin and, therefore, prevents uterine production of luteolytic pulses of PGF. This may explain why endometrial receptors for oxytocin remain low in pregnant ewes and cyclic ewes receiving intrauterine infusions of oTP-1 between days 12 and 14 (Bazer et al., 1991). The PGE_2 levels in utero-ovarian vein blood increase about fourfold between days 12.5 and 14.5 of pregnancy and may reflect an increased output of PGE_2 by the endometrium and/ or conceptus. Although PGE_2 is not the antiluteolytic hormone of pregnancy, it may facilitate maternal recognition of

pregnancy by exerting a luteal protective effect. oTP-1 does not stimulate uterine secretion of PGE_2.

The current hypothesis contrasts events associated with luteolysis in cyclic ewes and maternal recognition of pregnancy. In cyclic ewes, endometrial estrogen and progesterone receptor levels are high between estrus and day 12, and then progesterone receptors decrease, while estrogen receptors increase. With loss of progesterone receptors and increasing numbers of estrogen receptors, endometrial synthesis of oxytocin receptors begins, possibly enhanced by ovarian estrogens, and the endometrium becomes responsive to oxytocin released from the corpora lutea and/ or posterior pituitary, resulting in episodic release of luteolytic pulses of PGF. In pregnant ewes, oTP-1 may stabilize the progesterone receptor and/or prevent increases in estrogen receptors to inhibit oxytocin receptor synthesis. Consequently, oxytocin is unable to stimulate episodic secretion of PGF, and a functional corpus luteum persists in pregnant ewes.

Cow

The uterine luteolysin is $PGF_{2\alpha}$ and maternal recognition of pregnancy is believed to occur between days 16 to 19 of pregnancy in cows (Thatcher et al., 1989). Peripheral plasma 15 keto-13,14 dihydro $PGF_{2\alpha}$ (PGFM) provides a reliable means for studying secretion of $PGF_{2\alpha}$ by the bovine uterus. In nonpregnant cows, episodic release of PGFM is closely correlated with luteolysis. In pregnant cows, however, PGFM levels are markedly reduced and corpus luteum maintenance results. A three- to fourfold increase in PGFM can be detected by 6 hours after an IV injection of 3 mg estradiol on day 13 of the estrous cycle, but this response is significantly reduced when estradiol is injected on days 18 and 20 of pregnancy. The interval between estrous periods is increased from 20 ± .8 days, when bovine conceptuses are removed on day 15, to 25 ± 1 days, when the conceptus is removed on day 17. Intrauterine infusion of bovine conceptus homogenates also extends the interestrous interval.

The bovine conceptus produces a number of relatively low molecular weight acidic proteins, which include bovine trophoblast protein-1 (bTP-1) which, like oTP-1, is a Type I conceptus interferon. Introduction of the total array of bovine conceptus secretory proteins or a preparation highly enriched in bTP-1 into the uterine lumen of cyclic cows between days 15 and 21 extends corpus luteum life span (Thatcher et al., 1989). Bovine conceptus secretory proteins, when introduced into the uterine lumen, between days 15 and 18 inhibit uterine production of PGF in response to an estradiol injection on day 18. The model for maternal recognition of pregnancy in cows is very similar to that for sheep. Endometrium of pregnant cows is unresponsive to estradiol- and oxytocin-induced uterine production of PGF and

has very low levels of oxytocin receptors on days 14 to 21 compared to cyclic cows (Fuchs et al., 1990). In addition, endometrium of pregnant cows produces an endometrial prostaglandin synthetase inhibitor (EPSI), which specifically decreases production of PGF. There is no evidence that endometrium of pregnant ewes produces EPSI. Bovine conceptuses also produce PGE_2, which may play a luteal protective role in maintenance of corpus luteum function.

Mare

The uterine luteolytic substance in mares is $PGF_{2\alpha}$ and the conceptus appears to inhibit production of $PGF_{2\alpha}$ by the uterine endometrium (Sharp et al., 1984). In the cycling mare, $PGF_{2\alpha}$ concentrations in uterine venous plasma and uterine flushings increase from day 8 to days 14 to 16, when luteolysis occurs and plasma progesterone levels decline. The amount of $PGF_{2\alpha}$ bound by luteal receptors is maximal on day 14 of the cycle and day 18 of pregnancy. Since the mare's corpus luteum can apparently respond to circulating $PGF_{2\alpha}$ during pregnancy, the conceptus must evoke some antiluteolytic mechanism. Pregnant mares have little $PGF_{2\alpha}$ in uterine fluids; $PGF_{2\alpha}$ in uterine venous plasma is reduced, and PGFM in peripheral plasma shows no episodic pattern of release (Sharp et al., 1984). However, in vitro, endometrial tissue from both pregnant and nonpregnant mares actively produces $PGF_{2\alpha}$. In the presence of the conceptus, however, endometrial production of $PGF_{2\alpha}$ is markedly reduced.

The equine conceptus migrates within the uterus from one uterine horn to the other 12 to 14 times per day between days 12 to 14 of pregnancy, possibly to inhibit endometrial $PGF_{2\alpha}$ production and thereby protect the corpus luteum. The equine conceptus does suppress $PGF_{2\alpha}$ production by the endometrium, but the agent has not been identified (Sharp et al., 1989). The equine conceptus also produces increasing amounts of estradiol between days 8 and 20 of gestation. A similar trend, but of greater magnitude, was found for estrone. Attempts to prolong the corpus luteum life span in mares by injecting estrogens have provided conflicting results.

Horse conceptuses secrete three major proteins between days 12 and 14 of pregnancy with molecular weights of greater than 40,000, 50,000 and 65,000. However, the role(s) of these proteins is not known. Estrogens and/or conceptus secretory proteins may provide the maternal recognition of pregnancy signal in the mare by directly or indirectly inhibiting endometrial $PGF_{2\alpha}$ production.

REFERENCES

Austin, C.R. (1951). Observations on the penetration of the sperm into the mammalian egg. Aust. J. Sci. Res. Ser. B. 4, 581–589.

Bazer, F.W. and First N.L. (1983). Pregnancy and parturition. J. Anim. Sci. Suppl. 2, 57 425–460.

Bazer, F.W., Sharp, D.C., Thatcher, W.W. and Roberts, R.M. (1981). Comparative approach to mechanisms in the maintenance of early pregnancy. *In* Reproductive Processes and Contraception. K.W. McKerns (ed.). New York, Plenum Press, pp. 581–618.

Bedford, J.M. (1983). Significance of the need for sperm capacitation before fertilization in Eutherian mammals. Biol. Reprod. 28, 108–120.

Biggers, J.D., Leonov, B.V., Baskar, J.F. and Fried, J. (1978). Inhibition of hatching of mouse blastocysts *in vitro* by prostaglandin antagonists. Biol. Reprod. 19, 519–533.

Bindon, B.M. and Piper, L.R. (1984). Endocrine differences in ovine prolificacy. *In* Proc. 10th Int. Congress on Animal Reprod. and Artif. Insem., Urbana-Champaign, IL, Vol. IV, p. 17–26.

Boland, M.P., Nancarrow, C.D., Murray, J.D., Scaramuzzi, R., Sutton, R., Hoskinson, R.M. and Hazelton, I.G. (1986). Fertilization and early embryonic development in androstenedione-immunized Merino ewes. J. Reprod. Fertil. 78, 423–431.

Bolton, V.N., Oades, P.J. and Johnson, M.H. (1984). The relationship between cleavage, DNA replication and gene expression in the 2-cell mouse embryo. J. Embryol. Exp. Morph. 79, 139–163.

Brown, R.W., Hungerford, J.W., Greenwood, P.E., Bloor R.J., Evans, D.F., Tsonis, C.G. and Forage, R.G. (1990). Immunization against recombinant bovine inhibin α subunit causes increased ovulation rates in gilts. J. Reprod. Fertil. 90, 199–205.

Chang, M.C. (1951). Fertilizing capacity of spermatozoa deposited into fallopian tubes. Nature (London) 168, 697.

Collas, P. and Robl, J.M. (1990). Factors affecting the efficiency of nuclear transplantation in the rabbit embryo. Biol. Reprod. 43, 877–884.

Crosby, I.M., Gandolfi, F. and Moor, R.M. (1988). Control of protein synthesis during early cleavage of sheep embryos. J. Reprod. Fertil. 82, 769–775.

Ducibella, T. (1977). Surface changes in the developing trophoblast cell. *In* Development in Mammals. Vol. 1. M.H. Johnson (ed.). North Holland, Amsterdam, pp. 5–30.

Fuchs, A.R., Behrens, O., Helmer, H., Liu, C.-H., Barros, C.M. and Fields, M.J. (1990). Oxytocin and vasopressin receptors in bovine endometrium and myometrium during the estrous cycle and early pregnancy. Endocrinology 127, 629–637.

Harney, J.P. and Bazer F.W. (1989). Effect of porcine conceptus secretory proteins on interoestrous interval and uterine secretion of prostaglandins. Biol. Reprod. 41, 277–284.

Hunter, R.H.F. (1976). Sperm–egg interactions in the pig: monospermy, extensive polyspermy, and the formation of chromatin aggregates. J. Anat. 122, 43–59.

Killeen, I.D. and Moore N.W. (1970). Fertilization and survival of fertilized eggs in the ewe following surgical insemination at various times after the onset of oestrus. Aust. J. Biol. Sci. 23, 1279–1287.

Kimelman, D., Abraham, J.A., Haaparanta, T., Palisi, T.M. and Kirschner, M.W. (1988). The presence of fibroblast growth factor in the frog egg: its role as a natural mesoderm inducer. Science 242, 1053–1056.

King, G.J., Atkinson, B.A. and Robertson, H.A. (1982). Implantation and early placentation in domestic ungulates. J. Reprod. Fertil. Suppl. 31, 17–30.

King, W.A., Niar, A., Chartrain, I., Betterridge, K.J. and Quay, P. (1988). Nucleolus organizer regions and nucleoli in preattachment bovine embryos. J. Reprod. Fertil. 82, 87–95.

Leith, G.S. and Ginther, O.J. (1984). Intrauterine mobility of the early equine conceptus. Proc. 10th Int. Congress on Animal Reprod. and Artif. Insem. Urbana-Champaign, IL, Vol. II, p. 118.

Linder, G.M. and Wright, R.W. (1978). Morphological and quantitative aspects of the development of swine embryos *in vitro*. J. Anim. Sci. 46, 711–718.

McCracken, J.A., Schramm, W. and Okulicz, W.C. (1984). Hormone receptor control of pulsatile secretion of $PGF_{2\alpha}$ from the ovine uterus during luteolysis and its abrogation in early pregnancy. Anim. Reprod. Sci. 7, 31–55.

McLaren, A. (1974). Fertilization, cleavage and implantation. *In* Reproduction in Farm Animals. E.S.E. Hafez (ed.). Philadelphia, Lea & Febiger.

Menino, A.R., Dyk, A.R., Gardiner, C.S., Gorbner, M.A., Kaaekuahiwi, M.A. and Williams, J.S. (1989). The effects of plaminogen on *in vitro* ovine embryo development. Biol. Reprod. *41*, 899–905.

Papaioannou, V.E. and Ebert, K.M. (1986). Comparative aspects of embryo manipulation in mammals. *In* Experimental Approaches to Mammalian Embryonic Development. J. Rossant and R.A. Pedersen (eds.). New York, Cambridge University Press.

Papaioannou, V.E. and Ebert K.M. (1988). The preimplantation pig embryo: cell number and allocation to trophectoderm and inner cell mass of the blastocyst *in vivo* and *in vitro*. Development *102*, 793–803.

Perry, J.S. (1981). The mammalian fetal membranes. J. Reprod. Fertil. *62*, 321–335.

Renard, J.P., Babinet, B. and Barra, J. (1991). Participation of the paternal genome is not required before the eight-cell stage for full-term development of mouse embryos. Dev. Biol. *143*, 199–202.

Schultz, G.A. (1986). Utilization of genetic information in the preimplantation mouse embryo. *In* Experimental Approaches to Mammalian Embryonic Development. J. Rossant and R.A. Pedersen (eds.). New York, Cambridge University Press.

Sharp, D.C., McDowell, K.J., Weithenauer, J. and Thatcher, W.W. (1989). The continuum of events leading to maternal recognition of pregnancy in mares. J. Reprod. Fertil. Suppl. *37*, 101–107.

Simmen, F.A. and Simmen, R.C.M. (1991). Peptide growth factors and proto-oncogenes in mammalian conceptus development. Biol. Reprod. *44*, 1–5.

Suarez, S.S., Drost, M., Redfern, K. and Gottibe, W. (1990). Sperm motility in oviduct. *In* Fertilization in Mammals. B.B. Bavister, J. Cummins and E.R.S. Roldan (eds.). Serono Symposium. Norwel, MA, Adams Publishing Group Ltd.

Surani, M.A.H. and Barton, S.C. (1983). Development gynogenetic eggs in the mouse: implications for parthenogenic embryos. Science *22*, 1034.

Sutherland, A.E., Speed, T.P. and Calarco, P.G. (1990). Inner cell allocation in the mouse morula: the role for oriented division during fourth cleavage. Dev. Biol. *137*, 13–25.

Thatcher, W.W., Hansen, P.J., Gross, T.S., Helmer, S.D., Plante, C. and Bazer F.W. (1989). Antiluteolytic effects of bovine trophoblast protein-1. J. Reprod. Fertil. *37*, 91–99.

Van Neikerk, C.H. and Gerneke, W.H. (1966). Persistence and parthenogenetic cleavage of tubal ova in the mare. Onderstepoort J. Vet. Res. *33*, 195–232.

Warner, C.A., Gollnick, S.O. and Goldbard, S.B. (1987). Linkage of the preimplantation-embryo development (ped) gene to the mouse major histocompatibility complex (MHC). Biol. Reprod. *36*, 606–610.

Wassarman, P.M. (1990). Profile of a mammalian sperm cell receptor. Development *108*, 1–17.

Wegmann, T.G., Anthanassakis, I., Guilbert, L., Branch, D., Dym, M., Menu, E. and Chaouat, G., (1989). The role of M-CSF and GM-CSF in fostering placental growth and fetal survival. Transplant. Proc. *20*, 566–573.

Willadsen, S.M., Janzen, R.E., McAlister, J.J., Shea, B.F., Hamilton, G. and McDermand, D. (1991). The viability of late morula and blastocysts produced by nuclear transplantation in cattle. Theriogenology *35*, 161–170.

Yanagimachi, R. (1981). Mechanisms of fertilization in mammals. *In* Fertilization and Embryonic Development *In Vitro*. L. Mastroianni, Jr. and J.D. Biggers (eds.). New York, Plenum.

Young, K.H., Kraeling, R.R. and Bazer, F.W. (1989). Effects of prolactin on conceptus survival and uterine secretory activity in pigs. J. Reprod. Fertil. *86*, 713–722.

9
Gestation, Prenatal Physiology, and Parturition

M.R. Jainudeen and E.S.E. Hafez

GESTATION

With the exception of *Monotremata*, mammals are viviparous, i.e., embryonic and fetal development is completed within the uterus. This period of intrauterine development is termed *pregnancy* or *gestation* and is concerned primarily with the nutrition of the growing fetus and the maternal adaptations directed to this end.

Length of Gestation

Length of gestation is calculated as the interval from fertile service to parturition (Table 9–1). The duration of gestation is genetically determined, although it can be modified by maternal, fetal, and environmental factors (Fig. 9–1).

Maternal Factors. The age of the dam influences the duration of pregnancy in different species. A 2-day extension from the norm occurs in the 8-year-old ewe. Young heifers carry their calves for a slightly shorter period than older heifers.

Fetal Factors. An inverse relation between the duration of gestation and litter size is well-documented in several polytocous species except the pig. Multiple fetuses in monotocous species also have shorter gestation periods. Twin calves are carried 3 to 6 days less than single calves. Interaction between fetal and placental sizes may influence gestation in the horse. The sex of the fetus may also determine gestation length; male calves and foals are carried 1 to 2 days longer than females.

TABLE 9–1. Differences in Gestation Periods of Farm Mammals

Animal	Average (Range)
Cattle (dairy breeds)	
Ayrshire	278
Brown Swiss	290 (270–306)
Dairy Shorthorn	282
Friesian	276 (240–303)
Guernsey	284
Holstein-Friesian	279 (262–309)
Jersey	279 (270–285)
Swedish-Friesian	282 (260–300)
Zebu (Brahman)	292 (271–310)
Cattle (beef breeds)	
Aberdeen-Angus	279
Hereford	285 (243–316)
Beef Shorthorn	283 (273–294)
Sheep	148 (140–159)
Swine	
Domestic	114 (102–128)
Wild Pig	(124–140)
Horse	
Arabian	337 (301–371)
Belgian	335 (304–354)
Clydesdale	334
Morgan	344 (316–363)
Percheron	(321–345)
Shire	340
Thoroughbred	338 (301–349)

The duration of pregnancy may be influenced by the endocrine functions of the fetus.

Genetic Factors. The small variations in pregnancy duration among breeds (Table 9–1) may be due to genetic, seasonal, or local effects. The extreme, expression of genetically prolonged gestation, is known among dairy cows that carry a fetus homozygous for an autosomal recessive gene.

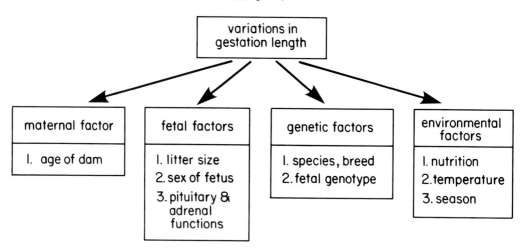

FIG. 9–1. Schematic representation of variations in length of gestation due to maternal, fetal, genetic, and environmental factors. Whereas many of these factors within a species cause minor variations, hypofunction of the pituitary–adrenal axis of the fetus is associated with prolonged gestation in the ewe and cow.

The influence of equine fetal genotype on gestation length can be demonstrated in hybrids between the horse and the donkey. In these matings, the gestation length is closer to the paternal than to the maternal component of the fetus. For example, the duration of pregnancy of a mare carrying a foal sired by a stallion is 320 to 360 days. Mares covered by a jack donkey, and therefore carrying hybrid mule foals, tend to exhibit the longer gestation of the donkey (360 to 380 days), whereas jenny donkeys carrying hinny foals as a result of mating with a stallion have a shorter gestation, similar to that of the horse. This influence may be mediated either through a hormonal mechanism or may merely reflect the influence of fetal size.

Breed of embryo determines the length of gestation in cattle (King et al., 1982). This has been established by transferring the embryos from breeds with shorter gestation length than the donor's and vice versa. Genetic factors are also responsible for differences in gestation length between mutton and wool breeds of sheep.

Environmental Factors. Of the environmental factors, season may influence the duration of gestation. Foals conceived in late summer and autumn have significantly shorter gestation periods than those conceived at the start of the breeding season in early spring. Gestation lengths are shorter by approximately 4 days for well-fed mares as opposed to those on a maintenance ration.

MATERNAL PHYSIOLOGY IN PREGNANCY

Early pregnancy is marked by processes that prolong the life span of the cyclic corpus luteum. These processes suggest a maternal recognition of pregnancy.

Reproductive Organ Changes

Vulvar and Vaginal Changes. During the latter half of gestation, changes occur in the genital tract, particularly in the vulva and vagina. The vulva becomes highly edematous and vascular. These vulval changes are more obvious in cattle than in horses and occur around the fifth month of gestation in heifers and the seventh in cows. The vaginal mucosa is pale and dry during most of gestation but is edematous and pliable toward the end of pregnancy.

The Cervix. During gestation, the developing fetus is retained within the uterus by tight closure of the external os of the cervix and a secretion of a highly viscid mucus that seals the cervical canal. This so-called mucous plug of pregnancy liquefies prior to parturition and is discharged in strings.

Uterine Changes. As pregnancy progresses, the uterus undergoes gradual enlargement to accommodate the growing fetus, but the myometrium remains quiescent, thereby preventing premature expulsion. Three phases can be identified in the adaption of the uterus: proliferation, growth, and stretching; the duration of each varies with the species. The mechanisms that permit the enormous increase in size are unknown but are probably hormonal.

Ovarian Changes. The corpus luteum regresses in a nonfertile estrous cycle; it persists as the corpus luteum of pregnancy (corpus luteum verum), and as a result, estrous cycles are suspended. Some cows, however, may show estrus during early pregnancy, which is due to follicular activity in the ovaries. As many as 10 to 15 follicles develop in mares between the 40th and 160th day of pregnancy. These follicles luteinize to form accessory corpora lutea.

The corpus luteum of pregnancy in the cow persists at a maximal size throughout pregnancy, but in the mare, both the primary as well as the accessory corpora lutea regress by the seventh month of pregnancy.

Pelvic Ligaments and Pubic Symphysis. Relaxation of the pelvic ligaments occurs gradually during the course of pregnancy but becomes more rapid with approaching parturition. This relaxation is more noticeable in the cow and ewe than in the mare and is related to high levels of estrogens in late pregnancy and to the action of relaxin. The caudal part of the sacrosciatic ligament is cordlike in the nonpregnant cow but becomes more re-

laxed and flaccid as parturition approaches.

Hormones of Pregnancy

Maintenance of Pregnancy. Progesterone is the key hormone necessary for maintenance of pregnancy. The corpus luteum (CL) persists throughout pregnancy in all farm animals except the horse. Thus, farm species can be classified according to the source of progesterone during the latter half of pregnancy as placenta dependent (mare, ewe) or CL dependent (cow, goat, and sow) (Fig. 9–2).

Blood and Urinary Concentrations of Hormones. Species differences occur in the urinary excretion of estrogens (Table 9–2). In the mare, plasma estrogen con-

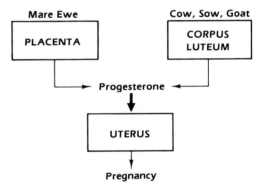

FIG. 9–2. Progesterone secreted by the corpus luteum is essential for the maintenance of early pregnancy in all farm species. The ovaries, however, can be removed (ovariectomy) during the latter half of pregnancy without interrupting pregnancy in the mare and ewe because the placenta produces progesterone in these species.

TABLE 9–2. **Estrogen and Related Compounds in the Urine During Pregnancy**

Female	Estrone	17β-Estradiol	17α-Estradiol
Cow	+	−	+
Ewe	−	−	+
Goat	−	−	+
Mare*	+	+	+
Sow	+	−	−

* Mare's urine also contains equilin, equilenin, 17α- and 17β-dihydroequilenin.

centrations (Fig. 9–3) remain low during the first 3 months of pregnancy, then rise steadily to reach a peak between the ninth and eleventh months, thereafter declining rapidly to term. In the sow, total urinary estrogen (estrone) rate shows an increase between the second and fifth weeks of gestation, a decline between the fifth and eighth weeks, and a rapid increase to a peak at the time of parturition, which declines rapidly thereafter. In the cow, maximal excretion of 17β-estradiol, and to a lesser degree estrone, occurs at 9 months of gestation.

The blood progesterone level remains constant throughout pregnancy in the ewe and cow and attains a high level early in pregnancy in the sow. Pregnanediol, the urinary metabolite of progesterone in the mare, has not been detected in other farm species. In the mare, progesterone concentration (Fig. 9–3) up to day 35 reflects secretion by the primary corpus luteum.

A rise in the level then occurs with the development of the secondary corpora lutea, and this concentration is maintained until the secondary corpora lutea begin to regress at day 150, at which time the placenta is sufficiently developed to take over this role. Subsequently, the plasma progestagen level remains low, but during the last 2 months of gestation, contrary to previous views, the level rises steadily to reach a second peak that is significantly higher than previous concentrations.

Between 40 and 130 days of gestation, high concentrations of equine chorionic gonadotrophin (eCG) (referred to as *pregnant mare serum gonadotropin*, or *PMSG*) are present in maternal but not in fetal blood. eCG, which is secreted by trophoblastic cells and not by the endometrium as was previously believed, luteinizes follicles and maintains the function of the secondary corpora lutea.

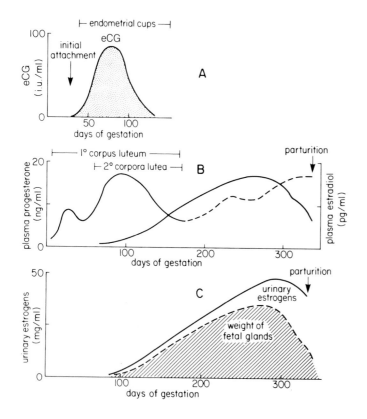

FIG. 9–3. The relationship of the changes occurring in the uterus and ovaries of the mare and the fetal gonads to endocrine events during pregnancy. *A*, The level of eCG reflects the functional activity of the endometrial cups. *B*, With the regression of the primary (1°) and secondary (2°) corpora lutea during pregnancy, the plasma progesterone level drops but pregnancy is maintained by placental progestagens (———). *C*, The fetal gonads respond to the increased secretion of estrogens by the fetomaternal unit by increasing in size and weight. Note that at parturition, the progestagen level continues to remain high while estrogen levels drop. (Adapted from Hay & Allen (1975). J. Reprod. Fertil. Suppl. *23*, 557; Squires et al. (1974). J. Anim. Sci. *38*, 759; Nett et al. (1973). J. Anim. Sci. *37*, 962.).

Because endometrial cups are of fetal rather than maternal origin, fetal genotype exerts a significant effect on endometrial cup development and the resulting secretion of eCG. For example, domestic horse females (*Equus caballus*) that are bred to donkey males (*Equus asinus*), producing hybrid mule fetuses, have lower peak eCG concentrations, and the period of eCG secretion is shorter than in mares carrying horse fetuses.

Maternal Adaptations

During the course of pregnancy, the mother makes metabolic and growth adjustments to provide an adequate supply of nutrients for the development of the fetus. Maternal body composition, feed intake, energy consumption, and metabolism are altered during pregnancy, but the mechanisms responsible are not fully established. Recent evidence has implicated insulin-like growth factors (IGFs) and their binding proteins as playing important roles in maternal adaptation, which guarantees an adequate supply of substrates to the developing fetus (Owens, 1991).

PLACENTA

A unique feature of early mammalian development is the provision of nutrients from the maternal organism by way of the placenta. The placenta is an apposition or fusion of the fetal membranes to the endometrium to permit physiologic exchange between fetus and mother. The placenta differs from other organs in many respects. It originates as a result of various degrees of fetal–maternal interactions and is connected to the embryo by a cord of blood vessels. The size and functions of the placenta change continuously during the course of pregnancy, and the organ is eventually expelled. For the fetus, the placenta combines in one organ many functional activities that are separate in the adult.

Placental Development

Fetal Membranes. The morphogenesis of the placenta during early gestation is closely related to those extraembryonic or fetal membranes that are differentiated into the yolk sac, amnion, allantois, and chorion (Table 9–3). The fetal membranes participate in the formation of the placenta, either separately or in certain combinations and give rise to three basic types of placentation, which differ in regard to the identity of the fetal membranes involved: chorionic, chorioallantoic, and yolk sac placentation. Among these types, the chorioallantoic placentation is characteristic of all farm animals (Perry, 1981). By fusion of the outer layer of the allantois to the chorion in the chorioallantoic placenta, the fetal vessels in the allantois come into close apposition to the umbilical arteries and veins located in the connective tissue between the allantois and chorion (Fig. 9–4).

Chorionic Villi. A feature of the chorioallantoic placenta is the highly increased area at the feto–maternal junction, either by the formation of chorionic villi protruding into uterine crypts or by the formation of chorionic labyrinths. The chorionic villi consist of vascular mesenchymal cones surrounded by cuboidal trophoblastic and giant binucleate cells. These either penetrate directly into the endometrium or simply interdigitate with vascular foldings of the endometrial surface (e.g., as in farm animals). The function of the villi is to bring the fetal (allantoic) vessels into proximity with the maternal blood vessels.

Classification of Placenta

The placenta may be classified according to morphology, microscopic characteristics of the maternal–fetal barrier, and loss of maternal tissue at birth (Table 9–4).

Gross Shape. The definitive shape of the placenta is determined by the distribution of villi over the chorionic surface (Fig. 9–5). In ruminants, the fetal cotyledons fuse with caruncles or specialized projections of the uterine mucosa to form placentomes or functional units. The caruncles

TABLE 9–3. The Fetal Membranes of Farm Animals

Membrane	Origin	Functions
Yolk sac	Early entodermal layer	Vestigial
Amnion	Cavitation from inner cell mass	Encloses fetus in a fluid-filled cavity
Allantois	Diverticulum of hindgut	Blood vessels connect fetal with placental circulation
		Fuses with chorion to form the chorioallantoic placenta
Chorion	Trophoblastic capsule of blastocyst	Encloses embryo and other fetal membranes
		Intimately associated with lining of uterus to form placenta
Umbilical cord	Amnion wraps about the yolk stalk	Encloses allantoic vessels and acts as the vascular link between mother and fetus

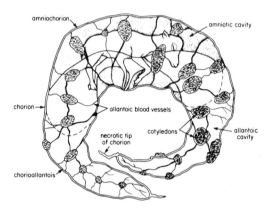

FIG. 9–4. Diagram of the fetal membranes of a 105-day fetal calf to show the allantoic and amniotic cavities. The cotyledons are distributed over the chorioallantoic membrane and the amniochorion.

are convex in the cow and concave in the ewe and goat (Fig. 9–5). In early pregnancy in the mare and sow, the placenta consists of a simple apposition of fetal and maternal epithelia, but between 75 and 110 days of gestation in the mare, the complex folding and branching of the two surfaces give rise to the formation of microcotyledons.

Endometrial cups are a unique feature of the equine placenta. They are discrete, raised areas of a few millimeters to several centimeters in diameter and arranged in a circular fashion at the caudal portion of the gravid uterine horn. These cups are formed by the invasion of the endometrium by a band of specialized trophoblastic cells (chorionic girdle) that peel off the fetal membranes by day 38. The endometrial cups are the source of the chorionic gonadotropin (eCG) present in high concentrations in the blood of mares between 40 and 130 days of gestation (Allen et al., 1973).

In sheep, placentomes ranging between 90 and 100 are evenly distributed between the pregnant and nonpregnant horns. In cattle, 70 to 120 placentomes develop around the fetus and progress toward the distal limit of the chorioallantois in the nongravid horn (Fig. 9–4). During pregnancy, these placentomes enlarge to several times their original diameter. Normally, the chorioallantois extends into the nongravid horn, but the degree to which

TABLE 9–4. Classification of Chorioallantoic Placentas

	Classification		
Species	Chorionic Villous Pattern	Maternal–Fetal Barrier	Loss of Maternal Tissue at Birth
Pig	Diffuse	Epitheliochorial	None (nondeciduate)
Mare	Diffuse and Microcotyledonary	Epitheliochorial	None (nondeciduate)
Sheep, goat, cow, buffalo	Cotyledonary	Epitheliochorial	None (nondeciduate)
Dog, cat	Zonary	Endotheliochorial	Moderate (deciduate)
Man, monkey	Discoid	Hemochorial	Extensive (deciduate)

A

diffuse placenta

mare   pig

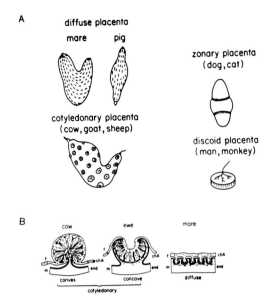

zonary placenta
(dog,cat)

cotyledonary placenta
(cow,goat,sheep)

discoid placenta
(man,monkey)

B

cow   ewe   mare

convex   concave   diffuse

cotyledonary

FIG. 9–5.   *A*, The distribution of chorionic villi
as the basis of classifying placental shape. *B*,
Epitheliochorial placenta of mare, ewe and
cow. The placenta of mare is diffuse and microcotyledonary; those of the ewe and cow are
cotyledonary. *chA*, Chorioallantois; *end*, endometrium; *F*, fetal; *M*, maternal. (Redrawn from
Silver et al. (1973). *In* Proceedings of Sir Joseph
Barcroft Centenary Symposium, K.S. Comline
et al. (eds.). Cambridge, Cambridge University
Press.)

the caruncles hypertrophy is usually less
than that in the gravid horn.

The chorionic sacs of adjacent pig fetuses are in apposition, and chorionic attachment between one or more fetuses is
encountered frequently. Though there is
a high incidence of chorionic fusion during
multiple pregnancy, vascular anastomosis
between allantoic circulations rarely occurs in sheep. In contrast, a high incidence
of vascular anastomosis is encountered between twin bovine fetuses, giving rise to
the well-known intersexual condition of
freemartinism.

Placental Barrier

The membranes separating the fetal
and maternal circulations are collectively
known as the *placental barrier.* This bar-

rier is named according to the maternal
and fetal tissues actually in contact, in the
order from maternal to fetal tissues.

The ultrastructural features of the junctional zone between fetal and maternal
tissues of the epitheliochorial placenta
show an interdigitation of fetal and maternal microvilli with little direct contact between fetal and maternal cell membranes.
Wide structural variations occur in the
epitheliochorial placenta of farm species.
For example, the uterine epithelium
forms a partial syncytium in the ewe and
large binucleate cells in the chorionic epithelium of the cow and ewe (Steven,
1975).

Placental Circulation

In the placenta, two circulations are parallel to the fetal and maternal circulations,
but the fetal and the maternal blood do
not intermingle in the epitheliochorial
placentas of farm animals.

Uterine Blood Flow. The maternal
blood supply to the placenta is derived
from the uterine arteries and veins. As gestation advances, the rate of uterine blood
flow increases in sheep and is related to
fetal weight. About 84% of the total uterine flow near term passes to the placentomes; the remainder supplies the endometrial and myometrial layers of the
placenta.

Umbilical Blood Flow. The umbilical
arteries bring blood from the fetus to the
placenta, and the umbilical veins return
blood from the placenta to the fetus. Most
of the umbilical blood flow is distributed
to the cotyledons, while only 6% supplies
the chorioallantois.

The rate of umbilical flow increases with
advancing pregnancy to meet the growing
demands of the fetus. The overall increase
in umbilical flow is achieved by a decreased umbilical vascular resistance earlier in pregnancy and by an increased arterial blood pressure later.

Placental   Microcirculation. Various
theoretical models have been proposed to
explain the direction of maternal and fetal

blood flow in the placenta. Blood flow in adjacent maternal and fetal vascular channels could be countercurrent, concurrent, crosscurrent (multivillous), or pool. In the pool flow, maternal blood enters a large space in which it is exposed to fetal capillaries.

The pattern of blood flow in the ovine placenta is either crosscurrent or a mixture of crosscurrent and countercurrent. In the mare, the microcotyledons, like the cotyledons of the sheep and cow, are highly vascularized. Long, straight arteries pass between the uterine glands to the endometrium, where they branch (Fig. 9–6). On the fetal side, the chorionic villi are supplied by branches of the umbilical arteries and veins. The blood flow in the fetal capillaries is from the tip to the base of each villus and is opposite to the flow in the maternal capillaries (countercurrent).

Placental Functions

The placenta performs many functions and substitutes for the fetal gastrointestinal tract, lung, kidney, liver, and endocrine glands. In addition, the placenta separates the maternal and fetal organisms, thus ensuring the separate development of the fetus (Fig. 9–7).

Placental Transport.   The blood of the fetus and dam never come into direct contact, yet the two circulations are close enough at the junction of the chorion and endometrium for oxygen and nutrients to

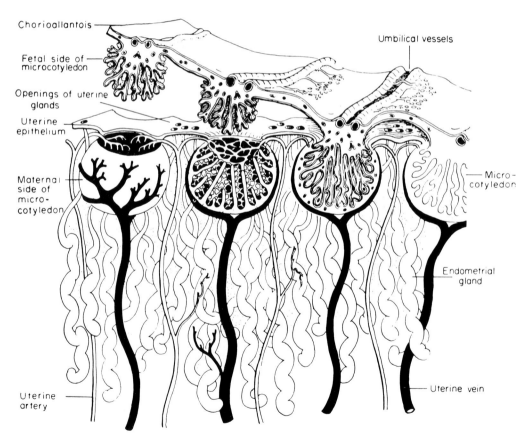

FIG. 9–6.   Diagram of the mature equine placenta illustrating the structure of the microcotyledons, which are formed between 75 and 100 days of gestation. (From Steven and Samuel, (1975) J. Reprod. Fertil. Suppl. *23,* 580.)

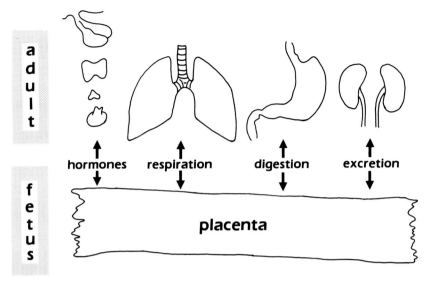

FIG. 9–7. The functions of the placenta. The placenta combines in one organ many activities of the fetus—hormones, respiration, digestion and excretion—that are separate in the adult.

pass from maternal to fetal blood, and waste products in the opposite direction.

Gases. Many similarities exist between the gas exchange across the placenta and that across the lungs. The major difference, however, is that in the placenta it is a fluid-to-fluid system, whereas in the lung it is a gas-to-fluid system. The umbilical arteries carry unoxygenated blood from the fetus to the placenta, while the umbilical veins carry oxygenated blood in the reverse direction.

The efficiency of oxygen exchange varies depending on the system. It is maximal in the countercurrent systems and minimal in the concurrent system. The efficiency of the multivillous system is intermediate between the previously mentioned systems.

Carbon dioxide diffuses freely from the fetal to the maternal circulation and is facilitated by certain physiologic mechanisms. For example, fetal blood has a lower affinity for CO_2, than maternal blood during placental oxygen transfer. This favors the diffusion of CO_2 from fetal to maternal blood.

Nutrients. The placenta permits the transport of sugars, amino acids, vitamins, and minerals to the fetus as substrates for fetal growth. Placental transport of nutrients is based on net flux from either mother to fetus or in the opposite direction. It can be due to a concentration difference or of unidirectional carrier-mediated transport. Many nutrients such as glucose, amino acids, electrolytes, and vitamins are transported by carrier systems located in the trophoblast (Schneider, 1991).

Placenta contains large amounts of glycogen synthesized mainly from maternal glucose. Fetal fructose is produced by the placenta from glucose, and its function in the fetus is obscure. Fructose comprises about 70 to 80% of the sugar in fetal blood, while glucose is predominant in maternal blood. Fetal fructose values are correlated with maternal glucose levels, and the maintenance of high fetal concentrations might be an indicator of placental function. Free fatty acids (FFA) are transported across the placenta by simple diffusion. The maternal and fetal levels of FFA are closely correlated in the horse but FFA transfer across the ruminant placenta is minimal.

Proteins as such are not transferred. Amino acids cross readily against a concentration gradient and are found in higher concentrations in fetal than in maternal plasma. Immunoglobulins are transmitted in man and some animals but not in farm animals. This difference may be related to structural differences in the various placental types.

The lipid soluble vitamins (A, D, and E) are impeded by the placenta; thus at birth the concentrations of these are lower in the fetus than in the mother. Water soluble vitamins (B and C) cross the placental barrier more readily than those that are lipid soluble. Polypeptides cross the placenta slowly. Although iodine crosses the placenta readily in sheep, there is little or no transfer of thyroid hormones or thyroid-stimulating hormone. Insulin also probably crosses only slowly and in insignificant amounts.

Cortisol is transferred from mother to fetus in many species but not in goats and sheep. The unconjugated steroids, progesterone and estrogens cross the placental barrier readily. Many steroids undergo enzymic alteration in moving across the placenta, and such alterations play a major role in their transport.

Hormones. The placenta is a transient endocrine organ like the CL. It secretes both trophic and steroid hormones that are released into the fetal as well as the maternal circulations. The concept of a fetoplacental unit was proposed to explain the various mechanisms by which large amounts of progesterone and estrogens are produced during pregnancy. Both the placenta and the fetus lack certain enzymatic functions that are essential for steroidogenesis, but enzymes absent from the placenta are present in the fetus and vice versa. Thus, by sequential integration of the fetal and placental steroidogenic functions, the fetoplacental unit can elaborate most, if not all, hormonally active steroids.

Some species (ewe and mare) and not others (cow, goat, and sow) are capable of synthesizing sufficient amounts of progesterone to maintain pregnancy by using acetate and cholesterol derived from the maternal circulation. During the latter half of gestation, a high rate of estrogen production occurs in the placentas of the mare, cow, sow, and ewe. The placenta relies on fetal cortisol to induce activity of the placental enzymes and thus synthesize estrogen from progesterone.

Placental lactogen (PL), also known as chorionic somatomammotropin, is a peptide hormone of pregnancy found in many mammalian species and reported to have trophic and growth hormone-like effects in both mother and fetus.

Mother–Fetus Immunologic Relationship

Fetus as an Allograft. The presence of a developing fetus in the intrauterine environment poses a serious problem. The fetus inherits from the father genetic characteristics that are foreign to the mother and therefore may be considered as an allograft or tissue from a different individual of the same species. If the donor has antigens not possessed by the recipient, the recipient will usually reject the transplanted tissue. Antigens that provoke rejection are termed *transplantation* or *histocompatibility antigens*. The rejection is usually mediated by T-lymphocytes rather than by antibodies (Fig. 9–8). These transplantation antigens are present on the cell surface and are directly exposed to the T-lymphocytes of the recipient circulatory system.

The fetus does provide antigenic challenge to the maternal immune system that should be capable of eliciting immunologic rejection reactions, but unlike the immunologic destruction of allografts in other parts of the organism, the placenta is not rejected until parturition, a period far in excess of the time taken to elicit an allograft reaction (usually in 2 to 3 weeks). The failure of maternal tissue to reject the placenta has puzzled immunologists and has led to many theories to explain the unique relationship between mother and

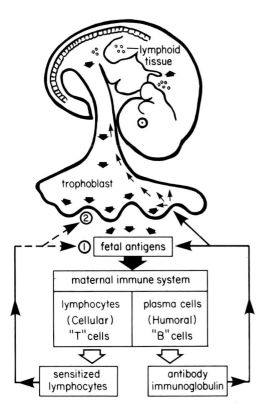

lymphoid tissue

trophoblast

② ① fetal antigens

maternal immune system	
lymphocytes (Cellular) "T" cells	plasma cells (Humoral) "B" cells
sensitized lymphocytes	antibody immunoglobulin

FIG. 9–8. Processes occurring to protect the fetus from an immunologic attack by the sensitized lymphocytes of the mother. Antigens present on the trophoblast or fetal cells sensitize the maternal immune system giving rise to antibodies and sensitized lymphocytes. The action of killer cells (sensitized lymphocytes) on the fetoplacental unit may be blocked by: (1) "immunologic enhancement" involving the combination of humoral antibodies with sites on the trophoblast cells thereby blocking the sensitized lymphocytes reaching these cells; and (2) synthesis of unique proteins and steroid hormones produced by the trophoblast.

The exact nature of the immunoregulatory mechanisms is highly controversial, and there is no simple explanation for the immune coexistence between mother and fetus. The key to the maintenance of pregnancy may reside in the trophoblast (Billington, 1989). Antigens present on trophoblast or fetal cells presumably sensitize the maternal immune system (Fig. 9–8), giving rise to antibodies and sensitized lymphocytes. However, trophoblast tissue acts as a barrier, preventing the entry of maternal lymphocytes to the fetus. This protection from a maternal immunologic attack might be due to the unique structure of the trophoblastic cell surface (sialomucin) and/or synthesis of factors that render it insensitive to an antibody- or cell-mediated immunologic lysis.

During the 1980s, true interspecific pregnancies, in which the conceptus and female carrying the pregnancy are of different species, have been produced through embryo manipulation and transfer. These pregnancies were used to study the mechanisms that allow the fetal allograft to survive without immunologic rejection (Anderson, 1988). Experiments of the equine model (domestic horse and donkey) and the bovid model (domestic goat and sheep) have revealed the presence of an immunologic barrier that restricts interspecific pregnancy. Apparently, however, there are species differences in the manifestation of the barrier. A cell-mediated immunologic response may be necessary for preventing trophoblastic rejection in the equine model, whereas inadequate interaction of the trophoblast with the endometrium, instead of the immunologic response, may be important in the bovid model (Anderson 1988). Several mechanisms must also exist for protection of preimplantation embryos from the destruction of the maternal immune system. One such mechanism at the cellular level might be the zona pelluicda, acting as a physical barrier between the mother and fetus (Warner et al., 1988).

fetus. Detailed discussion of the many theories proposed to explain this phenomenon may be found in several reviews (Anderson, 1988; Beer and Sio, 1982; Cooper, 1980; Hogarth, 1982). The following theories have been proposed: The fetus is antigenically immature; maternal immunologic activities are reduced or suspended during pregnancy; the uterus is an immunologically privileged site; and a maternal–fetal physical barrier is present.

PRENATAL PHYSIOLOGY

Prenatal Periods

The prenatal development of farm animals may be divided into three main periods. The ovum period culminates with the initial attachment of the blastocyst but is before the establishment of an intraembryonic circulation. The embryonic period extends from day 15 to day 45 of gestation in the cow, day 12 to about day 34 in the sheep, and day 12 to day 60 in the mare. In this period, rapid growth and differentiation occur, during which the major tissues, organs and systems (Fig. 9–9) are established and the major features of external body form are recognizable. The fetal period extends from about day 34 of gestation in sheep, day 45 in cattle, and from day 60 in horses until birth. This period is characterized by growth and changes in the form of the fetus.

Fetal Nutrition and Metabolism

Whereas the blastocyst and the early embryo are nourished by endometrial fluid, the fetus receives its supply of nutrients from the maternal circulation across the placenta. The fetus may be regarded as a parasite living within the mother, and it has priority in the event of insufficient maternal nutrition so that its development can proceed unimpaired. It needs carbohydrates, proteins, vitamins, and minerals for maintenance, differentiation, and subsequent development and growth.

The fetus receives a continuous supply of glucose from its mother through the placenta. Glucose is the major metabolic fuel for the fetus. Toward the end of the gestation, the normal fetus accumulates glycogen in its liver and skeletal muscles to assist it in overcoming the transitional period after birth until efficient suckling is established. Although fructose comprises about 70 to 80% of the sugar in the blood of fetal ungulates (cattle, sheep, goats), its use is negligible, except when blood glucose levels are low. In ruminant fetuses, acetate, lactate, and amino acids may be important energy substrates.

The fetus synthesizes all its proteins from the amino acids derived from the mother; proteins are used mainly for synthesis rather than oxidation or gluconeogenesis.

Throughout gestation, the retention of calcium, phosphorus, and iron increases relative to fetal body weight. The fetus has the unique ability to deplete maternal skeletal stores of calcium if feeds are low

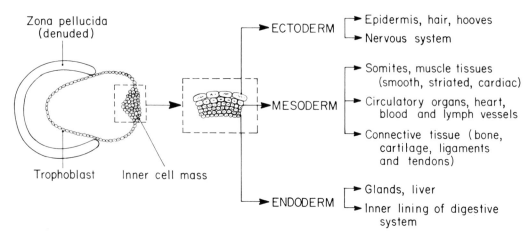

Fig. 9–9. The derivation of various body organs by progressive differentiation and divergent specialization. The origin of all fetal organs can be traced back to the primary germ layers that originate from the inner cell mass.

in calcium. Iron is used for hemoglobin synthesis, but little is known about its distribution and metabolism.

Fetal Growth

Growth Rate. As it grows from the spherical fertilized ovum to the full-term fetus, the embryo not only increases in size and weight but also undergoes many changes in form. The rate of growth—that is, the percentage increase in weight and dimensions per unit of time (relative growth)—is most rapid in the earlier stages and declines as gestation advances, whereas the absolute increment per unit of time (absolute growth) increases exponentially, reaching a maximum during late gestation. In cattle, over one half of the increase in fetal weight occurs during the last 2 months of gestation. At term, the weight of the fetus contributes to approximately 60% of the total weight of the conceptus.

The growth rates of the fetus and its component organs and tissues vary during different stages of intrauterine life. For example, during early fetal development, the cephalic region grows rapidly and, consequently, the fetal head is disproportionately large. Later in gestation, cephalic growth slows. At birth, the head and limbs are relatively more developed than the muscles.

Factors Affecting Fetal Growth. The rate of fetal growth depends primarily on the feed supply and the ability of the fetus to use the feed (Fig. 9–10). Species, breed, and strain differences in fetal size are due to differences in the rate of cell division, which is determined genetically. Thus, there is close integration between the feed supply to the fetus (environmental factors), the rate of cell division (genetic factors), and hence, the rate of growth.

Genetic Factors. Holstein fetuses at birth weigh about 35% more than Jersey calves and about 15% more than the average dairy calf. Similarly, Romney sheep fetuses grow faster than Merino fetuses. The maternal contribution to variability

in fetal size is greater than the paternal contribution.

Environmental Factors. These include size, parity, and nutrition of the mother, litter size, placental size, and climatic stress. Of these factors, maternal size is important. The size of the young at birth from reciprocal crosses between the large Shire horses and the small Shetland ponies depends mainly on the size of the mother. The size of the sire only begins to exert influence on growth after birth. Similar observations have been made in cattle and sheep.

Maternal nutrition exerts an important influence on fetal growth, notably in sheep. Undernutrition of the ewe during the latter part of gestation leads to the production of stunted lambs, even though a normal level of nutrition was present earlier. Conversely, a reversed type of feeding program results in normal-sized lambs.

In polytocous species such as the pig, during early gestation, feed and uterine accommodation are adequate, but in the later stages, the number of fetuses sharing the uterine blood supply can have a profound influence on their size at birth. The length of gestation in the pig is not reduced by increases in litter size, suggesting that the small birth weight with large litters must be related to the availability of nutrition to individual fetuses. In monotocous species, notably cattle, twin fetuses are generally smaller than single fetuses, probably because the length of gestation is reduced. In sheep, fetal weight is related to placental weight. In several species including human, the difference in fetal size between singletons and twins in late pregnancy is not wholly accounted for by the difference in placental weight.

High ambient temperature during pregnancy affects fetal size. Exposure of pregnant ewes to heat stress reduces fetal growth, the degree of reduction being proportional to the length of exposure. This dwarfing is a specific effect of temperature and is not due to reduced feed intake during pregnancy.

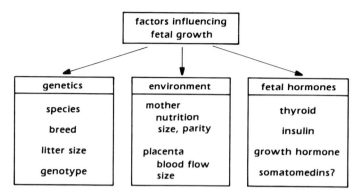

FIG. 9–10. Summary of factors influencing fetal growth. Species and breed differences in fetal size are due to differences in the rate of cell division that is determined genetically. The rate of fetal growth depends on the intrauterine environment. Fetal hormones may influence fetal growth. Somatomedins are insulin-like growth factors that stimulate growth of fetal cells *in vitro*, but their role in the fetus is unknown.

Fetal Hormones. Fetal hormones are likely to influence fetal growth (Colenbrander et al., 1984; Jost, 1979). Growth hormone can stimulate fetal growth, but there is no evidence that it is essential for fetal growth.

Insulin is of importance in fetal growth and exerts its effects through an increase of energy substrate availability and stimulates placental growth. The fetal thyroid is dispensable in some species (rabbit, human), whereas in others (monkey, sheep) its absence results in delayed skeletal and muscular maturation.

Insulin-like Growth Factors. The insulin-like growth factors (IGF-I and -II) or sommatomedins are polypeptide hormones similar to insulin. They occur in fetal and placental tissues (Falconer et al., 1991). IGF-II appears not only to mediate fetal growth according to the availability of glucose but also, acting in concert with placental hormones, regulates the metabolic activities of the mother so that a continuous supply of substrates for fetal development is available (Owens, 1991).

Fetal Circulation

The fetal circulation (Fig. 9–11) is essentially similar to that of the adult except that oxygenation of blood occurs in the placenta rather than in the lungs. The fetal circulation also has several shunts or bypasses that direct oxygenated blood to the tissue. A major portion of the blood in the

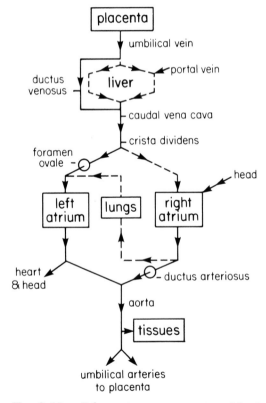

FIG. 9–11. Schematic representation of fetal circulation. The ductus venosus, crista dividens, foramen ovale, and ductus arteriosus act as shunts directing oxygenated blood away from the liver, right ventricle, and functionless lungs, respectively.

umbilical vein is shunted through the ductus venosus in the liver into the caudal vena cava to avoid metabolism in the liver. A ductus venosus, however, never develops, and the umbilical venous blood passes through the liver sinusoids in the pig and the horse.

The crista dividens projects from the border of the foramen ovale and separates the caudal vena cava flow into two streams before the atria are reached; the stream from the ductus venosus is guided through the foramen ovale largely into the left atrium, thereby directing oxygenated blood to the head and developing the left ventricle in the neonatal period. The ductus arteriosus shunts most of the pulmonary arterial blood flow into the aorta and away from the functionless lungs. The two umbilical arteries originate from the caudal end of the descending aorta and carry blood to the placenta.

The higher blood pressure in the right side of the fetal heart than in the left side keeps the foramen ovale patent. Likewise, this pressure difference causes the blood to flow from the pulmonary artery into the aorta by way of the ductus arteriosus.

In general, heart rates are higher in the fetus than in the adult. Fetal heart rates differ in various species as well as at different stages of gestation within each species. The fetal heart rate ranges from 170 to 220 beats per minute in sheep and from 120 to 140 beats per minute in cattle.

Fetal Fluids

Origin. The origin of fetal fluids (amniotic and allantoic) and the secretions that contribute to them are complex (Table 9–5). There are at least four sites at which absorption and secretion might occur: the respiratory, urinary, and digestive systems and also the fetal skin. In the fetal lamb, urine formed by the mesonephros passes into the allantoic cavity through the urachus until about 90 days of gestation. Thereafter, urine passes in increasing quantities into the amniotic sac, which is due to occlusion of the urachus and patency of the urethra. Thus fetal urine forms a major source of amniotic fluid in the latter part of pregnancy in sheep.

Other sources may influence the amount and composition of amniotic fluid in other species, for example: secretions from fetal salivary glands, buccal mucosa, lungs, and trachea; and dynamic interchange between maternal, fetal, and amniotic fluid compartments. In the pig, the initial accumulation of allantoic fluid is the result of the secretory activity of the allantoic membrane; later in gestation, however, the fetal urine provides most of the allantoic fluid (Table 9–5).

A rapid exchange of water occurs between the maternal circulation, the fetal circulation, and the amniotic fluid with a new water circulation: mother to fetus to amniotic fluid to mother. The fetus also removes fluid by swallowing or by drawing amniotic fluid into the fetal lungs during respiratory movements.

Volume. The relative volumes of fluid in the amniotic and allantoic cavities show much fluctuation during pregnancy. These variations probably reflect the contributions of the fetal and maternal compartments. The control of the fluid compartments is probably regulated by the fetal endocrine system and the fetal kidneys. Fetal fluids increase throughout gestation in all species, but in the pig they tend to decline at term. The volume of allantoic fluid is relatively higher than amniotic fluid during pregnancy, the exception being the ewe at midgestation.

Functions. Amniotic fluid is not a stagnant pool but rather a vital fluid bathing the fetus and performing several functions (Table 9–5). Allantoic fluid, composed of hypotonic urine, maintains the osmotic pressure of the fetal plasma and prevents fluid loss to maternal circulation. In the pig, the chorioallantoic membrane possesses secretory properties, and it is capable of actively removing sodium from the allantoic cavity, thereby maintaining the allantoic fluid hypotonic relative to bladder or serum.

TABLE 9–5. Origin, Composition, and Functions of Fetal Fluids in Farm Animals

Fluid	Origin	Composition	Functions
Amniotic	Fetal urine Secretions from respiratory tract and buccal cavity Maternal circulation	A solution with suspended particulate material Low levels of K^+, Mg^{++}, glucose creatinine, uric acid and urea High levels of Na^+, Cl^-, P^{+++} and fructose Enzymes, iron, amniotic plaques, cells	Protects fetus from external shock Prevents adhesion between fetal skin and amniotic membrane Assists in dilating cervix and lubricating birth passages during birth
Allantoic	Fetal urine Secretory activity of allantoic membrane	Ultrafiltrate Low levels of Na^+, Cl^-, P^{+++}, glucose High levels of K^+, Mg^{++}, Ca^{++}, fructose, creatinine, uric acid, and urea	Brings allantochorion into close apposition with endometrium during initial steps of attachment Stores fetal excretory products not readily transferred back to the mother Helps to maintain osmotic pressure of fetal plasma

Composition. Amniotic and allantoic fluids contain metabolic constituents, electrolytes, enzymes, hormones, cells, and other structures.

In ruminants, the inner lining of the amnion, particularly near the umbilicus, contains numerous raised, discrete, round foci called *amnionic plaques,* which are rich in glycogen and disappear late in gestation. Amniotic fluid also contains cells that may be used for a prenatal diagnosis of sex. *Hippomanes* are smooth, discoid, rubberlike, amber masses floating in the allantoic fluid and are probably aggregations of fetal hair and meconium.

PARTURITION

Parturition, or labor, is defined as the physiologic process by which the pregnant uterus delivers the fetus and placenta from the maternal organism.

Signs of Approaching Parturition

Most signs of approaching parturition relate to changes in the pelvic ligaments, enlargement and edema of the vulva, and mammary activity. These signs are useful as a guide, but they are too variable for an accurate prediction of the date of parturition.

Obvious enlargement of the mammary gland occurs in all farm species. The teats become swollen and secretions may escape through the teat orifice. In the mare, colostrum oozes from the teat orifice, forming a bead of waxing material at each teat orifice. Waxing occurs in most mares between 6 to 48 hours before foaling and is replaced by drips or streams of milk 12 to 24 hours later.

Nest building is a feature of impending parturition in polytocous species such as the pig, but an expression of this behavior may be suspended in intensive management systems. Cattle and sheep under grazing systems remain with the herd but seek isolation just before the onset of parturition.

Initiation of Parturition

Parturition is triggered by the fetus and is completed by a complex interaction of endocrine, neural, and mechanical factors (Table 9–6), but their precise roles and interrelationships are not fully understood.

Several reviews have discussed the control of parturition in farm animals or in individual species such as sheep (Liggins et al., 1973), goat (Thorburn, 1979), cattle (Hoffman et al., 1979), pig (First and Bosc, 1979), and horse (Allen and Pashen, 1981).

TABLE 9–6. Some Theories on the Initiation of Parturition

Theory	Possible Mechanism(s)
Fall in progesterone concentration	Blocks myometrial contractions during pregnancy; near term the blocking action of progesterone decreases
A rise in estrogen concentration	Overcomes the progesterone block of myometrial contractility and/or increases spontaneous myometrial contractility
Increase of uterine volume	Overcomes the effects of progesterone block of myometrial contractility
Release of oxytocin	Leads to contractions in an estrogen-sensitized myometrium
Release of prostaglandins ($PGF_{2\alpha}$)	Stimulates myometrial contractions; induces luteolysis leading to a fall in progesterone concentration (corpus luteum-dependent species)
Activation of fetal hypothalamic-pituitary-adrenal axis	Fetal corticosteroids cause a fall in progesterone, a rise in estrogen, and a release of $PGF_{2\alpha}$. These events lead to myometrial contractility

Mechanics of Parturition

Successful parturition depends on two mechanical processes: the ability of the uterus to contract and the capacity of the cervix to dilate sufficiently to enable the passage of the fetus (Fig. 9–12).

Myometrial Contractions. The activity of the uterine muscle (myometrium) is under the influence of progesterone, which ensures an environment conducive to the developing fetus. Myometrial contractions of low amplitude and frequency occur during the major part of gestation, and at the onset of parturition, these are replaced by the expulsive form characteristic of delivery. The biochemical mechanisms controlling contractions in the myometrium are similar to those in smooth muscle.

There is controversy as to the roles of estrogen and progesterone in controlling uterine activity during gestation and parturition (Table 9–6). These hormones influence uterine motility through the release of $PGF_{2\alpha}$; the latter interacts with the smooth muscle adenyl cyclase system to lower cAMP levels and cause myometrial contractions.

Dilation of Cervix. A major function of the cervix during pregnancy is to retain the growing conceptus within the uterus. The cervix is firmer and more rigid than the uterine wall, which is due to the higher content of connective tissue (collagen) in the cervix. Dilation of the cervix is due more to changes in the physical characteristics of cervical collagen ("ripening") than to increased intrauterine pressure. This is

UTERUS   CERVIX

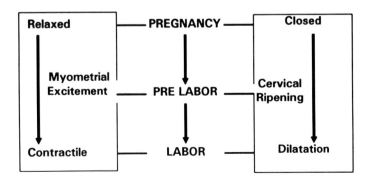

FIG. 9–12. Roles of the uterus and cervix during pregnancy and labor. During the prelabor stage, the myometrium loses its inhibitions and generates contractility, whereas the cervix "ripens" and dilates, permitting the normal onset of labor. (Redrawn from Calder, A.A. (1990). Reprod. Fertil. Dev. 2, 553.)

clearly evident in species such as sheep, goats, and cattle that have a rigid cervix (Fitzpatrick and Dobson, 1979). A few hours before labor contractions commence, the cervix softens, becomes more compliant, and gradually dilates. Ripening of the cervix is hormone dependent and may be influenced by factors such as the elevated levels of estrogens, secretion of relaxin (pig), and $PGF_{2\alpha}$ at the onset of parturition.

Initiation of Parturition

Fetal Mechanisms. One of the exciting discoveries in reproductive biology is that the fetus, not the mother, dominates the mechanisms stimulating the onset of parturition in most mammalian species.

Congenital fetal abnormalities occurring in prolonged gestation in sheep and cattle led to the recognition of the fetal role in the initiation of parturition. Subsequent experimental studies in farm species have provided convincing evidence that the fetus coordinates the events leading to the initiation of its own delivery (First and Lohse, 1984).

The fetus possesses a number of mechanisms to ensure that the myometrium remains quiescent so that its development in utero is unhindered. The placental production of progesterone imposes a conduction block on the myometrium (Table 9–6). A significant increase in the fetal plasma concentration of cortisol occurs during the final stages of gestation in sheep, which is due to a signal originating in the fetal hypothalamic–pituitary axis; whether it is adrenocorticotropic hormone (ACTH) or some other trophic stimulus from the fetal pituitary has not been established. Thorburn (1991) has postulated that the increasing metabolic demands on the placenta during the phase of rapid fetal growth (last trimester) stimulate placental production of prostaglandin E_2, which in turn activates the fetal hypothalamic-pituitary-adrenal axis, leading to a rise in concentration of fetal cortisol (Fig. 9–13).

A similar rise in fetal cortisol secretion triggers parturition in goats, cattle, and pigs (Thorburn et al., 1977). Some increase in adrenal activity probably occurs in the equine fetus near term, but the spectacular rise in fetal plasma cortisol concentration before birth does not occur.

The mechanisms that follow the release of cortisol differ among species depending on the source of progesterone maintaining the pregnancy. In sheep, cortisol stimulates the placenta to convert progesterone to estrogen. The elevated levels of estrogen stimulate secretion of $PGF_{2\alpha}$ and development of oxytocin receptors. In CL-dependent species, cortisol in addition to the synthesis of estrogen causes a release of $PGF_{2\alpha}$ from the endometrium, which in turn causes regression of the corpora lutea.

Maternal Mechanisms. The maternal contribution, although less dramatic than those of the fetus, is clearly evident in the timing of birth. For example, the predilection of the mare to foal during the hours of darkness and the ability to postpone birth until she is undisturbed is well recognized. Anxiety, stress, or fear prolongs the act of parturition in several species through a decrease in myometrial contractility induced by a release of epinephrine. Management routines such as feeding may also influence the time of parturition in cattle, horses, and sheep. Thus, it is reasonable to conclude that the fetus determines the day of parturition, whereas the mother decides the hour of parturition.

Labor

Labor commences with the onset of regular, peristaltic uterine contractions accompanied by progressive dilation of the cervix.

Stages of Labor. For descriptive purposes three stages of labor may be recognized: (a) dilation of the cervix, (b) expulsion of the fetus, and (c) expulsion of the placenta (Table 9–7). The time required for the expulsion of the fetus is the shortest of the three stages in monotocous species (Table 9–8).

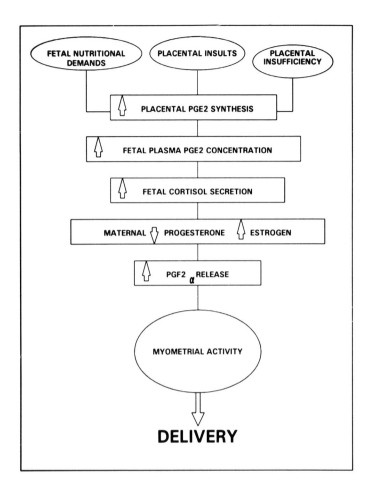

FETAL NUTRITIONAL DEMANDS   PLACENTAL INSULTS   PLACENTAL INSUFFICIENCY

PLACENTAL PGE2 SYNTHESIS

FETAL PLASMA PGE2 CONCENTRATION

FETAL CORTISOL SECRETION

MATERNAL PROGESTERONE   ESTROGEN

PGF2$_{\alpha}$ RELEASE

MYOMETRIAL ACTIVITY

DELIVERY

FIG. 9–13. Placental–nutritional model for parturition in sheep. Fetal nutrient demands and placental insults or insufficiency increase placental PGE$_2$, leading to high levels of PGE$_2$ in the fetal circulation and a rise in fetal cortisol secretion. Fetal cortisol alters the progesterone-estrogen ratio in maternal blood, increasing PGF$_{2\alpha}$ release from the maternal placenta, which in turn leads to myometrial contractility and parturition. (Adapted from Thorburn, G.D. (1991). Reprod. Fertil. Dev. *3*, 277.)

Forces of Delivery. Myometrial contractions start at the apex of the cornua in monotocous species, and in the pig they begin at both ends of the uterine horns and subsequently are propagated toward the cervix or in the opposite direction. The "bellows" effect in the pig (Taverne, 1982) reduces the distance traversed by succeeding piglets and avoids a pile of piglets at the cervix. During the first stage, uterine contractions are painful, causing restlessness and signs of abdominal discomfort. As the fetus progresses through the cervix, the allantochorion ruptures, releasing a urine-like fluid that marks the end of the first stage of labor.

The distention of the cervix and vagina by the conceptus initiates the neurohumoral reflex (Ferguson's reflex), which produces the expulsive force of abdominal muscular contractions (straining) and the release of oxytocin, which in turn accentuates myometrial contractions. The combined forces of intra-abdominal and intra-uterine pressure mark the beginning of the second stage of labor. Straining consists of a few contractions followed by a few minutes of rest. The fetus enclosed in the amnion is propelled through the birth canal and appears at the vulva. As straining continues, the amnion ruptures. The greatest effort is associated with the emergence of the head and chest. All farm species assume lateral recumbency with limbs extended during delivery. The umbilical cord breaks as the neonate or the dam moves.

TABLE 9–7. Stages of Labor and Related Events in Farm Animals

Stage of Labor	Mechanical Forces	Period	Related Events
I Dilation of Cervix	Regular uterine contractions	Beginning of uterine contractions until cervix is fully dilated and continuous with vagina	Maternal restlessness, elevated pulse and respiratory rates Changes in fetal position and posture
II Expulsion of fetus*	Strong uterine and abdominal contractions	From complete cervical dilation to end of delivery of fetus	Maternal recumbency and straining Rupture of allantochorion and escape of fluid from vulva Appearance of amnion (water-bag) at vulva Rupture of amnion and delivery of fetus
III Expulsion of placenta	Uterine contractions decrease in amplitude	Following delivery of fetus to expulsion of placenta	Maternal straining ceases Loosening of chorionic villi from maternal crypts Inversion of chorioallantois Straining and expulsion of fetal membranes

* In polytocous species (sow) and twin-bearing species (sheep and goat), this stage cannot be separated from the next stage (third).

TABLE 9–8. Average Duration of the Three Stages of Labor in Farm Animals (Hours)

	Stage of Labor		
	I	II	III
Animal	Dilation of Cervix	Expulsion of Fetus(es)	Expulsion of Placenta(s)
Mare	1–4	0.2–0.5	1
Cow, buffalo	2–6	0.5–1.0	6–12
Ewe	2–6	0.5–2.0	0.5–8
Sow	2–12	2.5–3.0	1–4

Rhythmic uterine contractions originating at the apex of the uterine horn continue after birth (third stage) and cause the inversion of the chorioallantois in ruminants. The presence of the detached placenta within the birth canal then initiates further straining and expulsion of the placenta. The expulsion of the placenta is rapid in the mare but is slower in ruminants as a result of the cotyledonary type of placentation. The placentas of adjacent piglets are usually fused and often expelled as one or more masses interspersed with the birth of piglets. The largest mass of placenta, however, is usually expelled 3 to 4 hours after the delivery of the last piglet.

Induction of Parturition

There is interest in the induction of parturition as a management tool, particularly for cattle and pigs. Exogenous glucocorticoids can be used to induce parturition in cattle, goat, and sheep but not in the horse or pig. $PGF_{2\alpha}$ induces parturition in the pig, goat, and cattle because they depend on the CL for progesterone during pregnancy.

Perinatal Adaptions

The fetus, which depended on the placenta for respiration, nutrition, and excretion, makes a complex series of structural and physiologic adjustments for extrauterine life. During birth, the fetus faces several hazards such as asphyxia or trauma, which may be fatal or reduce the neonate's ability to survive (Randall, 1984).

Cardiovascular Changes. During fetal life, the cardiovascular system is modified to bypass the unexpanded lungs. Thus, when the placenta functions as the respiratory organ, the lungs are in parallel with the systemic circulation; the foramen ovale allows blood to pass from the right auricle to the left, and the ductus arteriosus shunts blood from the pulmonary artery to the aorta.

With the cessation of the umbilical circulation and the commencement of lung ventilation at birth, the flow in the ductus arteriosus is reversed and ceases. The closure of the ductus arteriosus is one of the most important adjustments for extrauterine life and allows the flow of blood through the lungs during each circuit of the body.

The rapid decline in blood pressure in the right auricle, resulting from the interruption of the umbilical flow and the increasing left auricular pressure, causes closure of the foramen ovale within a few hours in the foal and toward the end of the first week of life in the lamb.

Lung Maturation. After the neonate is cut off from the placenta, its survival depends on the rapid establishment of efficient gaseous exchange in the lungs. This requires the maintained expansion of the lungs, rhythmic respiratory movements, and alterations in blood flow to adult patterns. Lung expansion is facilitated by secretion of a surface active material (surfactant), which reduces the surface tension within the alveoli.

Thermoregulatory Adjustments. At birth the neonate must make thermoregulatory adjustments to fluctuating environmental conditions, in contrast to the relatively constant temperature and nutrient supply present *in utero* during pregnancy. The efficiency of such adjustments depends primarily on the degree of physiologic immaturity of the species at birth, the glycogen reserves, and the presence of brown adipose tissue. Swine and sheep are particularly susceptible to low ambient temperatures; the rectal temperature of lambs falls 2 to 3° C, while that of piglets declines 2 to 5° C in the first hour after birth.

The neonate is not well adapted to withstand high temperatures early in life, lambs and calves being especially susceptible. For example, lambs between 2 and 7 days of age cannot survive longer than 2 hours at 38°C or more than 3 hours of solar radiation exposure.

Energy Metabolism After Birth. During the period between birth and suckling, the neonate depends on its own resources of glycogen stored in the liver and skeletal and cardiac muscles for energy metabolism. The rapid fall in liver glycogen concentration after birth suggests that it is mobilized rapidly to maintain the blood glucose levels.

Immune Status. The offspring is born without a supply of maternal antibodies or immunoglobulins in its blood. During prenatal life, the fetus synthesizes little or no antibodies. It acquires antibodies from its mother (passive immunity) while it is still in utero (rat, rabbit, and human), or the antibodies are secreted by the mammary glands and acquired by suckling (farm animals). This difference may be related to the impermeability of the epitheliochorial placenta of farm animals to maternal antibodies. Immediately after birth, however, immunoglobulins are transferred to the newborn by way of the colostrum; the small intestine is permeable to immunoglobulins for a period of 24 to 36 hours after birth.

PUERPERIUM

While nursing one or more offspring, the postpartum female makes a series of physiologic and anatomic readjustments both in the uterus and ovaries for the restoration of her reproductive capacity (Fig. 9–14). The *puerperium*, or the postpartum period, is broadly defined as the period extending from delivery until the maternal organism has returned to its normal nonpregnant state. Since early rebreeding is often practiced in horse and cattle, a more suitable definition of puerperium would be the interval between parturition and the occurrence of the first estrus

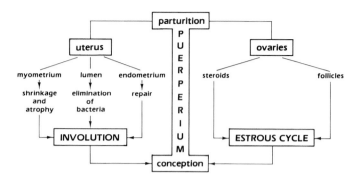

FIG. 9–14. Diagram depicting the various processes occurring in the uterus and the ovaries. Involution and resumption of the estrous cycle occur during the puerperium before another pregnancy can be established.

("open" period) at which conception can occur. In a seasonal breeder such as sheep, postpartum ovarian cycles are suspended until the next breeding season.

Involution of Uterus

The restoration of the uterus to its normal nonpregnant size and function after parturition is termed *uterine involution*. It depends on myometrial contractions, elimination of bacterial infection, and regeneration of the endometrium (Fig. 9–13).

Lochia, or the uterine discharge that normally occurs during the puerperium, is composed of mucus, blood, shreds of fetal membranes, and maternal tissue and fetal fluids. Lochia ceases by the first week after parturition. The expulsion of lochia and reduction of uterine size are caused by myometrial contractions. This is due to a sustained release of $PGF_{2\alpha}$ after parturition, which increases uterine tone and thus promotes involution. The duration of release of $PGF_{2\alpha}$ is longer in species with a cotyledonary type of placenta (cow, goat, buffalo) than in those with a diffuse type (horse, pig) (Kindahl et al., 1984).

The sterile conditions of the uterus that prevailed during pregnancy are disrupted at parturition. Both pathogenic and nonpathogenic bacteria enter the uterus through the dilated cervix and rapidly multiply in a favorable uterine environment. The normal uterus possesses defense mechanisms that include a massive infiltration of lymphocytes to counteract this bacterial invasion. The increased myo-metrial activity with the onset of estrogenic activity in the ovaries further assists the uterus in eliminating the infection through the cervix. The time needed to clear the uterus of bacteria depends on the extent of contamination at parturition, retention of fetal membranes, and the production of estrogen.

Regeneration of the endometrium is completed earlier in species with a diffuse placenta than those with a cotyledonary placenta. The endometrium is fully regenerated between the second and third week in the horse and pig and between the fourth and fifth week in ruminants.

Resumption of Estrous Cycles

Estrus and ovulation are usually suspended during lactation (postpartum anestrus) in several mammalian species, but the inhibitory effects of lactation have been partially or completely overcome in farm animals through selection, improvements in nutrition and weaning. Postpartum ovarian function has received considerable attention in cattle because of the production target of a calf per cow each year. Several reviews are available on the postpartum endocrinology of cattle (Lamming, 1982; Malven, 1984), sheep (Novoa, 1984), and buffalo (Jainudeen, 1984).

In cattle, the CL of the previous pregnancy regresses rapidly after parturition. The first ovulation is often not preceded by overt estrus. In cattle, the acyclic period is generally shorter in dairy cows than in suckled beef cows. By day 50 postpartum, about 95% of dairy cows will resume ovarian cycles, as compared with about 40% of beef cows (Peters and Riley, 1982). Suckling and increasing the frequency of milking (four milkings vs. two milkings per day) prolong this interval, whereas removal of the calf from the mother shortens it.

Most mares exhibit a foal heat within 6 to 13 days postpartum. It is a routine practice to breed mares at the foal heat despite the lower conception rates and higher incidence of nonviable foals and abortions.

Sows frequently exhibit an anovulatory estrus 3 to 5 days after farrowing, but estrus and ovulation are generally inhibited throughout lactation in most animals. Removing the piglets or weaning them at any time induces estrus and ovulation with 3 to 5 days.

Acyclicity during the postpartum period may be due to inhibition at several levels of the hypothalmo-pituitary-ovarian axis (Peters and Lamming, 1990). Ovarian activity may be blocked by preventing the release of gonadotropin-releasing hormone (hypothalamus), follicle-stimulating hormone, and luteinizing hormone (LH) (anterior pituitary) or ovarian follicles to respond to gonadotropin stimulation. Most evidence suggests that postpartum acyclicity is caused by a failure of GnRH release, resulting in a deficient secretion of gonadotropins.

The most consistent endocrine event preceding the first postpartum ovulation is the appearance of a pulsatile pattern of luteinizing LH in sheep, pigs, and cattle. Also, a small increase in progesterone secretion precedes the first postpartum estrus in cattle and sheep. Suckling or the act of milking apparently inhibits the release of GnRH necessary for restoration of the pulsatile pattern of LH release.

REFERENCES

Allen, W.R., Hamilton, D.W. and Moor, R.M. (1973). Origin of equine endometrial cups. (II) Invasion of the endometrium by trophoblast. Anat. Rec. *177*, 485.

Allen, W.R. and Pashen, R.L. (1981). The role of prostaglandins during parturition in the mare. Acta Vet. Scand. Suppl. *77*, 279.

Anderson, G.B. (1988). Interspecific pregnancy: barriers and prospects. Biol. Reprod. *38*, 1.

Beer, A.E. and Sio, J.O. (1982). Placenta as an immunological barrier. Biol. Reprod. *26*, 15.

Billington, W.D. (1989). Maternal immune response to pregnancy. Reprod. Fertil. Dev. *1*, 83.

Colenbrander, B., Garssen, G.J., Meijer, J.C. and Spencer, G.S.G. (1984). Interaction of hormones and growth factors. Proc. 10th Int. Congress on Animal Reprod. and Artif. Insem. Urbana-Champaign, IL, Vol. IV, pp. v–xvii.

Cooper, D.W. (1980). Immunological relationships between mother and conceptus in man. *In* Immunological Aspects of Reproduction and Fertility Control. J.H. Hearn (ed.). England, MTP Press.

Falconer, J., Davies, JJ., Zhang, H.P. and Smith, R. (1991). Release of insulin-like growth factor I by the sheep placenta *in vitro*. Reprod. Fertil. Dev. *3*, 379.

First, N.L. and Bosc, M.J. (1979). Proposed mechanism controlling parturition and induction of parturition in swine. J. Anim. Sci. *48*, 1407.

First, N.L. and Lohse, J.K. (1984). Mechanisms initiating and controlling parturition. Proc. 10th Int. Congress on Animal Reprod. and Artif. Insem. Urbana-Champaign, IL, Vol. IV, pp. v–xxxi.

Fitzpatrick, R.J. and Dobson, J. (1979). The cervix of the sheep and goat at parturition. Anim. Reprod. Sci. *2*, 209.

Hoffmann, B., Wagner, W.C., Hixon, J.E. and Bahr, J. (1979). Observations concerning the functional status of the corpus luteum and the placenta around parturition in the cow. Anim. Reprod. Sci. *1*, 253.

Hogarth, P.J. (1982). Immunological Aspects of Mammalian Reproduction. Glasgow, Blackie & Son.

Jainudeen, M.R. (1984). Reproduction in the water buffalo: postpartum female. Proc. 10th Int. Congress on Animal Reprod. and Artificial Insem. Urbana-Champaign, IL, Vol. IX, pp. xiv–42.

Jost, A.J. (1979). Fetal hormones and fetal growth. *In* Fetal Endocrinology. T. Zondek and L.H. Zondek (eds.). New York, S. Karger.

Kindahl, H., Fredricksson, G., Madej, A. and Edqvist, L.E. (1984). Role of prostaglandins in uterine involution. Proc. 10th Int. Congress on Animal Reprod. and Artif. Insem. Urbana-Champaign, IL, Vol. IX, pp. xi–9.

King, J.W., Seidel, G.E., Jr. and Elsden, R.O. (1982). Factors affecting gestation length in bovine transfer recipients. Theriogenology *17*, 92.

Lamming, G.E. (1982). Endocrine regulations of post partum function. *In* Factors Influencing Fertility in the Postpartum Cow. H. Karg and E. Schallenberger (eds.). Brussels, Martinus Nijhoff Publishers.

Liggins, G.C., Fairclough, R.J., Grieves, S.A., Kendall, J.Z. and Knox, B.S. (1973). The mechanism of initiation of parturition in the ewe. Recent Prog. Horm. Res. *29*, 111.

Malven, P.V. (1984). Pathophysiology of the puerperium: definition of the problem. Proc. 10th Int. Congress on Animal Reprod. and Artif. Insem. Urbana-Champaign, IL, Vol. IV, pp. iii–1.

Novoa, C. (1984). The postpartum ewe. Proc. 10th Int. Congress on Animal Reprod. and Artif. Insem. Urbana-Champaign, IL, Vol. IV, pp. vii–24.

Owens, J.A. (1991). Endocrine and substrate control of fetal growth: placental and maternal influences and insulin-like growth factors. Reprod. Fertil. Dev. *3*, 501.

Perry, J.S. (1981). Mammalian fetal membranes. J. Reprod. Fertil. *62*, 321.

Peters, A.R. and Lamming, G.E. (1990). Lactational anoestrus in farm animals. *In* Oxford Reviews of Reproductive Biology. Vol. 12. S.R. Milligan (ed.). New York, Oxford University Press.

Peters, A.R. and Riley, G.M. (1982). Milk progesterone profiles and factors affecting post partum ovarian activity in beef cows. Animal Production. *49*, 335.

Randall, G.C.B. (1984). Perinatal adaptation. Proc. 10th Int. Congress on Animal Reprod. and Artif. Insem. Urbana-Champaign, IL, Vol. IV, pp. v–43.

Schneider, H. (1991). Placental transport function. Reprod. Fertil. Dev. *3*, 345.

Steven, D. (1975). Anatomy of the placental barrier. *In* Comparative Placentation. D.H. Steven (ed.). New York, Academic Press.

Taverne, M.A.M. (1982). Myometrial activity during pregnancy and parturition in the pig. *In* Control of Pig Reproduction. D.J.A. Cole and G.R. Foxcroft (eds.). London, Butterworths.

Thorburn, G.D. (1979). Physiology and control of parturition: reflections on the past and ideas for the future. Anim. Reprod. Sci. *2*, 1.

Thorburn, G.D., Challis, J.R.C. and Currie, W.B. (1977). Control of parturition in domestic animals. Biol. Reprod. *16*, 18.

Thorburn, G.D. (1991). The placenta, prostaglandins and parturition: a review. Reprod. Fertil. Dev. *3*, 277.

Warner, C.M., Brownell, M.S. and Ewoldsen, M.A. (1988). Why aren't embryos immunologically rejected by their mothers? Biol. Reprod. *38*, 17.

10
Reproductive Behavior

E.S.E. Hafez

The behavior of animals plays an important role in reproduction, affecting both the success of mating and survival of the young. Behavioral patterns associated with courtship and copulation, birth, maternal care, and suckling attempts of the newborn have a dramatic quality that has attracted students of mammalian behavior (Fig. 10–1).

This chapter deals with patterns that have been muted by domestication and restricted or modified by conditions imposed in accordance with husbandry requirements. These requirements include confinement in paddocks, yard, or indoor pens; segregation of sexes; controlled mating; cesarean delivery; enforced weaning; imposed proximity with other individuals;

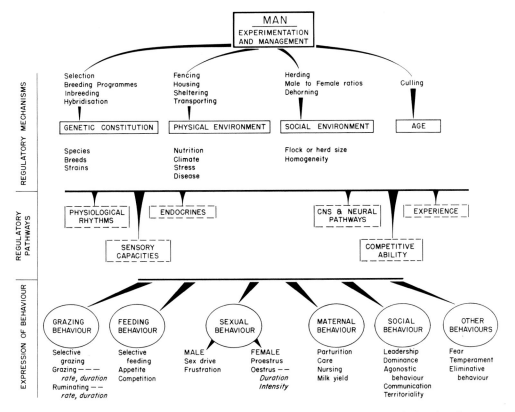

FIG. 10–1. The interaction between physical and social environment and the development of reproductive and other behaviors in farm animals.

237

and the inescapable presence of humans, dogs, and machinery.

SEXUAL BEHAVIOR

Various patterns of courtship, display, motor activities, and postures are directed to bring the male and female gametes together to ensure fertilization, pregnancy, and propagation of the species. The coordination of motor patterns leading to insemination of the female has been achieved by the evolution of an orderly series of responses to specific stimuli. Each response becomes a stimulus in turn, and thus leads to other responses and stimuli, a phenomenon known as a behavioral chain or sequence.

Promiscuous sexual behavior in animals is an advantage in domesticating a species and also in carrying out a breeding program based on the use of a few desirable sires. Because any female can be mated to any male, the chances of a suitable pairing are greatly increased over those possible when pair-bonds between male and female must first be established.

Psychosocial Aspects of Reproduction

The encounter of sexual partners is the first step of reproductive behavior. In free-living animals, this occurs largely under the influence of pre-existing social structure and the territorial or home range behavior of males and females, and leads to an organized pattern of reproduction that varies with the sociospatial or territorial characteristics of the species. In the roe deer and muntjak antelope, males and females live in a limited area, the boundaries of which are defended against any intruder of the same sex. The territories of males and females are overlapping, with permanent association between potential sexual partners. In other species, as in the wild rabbit and beaver, the territory is occupied by a permanent couple or harem, and the male avoids any encounter outside his territory. This pattern persists under artificial environments. For example, male rabbits breeding in cages display sex-

ual behavior toward receptive females only after the male occupies the cage for a sufficiently long time to consider it as his territory. Territorial behavior is intensified during the season of reproduction and in fact in many species such as the seal it exists only at that time.

Under feral conditions, farm animals do not defend defined territories against intruders, but herds and flocks tend to occupy a "home range." The basic unit is matriarchal, consisting of a female, her adult female offspring and their immature young. Such a matriarchal herd is remarkably stable. It persists after a temporary dispersion of its members, or mixing in large groups of several hundreds of individuals (African antelopes, bisons). This stability is the consequence of strong inter-individual bonds resulting from contacts occurring during infancy. Experimentally, cows reared together from birth form such a stable group even in the middle of a large herd. Such a bond, limited to the dams and their female offspring, could be the basis of the social organization in ungulates.

Increasing population density may led to abnormal behavior such as tail biting, cannibalism and an increased level of aggression. Such abnormal behavior may be detrimental in that the performance of individual animals with low social status in the group would decline because of stress (Randolph et al., 1981).

In horses, each matriarchal herd is the permanent harem of a dominant stallion, whereas younger males form a permanent "bachelor" herd (Klingel, 1967). In other species, the males either aggregate in groups (feral sheep and goats) or even stay solitary, with occasional contacts with animals of the same species (bisons, wild pigs) (Fig. 10–2). In such cases, the herds of males are only temporary associations in which the interindividual bonds are loose.

The pig's characteristic body odor is produced by skin gland secretions. The carpal glands are well differentiated on the front legs (Fig. 10–3). In the male, secretions of the preputial pouch, which give pork its

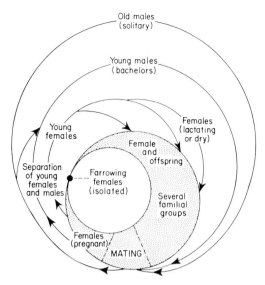

FIG. 10–2. Diagram of the evolution of the social organization in pigs. (By Dr. J.P. Signoret.)

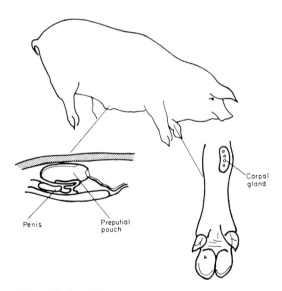

FIG. 10–3. The specialized scent or musk glands of the pig. Carpal glands occur in both sexes. Preputial glands occur only in the boar and are responsible for this odor. (Photo Courtesy of Dr. J.P. Signoret.)

"boar" odor are involved in sexual behavior.

Sequence of Sexual Behavior

The motor patterns of courtship behavior are stereotyped and are not altered by experience, which acts mainly on the latency and efficiency of mating (Table 10–1). The components of copulatory patterns are sexual arousal, courtship (sexual display), erection, penile protrusion, mounting, intromission, ejaculation, dismounting, and refractoriness (Fig. 10–4). The duration of courtship and copulation varies with the species; both events are shorter in cattle and sheep than in swine and horses.

Male. In the male, sniffing and licking the female are the most frequent patterns, suggesting an important function of chemical communication through olfaction. Except in swine, the male of domestic ungulates smells the female's urine and then raises his head, with lips curled, in the ritualized "Flehmen" reaction. In sheep, goats and cattle, tactile stimulation of the female is made by nuzzling and licking the perineal region, whereas with the horse, the stallion often bites the female's neck, and with swine the boar noses her flanks.

Female. In most species, the estrous female shows increased motor activity, becoming restless and moving at the slightest disturbance. Receptive cows and goats exhibit increased frequency of nonspecific bellows or bleats, whereas the sow utters a typical estrous grunt. Cows, goats, and sows tend to mount and to be mounted by other females but this is exceptional in ewes and mares. In the presence of a male, the female sniffs at his perineum or scrotal region. Mutual sniffing leads both animals to circling motions in a reverse parallel position. Receptive sows also display interest in the boar's head. Frontal contact between the estrous cow or sow and the boar may be associated with "mock fighting." Estrous mares tend to urinate frequently in the presence of a stallion.

TABLE 10–1.   **Patterns of Male Sexual Behavior**

Animal	Aspect Measured	Technique	Comments
Sheep	Latency of successive ejaculates; total number of ejaculates as a measure of sex drive.	Libido measured by time required to produce successive ejaculates and by number of ejaculates in 30 min. period; rams run with ewes in panel pens or small pastures.	Stress on nonbehavior aspects, e.g., semen analyses, lambing records; no component study of ram behavior.
Cattle	Latency to ejaculation; frequency; stimulus satiation, recovery period; reaction to new stimulus situation.	Standardized test periods, artificial vagina; constant stimulus animals. Responses measured in time and frequency scores; new stimulus animals.	Animals must be trained to collection room procedures. Concept of stimulus pressure is presented.
Cattle	Ejaculatory response.	Artificial ejaculation using transparent artificial vagina; electroejaculators.	For study of physiology of ejaculation; measurement of thrust and penis lengthening; drug effects on response, etc.
Cattle	Variability in sexual performance; age effects; heritability; effect of inbreeding.	Sex drive index devised on basis of performance of sexual pattern. Bulls exposed and measured 3 times with natural mating.	Inbreeding coefficient determinations for 3 or 4 generations to measure influence of inbreeding and heritability of performance. Selection of measurable features of behavior to study cause of variation.
Horse	Erection reflex time; effect of elimination of vision and suppression of olfaction on erection and leap reflexes.	Comparison of young and experienced "old" stallions in tests with blindfold; blindfold, nose mask and odoriferous substances.	Young stallions apathetic to dummy presentations, whereas older stallions responded with normal sexual behavior.

Denenberg and Banks, 1969.

When approached and stimulated by the male, the female domestic ungulate assumes a mating posture. This entails immobilization, often accompanied by tail deviation, and some minor species-specific features such as turning the head back in the goat and ewe, cocking the ears in the sow, and exposing the clitoris in the mare.

Mating.   The posture of the sexually receptive female terminates courtship behavior by allowing mating to take place. The female stands immobile, and the male mounts and ejaculates (Fig. 10–5).

Mounting.   In the presence of a proestrous female, the male attempts several mounts; the penis become partially erect and protrudes from the prepuce. These mounts are usually unsuccessful. During this activity, the male, especially the bull, excretes "dribblings" of accessory fluid, derived from the Cowper's gland and differing from the seminal plasma emitted from the vesicular glands during ejaculation. If the female is receptive, however, copulation may occur rapidly. The male rests his chin on the female and she in turn responds by "standing." The male then mounts, "fixes" his forelegs around the female, grasps her firmly and performs rhythmic pelvic thrusts (see Fig. 10–5).

The mounting reactions of the male, which are released by a simple visual stimulus, may explain the abnormal mounting and homosexuality frequently observed in swine. Frequently, boars reared in pairs or all-male groups form stable homosexual relationships. Such relationships persist for many months, although members repeatedly copulate with females. The identity of the active and passive partner is maintained. The behavior pattern of the aggressor is the same as the pattern that occurs in normal heterosexual copulation and may include rectal intromission and ejaculation while the passive male stands quietly. If such pairing is well established,

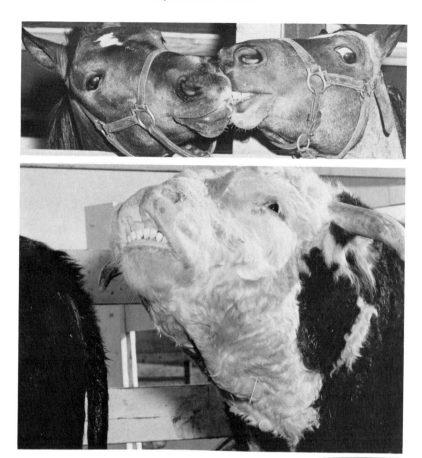

FIG. 10–4. Patterns of precopulatory courtship in horses and cattle.

homosexual coitus occurs even in the presence of estrous females.

Intromission. At mounting, the abdominal muscles of the male, particularly the rectus abdominis muscles, contract suddenly. As a result, the pelvic region of the male is quickly brought into direct apposition to the external genitalia of the female. The boar, with the penis partially out of the prepuce, thrusts his pelvis until the tip of the penis penetrates the vulva; only then is the penis fully unsheathed and intromission accomplished.

When intromission is vaginal, the boar seldom withdraws or dismounts and ejaculation occurs. A series of pelvic thrusts may occur after a rectal intromission, but the penis is most often withdrawn without ejaculation. Abortive ejaculation may take place if the sow refuses intromission or if the boar fails to penetrate either orifice.

Among farm animals, the boar has the longest ejaculation time. Copulation is performed within 3 to 20 minutes with an average of 4 to 5 minutes. The female generally remains completely immobile until the boar dismounts (Fig. 10–6). The female sometimes moves at the end of copulation, but this seldom disturbs ejaculation. After mating, the sow remains by the boar and often licks the flocculent discharge that accumulates on his penis.

The stallion oscillates the pelvis several times, resulting in engorgement of the penis with blood and making it rigid for maximal intromission. In contrast, ejaculation

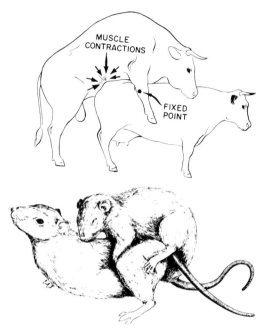

FIG. 10–5. Species differences: copulatory posture in cattle and rodents.

in several species of rodents is preceded by a series of mounts and intromissions.

Ejaculation. Semen is ejaculated near the os cervix in the case of cattle and sheep, into the uterus in swine and partially into the uterus in horses. Abortive ejaculations may occur if the female refuses intromission or the penis fails to penetrate the vulva. In the ram, the goat, and the bull, an intense generalized muscular contraction takes place at ejaculation. Often, the force is so strong in the bull that the hind legs of the male leave the ground, giving the appearance of an active leap. During ejaculation itself, the boar is quiet, presenting only slight rhythmic contractions of the scrotum; such periods of immobility are followed by some thrusts at irregular intervals. After ejaculation, the male dismounts, and the penis is soon retracted into the prepuce.

Refractoriness. Most males show no sexual activity immediately following copulation. The duration of the refractory period is highly variable and increases gradu-

ally when several copulations are allowed successively with the same female.

Frequency of Copulation. The frequency of copulation varies with the species, the breed, the ratio of males and females present, available space, period of sexual rest, climate, and nature of sexual stimuli. The maximal number of ejaculations is higher in bulls and rams than in stallions and boars: some bulls have been observed to copulate over 80 times within 24 hours or 60 times within 6 hours; an average of 21 copulations before exhaustion was observed.

After a long sexual rest, a ram may copulate up to 50 times on the first day after joining with the ewes, but this frequency is greatly reduced on subsequent days. The goat, the stallion, and the boar reach exhaustion after a less number of ejaculations than in the ram and bull (Table 10–2).

Duration of Estrus. The duration of estrus is influenced by species, breed, climate, and management. Estrus is limited to about a day in sheep and cattle but to longer periods in the sow and the mare (Table 10–2). In species in which the period of sexual receptivity is short, ovulation takes place after its end, but in species that remain receptive for long periods, ovulation occurs during estrus.

MECHANISMS OF SEXUAL BEHAVIOR

The physiologic signal that originates sexual motivation is the gonadal steroid balance. Transmitted by the blood flow, the hormones activate the central nervous system. The humoral signal is transformed into sexual motivation, or sex drive. The motor patterns of copulatory activity are programmed according to pre-existing species-specific neuronal circuits.

The behavioral interactions leading to copulation can be divided into four major phases: mutual searching for the sexual partner; identification of the physiologic state of the partner; the sequence of behavioral interactions resulting in the adoption of the mating posture by the female;

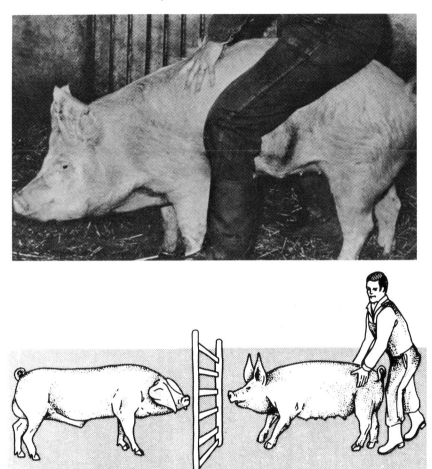

FIG. 10–6.   Among the farm species, sexually receptive female pigs are identified most easily: those that are in estrus will respond to pressure on the back, especially in the presence of a mature male; by immobility, arching of the back, and "pricking" of the ears. This test is not applicable in cows and sheep in which species estrus is best identified with a teaser male. (Hunter, R.H.F. (1982). Reproduction of Farm Animals. New York, Longman.)

and the mounting reaction of the male leading to copulation.

The "mating stance" of the sow—clear, long lasting and easy to release by an experimenter—is especially suitable for a study of releasing mechanism. During the "standing reaction," the receptive sow is absolutely immobile, arches her back, and cocks the ears, and this reaction may be exhibited when an estrous female is touched on the back (Fig. 10–6). Only 48% of estrous gilts, however, will "stand" in the absence of the male. Broadcasting tape-recorded "courting grunts" is similarly effective in 50% of previously negative females. Thus, the stimuli emitted during precopulatory interactions facilitate the release of the female's postural response.

Females in the mating stance are mounted immediately, and this reaction seems to be released mainly by visual and tactile clues. A restrained female, although not in estrus, is immediately mounted even by a sexually experienced bull or ram. Similarly, a ram does not copu-

TABLE 10–2. Patterns of Mating in Farm Mammals

	Cattle	Sheep	Goat	Swine	Horse
Duration of estrus	15 hrs (5 to 30)	24 hrs (12 to 50)	32 hrs (24 to 96)	50 hrs (24 to 72)	7 days (2 to 10 days)
Time of ovulation	4 to 15 hrs after onset of estrus	30 hrs after onset of estrus	30 to 36 hrs after onset of estrus	40 hrs after onset of estrus	24 to 48 hrs before end of estrus
Male anatomy					
Penis	Fibroelastic	Fibroelastic with filiform process		Fibroelastic spiral tip	Vascular–muscular
Scrotum		Pendulous		Close to body	
Mating					
Duration		Brief (a second or less)		5 minutes	40 seconds
Site of semen ejaculation		Near os cervix		Cervix and uterus	Uterus
Number of ejaculations to exhaustion, average	20	10	7	3	3
Maximum	60 to 80	30 to 40	14	8	20

Alexander et al., 1980.

late selectively with an estrous ewe when presented with two restrained anestrous females. Sexual reactions of the male toward stimuli other than those emanating from the female are common. For example, the bull or the boar reacts rapidly to a restrained male or to a dummy.

The sexual releaser for mounting may be the overall shape of the female and her immobility. The other visual, olfactory, or acoustic information from the estrous female may be of minor but complementary importance (Fig. 10–7).

Cortex and Sensory Capacities

Deprivation of sensory capacity can inhibit sexual behavior, reduce the ability to detect the partner and/or impair orientation. Inexperienced males are impaired to a greater degree than experienced ones. If one sense is inhibited, another sense that is ordinarily used to a lesser degree may be augmented. Thus, elimination of the stimuli to visual receptors in males results in the use of tactile and olfactory receptors. Copulation in domestic mammals is not suppressed with the elimination of vision, smell, or hearing provided contact with the partner has been established. Tactile stimuli are involved in the organi-

zation of postural responses of copulation (e.g., immobilization of the estrous sow and lordosis in the estrous rat in response to flank palpation).

Neural Mechanisms of Erection and Ejaculation

Erection is predominantly under the influence of the parasympathetic system. The parasympathetic nerves in the bull, which supply the external genitalia, arise from the sacral segments of the spinal cord.

The copulatory patterns of the male are primarily governed by the neuromuscular anatomy and blood supply of the penis. The bull, ram, and boar have a fibroelastic penis that is relatively small in diameter and rigid when non-erect. Although the penis becomes more rigid on rapid erection, it enlarges little, and the amount of contractile tissue is limited. Protrusion is effected mainly by straightening the S-shaped flexure and relaxation of the retractor muscle (Fig. 10–8).

On the other hand, the stallion has a typical vascular penis with no sigmoid flexure. The function of the penis as an organ of intromission depends on the power of erection as a result of sexual excitement.

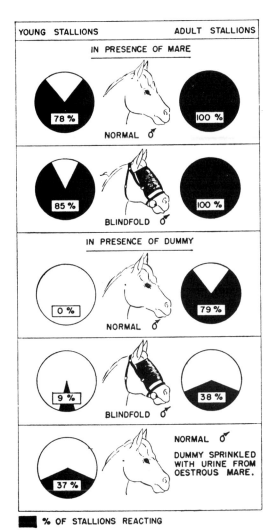

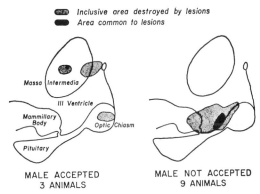

FIG. 10–8. Effect of hypothalamic lesions on estrous behavior in the ewe. The male was accepted when the lesions were in the massa intermedia or in the optic chiasm of the hypothalamus. (Clegg et al. (1958). Endocrinology *62*, 790.)

FIG. 10–7. Effect of sexual experience on copulatory responses of stallions under normal and experimental conditions. Young stallions did not react sexually to the dummy. The percentage of adult stallions that showed sexual responses to the dummy was lower in blindfolded stallions. In young stallions, sexual response was increased toward the dummy when it was sprinkled with urine from an estrous mare. (Adapted from data by S. Wierzbowski.)

The size, shape, and length of the penis vary greatly between the flaccid and the erect state (Fig. 10–9).

Intromission and ejaculation are elicited by tactile stimuli (warmth of vagina and slipperiness of mucus) acting on the penile receptors. The penis of the bull and the ram is sensitive to temperature, whereas that of the stallion is more sensitive to pressure exerted by the contractions of the vaginal walls. In the board, the corkscrew-shaped tip of the penis is engaged in the cervix during mating. The pressure exerted by this is sufficient to elicit ejaculation even without any thermal stimulation.

FACTORS AFFECTING SEXUAL BEHAVIOR

The patterns and intensity of sexual behavior are affected by genetic, physiologic, and environmental factors as well as previous experience.

Genetic Factors

Breed and strain differences in libido are frequently observed. Males of dairy breeds are more active than beef males, whereas Brahman bulls are sluggish. Yorkshire boars are easier to train for semen collections than Durocs. More differences in the pattern of sexual behavior occur between pairs of identical twin bulls than between members of the pair (Fig. 10–10). Breed differences in the duration of estrus in sheep and pigs may be partly due to differences in ovulation rates. Individual

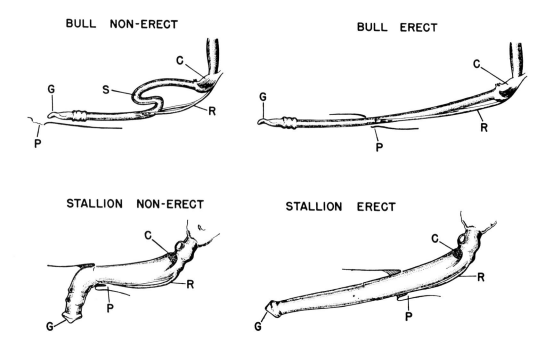

BULL NON-ERECT

BULL ERECT

STALLION NON-ERECT

STALLION ERECT

FIG. 10–9. Diagram of the anatomy of fibroelastic type penis (bull) and a vascular–muscular type penis (stallion) in the nonerect and erect positions. The anatomy of the penis determines, to a great extent, the ejaculatory responses of the species. C, cavernous muscle; G, glans; P, prepuce; R, retractor penile muscle; S, sigmoid flexure.

differences in the amount of sexual stimulation required to elicit "immobilization reaction" in the sow are independent of sexual experience.

Environmental Factors

The effect of external stimulation on sexual behavior is more pronounced in the male than in the female.

Effect of Novelty of Stimulus Females (Coolidge Effect). Sexual activity of the male increases when new females in the herd become receptive. If four receptive ewes are available, the ram mates three times as much as he does when only one ewe is in estrus. The enhancing effect of a new stimulus animal should be kept in mind under modern husbandry conditions. For instance, changing the teaser cow is an effective way to increase sexual behavior of a sluggish male.

Nonspecific Stimuli. Nonspecific external stimuli may lead to sexual activity during the refractory period that follows ejaculation in males of low libido. In the rat, both painful stimuli such as an electric shock and gentle handling increase the frequency of ejaculations and reduce the postejaculatory interval. Changing the place of semen collection by moving the teaser animal, or "encouraging" the bull, are all effective in sluggish bulls.

Presence of Other Animals. The presence of other males while teasing a female or copulating improves sexual libido of the male. Social hierarchy, however, may interfere with sexual activity when several males compete for one receptive female. The dominant male performs most of the copulations and restricts the sexual performance of his subordinates. When females are in excess, however, dominant males cannot effectively control the activity of their inferiors. Adult rams usually dominate or "boss" yearling rams, and the degree of their dominance is greater than

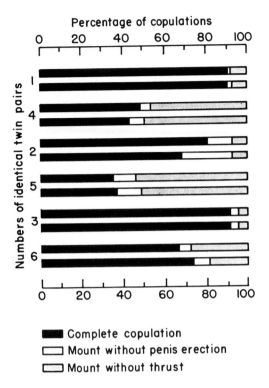

Percentage of copulations

Numbers of identical twin pairs

Complete copulation
Mount without penis erection
Mount without thrust

FIG. 10–10. Ejaculatory behavior in identical twin dairy bulls showing percentage distribution of complete copulations, mounts without penis erection and mounts without thrust. Note the great similarities in the ejaculatory pattern of the twin brothers and the great variability between the twin pairs. (Adapted from Bane, A. (1954). Acta Agric. Scand. *4*, 95.)

the dominance of yearling rams over other yearlings. Unfortunately social dominance is not correlated with fertility of males. Thus a "bossy" male who is infertile or diseased may depress the conception rate of the entire herd. The size of the pasture also affects the competition among males and the number of copulations per female.

Season and Climate. Seasonal variations in sexual behavior of sheep, goats, and horses are mostly due to seasonality of pituitary function controlling the secretion of gonadal hormones. Seasonal changes are also reported in the responsiveness of ovariectomized ewes and sows to exogenous hormones, showing a direct effect of the season on the responses of

the nervous system. The intensity of sexual behavior is reduced in hot climates. The plane of nutrition per se does not seem to affect sexual behavior. However, any physical trouble may seriously affect sexual expression (e.g., inflammation of the hooves or joints, change in teeth, eczema, pains from accidents, or certain diseases).

Effect of Experience

The efficiency of copulation of males and females is improved by experience. Individual contacts before puberty can have an organizing effect on subsequent sexual performance. Social deprivation during infancy drastically impairs adult sexual behavior in primates. In other mammals, the female's sexual behavior does not appear modified by deprivation of social contacts. However, social deprivation during ontogeny may account for some cases of sexual inhibition of domestic males. In boars and rams, rearing in isolation or in unisexual groups has a detrimental effect on subsequent libido. Young, inexperienced males are usually awkward during their first contact with a receptive female: they approach hesitantly, spend a long time exploring the genitalia, mount with erection, descend, and try to mount again. Erection and ejaculation are weak, and the volume of semen is small. After the first ejaculation, the motor patterns are rapidly organized and normal mating efficiency is reached.

Uterine Motility and Sperm Transport. Sterile matings with a vasectomized male stimulate sperm transport in the rabbit but not in sheep. Stimulation of the genitalia or precoital stimuli cause contraction of the cervix and uterus of the ewe and the cow, as a result of the release of oxytocin. Vaginal distention and precoital stimulation cause maximal oxytocin release in sheep and goats. Oxytocin release often occurs before actual coitus has taken place.

Effect of Male on Anestrous Females. Many domestic females undergo periods of anestrus. By the end of seasonal anestrus in sheep and goats, the introduction of the male results in an earlier and synchronized appearance of estrous cycles. Even the Merino sheep, which is reputed to breed throughout the year, ovulates and breeds spontaneously for only a restricted period during autumn. The peak of estrus observed 17 to 18 days following the introduction of the male represents in fact the second cycle, and this allows normal fertilization.

An androgen-dependent pheromone from the male is responsible for similar synchronization of estrus in mice and possibly in sheep. Neither sight nor contact is necessary for the synchronization of the first estrus of the breeding season in sheep.

Nursing the young delays estrus compared with milking in cows and ewes. The presence of the ram results in an earlier postpartum estrus in nursing ewes, making the postpartum estrus similar in dry and milked females.

The introduction of the boar shortly before spontaneous puberty in a group of previously isolated gilts results in earlier onset of estrus.

Male

Precoital stimulation affects both composition of the ejaculate and androgen secretion. A period of restraint for 2 to 20 minutes causes an increase in semen volume and concentration and number of sperm in bulls, with sperm motility being unaffected. False mounts cause further increases in semen characteristics. The presence of another bull, changing the teaser, or using the bull as a teaser prior to collection has no such augmenting effect on semen characteristics despite a great increase in sexual excitement. Thus, the stimuli that influence semen composition differ from those that cause sexual excitement.

ABNORMAL SEXUAL BEHAVIOR

Homosexuality, hypersexuality, hyposexuality, and autoerotic behavior are not uncommon. These syndromes may be due to genetic factors, disturbance in the endocrine or nervous systems, or faulty management. Unadapted sexual reactions are more frequent among domestic animals and under conditions of captivity in the zoo than in the wild. *Homosexuality* refers to sexual behavior among males, particularly at puberty and when young males are housed together. The stimuli eliciting the male's sexual response are essentially visual. A releaser of an appropriate shape and size presented to a highly motivated male may elicit mounting. An immobile anestrous female, another male, or an inanimate object may release sexual reactions. Most homosexual males in sex-segregated groups become heterosexual when placed with females and again homosexual when segregated.

Hypersexuality in males consists of increased sexual excitement, increased frequency of copulation, and attempted copulations with young males and females of the same or different species. Hyposexuality is characterized by abnormalities in the ejaculatory pattern. Certain males may fail to ejaculate in spite of protrusion of erection, whereas others cannot mount or exhibit no sexual desire for varying periods of time.

In Belgian stallions, failure to ejaculate may be manifested in the first breeding season or at the peak of any successive season. In some cases, ejaculation is inhibited when semen is collected by an artificial vagina, but no inhibition occurs with natural mating. Such inhibition is temporary and is mainly due to faulty application of the artificial vagina. Another anomaly is the incomplete intromission and the lack of pelvic oscillations after intromission. This irregularity, which is partly hereditary, may appear in young stallions at the onset of their sexual life and may persist during the following years.

Excessive biting of the mare during copulation may be associated with disturbances in the copulatory mechanisms when the stallion performs the usual pelvic oscillations without ejaculation or with incomplete erection. Excessive biting of the mare may be caused by inhibition.

Autoerotic behavior refers to self-arousal of sexual responses, which is called *masturbation* in males. The motor patterns vary with the species. The stallion rubs his rigid erected penis against the hypogastrium (anterior median of the abdomen) and lowers the loin region rapidly. This is followed by several forward movements of the pelvis, resulting in abortive ejaculation. Masturbation is less common in rams and most common among bulls on high protein ration (e.g., bulls prepared for shows). As a result of such diets, the peripheral mucosa of the penis become more sensitive to tactile stimulation.

The most common abnormal female behavior is nymphomania in cattle.

"Split" estrus and prolonged estrus are common in mares. In split estrus, the manifestation of estrus ceases for a short period followed by recurrence of sexual receptivity during what is evidently one full estrous period. Prolonged estrus may last from 10 to 40 days. The prolonged estrus usually occurs in mares that have failed to conceive or have aborted and those used for heavy draught.

MATERNAL AND NEONATAL BEHAVIOR

The behavioral events at birth and shortly afterward (Table 10–3) have an important influence on the survival of the newborn and hence on the successful outcome of reproductive processes. This is especially true when the initial suckling and development of a bond between mother and young occur in the outdoor environment, often under adverse conditions such as inclement weather and the presence of predators, or in artificial conditions of close confinement indoors.

Several experimental approaches have been used to evaluate maternal behavior such as (a) whether each young is suckled, (b) whether each young is groomed (licked) by its mother, (c) frequency of suckling or attempting to suckle alien mothers, and (d) other mother–offspring

interactions relevant to weaning and development under intensive management conditions (Price et al., 1981).

Some standard practices interfere with the formation of maternal bonds between dams and offspring. Early separation of newborn young from the mother, as in dairy cattle practice or in the production of gnotobiotic piglets, induces modifications in the behavior of young animals. In most species of wild bovids, parturient females leave the nursery herd and seclude themselves during parturition and the immediate postnatal period. Most management procedures preclude this possibility and increase the likelihood of interference by other herd members. Lamb stealing is a common and deleterious consequence of housing together large numbers of pregnant ewes. Early weaning and artificial feeding adversely affect the suckling behavior of young lambs and piglets.

Suckling

Milk is let down in response to suckling, massage of the udder, or injection of posterior pituitary hormone. Suckling excites a nervous reflex that augments secretion of hormones from the posterior pituitary. Fright or adrenaline injections inhibit milk letdown.

The young may reach the udder within a few seconds after birth, while the umbilical cord is still attached. They express the suckling response as soon as their noses make contact with other objects. Piglets that are milk-fed and reared in the laboratory must be cared for individually during the first week. If two or more are joined together at birth, they will suckle each other on any available soft part.

Parent–Young Interactions

After birth, the young are able to move about almost immediately and react to a variety of objects as surrogate (substitute) mothers. During this imprinting period, the young normally establish a species-bond to their own species and as adults

TABLE 10–3. **Maternal and Neonatal Behavior in Domestic Ungulates—Semiquantitative Comparison of Species**

	Sheep	Goats	Cattle	Horses	Swine
Prepartum behavior					
Restless	+		+	+	+
Seeks isolation	±	Probably the	±	(?)	+
Milk ejection	−	same as sheep	±	±	−
Builds nest	−		−	−	+
Delivery of placenta					
Time from delivery of young to delivery of placenta (approximate hours)	Several	Several	Several	1(?)	Several
Eating of placenta by dam	±	±(?)	±	−	±
Time for dam to stand up after birth (if not already standing) (approx. min.)	<1	<1	<1	10	3
Maternal solicitude for alien	−	(?)	±	(?)	+
Abnormal maternal behavior					
Desertion of young	+		+	(?)	+
Moves from suckling	+	Probably the	+	+	NA
Attacks young	+	same as sheep	+	+	NA
Cannibalism	−		−	−	NA
Frequency of suckling (times per day approximately)					
First 4 days	30	(?)	4(?)	(?)	10
Midlactation	15	(?)	3(?)	(?)	25

direct their sexual behavior toward species members.

Recognition of young is established in sheep and goats soon after parturition, and other young may be adopted at that time. Continuous contact is important and females may reject their own lambs or kids if separated from them for more than a few hours immediately after parturition.

During and immediately following birth, the mothers chew and lick the placenta and its components (a phenomenon called *placentophagy*). The mother may consume parts of it and groom the neonate. Licking or maternal grooming has various functions. The maternal stimulation facilitates the development of successful suckling orientations in the offspring. Suckling by the neonate, in turn, likely has a stimulating influence on the mother in that it reduces tension in the udder and provides the occasion for further licking of the neonate. The response patterns of the mother and offspring rapidly become mutually dependent. At the time of parturition, licking has a hygienic function in addition to stimulating the young to stand

and eventually suckle. The mother may "label" her offspring by maternal grooming at this time, thus, providing a mechanism for offspring discrimination. Later, as the young mature, the hygienic significance of grooming is gradually replaced by social functions relating to the establishment and maintenance of a social bond or attachment between mother and young. Removal of the offspring from the maternal animal leads, under some conditions, to the later rejection of the neonate. The maternal animal may reject her own offspring, if it is removed at birth and kept away for several hours. A very rapid social attachment is formed between mother and neonate. Kids that have been removed from the dam immediately following parturition and maintained in isolation for a period as brief as 1 hour are later rejected. Maternal rejection, however, is not an inevitable consequence of early separation of the newborn lamb from its mother. Strong maternal–young attachments form in sheep even when postpartum interaction is delayed for a period of up to 8 hours after birth.

Maternal Behavior in Sheep

Prepartum Behavior

Ewes tend to cease grazing within an hour or so before lambing and wander about as if searching for a lamb. Parturition, at least in Merinos, usually begins while the ewe is with the flock, and the lambing ewe is left behind as the flock grazes on.

Role of Fetal Fluids. The birth site appears to be determined fortuitously by where the placental fluids are first spilled. These fluids are attractive to ewes near the time of lambing and the ewe usually remains at the site of spillage, licking and pawing the ground. The fluids appear to play a critical role in attracting the ewe to her newborn lamb. Ewes that have not yet lambed are attracted to the fluids and to newborn lambs of other ewes, leading to "lamb stealing." This adoption sometimes results in lambs being left without maternal care, and the rearing of lambs by ewes that are not their natural mothers.

Lambing

There is no consistent peak of lambing at any particular time of the day. Behavior during parturition largely depends on the ease of the process, but generally, the initial restlessness is broken by periods of lying with abdominal straining. Most lambs are born with head and forefeet foremost. Lambing usually occurs while the ewe is recumbent, but it can also occur while the ewe is standing; most ewes are on their feet within a minute after birth. The umbilical cord is broken simply by stretching. The fetal placenta, or "afterbirth," is delivered 2 to 5 hours later and is frequently eaten by some breeds, but rarely by others.

The duration of birth varies widely within the one flock. Sometimes an extended birth is associated with a single lamb being too large for the vagina, with twins being impacted in the vagina or with an abnormal presentation resulting in an increase in the effective diameter of the lamb. Birth also tends to be protracted in ewes lambing for the first time or in ewes debilitated by ill-health or undernutrition. Protracted labor can exhaust the ewe and have adverse effects on maternal behavior and the viability of the lamb.

Twin births are usually more rapid than single births because twins are usually smaller than singles, but the interval between delivery of twins varies widely from a few minutes to an hour or more.

Postpartum Behavior

Vigorous licking (grooming) and eating of any amniotic and allantoic membranes adhering to the lamb usually commence immediately after birth. During this phase of intense olfactory and gustatory contact, which persists for little more than an hour, the ewe learns to distinguish her own lamb from aliens, which are soon rejected by vigorous butting. Experiments with lambing ewes in which the olfactory bulbs have been destroyed confirms that this attraction is largely olfactory. However, maternal behavior is not abolished by destroying the sense of smell. Other factors, such as warmth and movement, may be important in maintaining the attraction of the mother to the newborn lamb; ewes rapidly lose interest in an immobile, chilled lamb. This "critical period" of attachment of the ewe to the lamb is short; if the lamb is removed at birth, it will be rejected by the ewe if presented to her 6 to 12 hours later.

Grooming of the lamb by the ewe may remove some of the 0.5 kg of fluid present in the coat at birth, so reducing heat loss. Grooming may also play an important role in stimulating the lamb to stand and suckle for the first time.

Maternal behavior appears to be under endocrine control; it can be induced in sheep under the influences of a rapidly declining progesterone level and rapidly increasing estrogen level, conditions that normally apply around birth.

Finding the Teats for the First Time. Most lambs are standing within 15 minutes of birth, and with increasing coordination make exploratory approaches to the ewe, moving from the head along her side and nosing into body angles. During the initial approaches, the ewe tends to keep the lamb in front of her head to facilitate grooming, but within an hour or two, most ewes will allow the lamb to move toward the udder.

Both maternal orientation and grooming appear to facilitate the lamb's finding the teats for the first time, but neither is essential. The teats seem to be found by trial and error. For example, in goats the teats are found with equal success whether the udder is in the normal position or has been grafted onto the neck. Visual guidance is not essential, as lambs will suckle for the first time in a light-proof room; however, visual cues appear to facilitate suckling subsequently. There is no information on any role of odor.

Aberrant Behavior. Ewes that are exhausted by a difficult parturition may remain prone for some hours after birth and the lamb may stray. Some ewes lambing for the first time display little interest and abandon their newborn lambs. Other forms of misbehavior in inexperienced ewes include butting the newborn lamb as it moves, and a tendency to move to maintain the initial head-to-head orientation. When these behavioral patterns persist, the lamb's chances of finding the teats and suckling can be reduced, since the teat-seeking activity declines rapidly from about 2 hours after birth in the absence of successful suckling. Some lambs, particularly after poor fetal nutrition, a long birth process, birth injury, or chilling, are slow to stand and suckle.

Aberrant patterns are more common with twin births than with single births, especially among Merinos. For example, if twins are born several meters apart, one lamb may be neglected and become lost or may be repelled as an alien if contact is remade after the critical receptive period of the ewe has passed; imprinting with one lamb does not guarantee acceptance of others in the same litter. Aberrant behavior in the postpartum period is a significant cause of lamb mortality.

Suckling

Ewes with lambs tend to form distinct groups away from the main flock, and for some days after birth, the ewes remain within earshot of their lambs. Accidental separation results in considerable agitation of both ewe and lamb, so it is important that there are effective mechanisms for reunion of the two.

Mutual Recognition by Ewes and Lambs. The means whereby ewes and their lambs recognize each other have been the subject of much research. The experiments were largely based on manipulation of the cues to recognition provided by the partner (Alexander, 1977). Voices were blocked by local anesthesia, and visual cues were removed by screening or altered by dusting pigments into the coat, or by shearing. The effects were observed in a small enclosure when a ewe and a lamb were simultaneously released from opposite ends.

The experiments showed that ewes are attracted by a lamb's bleat and the attraction is particularly strong for the lamb's own mother, but it is not essential for a ewe to hear her lamb's voice for her to accept it. The appearance of the lamb is of paramount importance; for example, if lambs are disguised by blackening or coloring, many ewes actively avoid the approaches of the disguised lamb when initially presented with it, even if the lamb is the ewe's own. Similar experiments with blackening various parts of the lamb show that critical visual cues emanate (Fig. 10–11). The scent of the lamb is also important but only at close quarters. Scent appears to be the final criterion by which a ewe identifies a lamb as her own.

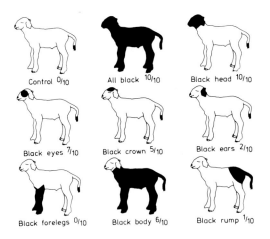

FIG. 10–11. The effect of blackening various regions of lambs' bodies on the incidence of hesitation or dodging away by their dams when confronted with their partially blackened lamb for the first time. The number of ewes reacting out of the 10 tested with each treatment is indicated. (Adapted from G. Alexander and Shillito, R. (1977). Appl. Anim. Ethol. *3*, 137.)

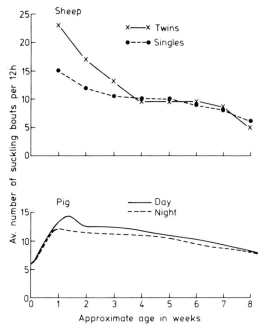

FIG. 10–12. Frequency of suckling bouts in sheep and pigs. Peak frequency is reached later in swine than in sheep. (From Ewbank, E. (1967). Anim. Behav. *15*, 251, and data of Niwa et al. (1951). Bull. Nat. Inst. Agric. Sci. Tokyo (Ser. G) *1*, 135.)

Initially, lambs are insensitive to identity cues provided by the mother, and they will attempt to suckle from any ewe. There is nonspecific attraction of ewe's voices initially, but the specificity increases with age. Visual cues become more important than auditory cues by the time the lamb is about 3 weeks old. Whether an odor from the ewe plays any role in recognition by the lamb is unknown.

Suckling Behavior. After the newborn lamb has achieved satiety, the frequency of suckling stabilizes at once or twice per hour (Fig. 10–12). During the first week, suckling is usually initiated and terminated by the lamb. Twin lambs may be suckled individually and more frequently than singles.

As the lamb becomes older and mutual recognition improves, ewes and lambs stray farther apart, and the ewe now tends to terminate suckling, although she may initiate suckling by approaching and calling the lamb. After a week or so, twins are not usually permitted to suckle unless both are present, so the ewe now recognizes

that she has two lambs. With advancing age of the lamb, the frequency and duration of suckling decline (Fig. 10–12). Under natural conditions, these changes culminate in weaning, with maternal solicitude being suddenly replaced by antagonistic behavior.

There is no fierce maternal protective behavior in sheep; the mere presence of the ewe appears to act as a deterrent to predators such as foxes and crows. Maternal care consists primarily of supplying milk exclusively for her own lamb. A small minority of ewes will allow an alien lamb to suckle, and some lambs become adept at stealing milk from an alien ewe; these abnormal patterns may be due to disruption of the normal sequence of events immediately after birth.

Maternal Behavior in Goats

Maternal and neonatal behavior of goats is similar to that of sheep. However, goats may be more efficient than sheep in recognizing that they have twins. Also, the doe spends more time vigorously grooming and orienting to the firstborn, so that the secondborn, which is usually the weaker of the two, has the greater opportunity to suckle. Kids' voices are initially similar, when analyzed by a sonagraph, and the does cannot distinguish between kids by auditory means until the sounds begin to diverge at about 4 days of age.

Maternal Behavior in Cattle

Both normal and abnormal behavioral patterns of the cow and calf are remarkably similar to those of sheep, although there are some points of difference. A day or two before calving, the cow may become restless and keep to a small isolated area, which she defends against other cows. Confinement and interference at this time can result in prolonged birth and poor calf survival. Cows tend to eat the afterbirth more frequently than do sheep. Most new calves take at least 45 minutes to stand and may take upward of 4 hours to suckle for the first time.

Suckling

Newborn calves begin to suckle within 2 to 5 hours after birth. Until a teat is located, the calf readily mouths and sucks any protuberance on the mother's body. The mother seems to help the calf find a teat by positioning her body appropriately and by licking, nuzzling, and nudging the calf.

Twinning in cattle does not affect the probability that a mother would nurse her offspring during morning and evening sessions. Twins are suckled longer than single calves, presumably because of suboptimal milk supply. Twins receive less grooming (licking) from their mothers than single calves.

Nursing involves both mother and calf. As mentioned, the cow initially helps the calf locate her teats. While the calf suckles, the mother licks its perineal and preputial areas, stimulating it to urinate and or defecate. Cows without calves or those that have recently calved but no longer possess young often show little interest in calves that may be present.

Frequently, females may give birth in the close company of pregnant conspecifics and mothers with newborn young. This may increase patterns of aberrant maternal behavior, i.e., abandonment of young, calf stealing, and cross suckling.

Non-nutritional sucking markedly increases in calves fed low-energy, low-protein diets, suggesting that it is related to the diet. Calves suckling their dams drink more than bucket-fed animals, among which the incidence of non-nutritional sucking is high. Non-nutritional sucking has important consequences, particularly if it continues into adult life. Such activity markedly decreases the dry-matter consumption of calves and retards growth. Hair balls commonly occur in the rumina of calves that exhibit non-nutritional licking behavior. These may attain a size of 3788 g and may be fatal if they block the entrance to the rumen and prevent eructation (Fig. 10–13).

Maternal Behavior in Horses

Approaching birth may be indicated by milk ejection and restlessness, but these signs are not confined to the immediate prepartum period. In mares, most births occur at night, but whether this is due to photoperiodic effects or routine husbandry procedures is not clear. Delays in parturition are attributed to human presence and interference, as well as to the presence of spectator groups of mares.

Abnormally long parturition is usually associated with malpresentation of the fetus, though aged mares may not sustain their efforts to foal. Mares tend to remain recumbent longer than sheep, often not standing until more than 10 minutes after birth. Most foals take an hour or more to maintain a stable stance, and most have

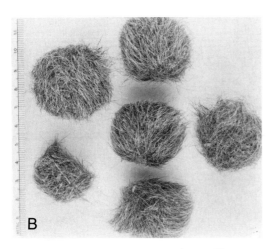

FIG. 10–13. Non-nutritional suckling in calves. Hair balls collected from the rumen of a 41-day old calf reared individually on the Nursette. The hair was accumulated by the calf licking itself.

suckled within 3 hours of birth. Grooming continues for several hours. Premature young are more common in horses than in ruminants, and the premature foal tends to be weak and slow to progress, although the suckling reflex is well developed.

Maternal Behavior in Pigs

Behavior in the pig with its large litters of small, almost naked young contrasts with that in other domestic ungulates. Appropriate behavior patterns are of particular importance in swine because of the susceptibility of the young to starvation, chilling, and accidental injury by the sow.

Prepartum Behavior

In the field the approach of parturition is indicated by characteristic nest-building activity, but in practice, sows are so restricted by the lack of nest-building material and by modern farrowing pens designed to protect the piglets that this activity is inhibited and the sows may become disturbed. As parturition approaches, characteristic vocalizations become evident and the "nest" area is defended as if piglets are present.

Farrowing

Parturition in the sow is most frequent after sunset. Though most domestic sows tolerate the presence of an observer at farrowing, some become highly disturbed. Sows normally farrow lying on one side, and delivery is accomplished with much less apparent effort than in other farm animals.

The rupture of the membranes and the voiding of the fetal fluids is not well-defined as in other ungulates. Most piglets are born partly covered with fetal membranes, and in contrast with the larger young of other ungulates, the piglet must escape from these without maternal aid or perish. The umbilical cord is broken by the piglet moving away from the vulva. At the end of delivery, the sow usually stands to urinate, and in the process of lying down again and also during earlier bouts of restlessness, the piglets are prone to be overlain and injured.

The average duration of farrowing is about 3 hours, but can range from a half to 8 hours or more. The interval between birth of individual piglets ranges from less than a minute to 3 or more hours, and piglets in the last half of the litter are prone to be stillborn, perhaps because of premature rupture of the cord and prolonged hypoxia.

Postpartum Behavior

Newborn piglets are almost immediately mobile. They rapidly find their way to the udder and may be suckling within 5 minutes; most have obtained milk within half an hour of birth. At this early stage, milk is available on demand, possibly because of continuous milk letdown due to circulating oxytocin associated with the birth process. Behavior of litters immediately after birth is variable, and piglets may be attracted to infrared heaters before moving to the udder. Attraction to heaters is probably undesirable at this early stage when a teat-order is being established but may be desirable subsequently in keeping piglets from being overlain by the sow. In the search for the teats, the piglets tend to concentrate on the pectoral region of the udder and explore vertical surfaces with their noses until a teat is contacted, grasped, and suckled. Piglets that do not find a functional teat soon after birth rapidly deplete their energy reserves in cold weather and die from hypothermia.

Suckling

Having suckled initially, the piglets tend to sample several teats in the same row as the teat first sucked; they locate these teats readily, having rapidly learned the appropriate orientation and teat height. Contact with another piglet may now result in fighting, in the form of pushing or biting with the sharp canine teeth.

The teat order tends to be unstable with large litters or with a poor milk supply. Identification of teats by piglets does not seem to be based on taste or smell. In small litters, some piglets have the regular use of adjacent teats, though one is usually preferred. There is clear preference for the anterior teats. Although their control is usually gained by the larger, dominant piglets, there appears to be no major advantage in suckling from them.

Suckling bouts are initiated by the sow, either spontaneously or by the piglets squealing or attempting to suckle. There is a distinctive food call, a series of soft grunts to which the litter rapidly becomes conditioned, and which initiates suckling. The bouts can be stimulated by a disturbance in the farrowing house or by suckling by a neighboring sow (Table 10–4). Suckling positions tend to be characteristic of the individual sow; the standing position is more common in feral than domestic pigs.

The food call initiates a period of intense udder massage lasting several minutes by the nose of the piglet; at the same time, a recumbent sow rotates her body to expose the teats. The grunt frequency increases to a peak, and the phase of active move-

TABLE 10–4. Nursing and Suckling Behavior in Swine

Suckling Pattern	Values
Time taken by sow to lie down after piglets enter the pen (sec)	11–17
Suckling frequency (periods/day)	18–28
Interval between sucklings (min)	51–63 (up to 160 is rare)
Duration of nursing (min)	4–8
Duration of suckling (sec)	
Nosing phase	55–140
Quiet phase	16–23
True suckling	13–37
Milk consumption of piglet/suckling period (g)	24–28
Milk consumption of piglet/day (g)	546–676
Milk consumption of piglet/lactation period (kg)	30–37

ment by the piglets is suddenly replaced by a quieter phase of milk letdown and suckling that lasts for only a minute or two. Piglets do not appear to discriminate between sows. Fostering is not difficult, and litters can be reared together, with piglets suckling more than one sow. Lactating sows may become aggressive if piglets are disturbed or threatened.

Behavioral Anomalies, Thermoregulation and Neonatal Mortality

Newborn piglets, with their small body size, sparse pelage, and skin wet with fluids are prone to chill in air temperatures as high as 20°C with a 5-km per hour wind, despite a vigorous thermogenic response. Young piglets huddle together or against the sow to minimize heat loss; feral piglets appear to be more cold-resistant than domestic piglets.

Improved thermoregulation in wild newborn pigs is partly due to extra pelage and to a more mature metabolic response to cold. Piglet mortality is attributed to infection, chilling, poor nutrition, and crushing. These ultimate causes of death may be secondary to inadequate development of energy stores prenatally and inactive metabolic pathways postnatally (Kas-

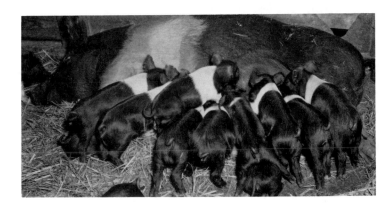

FIG. 10–14. Test order and suckling intervals in piglets.

ser et al., 1981). Deaths from direct or indirect effects of chilling are common in unheated farrowing houses, but the resistance to cold increases during the 2 or 3 days that piglets would remain in the nest. Piglets exposed to cold spent more time in behavioral thermoregulation than in suckling. Behavioral thermoregulation causes a reduction in the amount of colostrum consumed. This phenomenon would represent a cold-induced decrease in the ingestion of colostral immunoglobulins. Alternatively, cold exposure may also reduce the capability of piglets to localize, internalize, and transport colostral immunoglobulins through the intestinal epithelial cells and into the blood (Kelly et al., 1982).

Sows occasionally kill and eat their young during parturition. If aggressive behavior is detected as farrowing approaches, the piglets can be removed at birth and returned in relative safety after farrowing is complete, but cannibalism can also occur later in lactation.

Starvation accounts for nearly half of the 10% mortality in liveborn domestic piglets. Young piglets will suckle anything that contacts their noses, including the maternal vulva and other piglets. The number of teats available is effectively reduced in some sows, particularly in older animals in which the teats can be hidden beneath the udder. Piglets that are dis-placed from their established position at the udder after the first day or two do not readily accept a vacant teat and may die.

REFERENCES

Alexander, G. (1975). Body temperature control in mammalian young. Br. Med. Bull. *31*, 62.

Alexander, G. (1977). Role of auditory and visual cues in mutual recognition between ewes and lambs in Merino sheep. Appl. Anim. Ethol. *3*, 65.

Alexander, G., Signoret, J.P., and Hafez, E.S.E. (1980). Sexual maternal and neonatal behavior. *In* Reproduction in Farm Animals, 4th ed. E.S.E. Hafez (ed.). Philadelphia, Lea & Febiger.

Bronson, F.H. (1984). Energy allocation and reproductive development in wild and domestic house mice. Biol. Reprod. *31*, 83–88.

Denenberg, V.H., and Banks, E.M. (1969). Techniques of measurement and evaluation. *In* The Behavior of Domestic Animals. E.S.E. Hafez (ed.). London, England, Bailliere, Tindall & Cassell.

Kasser, T.R., Martin, R.J., Gahagan, J.H., and Wangsness, P.J. (1981). Fasting plasma hormones and metabolites in feral and newborn pigs. J. Anim. Sic. *53*, 420–426.

Kelley, K.W., Blecha, F., and Regnier, J.A. (1982). Cold exposure and absorption of colostral immunoglobulins by neonatal pigs. J. Anim. Sci. *55*, 363–368.

Klingel, H. (1967). Soziale Organization and Verhalten freilebender Steppenzebras. Z. Tierpsychol. *34*, 580.

Price, E.O., Thos, J., and Anderson, G.B. (1981). Maternal responses of confined beef cattle to single versus twin calves. J. Anim. Sci. *53*, 934–939.

Randolph, J.H., Cromwell, G.L., Stahly, T.S., and Kratzer, D.D. (1981). Effects of group size and space allowance on performance and behavior of swine. J. Anim. Sci. *53*, 922–927.

III. reproductive failure

11
Reproductive Failure in Females

M.R. JAINUDEEN AND E.S.E. HAFEZ

Sterility is a permanent factor preventing procreation, and infertility or temporary sterility is the inability to produce viable young within a stipulated time characteristic for each species. This chapter examines the phases of the reproductive process that are most vulnerable and shows how hormonal imbalances or adverse environmental, genetic, and hereditary factors exert their influences (Fig. 11–1).

OVARIAN DYSFUNCTION

The two main functions of the ovary, the production of ova and secretion of ovarian hormones, are intimately related and directed toward successful reproduction.

Anestrus

Anestrus denotes a state of complete sexual inactivity with no manifestations of estrus. It is not a disease but a sign of a variety of conditions (Table 11–1). Although anestrus is observed during certain physiologic states—e.g., before puberty,

during pregnancy and lactation, and in seasonal breeders—it is most often a sign of temporary or permanent depression of ovarian activity (true anestrus) caused by seasonal changes in the physical environment, nutritional deficiencies, lactation stress, and aging (Fig. 11–2). Certain pathologic conditions of the ovaries or the uterus also suppress estrus.

Seasonal Anestrus. During seasonal anestrus, there are no cyclic changes in the ovaries and reproductive tract. The extent of seasonal anestrus varies with the species, breed, and physical environment and is more pronounced in sheep and horses than in cattle, pigs, and most laboratory mammals. The seasonal anestrus in sheep and goats in the temperate zone is mainly influenced by photoperiod and involves changes in tonic LH secretion. Although the sow and cow are polyestrous, there is evidence for a seasonal control of their reproductive efficiency. Anestrus in the mare occurs during the winter and

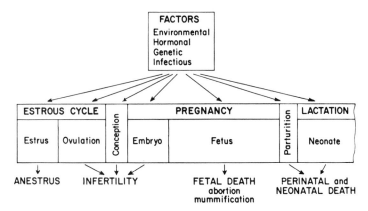

FIG. 11–1. Schematic representation of factors that adversely affect the reproductive process. Common types of reproductive failure are anestrus, infertility, fetal, perinatal, and neonatal deaths. Note that infertility may result from fertilization failure or embryonic mortality.

TABLE 11–1. **Abnormalities of Estrus**

Species	Abnormality	Causes	Physiologic Mechanisms
Cattle	Anestrus	Pyometra, mummification	Maintenance of corpus luteum
		Lactation	Suckling stimulus inhibits gonadotropin release
		Cystic ovaries	Deficiency of LH and/or GnRH
		Ovarian hypoplasia and freemartinism	Failure to produce ovarian estrogens
		Nutritional and vitamin deficiencies	Gonadotropin production by anterior pituitary
	Subestrus, silent estrus (quiet ovulation)	High lactation	Endocrine imbalance
	Nymphomania	Cystic ovaries	
Sheep	Anestrus	Season, lactation	Effect of photoperiod on gonadotropin secretion
Swine	Anestrus	Lactation	As for cattle
Horse	Anestrus	Season, diet, ovarian hypoplasia	As for sheep
	Prolonged estrus	Early in breeding season	Failure of follicles beyond 2 cm to develop that is due to inadequate endocrine stimulus
	Split estrus, silent estrus		
	Lack of estrus	Pseudopregnancy	Early pregnancy failure with persistence of corpus luteum
		Prolonged diestrus after foaling	Persistence of corpus luteum

GnRH = gonadotropin-releasing hormone

spring when daylight hours are short. The ovaries become small and hard, contain neither follicles nor corpora lutea, and there are low serum concentrations of LH, progesterone, and estradiol. Seasonal anestrus is due to a reduction in gonadotropin-releasing hormone (GnRH) secretion. With increasing daylight after winter solstice, GnRH secretion is stimulated, FSH is released, which in turn stimulates follicular development resulting in estrus and ovulation. Several methods are used to overcome seasonal anestrus including the daily administration of progesterone, artificial lighting (16 hours a day) and GnRH. Because of the disadvantages of artificial light treatment, the use of GnRH to advance the breeding season is being researched in several laboratories.

Anestrus During Lactation. In several species, ovulation and related reproductive activity are suppressed for a variable period after parturition and during lactation. The incidence and duration of anestrus vary greatly between different species and breeds and are also influenced by the season of parturition, level of milk production, number of young being nursed, and the degree of postpartum involution of the uterus.

Estrus and ovulation are completely suppressed during lactation in the sow, although this inhibition may be due to the suckling reflex and/or the presence of a litter rather than lactation per se. Weaning is followed by estrus and ovulation within 4 to 8 days. Normally, ovarian activity is reestablished in milked cows within 30 days postpartum (Lamming et al., 1981). On the other hand, the suckled cow and buffalo experience an extended postpartum period. During periods of high temperatures and on poor diets, Brahman cows that are nursing calves are particularly subject to anestrus. The duration of anestrus in cows nursing calves is longer than in similar cows milked twice daily; this suggests that nursing or frequency of milk removal may influence the pituitary gonadotropic activity.

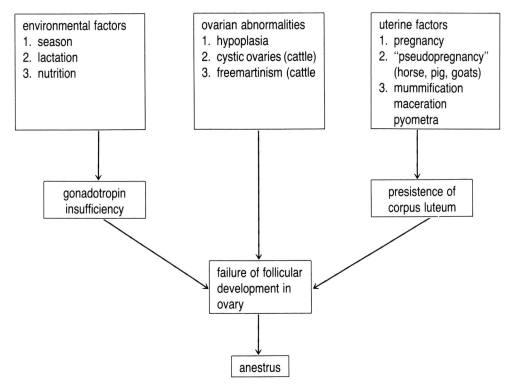

FIG. 11–2.   Scheme illustrating the possible causes leading to a failure of follicular development in the ovary and anestrus in farm animals. Note that pregnancy is an important cause for an absence of estrus.

In sheep, lactational anestrus lasts 5 to 7 weeks. Some ewes suckling lambs will come into estrus, but most ewes show estrus about 2 weeks after the lambs are weaned. Nutrition and season may modify the effects of suckling and lactation on resumption of postpartum ovarian activity. For example, anestrus is more pronounced at the end than at the start of the breeding season when nutrition is inadequate. Similarly, summer conditions may prolong the interval from weaning to first estrus in primiparous sows (Britt et al., 1983). Most foaling mares come into estrus within 5 to 15 days after foaling, but some nervous lactating mares may experience lactational anestrus as a result of psychologic disturbance rather than of the stress of lactation.

The endocrinology of lactational anestrus in farm animals has been extensively reviewed (Peters and Lamming, 1990). The initial block to cyclicity appears to be due to the inhibitory effects of steroids secreted during pregnancy at the hypothalamus and pituitary level being continued into the postpartum period. However, the hypothalamus begins to secrete enough GnRH to effect the release of FSH earlier than the release of LH. Follicular development occurs, leading to the negative feedback control by estradiol and the induction of the preovulatory LH surge. Suckling and undernutrition inhibit the tonic GnRH and LH secretion. Regular milking of dairy cows is less inhibitory to spontaneous LH release than the combination of milking and nursing (Carruthers et al., 1980). In addition, cessation of suckling in beef cows enhances the amount of LH released in response to LH-RH (Troxel et al., 1983). Alternatively, inhibition of

LH release may be caused by the high cortisol levels occurring during suckling or milk removal (Wagner and Li, 1982). New evidence suggests that an opioid-mediated mechanism may be responsible for the suckling-induced LH suppression in the suckled cow (Whisnant et al., 1986).

Anestrus That Is Due to Aging. Farm animals with the exception of the horse are rarely maintained into old age for economic reasons, and even more rarely given the opportunity to breed late in life. In rodents, the incidence of irregular or anovulatory cycles rises steadily with age, and even when the females are no longer fertile, mating frequently results in pseudopregnancy. Abnormal corpora lutea and ovaries lacking corpora lutea accounted for over 80% of cases of infertility in cows 14 to 15 years old. Regardless of the mechanism involved, anestrus that is due to aging probably alters the functional relationship of the hypothalamus-pituitary-ovarian axis.

Nutritional Deficiencies. Energy level has a significant effect on ovarian activity. Inadequate nutrition suppresses estrus in young growing females more than in adults. Low levels of energy lead to ovarian inactivity and anestrus in beef cows that are suckling calves and in sows after weaning. It may be possible to shorten the anovulatory period in primiparous beef heifers by increasing dietary energy intake during late gestation (Echternkamp et al., 1982), restricting suckling to once daily from 30 days postpartum to the first estrus (Randel, 1981), and early weaning or calf removal for 72 hours with or without exogenous progestagen (Walters et al., 1984).

In dairy cattle, interrelationships between energy balance and postpartum reproduction have been extensively reviewed by Butler and Smith (1989). It has been proposed that negative energy balance probably depresses ovarian activity by inhibiting pulsatile LH release. Low levels of glucose and insulin during early lactation may depress LH pulsatility secretion or act directly on the ovary to depress steroid secretion. On the other hand, release of endogenous opioids with increasing feed intake or other hormones associated with lactation could inhibit the pulsatile release of LH and depress ovarian function.

Deficiencies of minerals or vitamins cause anestrus. Phosphorus deficiency in range cattle and sheep causes ovarian dysfunction, which in turn leads to delayed puberty, depressed signs of estrus, and eventually cessation of estrus. However, neither estrous behavior nor blood levels of progesterone, estradiol, or LH measured around the time of estrus were altered in Holstein and Jersey heifers allotted to a phosphorus-deficient diet, despite a reduction in plasma inorganic phosphorus concentration (Hurley et al., 1982). Gilts or cows fed a manganese-deficient diet experience ovarian disturbances ranging from weak signs of estrus to anestrus. Vitamin A or E deficiencies may cause irregular estrous cycles or anestrus.

Stress. Environmental stresses such as climate, high population density, or excessive handling during the premating period may depress estrus, ovulation, and luteal function in ewe, sow, and cow. Environmental stress depresses ovarian function by acting at different sites and by diverse mechanisms (Armstrong, 1986). These stresses may disrupt the hypothalamohypophyseal system, resulting in disruption of the normal pattern of gonadotropin secretion, or may alter ovarian function either directly or indirectly through other organs. These metabolic alterations change the balance of feedback control of the hypothalamo-pituitary-ovarian system.

Abnormalities of the Ovary or Uterus. *Ovarian hypoplasia* occurs in Swedish mountain cattle. Affected animals have infantile reproductive tracts and never exhibit estrus. The morphology of the ovary differs from that of seasonal anestrus. Follicles of varying diameter up to the preovulatory size, which commonly are present in the ovaries of anestrous animals, are absent in ovarian hypoplasia. Ovarian hypoplasia tends to be associated with white coat color, being inherited as an autosomal recessive. Some mares with small inactive ovaries have abnormal sex chromosome complement (e.g., XO) as well as low plasma estrogen and high LH levels.

Freemartins, or heifers born co-twin to bulls, have poorly developed ovaries and fail to show estrus. *Cystic ovaries* in cattle may lead to a prolonged period of anestrus.

Uterine distention in cattle and swine that is due to pathologic conditions (e.g., pyometra, mucometra, fetal mummification, or maceration) or *pseudopregnancy* in the mare, sow, and doe is associated with a retention of the corpus luteum and therefore a suppression of the estrous cycle.

Pseudopregnancy in the pig is characterized by functional corpora lutea and a uterus containing either endometrial gland secretions or remnants of embryonic or fetal tissue. Injections of estrogens (embryonic luteotropin) toward the end of the luteal phase of the estrous cycle also induce pseudopregnancy in the sow. Pseudopregnancy in the doe is unrelated to mating. The abdomen of the doe enlarges as in pregnancy, but udder development and kidding fail to occur.

The term *cloudburst* is used when spontaneous discharge of a cloudy uterine fluid occurs around the expected time of parturition in animals that have been mated. Progesterone levels are elevated, making it difficult to differentiate this state from pregnancy; it can easily be diagnosed by real-time ultrasonography, however, whichdemonstrates the lack of placentomes in the fluid-filled uterus. The factors causing pseudopregnancy in the goat have not been established, but prolactin plays an important luteotropic role during pseudopregnancy in goats (Taverne et al., 1988). Both prostaglandin and repeated oxytocin treatments result in a decline in progesterone levels, es-

trous behavior, and the discharge of intrauterine fluid (Pieterse and Taverne, 1986), a condition that could be misdiagnosed as pregnancy. In all species, exogenous $PGF_{2\alpha}$ terminates pseudopregnancy as a result of persistence of the CL.

Prolonged diestrus, apparently unique to mares, results from spontaneous prolongation of the life of the cyclic corpus luteum beyond the normal 14 to 15 days and is a major cause of anestrus during the natural breeding season. Persistence of the corpus luteum may be attributed to a failure of $PGF_{2\alpha}$ release.

Atypical Estrus

Short estrus, prolonged estrus, "split" estrus, nymphomania, and "silent" estrus are not uncommon (Table 11–1). Estrus may be of short duration and without well-marked signs. It may be undetected in young animals without the presence of a teaser male, or it may occur during the night, particularly in cattle. Prolonged estrus, lasting from 10 to 40 days, without ovulation, characterizes the transition from seasonal anestrus to resumption of cyclic activity in mares during the breeding season. "Split" estrus or behavioral estrus interrupted by 1 or 2 days of sexual nonreceptivity is also observed in mares, especially at the start of the breeding season.

Nymphomania occurs more frequently in dairy cattle than in beef cattle and horses. Nymphomania is one of the signs of cystic ovaries in cattle. Nymphomaniac cows show intense estrous behavior persistently or at frequent but irregular intervals, depressed milk production, a frequent copious discharge of clear mucus from the vulva, edema and relaxation of the sacrosciatic ligaments, and a raised tail head. Nymphomaniac mares are excitable, vicious, and intractable. They will not tolerate the approach of another horse, nor will they stand for mating. The occurrence of ovarian cysts in the mare analogous to the condition in cows is doubtful, since in the mare ovariectomy has no effect on the abnormal behavioral pattern.

"Silent" estrus (quiet ovulation), or the occurrence of ovulation without overt estrus, occurs in all farm animals, particularly young animals and those on a submaintenance ration. It is suspected when the interval between two consecutive estrous periods is double or triple the normal length. A high incidence of silent estrus occurs in sheep during the first estrous cycle of the breeding season, apparently related to the absence of a corpus luteum from a previous cycle, and at the end of the breeding season, probably as a result of estrogen deficiency. Several silent estruses occur in beef cows and ewes that suckle young and in dairy cows milked three times daily. Silent estrus is frequently encountered in maiden mares and in mares with a foal at foot.

Ovulatory Failure

Ovulatory failure may be due to failure of the follicle to ovulate during a normal cycle or to cystic ovaries.

Anovulatory estrus is more common in swine and horses than in cattle and sheep. The animal shows normal behavioral estrus and the ovarian follicle reaches preovulatory size but does not rupture. Anovulatory follicles become partly luteinized and then regress during the estrous cycle, as does a normal corpus luteum.

Cystic ovarian disease or "cystic ovaries" is common in dairy cattle and swine but is rarely encountered in beef cattle or other species. The disease is a common endocrine abnormality in dairy cattle, particularly among high-producing dairy cows. Most ovarian cysts probably develop prior to the first ovulation postpartum since more ovarian cysts were detected in cows examined at 30 days postpartum than after breeding or after abnormal estrous behavior (Erb and White, 1981). Although some affected cows may exhibit intense mounting behavior (nymphomania), the majority fail to exhibit estrus (an-

estrus). One or both ovaries contain multiple small cysts or one or more large cysts. These are either follicular or luteal cysts. Follicular cysts undergo cyclic changes, i.e., they alternately grow and regress but fail to ovulate. Luteal cysts contain a thin rim of luteal tissue, also fail to ovulate, but persist for a prolonged period.

Concentrations of plasma progesterone are lower with follicular cysts than luteal cysts, but concentrations of estradiol show no relationship to the type of cyst. The levels of testosterone in affected cows are similar to those found during the estrous cycle (Kesler and Garverick, 1982). Some cows with cystic ovaries may show masculine characteristics. The cystic fluid is high in progesterone and low in estrogen, but these hormonal concentrations bear no relationship to the behavioral patterns (nymphomania or anestrus).

In swine, cystic ovaries are an important cause of reproductive failure and a major reason for culling, particularly older sows. Large multiple luteinized follicles are more common than small multiple cysts, and they contain progesterone. Estrous cycles that are irregular with prolonged periods between cycles may be mistaken for pregnancy (Wrathal, 1980).

Signs of estrus are pronounced, but nymphomania does not occur. It is not certain whether cystic ovaries in cattle and swine result from a failure of the ovulatory mechanism, from adrenal cortex hyperfunction, or from a disturbance in the hypothalamo–pituitary axis. In cattle, available evidence (see Kesler and Garverick, 1982) indicates that it may be caused by a failure in the LH-release mechanism. This failure is not due to a deficiency or release of GnRH but more to an insensitivity of the hypothalamic–pituitary axis to elevated levels of estradiol. The development of cystic ovaries in cattle has been related to high milk production, seasonal changes, hereditary predisposition, and pituitary dysfunction (Fig. 11–3). The cause and effect relationship between milk production and cystic ovarian disease is not clear, but

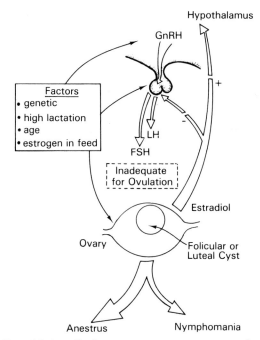

FIG. 11–3. Endocrine sequence, types of cysts, and behavioral manifestations associated with cystic ovarian disease in the cow. Inadequate secretion of LH results in ovulatory failure and formation of follicular or luteal cysts. Note that affected cows are either nymphomaniac or in anestrus.

the high milk yield may be a response to hormonal changes in cows with ovarian cysts rather than the cause of the disease (Kesler and Garverick, 1982). In dairy cattle, the development of cystic ovaries has been related to postpartum uterine infections. Endotoxins produced by microorganisms in the uterus may trigger the prostaglandin $F_{2\alpha}$ ($PGF_{2\alpha}$) release, which in turn stimulates the secretion of cortisol. The elevated cortisol levels suppress the preovulatory release of LH and lead to the development of cysts (Bosu and Peter, 1987). A relationship exists between cystic ovarian disease and heredity as the incidence has steadily declined in several herds after culling bulls whose daughters had cystic ovarian disease (Kirk et al., 1982). Cystic ovaries are also frequently encountered in dairy cows fed higher levels of nutrients and during the winter.

Several methods are available for the treatment of cystic ovarian disease in cattle. Manual rupture of the cyst by rectal palpation is one of the oldest methods. hCG and GnRH are equally effective for the treatment of follicular cysts, but GnRH, being of lower molecular weight, is less likely to stimulate antibody formation. Prostaglandin $F_{2\alpha}$ or its analogs are effective for treatment of luteal cysts. Progesterone injections or progesterone intravaginal devices may also restore ovarian cycles in cows with ovarian cysts.

DISORDERS OF FERTILIZATION

Disorders of fertilization include failure of fertilization and atypical fertilization.

Fertilization Failure

Fertilization failure may result from death of the egg before sperm entry, structural and functional abnormality in the egg or sperm, physical barriers in the female genital tract preventing gamete transport to the site of fertilization, or ovulatory failure and cystic ovaries, as discussed previously (Table 11–2).

Abnormal Eggs. Several types of morphologic and functional abnormalities have been observed in unfertilized eggs, e.g., giant egg, oval-shaped egg, lentil-shaped egg, and ruptured zona pellucida. Failure to undergo fertilization and normal embryonic development may be due to inherent abnormalities of the egg or to environmental factors. For example, fertilization is lower in animals exposed to elevated ambient temperature prior to breeding. In sheep, some of the conception failures at the beginning of the breeding season are associated with a high incidence of abnormal ova.

Abnormal Sperm. The physiologic significance of abnormal sperm in relation to fertilization failure has not been studied in animals other than cattle. Certain forms of male infertility are related to structural defects of the DNA protein complex.

Sperm aging and injury may cause alterations in the acrosomal cap. Acrosin, an

TABLE 11–2.   **Structural and Functional Causes of Fertilization Failure**

Cause	Abnormality	Affected Species	Mechanism Interfered With
Structural obstructions			
Congenital	Mesonephric cysts	More common in swine, sheep and cattle than in horses	Sperm transport
	Uterus unicornis		
	Double cervix		
Acquired	Tubal adhesions	All species, sheep and swine particularly	Egg pick-up, fertilization
	Hydrosalpinx		Egg transport
	Occluded uterine horns		
Functional			
Hormonal	Cystic ovaries	Cattle and swine	Ovulation
	Abnormal cervical and uterine secretions	Cattle; sheep on estrogenic pastures	Gamete transport
Management	Delayed insemination	In all species, horses and swine particularly	Death of egg
	Insemination too early	Cattle	Death of sperm
	Errors in estrus detection	Cattle	Fertilization failure

enzyme within the acrosome, appears to be important in the penetration of the zona pellucida of the egg. Acrosin inhibitors present in seminal plasma combine with acrosin only in spermatozoa with acrosomal damage and prevent defective spermatozoa from fertilizing the egg. In bull, ram and boar, a good correlation exists between fertility and acrosomal integrity.

Sperm aging during prolonged storage has been attributed either to a leakage of vital intracellular constituents such as cyclic AMP or to the formation of lipid peroxides from sperm plasmalogen when sperm are stored under anerobic conditions. Aging of spermatozoa in the male genital tract is typically accompanied by a declining fertility without resulting defects in the offspring, whereas aging of spermatozoa in the female genital tract is accompanied by a gradual decrease in the fertilizing capacity. Antigenic incompatibility between sperm and egg could lead to sperm rejection and fertilization failure.

Structural Barriers to Fertilization. Congenital or acquired defects of the female genital tract interfere with transport of the sperm and/or the ovum to the site of fertilization (Table 11–2). Con-

genital defects are the result of arrested development of the different segments of the Müllerian ducts (oviduct, uterus, and cervix) or of an incomplete fusion of these ducts caudally.

A classic congenital anomaly associated with the gene for white coat color is "white heifer disease" in cattle, in which the prenatal development of the müllerian ducts is arrested, and the vaginal canal is obstructed by the presence of an abnormally developed hymen. The degree and area of hypoplasia differ, so that various anomalies of the oviducts, uterus, cervix, and vagina are formed. This congenital anomaly can be differentiated from the freemartin syndrome by the presence of normal ovaries, vulva, and labia in the animals with white heifer disease. Acquired defects are caused by trauma or infection, particularly at time of parturition.

Reproductive failure occurs more in sheep than in cattle grazing on plants that contain compounds with estrogenic activity, e.g., subterranean clover *(Trifolium subterraneum)* and red clover *(Trifolium pratense)*. The estrogenic activity is due to plant isoflavones and related substances with hydroxyl groups (Fig. 11–4). The sub-

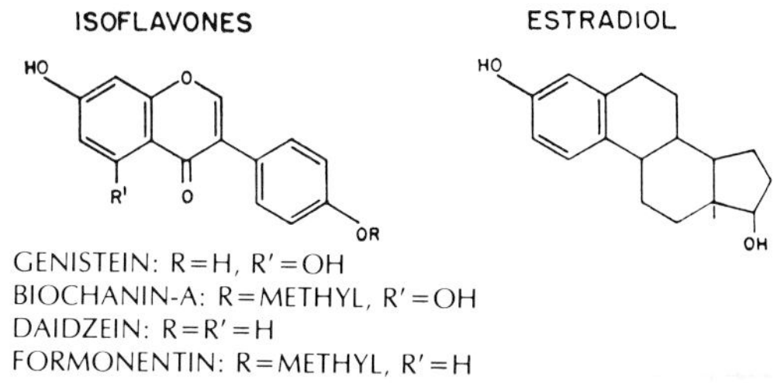

ISOFLAVONES · ESTRADIOL

GENISTEIN: R=H, R'=OH
BIOCHANIN-A: R=METHYL, R'=OH
DAIDZEIN: R=R'=H
FORMONENTIN: R=METHYL, R'=H

FIG. 11–4. The structures of plant estrogens (isoflavones) and estradiol. Isoflavones are found in many forage species of the family *Leguminosae;* formonetin has low estrogenic activity, whereas biochanin-A, genistein, and daidzein are metabolized in the rumen of the sheep to nonestrogenic compounds.

stance mainly responsible is the isoflavone formonetin, which is converted in the rumen of the sheep to equol, a weak estrogen. The other estrogenic isoflavones present in clovers (genistein and biochanin A) are converted to nonestrogenic metabolites in the rumen. Ewes grazing pastures with high levels of formonetin exhibit either temporary or permanent infertility but the mechanisms are distinctly different. Ewes grazed on estrogenic pastures around the time of joining shed fewer ova and have a reduced chance of conception. Fertility is improved within 3 weeks, when ewes are moved into nonestrogenic pastures. The pathologic changes in temporary infertility are due to actions of estrogen on the hypophyseal–ovarian axis and on sperm transport. Ewes grazed for several seasons on estrogenic pastures mate and ovulate, but fertilization rate is depressed as a result of failure of sperm transport caused by severe changes occurring in the cervix. The external genitalia become masculinized. These changes caused by estrogens have been considered to be an irreversible differentiation of the reproductive tract in the male direction (Adams, 1990).

Common anatomic abnormalities are adhesions of the infundibulum to the ovary or uterine horns; this interferes with the pick-up of the egg or causes a mechanical obstruction of one part of the repro-

ductive duct system. Bilateral or unilateral missing segments of the reproductive tract also cause anatomic sterility.

Atypical Fertilization

The complex process of fertilization is subject to several aberrations, namely, polyspermy, monospermic fertilization of an egg containing two female pronuclei, failure of pronucleus formation, and gynogenesis or androgenesis. Atypical fertilization may occur spontaneously as a result of aging of the gametes or elevation of environmental temperature. It has also been induced experimentally by x-rays or the administration of certain toxic substances.

The aging of the ovum is gradual, during which various functions are successively lost (Table 11–3). An early effect of egg aging is that the resulting embryo is not viable and is resorbed before birth. Further aging leads to abnormalities in fertilization, particularly involving the pronuclei. The biophysical and biochemical reactions associated with sperm entry into the egg become slower, a condition leading to increased polyspermy (entry of more than one sperm).

Polyspermy occurs in several species of laboratory and farm animals. In swine, a delay in copulation or injection of progesterone given 24 to 36 hours before ovulation leads to some eggs having more than two pronuclei. It is not clear whether these potential triploid embryos are caused by failure to extrude the second polar body or to polyspermy, which may result from failure of the block to polyspermy during ovum aging. The incidence of polyspermy increases when mating or insemination is delayed, resulting in triploid embryos that do not survive. This means that in horses and swine with a relatively long estrus, the timing of breeding in relation to ovulation is critical for normal fertilization and embryonic survival.

PRENATAL MORTALITY

Prenatal mortality, responsible for most gestation failures, can be divided into *em-*

TABLE 11–3. **Aging of Gametes and Atypical Fertilization**

Gamete	Mechanism	Abnormality
Sperm	Reduction or loss of DNA	Reduced viability of embryo
Egg	Incomplete maturation with failure to release the second polar body	Triploid embryo
	Inhibition of the block to polyspermy	Triploid or heteroploid embryo

bryonic and *fetal* mortality. A small percentage of prenatal loss is involved in the normal reproductive process and may be regarded as unavoidable.

Embryonic Mortality

Embryonic mortality denotes the death of fertilized ova and embryos up to the end of implantation. Approximately 25 to 40% of embryos are normally lost in farm species. Mortality is more common during the early than the late embryonic period (Table 11–4). Early embryonic mortality should be regarded as a normal process of eliminating unfit genotypes in each generation, particularly in large litters of swine and multiple pregnancies in cattle and sheep.

Approximately 25 to 40% of embryos in cattle, sheep, and swine are lost between the time of sperm penetration of the ovum and the end of implantation (Table 11–4). Most losses occur before or immediately following implantation, resulting in complete resorption of the conceptus. It is also noted in large litters of swine and during multiple pregnancies in cattle and sheep.

Embryonic mortality after natural breeding or artificial insemination accounts for the majority of reproductive failures in the bovine, with a mortality rate of up to 40% of all fertilized ova (Sreenan and Diskin, 1986). In cattle, because most embryonic deaths occur between days 8 and 16 during hatching of the blastocyst and implantation, cycle lengths are unaffected. In sheep, since most embryos die between days 9 and 15, infertile ewes may experience normal as well as prolonged cycles.

Caution should be exercised in using postservice cycle lengths to estimate the time of embryonic mortality. For example, an extended cycle length may be due to reasons other than embryonic mortality. Early embryonic deaths before regression of the corpus luteum are indistinguishable from failure of fertilization in that both

TABLE 11–4. **Causes of Embryonic Mortality**

Species	Period of Maximal Mortality		Possible Causes
	Days of Gestation	Stage of Development	
Cattle	8 to 16	Hatching of blastocysts and initiation of elongation and commencement of implantation	Progesterone deficiency; inbreeding; multiple pregnancy; blood group homozygosity; J-antigen in sera; parity; timing of inseminations; chromosomal aberrations
Sheep	9 to 15	Transition from yolk sac to allantoic placentation	Inbreeding; increasing maternal age; hemoglobin types; overfeeding; multiple pregnancy; high environmental temperature
Swine	8 to 16	Spacing of embryos; transuterine migration; maternal recognition of pregnancy	Inbreeding; chromosomal aberrations; overcrowding; overfeeding; increasing maternal age; high environmental temperature; transferrins
Horses	30 to 36	Corpus luteum of pregnancy regresses and accessory corpora lutea are formed; change from a yolk sac to an allantochorion placentation	Lactation; twinning; nutrition; chromosomal aberrations

cow and ewe return to estrus at the normal time. Death of one embryo in twin-ovulating ewes may be undetected, as pregnancy will continue. Thus, a better estimate may be obtained by examining embryos that have been collected by slaughter or *in vivo* flushing of the reproductive tract at different days after breeding. Loss of single embryos in sheep can be evaluated by counting the number of ovulations by laparoscopy.

Over two thirds of the reproductive wastage in the pig occur before 8 to 16 days of gestation (Wettemann et al., 1984). The effects of embryonic mortality on the estrous cycle of swine are determined by the number of embryos that survive and the stage of pregnancy. For example, if all embryos are lost by day 4 of gestation, the sow returns to estrus after a normal cycle length, but if one to four embryos survive beyond day 4, the pregnancy would still terminate but the next estrous period is delayed by 6 days. For pregnancy to continue beyond day 10 at least a total of 4 embryos must be present in both uterine horns, whereas for it to continue beyond 12 days, as few as 1 embryo is sufficient.

Normal and subfertile mares have similar fertilization rates, but subfertile mares have a higher embryonic loss rate before day 14 postovulation (Ball et al., 1987).

Causes

Embryonic mortality can be due to maternal factors, embryonic factors, or to embryonic–maternal interactions. Maternal failure tends to affect an entire litter, resulting in complete loss of pregnancy. In contrast, embryonic failure affects embryos individually, often leaving others in the litter unharmed. In other cases the maternal environment may be insufficient, allowing the support of only a few strong embryos. Embryonic loss is influenced by several factors (Fig. 11–5). Chromosomal aberrations and genetic factors contributing to embryonic mortality are discussed in Chapter 13.

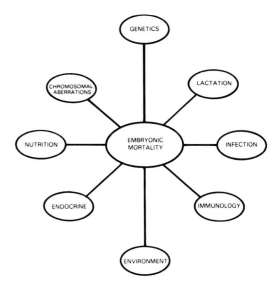

FIG. 11–5. Factors affecting embryonic mortality.

Endocrine Factors. Accelerated or delayed transport of the egg, as a result of estrogen–progesterone imbalance, leads to preimplantation death. An abnormally undersized conceptus might not be able to counteract the uterine luteolytic effect, with consequent regression of the corpus luteum and termination of pregnancy. In swine, as stated previously, at least four living blastocysts are needed by day 10 of pregnancy to counteract the uterine luteolytic effects.

A critical period of embryonic survival is the late blastocyst stage. Normally, the developing corpus luteum secretes progesterone, which acts on the female tract in close synchrony with the development of the embryos. The cause and effect relationship between luteolysis and embryonic deaths is controversial. Apparently, embryonic death in cattle is not caused by a progesterone deficiency during the luteal phase of the cycle; luteal regression follows rather than precedes embryonic mortality. However, a diminished response to circulating luteotrophic hormones may contribute to embryo mortality in subfertile cows (Shelton et al., 1990).

Lactation. During lactation, embryonic mortality occurs in cattle, sheep, and horses and is characterized by prolonged estrous cycles after breeding. Mating of mares at foal heat leads to early embryonic mortality, which has been attributed to reduced effectiveness of uterine defense mechanisms, stress of lactation, and incomplete regeneration of the endometrium. Sows bred after weaning at 7 days of lactation suffer high embryonic losses between days 9 and 20 of pregnancy.

Nutrition of the Dam. Caloric intake and specific nutritional deficiencies affect ovulation rate and fertilization rate, as well as cause prenatal death. In swine, high caloric intake or continuous unlimited feeding increases ovulation rate, thereby increasing the incidence of embryonic mortality before implantation. However, following implantation, fetal death is decreased by unlimited feeding. In sheep, full feeding before breeding also increases ovulation rate as well as embryonic death. Poor body condition of ewes at mating increases the incidence of embryonic mortality, whereas moderate feed restriction from day 20 to 100 of pregnancy is less likely to reduce lambing percentages. Undernutrition affects twin ovulators more than single ovulators because both embryos are lost in the former, while a single embryo survives in the latter. Thus, more twin than single ovulating ewes are barren. In the mare, the critical period for embryonic resorption is between 25 and 31 days after ovulation. No resorption occurs if mares are maintained on an adequate plane of nutrition until 35 days after service.

An amino acid (mimosine) extracted from the pasture legume *(Leucaena leucocephala)* caused both a lowered ovarian response to gonadotrophins and an increase in embryonic death.

Several common plants possess estrogenic activity, e.g., barley grain *(Hordeum vulgare)*, oat grain *(Avena sativa)*, the fruits of the apple *(Pyrus malus)* and cherry *(Prunus avium)*, the tuber of the potato *(Solanum tuberosum)*, and Bengal gram *(Cicer arietinum)*.

Age of Dam. A higher incidence of embryonic mortality is observed in gilts and in sows after the fifth gestation. In the ewe, the incidence of late embryonic loss is higher in ewe lambs and ewes over 6 years than it is in mature ewes which is due to factors associated with the embryo rather than the uterine environment.

Overcrowding in Utero. Because the degree of placental development is primarily influenced by the availability of space and vascular supply within the uterus, increasing the number of implantations decreases the vascular supply to each site and restricts placental development. This results in a high embryonic and fetal death rate and probably explains the higher incidence of embryonic mortality in cattle and sheep following twin rather than single ovulations. It should be noted, however, that uterine capacity does not limit the ability of the cow and ewe to carry twins, provided they are located in separate uterine horns.

In cattle and sheep with multiple ovulations, the number of embryos surviving is reduced to a fairly constant number ($2\frac{1}{2}$ to 3 embryos per female) within the first 3 or 4 weeks of pregnancy, which implies that embryonic loss increases as the number of ova shed increases. Mortality does not seem to be due to a deficiency of progesterone. In prolific breeds of sheep, late embryonic deaths occur in ewes with more than five ovulations.

Thermal Stress. Embryonic mortality increases in a number of species following exposure of the mother to elevated ambient temperatures, especially in tropical areas. In early stages of development, the embryo is directly affected by increased maternal body temperature as a result of thermal stress. The pig embryo is most susceptible to heat stress during the first 2 weeks of gestation, particularly during implantation. A greater incidence of embryonic deaths was noted among gilts exposed to high temperatures 8 to 16 days postbreeding than among those exposed during 0 to 8 days postbreeding.

The effects of thermal stress on the early embryo are not apparent until the later stages of its development. Fertilized eggs of sheep and cattle, when subjected to high temperatures either *in vitro* or *in vivo*, are damaged but continue to develop, only to die during the critical stages of implantation. Reduced fertility of summer heat-stressed dairy cows may result from decreased viability and developmental capacity of 6- to 8-day-old embryos (Monty and Racowsky, 1987; Putney et al., 1988) and may account for the well-documented seasonal reduction in the efficiency of artificial insemination (AI) during summer. Heat stress between days 8 and 17 of pregnancy may also alter the uterine environment as well as growth and secretory activity of the conceptus (Geisert et al., 1988).

Semen. A portion of all embryonic deaths is attributable to the male and the mating system. Genetic factors that are transmitted by the male to the embryo may be inherited, may arise from testicular tissue, or may occur in spermatozoa after they are released from the testis. The inherited genotype of the male may include a variety of genetic factors that lead to incompatibility and early embryonic loss. There may be incompatibility between spermatozoa and mother, between spermatozoa and egg, or between zygote and mother. Infertile matings by highly fertile bulls are primarily due to embryonic mortality, while those of bulls with low fertility are due to fertilization failure and embryonic deaths. In swine, semen stored for 3 days before insemination produced zygotes much more susceptible to early embryonic death, presumably owing to the reduced DNA content in aged spermatozoa.

Incompatibility. Immunologic incompatibilities may block fertilization (prezygotic selection), or cause embryonic, fetal, or neonatal death. In cattle, homozygosity for certain blood groups and certain substances related to transferrin (β-globulin) and J-antigen in sera are associated with increased embryonic loss as well as decreased fertilization rate.

Repeat Breeders

"Repeat-breeder" females return to service repeatedly after being bred to a fertile male. A repeat-breeder cow exhibits normal signs of estrus every 18 to 24 days but requires more than three services to become pregnant. Most embryonic losses occur at a much earlier time than previously believed. Embryos collected nonsurgically from repeat-breeder cows revealed that most embryonic abnormalities occur in the oviduct but are not apparent until about 6 to 7 days postservice or the blastocyst stage (Linares et al., 1980).

Both fertilization failure and embryonic deaths occur at a much higher rate than in normal cows 5 to 6 weeks postinsemination. The cause for loss of approximately 50% of the embryos during the first 3 weeks of pregnancy in repeat-breeder cows is obscure, although several factors have been suspected (Fig. 11–6).

The incidence of repeat-breeding is higher in dairy herds using artificial insemination rather than natural service. Errors in estrus detection may also contribute to repeat returns to service in dairy cows (O'Farrel et al., 1983). Embryonic mortality decreases with increasing parity up to the fifth pregnancy, then increases. Recent evidence suggests that the early development of bovine embryos is impaired in the uterine environment of repeat-breeder heifers (Albihn et al., 1989). The higher incidence of embryonic mortality in old cows may be due to a defective uterine environment. Repeat-breeding may also be due to numerical chromosomal abnormalities (refer to Chapter 13).

Repeat-breeding that is due to early embryonic mortality occurs in mares affected by contagious equine metritis. This contagious venereal disease is caused by *Taylorella equigenitalis* and is transmitted by carrier stallions.

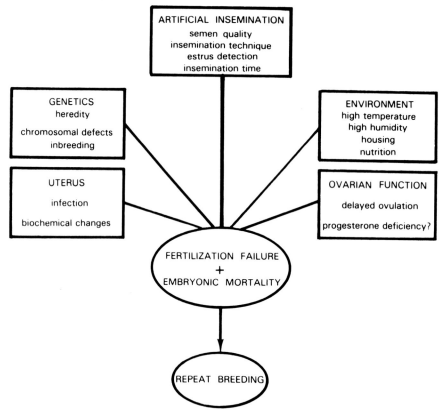

FIG. 11–6.　Causes of repeat-breeding in the cow.

Abortion

Abortion is termination of pregnancy with the expulsion of a fetus of recognizable size before it is viable, which is arbitrarily defined as 260 days for cattle, 290 days for horses, and 110 days for swine. Fetal death is not an essential prelude to abortion.

Abortions may be *spontaneous* or *induced, infectious* or *noninfectious.* Spontaneous abortion is more prevalent in cattle, particularly dairy cattle, than in sheep and horses. Noninfectious causes of spontaneous abortion may be genetic, chromosomal, hormonal, or nutritional factors (Table 11–5). Spontaneous abortion may also occur in animals bred immediately after puberty or immediately after parturition. Mares seem to be endocrinologically susceptible to abortion between the fifth and tenth months of pregnancy.

At least 90% of the human conceptuses that are chromosomally abnormal at fertilization will be lost spontaneously before 20 weeks gestation. Over two fifths of the cytogenetic abnormalities are associated with the presence of one extra chromosome (trisomy). Chromosomal abnormalities are known to cause embryonic losses in swine (see Chapter 13), but their importance in abortion in farm animals is unknown. A cytogenetic survey of aborted fetuses, stillbirths/neonatal deaths, and congenital defects in various domestic animals revealed an overall incidence of 8.7% chromosome anomalies, particularly mosaicism. Neither trisomy nor polyploidy were found (Berepubo and Long, 1983). Abortions are occasionally induced with high doses of estrogens, $PGF_{2\alpha}$, or glucocorticoids, particularly in young females

TABLE 11-5. Noninfectious Causes of Abortion in Farm Animals

Causes	Cow	Mare	Sow	Ewe or Doe
Chemicals, drugs, and poisonous plants	Nitrates Chlorinfated naphthalenes Arsenic Perennial broomweeds Pine needles	None	DicoumarinAlfatoxin Wood preservatives Creosote Pentachlorophenols	Lead, nitrate, locoweeds, lupines, sweet clover, onion grass, veratrum
Hormonal	High doses of estrogens, glucocorticoids, $PGF_{2\alpha}$ Progesterone deficiency	High doses of estrogens or cortisone (?)	High doses of estrogens or $PGF_{2\alpha}$	High doses of estrogens, cortisol or ACTH, $PGF_{2\alpha}$ Progesterone deficiency
Nutritional	Starvation, malnutrition Deficiencies of vitamin A or iodine	Reduced energy intake	Deficiencies of vitamin A, iron, and calcium	Lack of TDN or energy, deficiencies of vitamin A, copper, iodine and selenium
Genetic or chromosomal	Embryonic mortality Fetal anomalies	Fetal anomalies	Embryonic mortality Congenital or genetic lethal defects	Lethal genetic defects
Physical	Douching or insemination of pregnant uterus, stress (transport, fever, surgery)	Manual dilatation of cervix, natural service during pregnancy (?), rectal palpation of the very young blastodermic vesicle	Stress (transportation, fighting, injury) heat stress	Severe physical stress
Miscellaneous	Twinning, allergies, anaphylaxis	Twinning	Poor management	Twinning (?)

ACTH = adrenocorticotrophic hormone; $PGF_{2\alpha}$ = prostaglandin $F_{2\alpha}$; TDN = total digestive nutrients.

bred at an early age and in meat-producing animals.

Twin pregnancy is the most common cause of abortion in mares; over two thirds of twin pregnancies terminate in abortions. The inability of a mare to successfully carry twin fetuses to term may be related to placental insufficiency arising from competition between the placentae. This may lead to the death of one fetus and eventually to the abortion of both fetuses.

In the past, habitual abortions at 3 to $4\frac{1}{2}$ months of gestation in Angora goats were attributed to a hereditary defect of the anterior pituitary gland. These abortions are associated with two different syndromes (Wentzel, 1982). The first of these syndromes is related to nutritional stress. The hypoglycemia that occurs in the doe and fetus activates the fetal hypothalamic–pituitary axis and alters placental endocrine function. $PGF_{2\alpha}$, released by the placenta, causes the regression of the corpus luteum of pregnancy and expulsion of one or more recently dead fetuses. These losses may be reduced by improving the nutritional status of the does. The other syndrome, resulting from hyperactivity of the maternal adrenal cortex, leads to an excessive accumulation of fetal fluids over a prolonged period. The aborted fetus shows varying degrees of decomposition.

Abortion Caused by Infections. Several infectious agents that cause epidemics of abortion or a substantial number of abortions are described in the text. Other agents that are associated sporadically with abortion are listed in Table 11–6. The clinical signs, diagnosis and control of various reproductive infections that cause abortion are reviewed extensively by Kendrick and Howarth (1980).

Epizootic Bovine Abortion

Epizootic bovine abortion (EBA, foothill abortion) refers to a well-defined clinical condition that occurs principally in the foothills and mountain areas surrounding the Central Valleys of California. It occurs most commonly in beef cattle because these animals are most frequently pastured in the endemic areas. The highest incidence is in heifers, but older animals moved into endemic areas for the first time may subsequently abort. Usually a cow aborts only once, makes a complete recovery, and fertility is normal in subsequent gestations. The abortion rate may exceed 80% when large numbers of animals are exposed for the first time.

The cause is suspected to be a virus. The disease can be experimentally produced by feeding the tick *Ornithodoros coriaceus* on susceptible cattle during the second trimester of gestation.

Clinical Signs. Most abortions occur in the last third of pregnancy, and because most abortions are in beef cattle that are on a seasonal breeding program, there is a seasonal incidence of abortion. The mechanism for abortion under these circumstances is probably stress, which causes adrenal cortical hyperplasia, which in turn releases cortical hormones to initiate parturition.

No vaccine is available because the causative agent has not been identified. Adjusting the calving season so that the middle trimester of pregnancy does not coincide with the tick season has reduced the incidence of abortion. Animals that have experienced the disease will not abort again, and these should be maintained in the herd. There is no evidence that this disease spreads from cow to cow.

Equine Rhinopneumonitis (Viral Abortion, Equine Herpesvirus I Infection)

The equine herpesvirus I infection is primarily a disease of the upper respiratory tract. The horse first experiences exposure to this virus as a foal in the fall near weaning time. This epizootic disease in foals produces a massive exposure of mares that are in midpregnancy.

Abortion usually occurs after the eighth month of pregnancy and, because of seasonal breeding, most abortions occur between January and April. By far the most frequent cause of epizootics of abortion in

TABLE 11–6.   Causes of Sporadic Abortion

Cattle	Sheep	Horses	Swine
Parainfluenza$_3$ virus	Tick-borne fever	Equine viral arteritis	Foot and mouth disease
Bluetongue virus	Wesselsbron virus	Equine infectious anemia	Picorna viruses
Malignant catarrhal	Rift Valley fever	Dourine	Influenza
fever	Nairobi sheep disease	Piroplasmosis	Japanese B virus
Bovine viral diarrhea	Rinderpest		Hemagglutinating virus
Infectious bovine	Foot and mouth disease		African swine fever
rhinotracheitis	*Coxiella burnetti* (Q fever)		
Foot and mouth disease			
Rinderpest			
Tick-borne fever			
Bovine petechial fever			
Anaplasmosis			
Piroplasmosis			
Trypanosomiasis			
Toxoplasmosis			
Globidiosis			

(Kendrick and Howarth, 1980).

mares is the equine herpesvirus I, and this infection should be suspected until otherwise eliminated. Abortion from this infection rarely occurs in successive years, and in the absence of other control methods, it may not occur in a single band of mares for several years. Immunization is the best method of prevention.

Enzootic Abortion of Ewes

Enzootic abortion of ewes (EAE) occurs in many parts of the world and has been diagnosed in the western United States. The rate of abortion in a newly infected flock may be as high as 30%. In flocks experiencing a reinfection, the rate is less than 5%. Ewes abort during the last month of pregnancy. Abortions continue until normal lambing time, and some fetuses are expelled alive at term but are diseased. The causative agent of EAE is a member of the *Chlamydia* group. This disease must be differentiated from vibriosis.

Diagnosis of EAE depends on finding the elementary bodies of the infectious agent in smears from the cotyledon or from placental exudate. The disease produces immunity. A single infection produces life-time immunity, and the disease can be prevented by vaccination.

Fetal Mummification

Fetal mummification is characterized by fetal death, failure of abortion, resorption of placental fluids, dehydration of the fetus and its membranes, and involution of the uterus. It is more common in cattle and swine than in sheep and horses. The syndrome occurs mainly from the fifth to seventh months of gestation in all breeds of cattle. Affected cows conceive normally in the subsequent breeding period. Occasionally, bovine mummified fetuses are aborted spontaneously, but in most cases they are carried many months beyond the gestation period.

The mummification syndrome occurs in numerous pedigreed cows and in consecutive generations of cows bred to unrelated males. A high incidence of fetal mummification in the Jersey and Guernsey breeds also tends to support a hereditary influence. Twin-bearing ewes may abort a mummified fetus during late gestation and maintain the other lamb to full term, or they may deliver a mummified fetus attached to the placenta of a viable offspring.

Swine embryos that die in the first 6 weeks of gestation are completely resorbed. The fetuses that die during later stages are retained and expelled as mummified fetuses along with normal piglets at farrowing. Mummified fetuses are more prevalent in large than in small litters, in older sows than in gilts, and in some breeds than in others.

Mummification may be due to interference with the fetal blood supply, deficiency in placentation, anomalies in the umbilical cord of the fetus, or infection in the gravid uterus. Viruses causing stillbirths (S), mummification (M), embryonic death (ED) and infertility (I) in swine are termed *SMEDI viruses.* These viruses are an important cause of mummification in susceptible gilts and young sows. Transplacental infection leads to the establishment of the virus in one or two fetuses. These affected fetuses subsequently die after the infection has been transmitted to adjacent fetuses, which also die later.

The retention of a mummified fetus within the uterus could be due to a fetal influence on the endometrium, through suppression of the uterine luteolytic mechanism, causing persistence of the corpus luteum.

PERINATAL AND NEONATAL MORTALITY

Perinatal mortality refers to death of the offspring shortly before, during, or within the first 48 to 72 hours of life at normal term. Perinatal mortality, which includes stillbirths (born dead), accounts for most of the losses between birth and weaning. The extent of perinatal losses ranges from 5 to 15% in cattle and horses to 20 to 30% in sheep and pigs (Randall, 1984). Most losses occur within 72 hours of birth. Asphyxia, starvation, chilling, and congenital malformations are major contributing factors (Fig. 11–7). Species differences exist in the relative importance of these stresses. For example, trauma during prolonged or assisted birth occurs more frequently in cattle than in pigs, whereas asphyxiation may be more likely to occur in the pig as a result of premature rupture of the umbilical cord.

The use of drugs to induce parturition might adversely affect neonatal survival. For example, induction of parturition in the sow with $PGF_{2\alpha}$ before day 111 of gestation and in the cow with corticosteroids before day 265 of gestation may result in a higher incidence of perinatal mortality.

Stillborn piglets resemble live littermates, but their lungs do not float in water. One to two piglets in approximately one third of all litters are dead at birth with advancing parity, in extremes of litter size, and in litters in which the gestation period is less than 110 days. Two types of stillbirth occur in swine. In the first type, which is usually due to infectious causes, fetuses die prepartum, whereas in the second type, which is due to noninfectious causes, piglets die during parturition. The presence of meconium on the skin, in the mouth, and in the trachea of the piglet differentiates the latter from the former. A high incidence of piglet death is observed with uterine inertia, with prolongation of farrowing time or of the interval between births of piglets, in litters that contain less than four or more than nine piglets, and among piglets in the last third of the litter. These intrapartum deaths may be due to the low tolerance of piglets to anoxia and are usually associated with rupture of the umbilical cord prior to delivery. Since piglets suffer irreversible brain damage within 5 minutes after umbilical rupture or impeded umbilical flow, delivery must be completed rapidly.

In sheep, most losses between implantation and weaning occur during the perinatal period, as a result of starvation of the neonate, dystocia among lambs born to maiden ewes, ewes on poor pasture, or ewes with "clover disease."

Neonatal mortality—death of the neonate during the first few weeks of life—is related to heredity, environmental factors, nutrition, and infection. Several nutritional deficiencies may contribute to neonatal mortality (Table 11–7).

Respiratory distress syndrome (RDS) is characterized by a failure of the fetal lungs

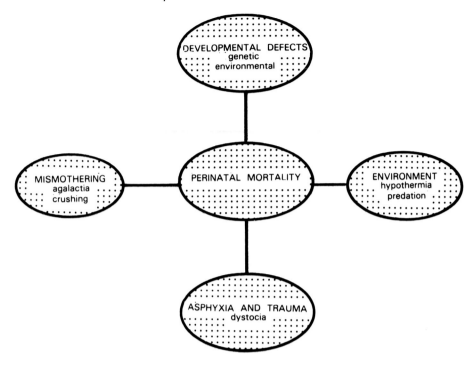

FIG. 11–7.   Factors affecting perinatal mortality.

TABLE 11–7.   **Neonatal Mortality That Is Due to Nutritional Deficiencies**

Disease	Species	Cause	Description
"White muscle" disease	Lambs and calves	Selenium deficiency	Acute and chronic forms, degeneration of cardiac and skeletal muscles, death
Hypomagnesemia	Milkfed calves	Decrease in serum Mg^{++}	Irritability, nervousness and tetany
Piglet anemia	Baby pigs during first week	Iron deficiency	Low hemoglobin levels in blood, weakness and prostration, inability to nurse
Goiter	Foals and lambs	Iodine deficiency	Enlargement of thyroids
Enzootic ataxia	Lambs	Copper deficiency	Locomotor incoordination leading to paralysis
Neonatal hypoglycemia	Newborn piglets	Low blood glucose	Loss of appetite, coma

to produce surfactant necessary to maintain the stability of the terminal air spaces of the lung after birth. RDS occurs in premature human infants and is invariably fatal. It has been reported in foals, calves, and piglets. Calves delivered by cesarian section near term or born before day 270 of gestation frequently develop RDS (Eigenmann et al., 1984). RDS in calves, as in the human infant, is caused by a deficiency of a surfactant (phospholipid), and its diagnosis is based on levels in the amniotic fluid of two phospholipids—lecithin and sphingomyelin.

Neonatal mortality may also be a result of long labor, poor maternal nutrition, weakness of the mother or the young, bacterial infection of the young through the umbilical cord, poor maternal behavior, or delayed onset of lactation. Exposure of the newborn pig to low environmental temperature leads to hypothermia, hypoglycemia, and death. Heat prostration and some deaths occur in newborn lambs exposed to high environmental temperature. Another source of danger to the neonate is the presence of mammalian or avian predators, such as the feral pig *(Suis scrofa)*, fox *(Vulpes vulpes)*, dingo *(Canis dingo)*, raven *(Corvus coronoides)*, wedge-tailed eagle *(Aquila audax)*, and sea eagle *(Haliaetus leucogaster)*.

DISORDERS OF GESTATION, PARTURITION, AND PUERPERIUM

Dystocia

Dystocia, difficult or obstructed parturition, may be due to fetal, maternal, or mechanical causes (Figs. 11–8 and 11–9).

Fetal Dystocia. This results from abnormalities in the presentation or position of the fetus and from postural irregularities of its head or limbs; it may be due to a relatively or absolutely oversized fetus,

and to fetal monstrosities. Fetal dystocia in common in certain breeds of dairy cattle, in cattle and sheep with multiple pregnancies, and in sows with small litters. Deviations of the head and flexion of the various joints in anterior presentation, flexion of both hindlimbs (breech) in posterior presentation, or twins may cause dystocia.

Maternal Dystocia. It is more frequent in dairy cattle and sheep than in horses and swine. It occurs frequently in primiparous animals and in animals with multiple young. The absence of uterine contractions or inertia may be primary or secondary. Primary uterine inertia that is due to excessive stretching is common in multiple pregnancy in cattle and in large litters in swine. Secondary uterine inertia is due to exhaustion of the uterine muscle secondary to obstructive dystocia. Failure of the cervix to dilate properly leads to "spasm" of the cervix in cattle.

Fetopelvic Disproportion. This is a disparity between the size of the fetus and the size of the pelvis of the dam. Fetopel-

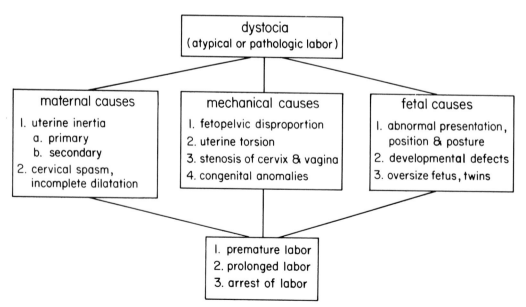

FIG. 11–8.   Schematic representation of maternal and fetal causes that lead to various forms of dystocia. Fetomaternal mechanical causes; abnormal fetal presentation, position, and posture; and maternal causes may lead to premature labor, prolonged labor, and arrest of labor.

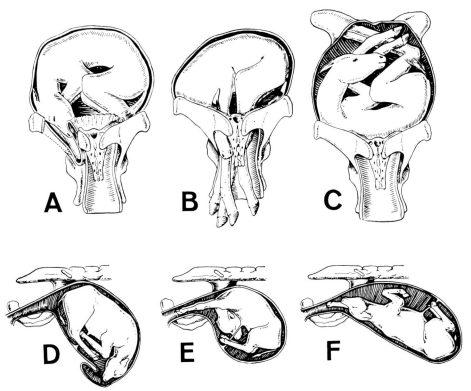

FIG. 11-9.   Malpresentation in horses *(A, B, C)* and cattle *(D, E, F)*. *A*, Ventrotransverse presentation with ventral displacement of the uterus. *B*, Ventrotransverse presentation; uterine body gestation. *(A, B* and *C* from Arthur (1964). Wright's Veterinary Obstetrics. London, Bailliere, Tindall & Cow. *D, E,* and *F* redrawn from U.S.D.A., Special Report (1942). Diseases of Cattle.)

vic disproportion is a common cause of dystocia in cows, ewes carrying single lambs, and sows with small litter size. It is uncommon in the mare. Anomalies of the soft parts of the reproductive passages or the bony pelvis are occasional causes of dystocia. One group of anomalies causes narrowing of the birth canal (e.g., abnormalities or fractures of the pelvis and stenosis or obstruction of the cervix, vagina or vulva), while another group of abnormalities prevents entry of the fetus into the birth passages (e.g., failure of the cervix to dilate or torsion of the uterus).

Fetopelvic disproportion accounts for about 30% of all bovine dystocia. The factors that contribute to fetopelvic disproportion are small pelvic area of the dam and large size of the calf. Dystocia that is due to fetopelvic disproportion may be reduced by matings planned to avoid disproportionately large calves in cows with small pelvic areas. Other measures include mating heifers by weight rather than age, reducing birth weights by using bulls of the same breed or a different breed known to sire smaller calves or selecting dams that have the ability to limit birth weight. Calving difficulty affects the future reproductive performance in cattle by increasing days open, days to first breeding, and number of services.

Retained Placenta

Retained placenta, or a failure of the fetal membranes to be expelled during the third stage of labor, is a common postpartum complication in ruminants, particularly in cattle. Retention of the placenta beyond 12 hours in cattle is considered pathologic and is primarily due to either uterine inertia or an inflammation of the placenta, which in turn results in a failure of the fetal villi to detach themselves from the maternal crypts (Arthur et al., 1982). Retained fetal membranes invariably accompany abortions in late gestation due to infections such as brucellosis, leptospirosis, and infectious bovine rhinotracheitis, premature births associated with twinning, and induced parturition with corticosteroids, obstructive dystocia, and cesarian operation.

Retained placenta occurs more frequently in dairy than beef breeds. Factors such as poor hygiene or the stresses affecting the dairy cow at time of calving, particularly "loose" type of housing, have been implicated. Since retained placenta leads to an infection of the uterus (metritis) and a delay in the involution of the uterus, the future fertility of the animal could be adversely affected. Controversy exists between removal and the more conservative method of leaving the fetal membranes *in situ*. Bolinder et al. (1988) reported that manual removal caused an immediate and large but short-lived increase in prostaglandin $PGF_{2\alpha}$ metabolite, which was probably due to the physical damage of uterine tissue. Manual removal also prolonged the interval from calving to first functional corpus luteum by 20 days. The mechanisms and therapy for retained fetal membranes in the cow have been extensively reviewed by Paisley et al. (1986).

Retention of the placenta in other ruminants such as buffaloes, sheep, or goats is less common than in cattle. In the mare, retention of placenta is thought to be a serious problem because it often leads to laminitis. It is usually treated by oxytocin injections with manual removal if it is not expelled by 24 hours after foaling.

Hydramnios and Hydrallantois

Hydramnios, the excessive accumulation of amniotic fluid, is less common than hydrallantois, the accumulation of allantoic fluid. Hydramnios, observed more often in cattle than sheep or swine, is associated with certain cranial abnormalities of the fetus. In these defective fetuses, swallowing is impaired, causing amniotic fluid to accumulate as gestation progresses. Fetuses of the Guernsey and Jersey breeds in prolonged gestation have hydramnios.

Hydrallantois occurs in cattle, especially in twin pregnancies, and it is characterized externally by an enormous enlargement of the abdomen after the sixth month of gestation. The syndrome has been attributed to fetal–maternal incompatibility and placental dysfunction. It has also been reported in horses after the seventh month of gestation and was associated with fetal abnormalities.

Multiple Pregnancy

In cattle, horses, sheep, and goats, the frequency of multiple pregnancies is higher than that of multiple births, owing to the high incidence of abortion and fetal resorption. In the cow, the sequelae of twinning include shortened gestation period, abortion, stillbirth, dystocia, and retained placenta. Economic losses are related to decreased fertility, neonatal mortality, decrease in birth weights of calves, longer calving intervals, and lower butter fat production. In addition, over 90% of the females born co-twin to a male are sterile (freemartins). Neonatal mortality in sheep is greater among twins than among singles. Ewes carrying twins are more susceptible to pregnancy toxemia (twin-lamb disease). In mares, a high percentage of twin fetuses are aborted.

Prolonged Gestation

Abnormally long gestations that are due to fetal abnormalities in cattle, sheep, and swine result from genetic and nongenetic factors.

There are two types of the syndrome in cattle, and each is governed by a single autosomal recessive gene. In the type seen in Holstein and Ayrshire breeds, the large fetuses have no facial abnormalities, and when delivered surgically, they are weak,

TABLE 11–8. Disorders of Gestation, Parturition, and Puerperium

Syndrome	Species	Causes	Description
Retained placenta	Cattle, buffalo, sheep, goat, horse, and pig	Dystocia, infections	Failure to expel placenta after parturition
Vaginal prolapse	Cattle and sheep	Excessive relaxation of pelvic ligaments, restricted exercise, twinning	Late gestation
Uterine prolapse	Cattle and sheep	Dystocia, placental retention	Follows parturition
Hydrops of fetal membranes	Cattle, sheep, and horses	Fetal anomalies, placental dysfunction, fetal–maternal incompatibility	Excessive accumulation of fluids within the amniotic or allantoic cavity
Twinning	Cattle, sheep, and horses	Spontaneous or induced	Abortion
Prolonged gestation	Cattle	Genetic and fetal abnormalities	Fetal death
	Sheep	Ingestion of teratogens in early pregnancy	Fetal death
	Swine	Genetic, in certain inbred lines	Fetal death
Respiratory distress syndrome	Calves, foals, and piglets	Deficiency of lung surfactant (phospholipid)	Failure of the fetal lungs to expand at birth

unable to nurse, and die in 6 to 8 hours from severe hypoglycemia. There is hypoplasia of the adenohypophysis and the adrenal cortex. The plasma progesterone level in a cow carrying an affected calf does not fall before parturition as it does in a normal cow. In the second type of syndrome, seen in the Guernsey and Jersey breeds, the fetuses are small, many exhibit facial abnormalities and hydramnios, they lack an adenohypophysis, and survive *in utero* for long periods past term but live for only a few minutes when delivered surgically. A summary of disorders of gestation and parturition appears in Table 11-8.

Uterine Infections

Postpartum uterine infections occur commonly in the cow and mare as sequela to retention of the fetal membranes and dystocia. *Endometritis* is the inflammation of the endometrium, whereas *metritis* involves the entire thickness of the uterus. *Pyometra* is the accumulation of purulent exudate within the uterus.

Most uterine infections affect the dairy cow, and of several bacteria that have been implicated, *Actinomyces pyogenes* is the most frequently encountered organism in the cow. $PGF_{2\alpha}$ is released in postpartum cows with either normal puerperium or with uterine infections, but higher levels persist for a longer period in cows with uterine infections. Apparently, bacterial infection and toxins stimulate the uterus to secrete abnormally higher levels of prostaglandins (Fredriksson et al., 1988), which delay the onset of cyclicity until the infection is cleared and the prostaglandin levels are low. Another possibility is that uterine infection may delay the initiation of folliculogenesis and suppress the rate of follicular growth in dairy cows during the early puerperium (Peter and Bosu, 1988) by inhibiting LH release. The inhibition is believed to be due to endotoxins produced by gram-negative bacteria in the postpartum uterus of the cow.

Ovarian activity during the early postpartum period exerts an important influence on the ability of the uterus to resist or eliminate bacterial infections. Both mare and cow can resist uterine infection during the estrogenic phase but are very susceptible during the progesterone phase, which is due to decreased leukocytic activity. If cows with uterine infection resume cyclicity relatively early in the postpartum period, pyometra is likely to occur when elevated levels of progesterone coincide with the presence of high numbers of pathogenic bacteria. Therefore, the practice of injecting cows with GnRH to induce cyclicity early in the postpartum period should be avoided, as it could lead to pyometra.

REFERENCES

Adams, N.R. (1990). Permanent infertility in ewes exposed to plant oestrogens. Aust. Vet. J. *67*, 197.

Albihn, A., Gustafsson, H., Rodriguez-Martinez, H. and Larsson, K. (1989). Development of day 7 bovine demi-embryos transferred into virgin and repeat-breeder heifers. Anim. Reprod. Sci. *21*, 161.

Armstrong, D.T. (1986). Environmental stress and ovarian function. Biol. Reprod. *34*, 29.

Arthur, G.H., Noakes, D.E. and Pearson, H. (1982). Veterinary Reproduction and Obstetrics. 5th Ed. London, Bailliere Tindall.

Ball, B.A., and Woods, G.L. (1987). Embryonic loss and early pregnancy loss in the mare. Compend. Cont. Ed. Pract. Vet. *9*, 459.

Berepubo, N.A. and Long, S.E. (1983). A study of the relationship between chromosome anomalies and reproductive wastage in domestic animals. Theriogenology *20*, 177.

Bolinder, A., Seguin, B., Kindahl, H., Bouley, D. and Otterby, D. (1988). Retained fetal membranes in cows: manual removal versus nonremoval and its effect on reproductive performance. Theriogenology *30*, 45.

Bosu, W.T.K. and Peter, A.T. (1987). Evidence for a role of intrauterine infections in the pathogenesis of cystic ovaries in postpartum dairy cows. Theriogenology *28*, 725.

Britt, J.H., Szarek, V.E. and Levis, D.G. (1983). Characterization of summer infertility of sows in large confinement units. Theriogenology *20*, 133.

Butler, W.R. and Smith, R.D. (1989). Interrelationships between energy balance and postpartum reproduction. J. Dairy Sci. *72*, 767.

Carruthers, T.D., Convey, E.M., Kesner, J.S., Hafs, H.D. and Cheng, K.W. (1980). The hypothalomopituitary gonadotropic axis of suckled and non-suckled dairy cows postpartum. J. Anim. Sci. *51,* 949.

Echternkkamp, S.E., Ferrel, C.L. and Rone, J.D. (1982). Influence of pre- and postpartum nutrition on LH secretion in suckled postpartum beef heifers. Theriogenology *18,* 283.

Eigenmann, U.J.E., Schoon, H.A., Jahn, D. and Grunert, E. (1984). Neonatal respiratory syndrome in the calf. Vet. Rec. *114,* 141.

Erb, N.H. and White, M.E. (1981). Incidence rates of cystic follicles in Holstein cows according to 15-day and 30-day postpartum intervals. Cornell Vet. *71,* 326.

Fredriksson, G., Kindahl, H., Alentus, S., Carlsson, U., Cort, N., Edqvist, L.-E. and Uggla, A. (1988). Uterine infections and impaired reproductive performance mediated through prostaglandin release. Proc. 11th Int. Congr. Animal Reprod. & AI, Vol. V, 81, Dublin, Ireland.

Geisert, R.D., Zavy, M.T. and Biggers, G.G. (1988). Effect of heat stress of conceptus and uterine secretion in the bovine. Theriogenology *29,* 1075.

Hurley, W.L., Edgerton, L.A., Olds, D. and Hemken, R.W. (1982). Estrous behavior and endocrine status of dairy heifers with varied intakes of phosphorus. J. Dairy Sci. *65,* 1976.

Kendrick, J.W. and Howarth, J.A. (1980). Reproductive infections. *In* Reproduction in Farm Animals. E.S.E. Hafez (ed.). Philadelphia, Lea & Febiger.

Kesler, D.J. and Garverick, H.A. (1982). Ovarian cysts in dairy cattle: a review. J. Anim. Sci. *55,* 1147.

Kirk, J.H., Huffman, M. and Lane, M. (1982). Bovine cystic ovarian disease: hereditary relationships and case study. J. Am. Vet. Med. Ass. *181,* 474.

Lamming, G.E., Wathes, D.C. and Peters, A.R. (1981). Endocrine patterns of the post-partum cow. J. Reprod. Fertil. Suppl. *30,* 155.

Linares, T., King, W.A. and Ploen, L. (1980). Observations on the early development of embryos from repeat breeder heifers. Nordisk Veterinaermedicin. *32,* 433.

Monty, D.E. Jr., Racowsky, C. (1987). In vitro evaluation of early embryo viability and development in summer heat-stressed, superovulated dairy cows. Theriogenology *28,* 451.

O'Farrel, K.J., Langley, O.H., Hartigan, P.J. and Sreenan, J.M. (1983). Fertilization and embryonic survival rates in dairy cows culled as repeat breeders. Vet. Rec. *112,* 95.

Paisley, L.G., Mickelsen, W.D. and Anderson, P.B. (1986). Mechanisms and therapy for retained fetal membranes and uterine infections of cows: a review. Theriogenology *25,* 353.

Peter, A.T. and Bosu, W.T.K. (1988). Relationship of uterine infections and folliculogenesis in dairy cows during early puerperium. Theriogenology *30,* 1045.

Peters, A.R. and Lamming, G.E. (1990). Lactational anoestrus in farm animals. *In* Oxford Reviews of Reproductive Biology, Vol. 12. S.R. (ed.). New York, Oxford University Press.

Pieterse, M.C., and Taverne, M.A.M. (1986). Hydrometra in goats: diagnosis with real-time ultrasound and treatment with prostaglandins or oxytocin. Theriogenology *26,* 813.

Putney, D.J., Drost, M. and Thatcher, W.W. (1988). Embryonic development in superovulated dairy cattle exposed to elevated ambient temperatures between days 1 to 7 post insemination. Theriogenology *30,* 195.

Randall, G.C.B. (1984). Perinatal adaptation. Proc. Int. Congr. Animal Reprod. & AI, Vol. IV, V-43. Urbana-Champaign, IL.

Randel, R.D. (1981). Effect of once-daily suckling on postpartum interval and cow-calf performance of first-calf Brahman × Hereford heifers. J. Anim. Sci. *53,* 755.

Shelton, K., Gayerie De Abreu, M.F., Hunter, M.G., Parkinson, T.J. and Lamming, G.E. (1990). Luteal inadequacy during the early luteal phase of subfertile cows. J. Reprod. Fertil. *90,* 1.

Sreenan, J.M. and Diskin, M.G. (1986). The extent and timing of embryonic mortality in the cow. *In* Embryonic Mortality in Farm Animals. J.M. Sreenan and M.J. Diskin (eds.). Boston, Martinus Nijhoff.

Taverne, M.A.M., Lavoir, M.C., Bevers, M.M., Pieterse, M.C. and Dieleman, S.J. (1988). Peripheral plasma prolactin and progesterone levels in pseudopregnant goats during Bromocryptine treatment. Theriogenology *30,* 777.

Troxel, T.R., Cmarik, G.F., Ott, R.S., Lock, T.F. and Kesler, D.J. (1983). The effect of method of GnRH and short-term calf removal on ovarian function and reproductive performance in postpartum suckled beef cows administered PGF$_{2\alpha}$ for estrous synchronization. Theriogenology *20,* 417.

Wagner, W.C. and Li, P.S. (1982). Influence of adrenal corticosteroids on pituitary and ovarian function. *In* Factors Influencing Fertility in the Post-Partum Cow. H. Karg and E. Schallenberger (eds.). The Hague, Martinus Nijhoff.

Walters, D.L., Burrel, W.C. and Wiltbank, J.N. (1984). Influence of calf removal on reproductive performance of anestrous beef cows. Theriogenology *21,* 395.

Wentzel, D. (1982). Noninfectious abortion in Angora goats. Proc. 3rd Int. Conf. on Goat Production and Diseases. Tucson, AZ.

Wettemann, R.P., Bazer, F.W., Thatcher, W.W. and Hoagland, T.A. (1984). Environmental influences on embryonic mortality. Proc. 10th Int. Congr. Animal Reprod. & AI, Vol. IV, XIII-26. Urbana-Champaign, IL.

Whisnant, C.S., Kiser, T.E., Thompson, F.N., and
   Barb, C.N. (1986). Influence of calf removal on
   the serum luteinizing hormone response to nal-
   oxone in the postpartum beef cow. J. Anim. Sci.
   62, 1340.

Wrathal, A.E. (1980). Pathology of the ovary and
   ovarian disorders in the sow. Proc. 9th Int.
   Congr. Animal Reprod. & AI, Vol. I, 223. Madrid,
   Spain.

12
Reproductive Failure in Males

M.R. JAINUDEEN AND E.S.E. HAFEZ

The fertility of a male is related to several phenomena: (1) sperm production; (2) viability and fertilizing capacity of the ejaculated sperm; (3) sexual desire; and (4) the ability to mate. The sterile male is readily identified, but the male with reduced fertility poses serious problems and causes economic losses to breeders and the artificial insemination (AI) industry. The purpose of this chapter is to review the functional aspects of male reproductive failure (Fig. 12–1). Genetic factors and chromosomal abnormalities associated with male reproductive failure are discussed in Chapter 13.

CONGENITAL MALFORMATIONS

Segmental Aplasia of the Wolffian Ducts. In this defect, small or large segments of one or both wolffian ducts (e.g., epididymis, vas deferens, or ampulla) are missing. Males with unilateral tubal deficiencies or occlusions often have normal fertility, but those with the bilateral condition are sterile. It is more common among the offspring of certain bulls that also exhibit this condition. It is characterized in cattle by a total or partial absence of one or both epididymides, but more often the right epididymis. Segmental aplasia of the epididymis is commonly associated with a localized accumulation of spermatozoa within an occluded epididymis, which is known as a *spermatocele*.

Cryptorchidism. The descent of the testes involves the abdominal migration to the internal inguinal ring, passage through the inguinal canal, and finally migration within the scrotum. In cryptorchidism, one testis or both testes fail to descend from the abdominal cavity into the scrotum.

Testicular descent in mammals results from swelling and subsequent regression of the gubernaculum. Early in this process, the gubernaculum extends from the caudal pole of the testis to the external inguinal ring. Traction that develops from swelling of the extra-abdominal portion of the gubernaculum draws the testis into the inguinal canal. Subsequent regression of the gubernaculum enables the testis to descend further into the scrotal position. Abnormal gubernacular development has been associated with cryptorchidism in swine.

The incidence of cryptorchidism is higher in swine and horses than in other farm animals. It is probably a hereditary defect transmitted by the male; it is dominant in the horse and recessive in other species. One or both testes may be located in the abdominal cavity or, more commonly, in the inguinal canal. The left testis is affected more often than the right testis in large type of horses, whereas either testis may be affected with approximately equal frequency in ponies. The rarity of cryptorchidism in older horses might be because some inguinal testis descend into the scrotum with advancing age.

Bilaterally cryptorchid animals are sterile owing to thermal suppression of spermatogenesis, whereas unilaterally cryptorchid animals have normal spermatogenesis in the scrotal testis. Unilaterally

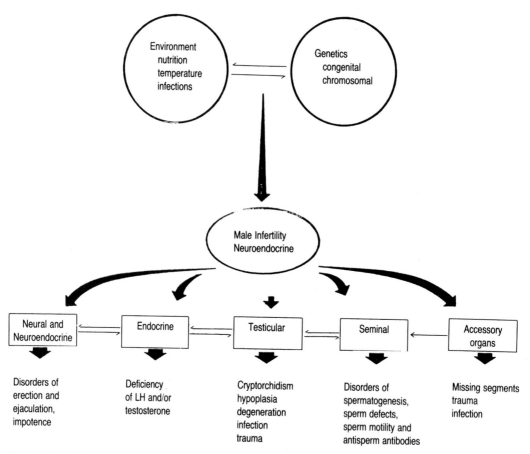

FIG. 12–1.   The various causes of reproductive failure in male farm animals.

cryptorchid animals are usually fertile but have reduced sperm concentrations; they display normal secondary sexual characteristics because their testes secrete testosterone at nearly normal levels because of elevated levels of LH.

The steroidogenic function of the cryptorchid testis is controversial. The cryptorchid testis has a lower ability than the normal scrotal testis in the ram and bull to secrete testosterone in response to exogenous gonadotropin. On the contrary, steroid production *in vitro* by Leydig cells was similar for both the abdominal and the contralateral scrotal testes in unilateral cryptorchid boars and stallions (Ryan and Raeside, 1984).

Despite the ability of a unilaterally cryptorchid male to reproduce, it should not be used for breeding because the trait can be transmitted to its offspring.

Testicular Hypoplasia. Hypoplasia of the testes, a congenital defect in which the potential for development of the spermatogenic epithelium is lacking, occurs in all farm animals, particularly in bulls of several breeds.

Inherited testicular hypoplasia is best known in Swedish Highland cattle and is caused by a recessive autosomal gene with incomplete (about 50%) penetrance. Testicular hypoplasia also occurs in other breeds of cattle, but a genetic basis has not been well documented, although a familial distribution has been noted (Galloway and Norman, 1976). Testicular hypoplasia also occurs in *Bos indicus,* particularly the Brahman and Brahman crossbred bulls.

Testicular hypoplasia is suspected only at puberty or later because of reduced fertility or sterility. One or both testes may be hypoplastic. In sterile bulls, the semen is watery and contains few or no spermatozoa. In less severe forms, semen, libido and the ability to serve are not affected, but sperm numbers may be reduced. Histologically, the seminiferous tubules are characterized by a lack of germinal elements, predominance of Sertoli cells, and a failure of spermatogenesis.

A hypoplastic testis is reduced in size. Although severe cases of testicular hypoplasia may be diagnosed by scrotal and testicular measurements, the less obvious cases are difficult to diagnose. Karyotype analysis may aid diagnosis, since a high incidence of chromosomal secondary constrictions is present in leukocyte cultures from the blood of bulls with testicular hypoplasia (Galloway and Norman, 1976).

As in the bull, testicular hypoplasia in boars and rams is characterized by small testes and semen with low sperm concentration (boar) or with a high percentage of abnormal spermatozoa (ram).

EJACULATORY DISTURBANCES

Ejaculatory disturbances are of two types: lack of sex drive or libido and failure to copulate, which encompasses disturbances in erection, mounting, intromission, or ejaculation.

Lack of Libido

Libido or sexual desire is an important aspect of male reproductive function. Lack of libido (*impotentia coeundi*) may be hereditary or may originate from psychogenic disturbances, endocrine imbalance, or environmental factors. Even though seminal characteristics may be satisfactory, fertility may be adversely affected as a result of poor libido.

Bull. Both libido and mating ability in bulls are influenced by genetic factors. Libido was found to be similar between monozygotic twin bulls under different managerial and nutritional systems. Lack of sexual desire is more frequent in some strains and breeds of cattle than in others, e.g., beef breeds and *Bos indicus* cattle.

Some bulls become apprehensive about sudden changes in the environment, such as changing the farm, the barn, the herdsman or the locality of semen collection. Since fear and apprehension are inimical to sexual expression, the intensity of sexual behavior declines until the bull becomes accustomed to the new situation. Inhibition may develop as a result of repeated frustration, faulty management, wrong techniques during semen collection, distraction during coitus, and too-rapid withdrawal of the teaser animal after copulation. Inhibition is characterized by refusal to copulate, incomplete erection, or incomplete ejaculation.

Bulls exhibit considerable differences in semen characteristics and libido. There is no association between libido and semen quality or scrotal circumference. Good quality semen can be collected with an electroejaculator from low libido bulls, but the method should not be used in AI programs because of the likelihood of disseminating genes associated with low libido. Poor libido is believed to be due to a deficiency in circulating androgens, but in Holstein bulls, the concentration of circulating testosterone is unrelated to libido or semen characteristics.

Stallion. Abnormal mating behavior in stallions is most often due to mismanagement at time of breeding. Overuse, rough treatment at service, or too-frequent ejaculation during winter may exert a detrimental effect on the behavior of young stallions. Pain resulting from injury at copulation or associated with mounting attempts is also a common cause of impotence. Seasonal variations in libido and the secretory and gametogenic activity of the stallion reproductive tract are mediated, at least in part, by the pattern of testosterone secretion. The greatest sperm output in stallions occurs during July, 2 months after the seasonal peak in plasma testosterone levels.

Rams. Despite the production of normal numbers of fertile sperm, rams may have low fertility because of their inability to breed sufficient numbers of ewes. This low-service frequency results from a lack of libido, poor dexterity, or interference from other rams.

Seasonal factors, such as daylight and temperature, influence the sexual performance of rams of different breeds under a wide variety of both natural and controlled experimental conditions. A decline in the hours of light generally appears to favor enhanced sexual performance, but evidence of such a relationship is conflicting. Ram fertility is also adversely affected during periods of high temperature.

Boar. Low libido in the boar is associated with obesity, heat stress, or too-high a plane of nutrition. Libido also may be seriously impaired by mismanagement of young boars during service.

Inability to Copulate

Physical disabilities may impede or prevent mating by causing failure in copulatory behavior, i.e., mounting, intromission, or ejaculation.

Failure to Mount. Inability to mount is a common disorder encountered in older bulls and boars. It is associated with locomotor dysfunction arising from dislocations, fractures, sprains, and osteoarthritic lesions of the hindlimbs and vertebrae. Degenerative changes in the articular surface of the stifle and hock joints and exostoses of the thoracolumbar vertebrae interfere with mobility and ability to mount, particularly in older bulls.

Failure to Achieve Intromission. This is a condition in which the penis fails to enter the vagina. It may result from insufficient protrusion of the penis from the sheath or deviation of the penis.

Phimosis, or stenosis of the preputial orifice that is due to congenital, traumatic, or infectious causes, may prevent the normal protrusion of the penis. The pendulous prolapse that occurs in *Bos indicus* breeds (Santa Gertrudis and Brahman), or the inherent tendency to preputial eversion that occurs in some polled *Bos taurus* breeds (Hereford and Aberdeen Angus), may lead to trauma, inflammatory changes, and eventually to preputial prolapse and phimosis (Fig. 12–2). At service, affected bulls are unable to protrude the penis more than 2 or 3 inches or even through the preputial orifice in more severe cases. The condition may be corrected by surgical amputation of the prolapsed preputial mucosa. Selective breeding and culling of *B. taurus* bulls with a predisposition to preputial prolapse may help to reduce the incidence.

Another serious cause of inability to protrude the penis is hematoma of the penis as a result of rupture of the corpus cavernosum of the penis (Fig. 12–2). It commonly occurs in bulls during coitus when the penis is thrust against the perineum of the cow. A hematoma develops distal to the sigmoid flexure, although some may be found proximally, and causes swelling, which may be palpated anterior to the scrotum.

Abnormal venous drainage of the corpus cavernosum in the bull could result in a penis too flaccid for intromission despite good libido. This is because erection in the bull is not, as commonly believed, due to the rigidity of the fibroelastic components of the penis and relaxation of the retractor penis muscle but mainly to the high pressures generated within the corpus cavernosum penis. This abnormality in the bull appears to be congenital, although it may be due to trauma of the tunica albuginea in older bulls (Ashdown et al., 1979).

Tumors of the glans penis may occasionally prevent protrusion of the penis. Fibropapillomas of viral origin are frequently noted on the glans penis of 2-year-old bulls. Affected bulls are reluctant to serve or are incapable of achieving intromission. Although spontaneous regression of the tumor can occur, surgical extirpation or vaccination with a tissue vaccine is employed to control the condition.

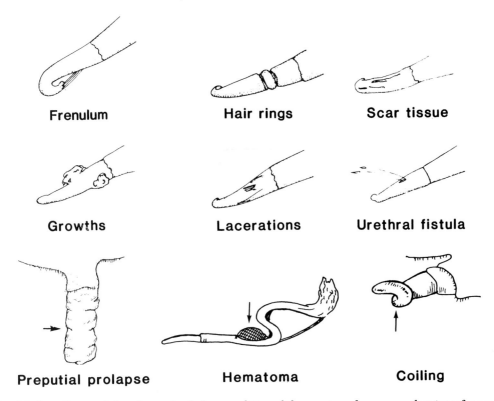

Fig. 12–2. Congenital and acquired abnormalities of the penis and prepuce that interfere with intromission in the bull and cause low conception rates. (Upper two rows redrawn from Sorensen, A.M. (1979). *In* Animal Reproduction: Principles and Practice. New York, McGraw-Hill.)

Congenital deformities of the penis or prepuce may render intromission difficult or impossible. One such deformity is the persistence of the frenulum commonly encountered in beef Shorthorn and Aberdeen Angus bulls (Fig. 12–2). In this condition, the frenulum attaches the ventral aspect of the glans penis to the preputial mucosa. At coitus, the deformity is noted as a ventral or downward deviation of the penis. Rarely, intromission may be accomplished. The deformity can be corrected by ligating and cutting the band of tissue. Three distinct types of congenital deviations of the penis are encountered in bulls. A spiral deviation of the penis occurs in most normal bulls after intromission. A similar spiralling occurs with the "corkscrew" type of penile deviation (Fig. 12–2), where the spiralling precedes intromission and prevents coitus. Less common

types of deviations of the penis are the ventral or "rainbow" deviation and the mild S-shaped deviation.

In the boar, abnormalities of the penis, e.g., persistent frenulum, penile hypoplasia, and enlargement of the preputial diverticulum, frequently result in a failure to achieve intromission and are the major causes of poor mating performance. With these defects, the boar is unable to erect his penis, to penetrate the vagina, or to lock it in the cervix.

Failure to Ejaculate. This condition is occasionally observed with bulls even when accompanied by vigorous thrust at intromission. Poor semen collection techniques, e.g., improper temperature or pressure within the artificial vagina, often cause failure of ejaculation in bulls used for AI purposes.

In the stallion, ejaculatory disorders, ranging from intromission without ejaculation to an abnormal copulatory pattern with or without occasional ejaculation, are frequently encountered. These disorders are probably caused by a functional disturbance of the nervous mechanisms that regulate the ejaculatory process. Unfamiliar surroundings, obesity, poor condition, or exhaustion resulting from frequent services may exert a detrimental effect on these nervous mechanisms.

FERTILIZATION FAILURE

Fertilization failure is an important cause of infertility in males that have normal libido and are capable of mating and ejaculating. This capacity or reduced capacity is related to defective semen characteristics or to errors in breeding techniques.

Diseases of Testes and Accessory Glands

Pathologic conditions of the testes, epididymis, and seminal vesicles (Table 12–1) may interfere with fertilization by disturbing spermatogenesis or sperm maturation, causing abnormal semen characteristics, or preventing the passage of spermatozoa from the testes to the urethra.

Heat Stress

Temperature is one of the important environmental factors modifying reproduction. Elevated body temperatures, during periods of high ambient temperature or pyrexia from disease, lead to testicular degeneration and reduce the percentage of normal and fertile spermatozoa in the ejaculate.

In several species, there are seasonal variations in the quality and fertility of semen. Bulls subjected to high environmental temperatures have reduced semen quality. Rams may retain a satisfactory level of fertility throughout the whole year, but in many instances, fertility is depressed when matings occur during the hot months of the year. Conception failure in ewes mated to heat-stressed rams is related more to failure of fertilization than to embryonic mortality.

When the scrotal contents of rams are heated to approximately 40°C for 1½ to 2 hours, a sharp increase in the proportion of morphologically abnormal spermatozoa occurs in the ejaculate 14 to 16 days later. Spermatozoa that are developing in the testis at the time of heating showed damage (e.g., dead and tailless spermatozoa), whereas epididymal spermatozoa are unaffected. Acrosomal damage is characterized by swelling, vesiculation, and eventual disintegration.

Seasonal variations occur in the fertility of boars, and levels are lowest immediately after the hottest months of the year. Volume of semen and total sperm per ejaculation from boars are greater during cool weather. Boars exposed to elevated ambient temperatures daily for 90 days show decreases in sperm concentration and motility, and increases in sperm abnormalities and acrosomal changes.

Exposure of boars for periods of 4 to 5 days to ambient temperatures above 35°C and to the diurnal variations prevailing in subtropical and tropical regions affects their semen quality but not semen volume. The adverse effects are evident 3 to 5 weeks later, particularly on sperm morphology (Cameron and Blackshaw, 1980). The high incidence of cytoplasmic droplets may be caused by the long-term effect of elevated ambient temperatures on the epididymis which, because of its unique location in the scrotum in the pig, is most sensitive to temperature (Stone, 1981).

Also, infectious diseases resulting in a febrile reaction are likely to affect the subsequent fertility of the boar for a 5- to 6-week period. The decrease in conception rate in artificially inseminated gilts maintained under elevated environmental temperatures is apparently due to embryonic mortality.

TABLE 12–1. Summary of Diseases of Male Reproductive Organs with Infertile Semen

Disease	Species Affected	Causes	Lesion	Seminal Changes
Testicular degeneration	Bull, ram	Thermal, localized or systemic infections; nutrition (vitamin A); vascular lesions; aging; obstructive lesions of the head of epididymis; noxious agents; hormonal factors	Testicular size reduced; fibrosis; disturbances in spermatogenesis; seminiferous tubules destroyed in advanced cases	Increase in immature and abnormal sperm with normal motility; later ejaculate is thin and watery due to reduction in sperm concentration; giant cells; azoospermia or necrozoospermia in severe cases
Orchitis	Bull, ram, boar	Brucellosis, tuberculosis	Inflammatory changes in testis leading to degeneration of seminiferous tubules	Asthenozoospermia; oligozoospermia; teratozoospermia; giant cells; erythrocytes and leukocytes; normal semen volume
Epididymitis	Bull, ram	Brucellosis; viral infections	Inflammation of epididymis; infiltration of lymphocytes and neutrophils; dead sperm and giant cells	Poor semen characteristics; semen contaminated by inflammatory exudate
Seminal vesiculitis	Bull	Brucellosis	Unilateral inflammation of seminal vesicles; glands enlarged and fibrosed	Purulent exudate in semen, normozoospermia, asthenozoospermia; lowered fructose content

(Adapted from R. Jubb and K. Kennedy (1970). Pathology of Domestic Animals. New York, Academic Press; Laing (1970). Fertility and Infertility in Domestic Animals. London, Bailliere Tindall and Cassell)

Breeding Techniques

Fertilization failure attributed to the male may result from poor breeding management or from faulty techniques in AI. Also, synchronization of estrus in cattle and sheep with progestational compounds, the ingestion of estrogenic pasture grass by sheep, or the imposition of stress during insemination may interfere with sperm transport and cause fertilization failure.

Breeding Management. Under natural mating programs, the frequency of service and the ratio of females assigned to each breeding male depend on the species, age, libido, fertility, and nutrition of the male; the duration of the mating season; the system of management; and the size of pasture or range.

Spermatogenesis is a continuous process, but frequent and repeated ejaculations adversely affect male libido and semen characteristics. Although libido returns to normal after a week of sexual rest, semen characteristics are not restored to normal for 6 weeks. Similarly, after a period of prolonged inactivity, semen characteristics and fertility remain low for the first few services.

Seasonal variations are especially important in seasonally breeding species such as stallions and rams; changes in the ratio of daylight to darkness are reflected in the quality and quantity of semen.

Infertility and Artificial Insemination. The male makes several contributions to reproductive failure in an AI program, e.g., defective semen, improper insemination techniques, or failure of sperm transport in the female tract. These and other factors affecting fertility in AI are considered in another chapter. Changes in the fertility of frozen semen during storage are important in the efficient use and design of AI programs.

Immunologic Factors

The ability of spermatozoa to induce antibodies has been recognized since the beginning of this century. Despite unsuccessful attempts to use immunity to spermatozoa as a method of male contraception, there is sufficient evidence to implicate sperm antibodies as a cause of human reproductive failure (Jones, 1980; Bronson et al., 1984). In contrast, relatively little is known or understood about immunologic infertility in domestic animals.

The antigenic components of semen originate in the testis, epididymis, vas deferens, and accessory glands. They can be broadly classified as those in the seminal plasma and those that are sperm bound. Spermatozoa carry a mixture of antigens, including sperm-specific antigens, histocompatibility antigens (i.e., those responsible for the rejection of tissue grafts), blood-group antigens, and other somatic tissue antigens. Sperm antigens may be antigenic within the male (autoantigens) or the female (isoantigens) reproductive system. Of the sperm antigens, those on the surface of the plasma membrane are probably responsible for the reproductive failure. To be effective, antibodies against spermatozoa must enter the seminal fluid or the cervical mucus following deposition in the female tract.

An autoimmune response is normally prevented by the relative isolation of the seminiferous tubules from the rest of the body—*blood–testis barrier.* If the barrier is breached, antisperm antibodies are produced that might attack sperm. Experimental allergic orchitis is an organ-specific autoimmune syndrome produced in experimental animals, such as the guinea pig, by the injection of autologous or homologous testis or sperm with Freund's complete adjuvant, which potentiates the immune response (Jones, 1980). The testicular damage results in germinal cell destruction and azoospermia (complete absence of sperm in the ejaculate) in the immunized animals. Similar treatment resulted in sperm agglutinins in bulls, but only one showed significant changes in semen characteristics (Wright, 1980). Autoantibodies against spermatozoa have been reported in the serum of infertile men. Antisperm antibodies are also found in the serum and seminal fluid of bulls, but there is no association between their presence and the classification of bulls as satisfactory or unsatisfactory potential breeders (Purswell et al., 1983).

Antisperm antibodies can prevent fertilization by immobilizing sperm, impairing sperm penetration of cervical mucus, inactivating acrosomal enzymes presumed essential for fertilization, inhibiting the attachment of spermatozoa to the zona pellucida or interfering with embryonic mortality (Menge, 1980). These effects of antibodies have been shown experimentally with isoimmunization of females of several species, including cattle, with sperm or sperm "plasma membrane" preparations. Rabbits inseminated with semen treated with antiserum against a sperm membrane autoantigen experienced a decrease in fertility as a result of the inability of the sperm to penetrate the zona pellucida (O'Rand, 1981). However, this effect may have been due to more than one mechanism because immune sera could have contained antibodies against different sperm antigens. This problem has been overcome with the development of monoclonal antibodies against sperm surface components of several laboratory species and man. Two such monoclonal antibodies showed a significant inhibition of postfertilization fertility in the rabbit (Naz et al., 1983).

Sperm antibodies have been implicated as a cause of repeat-breeding in cattle, but there was no evidence to indicate that antisperm antibodies were responsible for the reduced fertility in a group of repeat-breeder cows (Farhani et al., 1981).

Egg-yolk and milk used in semen extenders may also act as antigens. Antibodies against egg-yolk antigens have been detected in uterine mucus and tissue from cows that had been inseminated repeatedly (Griffin et al., 1971). When cows were inseminated with extenders containing egg-yolk, the fertility rate was lower in cows showing uterine titers to egg-yolk antigens than in cows not showing uterine titers.

NUTRITION AND MALE INFERTILITY

The effects of nutritional restrictions on fertility are more notable in the female than in the male. Nutritional deficiencies delay the onset of puberty and depress production and characteristics of semen in the male. The young and growing animal is much more susceptible to nutritional stress than the mature animal. In addition, nutrition affects the endocrine rather than the spermatogenic function of the testis. Common nutritional factors include caloric, protein, and vitamin deficiencies, but minerals or toxic agents may also be important.

Underfeeding. Despite the ability of a mature male to maintain sperm production and testosterone secretion under low levels of nutrition, the young male shows retarded sexual development and delayed puberty. This is due to suppression of endocrine activity of the testes and consequently to retardation of growth and secretory function of the male organs of reproduction. When mature bulls, rams, and boars are fed low-energy rations for prolonged periods, libido and testosterone production are affected much earlier than semen characteristics. The effects of undernutrition may be corrected in mature animals, whereas it is less successful in young animals because of the permanent damage caused to the germinal epithelium of the testis.

Obesity and overfeeding reduce libido and sexual activity in rams, boars, and bulls, particularly during hot weather.

Protein deficiency affects the young more than the mature male. Young bulls on a protein-deficient diet show decreases in libido and semen characteristics, whereas mature bulls, rams, and boars are rarely affected. Diets high in protein are not essential for optimal sperm production in the ram.

Vitamin Deficiencies. Dietary vitamin A or carotene deficiency leads to testicular degeneration in all farm animals. The effect of vitamin A on the testes is probably indirect and due to suppression of the release of pituitary gonadotropins. Injections of gonadotropic hormones or vitamin A will restore spermatogenesis, except in cases in which the damage to the testis is permanent. While bull calves maintained on a low vitamin A diet show degenerative changes in the germinal epithelium of the testis and azoospermia, mature bulls show no adverse effects in spermatogenesis.

Cattle are more resistant to vitamin A deficiency than swine. For example, night-blindness and incoordination of movement precede recognizable reduction in fertility of mature bulls, whereas testicular degeneration is one of the earliest signs of avitaminosis A in the mature boar. Vitamin E (tocopherol or wheat germ oil) is important for normal reproduction, but its role in the fertility of male farm animals is obscure.

Mineral Deficiencies. There is a paucity of information concerning the effects of trace mineral deficiencies on male reproductive functions. Iodine deficiency has been suspected as a cause of poor libido and semen characteristics in bulls. Also, improvement in sperm production and fertility have been noted following supplementary feeding of copper, cobalt, zinc, and manganese.

Toxic Agent. Plant estrogens exert adverse effects on male accessory organs, but infertility of sheep and cattle grazing on estrogenic pastures are related to changes in cervical mucus and to a failure of sperm transport in the female tract. Many chemicals, rare earth salts, and ionizing radiations interfere with spermatogenesis in a variety of mammalian species, but their contribution to male infertility remains to be established.

INFERTILITY AND CHROMOSOMAL ABERRATIONS

Chromosomal aberrations play an important role in human reproductive failure. From a breeding point of view, it is important to eliminate males that are affected by chromosomal aberrations, particularly those resulting in decreased fertility (Chapter 13).

REFERENCES

Ashdown, R.R., David, J.S.E. and Gibbs, C. (1979). Impotence in the bull: (1) Abnormal venous drainage of the corpus cavernosum penis. Vet. Rec. *104*, 423.

Bronson, R., Cooper, G. and Rosenfeld, D. (1984). Sperm antibodies: their role in infertility. Fertil. and Steril. *42*, 171.

Cameron, R.D.A. and Blackshaw, A.W. (1980). The effect of elevated ambient temperature on spermatogenesis in the boar. J. Reprod. Fertil. *59*, 173.

Farhani, J.K., Tompkins, W. and Wagner, W.C. (1981). Reproductive status of cows and incidence of antisperm antibodies. Theriogenology *15*, 605.

Galloway, D.B. and Norman, J.R. (1976). Testicular hypoplasia and autosomal secondary constrictions in bulls. 8th Internat. Congr. Animal Reprod. AI. Vol. IV, 710.

Griffin, J.F.T., Nunn, W.R. and Hartigan, P.J. (1971). An immune response to egg-yolk semen diluent in dairy cows. J. Reprod. Fertil. *25*, 193.

Jones, W.R. (1980). Immunological factors in male and female infertility. *In* Immunological Aspects of Reproduction and Fertility Control. J.P. Hearn (ed.). Lancaster, MTP Press.

Menge, A.C. (1980). Clinical immunologic infertility: diagnostic measures, incidence of antisperm antibodies, fertility and mechanisms. *In* Immunological Aspects of Infertility and Fertility Regulation. D. Dhindsa and G.F.B. Schumacher (eds.). New York, Elsevier North Holland.

Naz, R.K., Saxe, J.M. and Menge, C. (1983). Inhibition of fertility in rabbits by monoclonal antibodies against sperm. Biol. Reprod. *28*, 249.

O'Rand, M.G. (1981). Inhibition of fertility and sperm-zona binding an antiserum to the rabbit sperm membrane autoantigen RSA-1. Biol. Reprod. *25*, 621.

Purswell, B.J., Dawe, D.L., Caudle, A.B., Williams, D.J. and Brown, J. (1983). Spermagglutinins in serum and seminal fluid of bulls and their relationship to fertility classification. Theriogenology *20*, 375–381.

Ryan, P.L. and Raeside, J.I. (1984). Steroid production in Leydig cells from cryptorchid boars and stallions. Proc. 10th Int. Congr. Animal Reprod. & AI. Vol. III, 277. Urbana-Champaign, IL.

Stone, B.A. (1981). Thermal characteristics of the testis and epididymis of the boar. J. Reprod. Fertil. *63*, 551.

Wright, P.J. (1980). Serum spermagglutinins and semen quality in the bull. Aust. Vet. J. *56*, 10.

13
Genetics of Reproductive Failure

M.R. JAINUDEEN AND E.S.E. HAFEZ

Several abnormalities of male and female reproduction are genetically determined, although the precise genetic mechanism is not well understood. Genetic disorders may be either inherited or caused by chromosomal aberrations, abnormal fertilization, and mutation. Because reference is made to genetic mechanisms throughout this chapter, a brief review of some basic genetic concepts precedes a description of the genetic factors that cause abnormalities in the structure and functions of the reproductive system.

BASIC GENETIC CONCEPTS

Chromosomes

Chromosomes in every mammalian cell occur in pairs (*diploid*) except in gametes in which only one member of each pair is present (*haploid*). Each member of a pair is similar in size, shape, and proportion to its partner (*homologous chromosomes*). The diploid number (2n) of chromosomes is constant in normal individuals within a species. One pair of chromosomes in each cell is known as the *sex chromosomes* (XX in the female and XY in the male), whereas the nonsex pairs are known as *autosomes*. The gametes are haploid and contain half the number of chromosomes (n) with the X chromosome in the female (*homogametic sex*) and either an X or Y chromosome in the male (*heterogametic sex*).

The chromosome constitution of an animal may be determined during metaphase in actively dividing cells such as blood lymphocytes or skin fibroblasts. The

chromosomes are photographed and systematically displayed (karyotype) for study of their number, size, and morphology. Individual chromosomes may be identified by staining with quinacrine (Q-banding) or with Giemsa (G-banding). Chromosomes may be metacentric, submetacentric, acrocentric, or telocentric (Fig. 13–1), depending on the position of the centromere and the relative lengths of the arms.

Genes

The genetic material carried by the chromosome is divided into basic units known as *genes*. Each gene determines one or more characteristics or traits. A trait, which is determined by a gene, is said to be inherited as an autosomal or sex-linked trait. In addition, a trait may be dominant or recessive. Autosomal dominant traits affect both males and females.

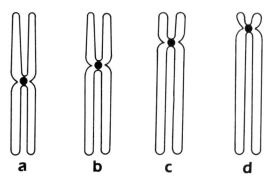

a   **b**   **c**   **d**

FIG. 13–1.   Chromosome types: *a*, metacentric; *b*, submetacentric; *c*, acrocentric; and *d*, telocentric.

They tend to vary considerably in their severity (expressivity) and rarely skip a generation (nonpenetrance). Autosomal recessive traits affect brothers and sisters (sibs), but parents are normal. Since no genes are found in the Y chromosomes, sex-linkage is synonymous with X-linkage. X-linked dominant traits are rare, whereas X-linked recessive disorders affect males but rarely females.

GENETIC MECHANISMS

Inherited Traits

Abnormalities of both structure and function of the reproductive system may be genetically determined. As most are the result of an interaction between environment and genotype, it is difficult to classify them strictly into inherited or acquired disorders. Breeding trials, e.g., daughter groups of sires under different environmental conditions, may be necessary to determine whether the defect is inherited or acquired. Most inherited abnormalities follow simple mendelian inheritance, a few are acquired as sex-linked, and others as polygenic traits.

Chromosomal Aberrations

Chromosomal aberrations may be divided into numerical and structural types (Table 13–1).

Numerical Aberrations. These arise from disturbances in the distribution of chromosomes or chromatids during meiosis or mitosis with the production of two types of individuals or cells, *euploid* and *aneuploid.* Euploids have chromosome numbers that are exact multiples of the haploid number (n) (Table 13–1). Polyploids are multiples higher than the diploid number and usually result from a failure of the cell to divide (cytokinesis) after the nucleus has divided (karyokinesis). Polyploidy may result from the fertilization of the ovum by more than one spermatozoa (polyandry) or from an ovum that failed to extrude the second polar body

(polygyny) by a single spermatozoa. Aging of gametes that is due to delayed fertilization may increase the incidence of polyploid embryos. True polyploids in animals appear to be lethal.

Aneuploids are individuals or cells having irregular chromosome numbers. They may be either *monosomic* $(2n - 1)$ or *trisomic* $(2n + 1)$. Aneuploid cells result from the failure of paired chromatids, usually one pair, to pass to opposite poles of the spindle at the anaphase of mitosis or meiosis. This is referred to as *nondisjunction,* resulting in trisomy in one cell and monosomy in the other. Occasionally, nondisjunction results from a failure of a chromatid, which moves slowly to the pole (anaphase lag), to be included in the nucleus of either daughter cell. In this situation, one daughter cell is a normal diploid and the other is a monosomic.

An animal that possesses two or more cell populations may either be a *mosaic* or a *chimera* (Table 13–1). Mosaicism or mixoploidy is commonly due to numerical differences and is usually due to nondisjunction at mitosis. A chimera results from a placental transfer or exchange of cells between dizygotic twins, particularly in cattle.

Structural Aberrations. These result from transverse breakage in one or more chromosomes with the subsequent reunion of the broken ends in such a way that the linear order of the genes is altered. These alterations may be brought about by the processes of deletion, inversion, and translocation (Fig. 13–2). The first two usually affect only single chromosomes, whereas translocations may involve one, two, or more chromosomes (Figs. 13–3 to 13–5).

A *deletion* is a structural change resulting in the breakage of a chromosome with a loss of genetic material. An *inversion* is a rearrangement of a chromosome so that the genes occur on the chromosome in an inverse order from their original sequence.

TABLE 13–1.   Definition of Common Types of Chromosomal Aberrations

Type of Aberration	Definition	Example	Animals
Numerical	Loss of gain of chromosomes		
Aneuploid	Loss (monosomy, $2n-1$) or gain (trisomy, $2n+1$) of one member of a homologous pair of chromosomes	63,XO	Mare
Polyploid	Gain of one (triploid, 3n), or two (tetraploid, 4n) sets of homologous chromosomes	65,XXY	Stallion
Mosaic	An animal possessing two or more cell populations (different karyotypes) derived from one zygote	60,XX/60,XY	Bull
Chimera	An animal possessing two or more cell populations (different karyotypes) derived from two or more zygotes	60,XX/60,XY	Heifer
Structural	Exchange of genetic material between nonhomologous chromosomes		
Reciprocal translocation	Breaks in two chromosomes and exchange of segments	38,XYt(7q−;11q+)	Boar
Robertsonian translocation	Centric fusion of two acrocentric chromosomes resulting in a metacentric or submetracentric chromosome	59,XYt(1p;2q)	Bull
Tandem fusion	Translocation resulting in a large acrocentric chromosome		
Deletions	Structural changes resulting in breakage of a chromosome and loss of genetic material		

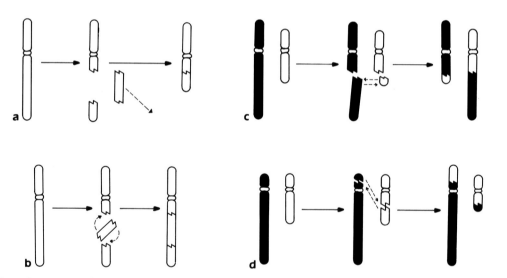

FIG. 13–2.   Development of structural aberrations of chromosomes: *a,* deletion; *b,* inversion; *c,* reciprocal translocation; and *d,* robertsonian translocation.

Translocation involves the simultaneous breakage of the arms of two nonhomologous chromosomes with exchange of the broken segments, forming two new chromosomes. Reciprocal translocations involve the mutual exchange of segments between two chromosomes. Robertsonian translocation or centric fusion is a type of reciprocal translocation that occurs between two acrocentric chromosomes.

Nomenclature. Chromosome abnormalities are stated (in order) by the num-

type	meiotic configuration during pairing of homologues	result

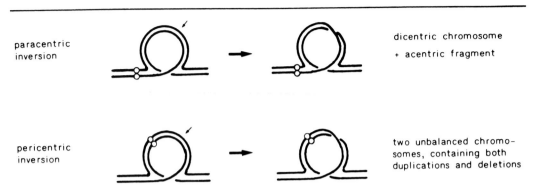

| paracentric inversion | | dicentric chromosome + acentric fragment |
| pericentric inversion | | two unbalanced chromosomes, containing both duplications and deletions |

FIG. 13–3. Examples of meiotic failures due to balanced chromosome aberrations. Failures resulting from paracentric and pericentric inversions. Simplified diagrams, only one chromatid of each chromosome, are shown. Since one of the homologues contains an inverted region, pairing with the normal homologue is feasible only by formation of a loop. If crossover takes place in this loop, various unbalanced chromosomes and dicentric and acentric fragments will be formed. The small arrow indicates the crossover point (Husslein et al., 1984).

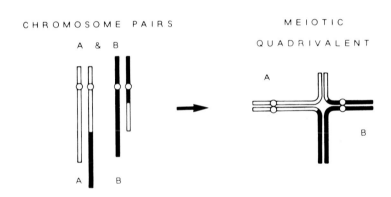

CHROMOSOME PAIRS

A & B

MEIOTIC

QUADRIVALENT

A

B

A   B

FIG. 13–4. Pairing of homologous chromosomes carrying reciprocal translocations during first meiotic division. Chromosome regions belonging to chromosome A are in white; those belonging to chromosome B are in black. Since all homologous regions tend to pair, a quadrivalent is formed during preparation for first meiotic division (Husslein, et al., 1984).

ber of chromosomes followed by the sex chromosome constitution and then the chromosomal aberration. The aberration is described using p and q for the short and long arms, respectively, of the chromosome; t is used for translocation (rep = reciprocal, rob = Robertsonian). The signs + and − are used to indicate loss of all or a portion of a chromosome. If it involves a whole chromosome, the sign is placed before the chromosome, whereas for a part of the chromosome it is placed after the chromosome (Table 13–1).

INHERITED ABNORMALITIES OF THE REPRODUCTIVE SYSTEM

Morphologic Defects

Morphologic defects of the reproductive system include cryptorchidism, gonadal hypoplasia, sperm defects, developmental abnormalities of the Mullerian ducts, and aplasia of the wolffian ducts (Table 13–2). Cryptorchidism occurs more frequently in boars and stallions than in other farm species. Bilateral cryptorchids

failure	diagram	result

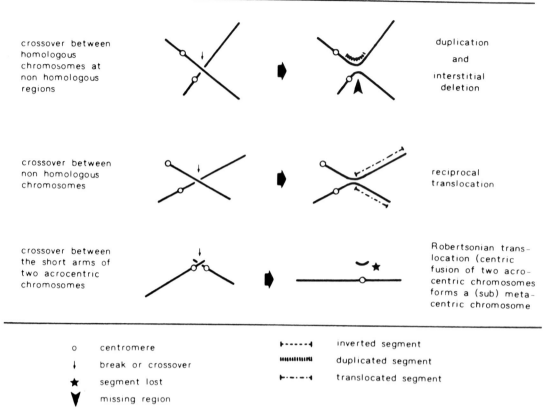

crossover between homologous chromosomes at non homologous regions — duplication and interstitial deletion

crossover between non homologous chromosomes — reciprocal translocation

crossover between the short arms of two acrocentric chromosomes — Robertsonian translocation (centric fusion of two acrocentric chromosomes forms a (sub) metacentric chromosome

o — centromere

↓ — break or crossover

★ — segment lost

▼ — missing region

▸-----◂ — inverted segment

⊪⊪⊪⊪⊪⊪ — duplicated segment

▸-·-·-◂ — translocated segment

FIG. 13–5. Origin of chromosome aberrations that are due to meiotic failures involving two chromosomes (either homologous or nonhomologous chromosomes). Duplication and interstitial deletions may result by crossover between homologous chromosomes at nonhomologous regions. The segment lost by one chromosome is inserted into the other homologous, resulting in duplication of the segment involved. Reciprocal translocation is due to exchange of chromosome segments between nonhomologous chromosomes after an irregular crossover event. In robertsonian translocation, two acrocentric chromosomes fuse by loss of the small short arms. Only one of the centromeres remains active (Husslein et al., 1984).

are sterile, whereas unilateral cryptorchids are fertile.

Swedish Highland cattle exhibit an inherited form of gonadal hypoplasia. Gonadal hypoplasia is a condition in which the testes or ovaries are totally or partially underdeveloped and lack germ cells. Affected bulls and cows are either sterile or have reduced fertility (Leipold et al., 1983).

Several structural defects of spermatozoa can cause sterility or subfertility of bulls (Table 13–3) by interfering with fertilization. Some of these sperm defects are inherited; however, the mode of inheritance is not clear because only a few animals and relatives of affected animals have been investigated. Development abnormalities of the mullerian duct system result in a structural barrier to fertilization in heifers, whereas aplasia of the wolffian duct in males may lead to sterility or infertility, depending on whether it is bilateral or unilateral.

TABLE 13–2. Some Inherited Abnormalities of Male and Female Reproductive Systems

Abnormality	Animals Affected	Mode of Inheritance	Reproductive Problem
Cryptorchidism	Boar	Sex-limited trait	Disturbance in spermatogenesis
	Stallion		
Gonadal hypoplasia	Bull	Recessive autosomal gene with incomplete penetrance	Sterility/infertility
	Cow		
Defects of müllerian duct system (white heifer disease)	Cow	Single recessive sex-limited gene for white coat	Sterility
Male pseudohermaphrodite	Goat	Dominant autosomal gene for hornlessness	Sterility
	Pig	Inherited (?)	Sterility
Sperm defects	Boar	Inherited (?)	Infertility
	Bull		
Cystic ovaries	Cow	Inherited (?)	Anestrus/nymphomania

TABLE 13–3. Some Inherited Sperm Defects Affecting Fertility of Cattle

Defect	Description of Defect	Fertility
Diadem effect	Nuclear pouch formation	Infertility
Knobbed sperm	Thickening of acrosome	Sterility
Decapitated	Ultrastructural abnormality in neck of sperm	Sterility
Sterilizing tail stump	Tail defect	Sterility
Dag defect	Strongly coiled main piece	Infertility
Pseudodroplet	Rounded or elongated thickening of midpiece	Sterility
Corkscrew	Tail defect	Infertility

Functional Disorders

Some functional disorders have a genetic predisposition. Susceptible animals develop the disorder only under certain environmental conditions, e.g., cystic ovaries and libido in cattle. Affected cows tend to produce a high proportion of daughters with the same condition. A sire effect has also been reported. In Sweden, the condition has been controlled by restricting the use of bulls with a high frequency of cystic ovaries among their daughters. Impotence in bulls may have a hereditary background because big differences exist between breeds in the frequency of impotence in Swedish bulls. These variations indicate that poor libido is largely conditioned by the genotype of the animal.

CHROMOSOMAL ABERRATIONS

Any chromosomal aberrations either transmitted in gametes or arising in embryos may result in phenotypic defects or may cause reproductive failure. Structural and numerical aberrations of either the sex chromosomes or the autosomes play an important role in reproductive failure in man and farm animals (Hare and Singh, 1979; Gustavsson, 1984). From a breeder's point of view, it is important to eliminate males that are affected by chromosomal aberrations, particularly those resulting in decreased fertility.

Congenital Malformations

Some malformations of the reproductive system present at birth (congenital) are caused by chromosomal aberrations, usually associated with the sex chromosomes.

Testicular Hypoplasia. Testicular hypoplasia associated with abnormal sex chromosome constitution (XXY) in man is known as Klinefelter's syndrome. The counterpart of this syndrome has been reported in infertile bulls, rams, and boars (Table 13–4).

Ovarian Hypoplasia. Monosomy of the X chromosome (XO) or Turner's syndrome in women occurs in mares. The condition is the result of nondisjunction during gametogenesis. The aneuploid zygote is formed when a normal ovum unites with a sperm that lacks either sex chromosome (Table 13–4). These mares (63,XO) are characterized by normal external genitalia, small stature, flaccid uterus, small inactive ovaries, complete absence of ovarian activity, and consequently, anestrus. It is an important cause of sterility in the mare (see Bruere, 1980). Mosaic mares (Table 13–4) have an erratic pattern of estrous cycles without ovulation; phenotypic females may have a history of anestrus or irregular estrous cycle activity. In general, they possess small uteri and small inactive ovaries devoid of follicular activity. Trisomy-X, associated with hypoplastic ovaries, has also been reported in mares with normal phenotypes and in the heifer.

Sterility and Infertility

Mosaicism (60 XX/60 XY) and chimerism (60 XX/60 XY) cause testicular hypoplasia in cattle and, depending on the severity of the condition, infertility or sterility. Chimeric bulls (Table 13–4) are born either as co-twin to heifers or as singletons, with the death of the female twin *in utero* (refer to the following section on freemartinism). The presence of XX germ cells in the testis of the bull twin does not lead to an excess of X-bearing spermatozoa, which would shift the sex ratio in favor of females (Long, 1979). Alternatively, these germ cells are nonviable and may result in infertility (Dunn et al., 1979).

Approximately 18% of repeat breeding heifers had numerical chromosomal abnormalities (Swartz and Vogt, 1983) that included tetraploid/diploid mosaics, chimeras, trisomy-X mosaics, and mixoploids (Table 13–4). Decreased fertility has been reported in heifers with Trisomy X and 1/29 translocation, in infertile heifers (Pinheiro et al., 1987), and in related cows heterozygous for the 1/29 chromosome translocation (Maurer and Vogt, 1988). These aberrations may be expected to cause infertility.

Translocations are of considerable interest in animal cytogenetics, since they are the most common forms of chromosomal rearrangements in farm animals (Bruere, 1980).

Prenatal Mortality

Chromosomal aberrations are important causes of most spontaneous abortions

TABLE 13–4. Reproductive Failure Associated with Chromosomal Aberrations

Reproductive Failure	Species	Chromosome Aberration	Karyotype
Testicular hypoplasia	Cattle	Trisomy-X	61,XXY
		Chimera	60,XX/XY
	Sheep	Trisomy-X	55,XXY
	Pig	Trisomy-X	39,XXY
Ovarian hypoplasia	Horse	Monosomy-X	63,XO
		Trisomy-X	65,XXX
		Mosaic	63,XO/64,XX
	Cattle	Trisomy-X	61,XXX
Repeat breeding	Cattle	Mosaic	60,XX/60,XY
		Mosaic	59,XO/60,XX
		Mixoploid	59,XO/60,XX/61,XXX
Infertility	Cattle	Robertsonian Translocation	59XY,t(1q;29q)
Embryonic mortality	Pig	Reciprocal Translocation	38,XY,t(7q−;11q+)
			38,XY,t(13q−;4q+)

(Data from Blue et al., 1978; Bongso et al., 1981; Bruere 1974; Chandley et al., 1975; Dunn et al., 1981; Gustavsson, 1984; Hancock and Daker, 1981; King et al., 1981; Norbert et al., 1976; Swartz and Vogt, 1983).

in women during the first trimester. Many of these chromosomal abnormalities include autosomal monosomies, triploidy, translocations (both reciprocal and robertsonian in one of the parents), inversions, and mosaics.

Chromosomal aberrations are related to embryonic mortality. Approximately 10% of pig blastocysts show chromosomal abnormalities such as triploidy and tetraploidy. A monosomy has been described in the pig (Gustavsson, 1984), which in many respects is similar to Turner's syndrome described in women in whom the genetic component is often lethal to the fetus and results in a spontaneous abortion. At least 14 reciprocal translocations have been recorded in the domestic pig (Gustavsson, 1984). Most of these are found in boars producing small litters. (Fig. 13–6).

In cattle, the 1/29 robertsonian translocation has been reported to increase the incidence of delayed returns to service (embryonic mortality) among the daughters of carrier bulls.

Intersexuality

An *intersex* is an animal with congenital malformations of sexual development that confuse the diagnosis of sex. Intersexes are broadly divided into three groups: true hermaphrodites, male and female pseudohermaphrodites, and freemartins, although some intersexes may fall into more than one group (Table 13–5).

True Hermaphrodites. These have various combinations of ovaries, testes, and ovotestes. There are varying degrees of bisexuality in the accessory sex organs, presumably depending on the hormone production by the embryonic gonad. True hermaphroditism occurs more frequently in pigs and goats than in cattle and horses. It would be expected that true hermaphrodites might be XX/XY mosaics. Some are, but the majority have a normal XX sex chromosome constitution.

Equine true hermaphrodites are rare. Two true hermaphrodites with chimerism had bilateral ovotestes, an underdeveloped penis, bilateral seminal vesicles, and uterine tissue (Table 13–5). Neither animal exhibited stallion-like behavior (Dunn et al., 1981). Probably the chimerism resulted from double fertilization or fusion of blastocysts, whereas the mosaicism resulted from a loss of a Y chromosome by anaphase lag in early embryonic XY cells.

Pseudohermaphrodites. In pseudohermaphrodites, there is a discrepancy between the external genitalia and the true gonadal sex. Thus, a male pseudohermaphrodite has testes but female external genitalia, whereas a female pseudohermaphrodite has ovaries and male external genitalia. Pseudohermaphrodites are more common than true hermaphrodites.

Male pseudohermaphrodites have undescended testes and varying combinations of male and female structures so that the external genitalia are often quite ambiguous. The sex chromosome complement may be XY or XX. As the development of the accessory genital organs depends on substances produced by the gonad, male pseudohermaphrodites could result from either a failure of normal production by the testes or from a lack of response to these substances by the target organs.

Testicular feminization syndrome in man (46 XY) is an example of a XY-male pseudohermaphrodite. In these cases, genetic and gonadal sex are male, but phenotypic, behavioral, and legal sex are female. A few cases similar to testicular feminization in man have been described in cattle (Table 13–5).

Male pseudohermaphrodites with XX sex chromosome constitution occur frequently in the goat and pig (Table 13–5). The condition is associated with a dominant autosomal gene for polledness in goats. The gonads consisting of testicular tissue are located within the abdomen or in the inguinal canal. All animals are genetic females, and the chromosomal complement may be 38,XX, 38,XX/XY or 38,XXY.

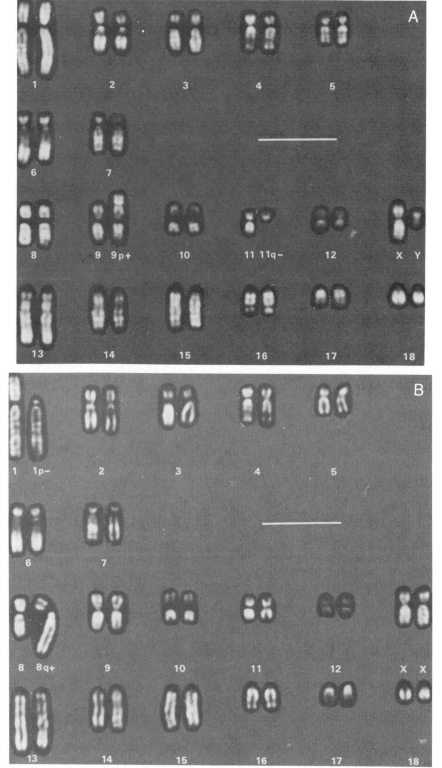

Fig. 13–6. *A,* Karyotype of a boar with the t(9p+;11q−) producing small litters but having normal sexual behavior and normal semen quality; *B,* Karyotype of the dam with the rcp(1p−;8q+) that produced the litter. (Gustavsson, I. et al. (1983). Occurrence of two different reciprocal translocations in the same litter of domestic pigs. Hereditas, *99,* 257.)

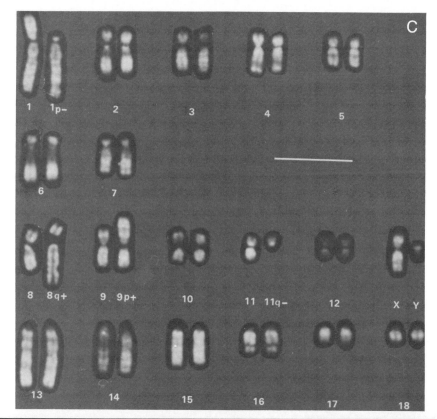

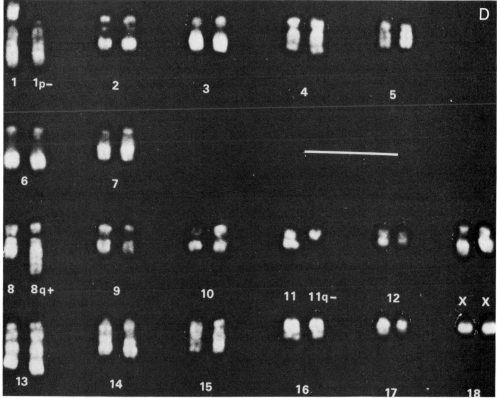

FIG. 13–6 (con't). *C,* The translocation rcp(lp−;8q+) from the dam was transmitted to all off-spring, whereas the translocation t(9p+;11q−) from the sire was found in only two offspring; and *D,* karotype of a chromosomally unbalanced embryo, der(11)t(9p+;11q−), rcp(lp−;8q+), recovered on day 21 of pregnancy. Scale indicates 10 μm. (Gustavsson, I. et al. (1983). Occurrence of two different reciprocal translocations in the same litter of domestic pigs. Hereditas, *99,* 257.)

TABLE 13–5. Chromosome Numbers and Reproductive Abnormalities in Intersexes

Syndrome	Species*	Karyotype	Gonads	External Genitalia	Sexual Behavior
True hermaphrodite	Goat	60,XX/60,XY; 60,XX	Ovotestes	Female	Female
	Pig	38,XX; 38,XX/38,XY	Ovotestes	Female	Female
		38,XY; 38,XX/39,XXY	Ovotestes	Female	Female
		37,XO/38,XX/38,XY	Ovotestes	Female	Female
	Horse	64,XX/64,XY; 63,XO/64	Ovotestes	Underdeveloped penis	Lack of male behavior
	Cattle	60,XX/60,XY; 60,XX/90,XXY	Ovary and ovotestis	Penis	Male
Pseudohermaphrodite					
Male	Goat	60,XX; 60,XY	Hypoplastic testes	Female	Male
		60,XX/60,XY			
	Pig	38,XX; 38,XX/XY	Testes	Female	Male
		39,XXYY			
	Horse	64,XX; 64,XX/64,XY	Retained testes	Enlarged clitoris and rudimentary penis	Male
	Cattle	60,XY; 60,XX/XY	Cryptorchid testes	Enlarged clitoris	Male
	†Cattle	60,XY	Abdominal testes	Female	Anestrus
	†Sheep (rare)	54,XY	Testes	Female	Anestrus
Female		2n,XX	Ovary	Male	?
Freemartin	Cattle	60,XX/XY	Ovotestes	Enlarged clitoris	Anestrus

* Species are arranged in descending order of incidence for each syndrome.
† Testicular feminization syndrome.
(Bishop, 1972; Dunn et al., 1981; Hare & Singh, 1979; Marcum, 1974)

Most intersexes in the horse are male pseudohermaphrodites. This condition has been confused with cryptorchidism because the testes are frequently retained. Affected animals have either an enlarged clitoris or a small penis located in the perineal region. The karyotypes are those of normal females or mosaics (Table 13–5). The testes contain no germ cells, and therefore affected animals are sterile.

Bovine Freemartinism. A freemartin results from the sexual modification of a female twin by the *in utero* exchange of blood from a male fetus (Fig. 13–7). The freemartin syndrome was known since ancient times. A freemartin is a genetic female at conception but becomes a 60,XX/XY chimera because of its hemopoietic and possibly gonadal tissues. The gonads of the freemartin, which range from modified ovaries to structures resembling testes, are intra-abdominal and rarely descend through the inguinal canal. There is no evidence of spermatogenesis, and testosterone appears to be the major steroid produced by the freemartin gonad.

Two theories have been advanced to explain freemartinism: the hormonal theory and the cellular theory. According to the *hormonal theory*, hormones from the male twin that reach the female through vascular anastomoses between the fused placentae cause masculinization of the female gonad. However, attempts to experimentally induce the freemartin syndrome have failed.

The *cellular theory* for the induction of freemartinism is based on the exchange blood forming cells and germ cells between the fetuses. As a result of this reciprocal exchange between dizygotic twins, identical erythrocyte antigen types occur in both twins and sex chromosome chimerism (60,XX/XY) appears in peripheral blood mononuclear leukocytes. The incidence of twinning in cattle is low. Approximately 92% of heterosexual twin females are freemartins. In the other cases, chorioallantoic vascular anastomes either fail to develop or occur after the critical stage in organogenesis.

Occasionally, a single-born animal is a chimera (Wijeratne et al., 1977). It is possible that one of the twins degenerates during early gestation and the surviving twin exhibits chimerism.

The freemartin syndrome generally refers to cattle but has also been described in other farm animals such as goats, sheep, and pigs.

Hybrids

Hybrids are the offspring resulting from the breeding of two closely related species, e.g., horse and donkey, cattle, and bison. Some interspecific hybrids are fertile, while others are subfertile and many are sterile. The hybrids of interest are those resulting from the crossing of domestic cattle (*Bos taurus*) with Zebu cattle (*Bos indicus*), cattle with bison (*Bison bison*), and the river-type buffalo (*Bubalus bubalis*) with the swamp-type buffalo (*B. bubalis*).

Both *B. taurus* and *B. indicus* have a diploid chromosome number of 60, consisting of 58 acrocentric autosomes and the sex chromosomes. There is one apparent difference between the karyotypes of the two species: The Y chromosome is acrocentric in *B. indicus* and submetacentric in *B. taurus*. Two forms of Y chromosomes are found in the hybrid, depending on the

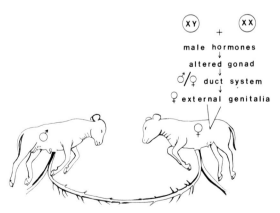

FIG. 13–7. Schematic illustration of the cause of the bovine freemartin.

TABLE 13–6.　Chromosomal Abnormalities at Different Developmental Stages

Stage	Cytogenetic Anomalies
Maternal gametogenesis	Somatic division of oogonia before onset of meiosis or during first or second meiotic division
Paternal gametogenesis	Mitotic divisions while male is *in utero* or during postpuberty; first or second meiotic division after puberty
Fertilization	Normal chromosomes with errors during fertilization; fertilization of a normal egg by two normal sperm
Zygote	Improper division of one or more chromosomes, anaphase lag, or nondisjunction; failure of cleavage of blastomeres or mosaic embryo

breed of sire used to establish the foundation stock (Potter et al., 1979). The hybrid cattle "line" based on Brahman bulls has an acrocentric Y chromosome, while cattle based on Africander bulls have a submetacentric Y chromosome.

Domestic cattle and bison have a chromosome number 2n = 60. The only chromosomal difference is that the Y chromosome is acrocentric in the bison but submetacentric in cattle. The F1 hybrid female is fertile, whereas the male is sterile. Catalos and beefaloes are offspring of parents with varying proportions of cattle and bison blood.

In many countries, crossbreeding programs are in progress to breed the swamp type of buffalo with semen of the river type of buffalo. The diploid chromosome numbers of the swamp and river type of water buffaloes are 48 and 50, respectively (Bongso and Jainudeen, 1979). The reduction in the diploid number in the swamp type by 2 is due to a tandem fusion of chromosome 9 to chromosome 4 (Di Berardino and Iannuzi, 1981). The F1 swamp × river hybrid possesses the intermediate karyotype of 2n = 49 with one of the fused chromosomes (4/9). However, unlike other interspecific hybrids possessing chromosome complements different from the parent species, both F1 males and females are fertile. Chromosomal anomalies appear to occur at different developmental stages (Table 13–6).

Equidae are remarkable for the large number of viable hybrids that are possible, even with wide chromosomal differences among species. Most of these interspecific hybrids are sterile. The hybrid mule (*Equus mulus mulus*, 2n = 63), produced by mating a male donkey (2n = 62) to a female horse (2n = 64), is usually sterile in both sexes.

A hybrid pregnancy that usually does not develop to term is that of the domestic sheep (*Ovis aries*, 2n = 54) and domestic goat (*Capra hircus*, 2n = 60).

REFERENCES

Bishop, M.W.H. (1972). Genetically determined abnormalities of the reproductive system. J. Reprod. Fertil. Suppl. *15*, 51.

Blue, M.G., Bruere, A.N. and Dewes, H.F. (1978). The significance of the XO syndrome in infertility of the mare. N.Z. Vet. J. *26*, 137.

Bongso, T.A. and Jainudeen, M.R. (1979). The karyotype of the cross-breed between the Murrah and Malaysian Swamp buffalo (*Bubalus bubalis*). Kajian Vet. *11*, 6.

Bongso, T.A., Jainudeen, M.R. and Lee, J.Y.S. (1981). Testicular hypoplasia in a bull with XX/XY chimerism. Cornell Vet. *70*, 376.

Bruere, A.N. (1974). Normal behaviour patterns and libido in chromatin-positive Kleinfelter sheep. Vet. Rec. *95*, 436.

Bruere, A.N. (1980). The application of cytogenetics to domestic animals. Vet. Ann. *20*, 29–40.

Chandley, A.C., Fletcher, J., Rossdale, P.D., Peace, C.K., Ricketts, S.W., McEnery, R.J., Thorne, J.P., Short, R.V. and Allen, W.R. (1975). Chromosome abnormalities as cause of infertility in mare. J. Reprod. Fertil. Supp. *23*, 377.

Di Berardino, D. and Iannuzi, L. (1981). Chromosome banding homologies in swamp and Murrah buffaloes. J. Heredity *72*, 183.

Dunn, H.O., McEntee, K. and Hansel, W. (1970). Diploidtriploid chimerism in a bovine true hermaphrodite. Cytogenetics *9*, 245.

Dunn, H.O., McEntee, K., Hall, C.E., Johnson, R.H. and Stone, W.H. (1979). Cytogenetics and reproductive studies of bulls born co-twin with freemartins. J. Reprod. Fert. *57*, 21.

Dunn, H.H., Smiley, D., Duncan, J.R. and McEntee, K. (1981). Two equine true hermaphrodites with 64,XX/64,XY and 63,XO/64,XY chimerism. Cornell Vet. *70,* 137.

Gustavsson, I. (1984). Cytogenetic evaluation and fertility. *In* Proc. 10th Int. Congr. Animal Reprod. AI., VI–1, Urbana-Champaign, IL.

Hancock, J.L. and Daker, M.G. (1981). Testicular hypoplasia in a boar with abnormal sex chromosome constitution (39 XXY). J. Reprod. Fertil. *61,* 395.

Hare, W.C.D. and Singh, E.L. (1979). Cytogenetics in animal reproduction. Animal Breeding Abstracts. Commonwealth Agriculture Bureaux, Farnham Royal, Slough, England.

Husslein, P., Schnedl, W. and Wagenbichler, P. (1984). Chromosome mutations and fetal wastage. *In* Spontaneous Abortion. E.S.E. Hafez (ed.). Lancaster, UK, MTP Press.

King, W.A., Gustavsson, I., Popescu, C.P. and Linares, T. (1981). Gametic products transmitted by rcp (13q−;14q+) translocation heterozygous pigs, and resulting embryonic loss. Hereditas *95,* 239.

Leipold, H.W., Huston, K. and Dennis, S.M. (1983). Bovine congenital defects. *In* Advances in Veterinary Science and Comparative Medicine. C.E. Cornelius and C.F. Simpson (eds.). New York, Academic Press.

Long, S.E. (1979). The fertility of bulls born twin to freemartins: a review. Vet. Rec. *104,* 211.

Marcum, J.B. (1974). The freemartin syndrome. Animal Breeding Abstracts *42,* 227.

Maurer, R.R. and Vogt, D.W. (1988). Decreased fertility in related females heterozygous for the 1/29 chromosome translocation. Theriogenology *30,* 1149.

Norberg, H.S., Refsdal, A.O., Garm, O.N. and Nes, N. (1976). A case report on X-trisomy in cattle. Hereditas *82,* 69.

Pinheiro, L.E.L., Almeida, Jr., I.L., Garcia, J.M. and Basrur, P.K. (1987). Trisomy X and 1/29 translocation in infertile heifers. Theriogenology *28,* 891.

Potter, W.L. and Upton, P.C. (1979). The Y-chromosome morphology of cattle. Aust. Vet. J. *55,* 539.

Swartz, H.A. and Vogt, D.W. (1983). Chromosome abnormalities as a cause of reproductive inefficiency in heifers. J. Hered. *74,* 320.

Wijeratne, W.V.S., Munro, I.B. and Wilkes, P.R. (1977). Heifer sterility associated with single-birth freemartinism. Vet. Res. *100,* 333.

IV. reproductive cycles

14
Cattle and Buffalo

M.R. JAINUDEEN AND E.S.E. HAFEZ

The domestic cattle (*Bos taurus, Bos indicus*) and buffalo (*Bubalus bubalis*), the African wild buffalo (*Syncerus caffer*), and the North American "buffalo" (*Bison bison*) are in the family Bovidae but belong to different genera and have different chromosome numbers.

Cattle and buffaloes were domesticated for draft, milk, and meat around the same period in history. The water buffalo, as the name denotes, has a predilection for water; several characteristics distinguish it from cattle. Many aspects of reproduction are similar in cattle and buffalo but indiscriminate extrapolation of reproductive phenomena and efficiency of cattle to the buffalo must be avoided.

CATTLE

Puberty

Female

Puberty is the age when first estrus accompanied by spontaneous ovulation occurs. One or more "quiet" ovulations may occur before heifers show overt signs of estrus in conjunction with ovulation, but the frequency of "quiet" ovulations can depend largely on the efficiency of estrus detection.

The age of first estrus in heifers varies considerably, mostly owing to breed and differences in growth rates. A low level of nutrient intake and slow growth delay puberty in heifers for weeks, and a high level of nutrition and rapid growth hasten puberty. The average age of puberty for groups of heifers on recommended levels of nutrition falls between 10 and 12 months for dairy breeds and between 11 months and 15 months for beef breeds. Zebu heifers attain puberty at 18 to 24 months. However, breed differences in age at puberty are not affected by nutrition. Season affects age at puberty. Winter conditions during the prepubertal period delays puberty. If heifers are provided with adequate nutrition, estrus normally recurs regularly after the pubertal estrus.

Male

Puberty in the male is the age at which the ejaculate contains sufficient spermatozoa to impregnate a cow. In cattle, it is when the first ejaculate contains 50 million spermatozoa with at least 10% progressive motility.

During calfhood, the penis is firmly adhered within the sheath by the preputial frenulum and cannot be extended; 2 to 4 months before puberty, partial protrusion of the penis occurs during mounting, followed by separation of the penis from the sheath and complete erection, and eventually by mating and ejaculation.

Cellular differentiation occurs gradually in the seminiferous epithelium of the testes during calfhood, with mature spermatozoa present in the seminiferous tubules by about 5 months of age. The testes produce increasing numbers of spermatozoa as puberty nears.

One of the earliest changes in the initiation of puberty in the bull is an increase in the frequency of pulsatile release of LH between 12 and 20 weeks. These LH discharges stimulate Leydig cells to secrete testosterone, which is needed for differentiation of Sertoli cells and spermatogenesis.

Breeds differ in age and bodyweight at puberty. Holstein bulls reached puberty earlier than Angus or Hereford bulls, with Charolais bulls falling between the others. Crossbred beef bulls generally reach puberty earlier than straightbred bulls. Zebu bulls reach puberty at a later age than most temperate breeds of cattle. This difference is presumably associated with the more rapid growth rate of crossbred bulls. After bulls reach puberty, the testes continue to grow and the number of sperm per ejaculate increases until 18 to 24 months of age in both beef and dairy bulls.

Breeding Season

Many wild species of bovidae are seasonal breeders with spring and summer being the most suitable times of the year for calving. During the course of domestication, both dairy and beef cattle were selected against seasonality, facilitating them to ovulate and conceive throughout the year. However, beef cows might still be sensitive to photoperiodicity. For example, beef cows exposed to longer photoperiods during late gestation and calving in the summer and fall resume ovarian cyclicity earlier than those calving in spring (King and Macleod, 1984; Peters and Riley, 1982).

Cyclic Changes

Morphologic, endocrine, and secretory changes occur in the ovaries and the tubular genitalia of the cow during the estrous cycle (Fig. 14–1). A knowledge of these changes is useful in estrus detection and synchronization, superovulation, and artificial insemination.

Several thousands of follicles are present in each ovary of the cow, but only one follicle ovulates per estrous cycle. Two waves of follicular activity occur during the bovine estrous cycle: The first occurs early in the cycle and the second at mid-

cycle. From the first wave, one small follicle (less than 5 mm) grows into a large follicle (greater than 10 mm) between the fifth and eleventh day, then it undergoes atresia. Although this follicle does not ovulate, it secretes similar levels of estradiol as an ovulatory follicle. From the second wave, large estrogen-producing follicles rapidly turn over (Matton et al., 1981; Staigmiller and England, 1982). Thus, at least one large follicle is present in the bovine ovary throughout the estrous cycle, and it apparently controls the fate of other follicles in the ovary.

Only one or two large follicles, present very near the onset of estrus, attain the final spurt of growth leading to mature Graafian follicles, capable of ovulation (Staigmiller and England, 1982).

The follicle collapses following ovulation. No hemorrhage occurs at this site; instead, the cavity gradually fills with luteal cells. The CL reaches maturity about 7 days after ovulation and functions for a further 8 or 9 days before it finally regresses.

Follicular growth, ovulation, and luteal function are regulated by the hypothalamic-pituitary-ovarian axis. The Graafian follicle secretes estrogens, particularly estradiol-17β. The rising levels of estradiol induce behavioral estrus and, combined with declining levels of progesterone, trigger the LH surge. If a mature follicle is present, this LH surge will cause ovulation about 24 hours later.

The physicochemical properties of cervical mucus are altered under the influence of estrogens. Alterations in viscosity, ferning, and electrical resistance are the basis for some methods of detecting estrus in cow (Table 14–1). Cervical mucus is less viscous on the day of estrus and hangs as a string of clear mucus from the vulva. Estrogen also dilates the cervix during estrus so that a catheter can be passed into the uterus more readily than at any other stage of the estrous cycle.

Estrogen improves the contractility or tonicity of the uterus. The uterus is flaccid

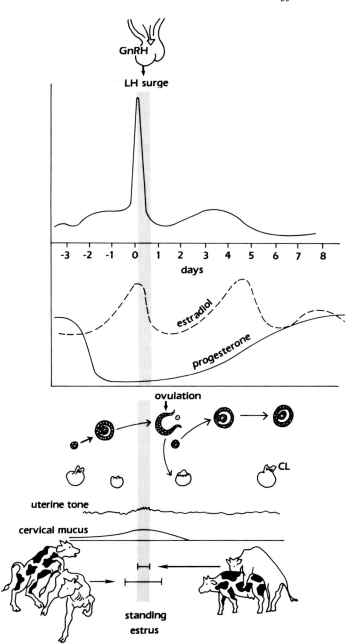

GnRH

LH surge

ovulation

CL

uterine tone

cervical mucus

standing
estrus

Fig. 14–1. The endocrine, physiologic, and behavioral changes associated with "standing estrus" (standing to be mounted) in the cow. During proestrus, the preovulatory follicle secretes increasing amounts of estradiol; at this time, the cow may ride other cows and begin to secrete cervical mucus. At the onset of estrus, peak levels of estradiol trigger a surge of LH that causes ovulation to occur about 10 to 12 hours after the end of estrus; uterine tone is maximum, and cervical mucus is copious and watery. While the growing corpus luteum secretes increasing amounts of progesterone, two waves of follicles occur, one at the early phase of the cycle and the other at midluteal phase. (Hormonal levels adapted from Hansel, W. and Convey, E.M. (1983) J. Anim. Sci. *57*, Suppl. 2, 404.)

and lacks tone during the luteal phase, whereas its tone peaks during estrus and then decreases after ovulation. Since uterine tone is a good indicator of estrus and can be detected by rectal palpation, it is used by most inseminators to verify if cows submitted for insemination are in estrus.

Estrogen increases vascular growth of the endometrium. The sudden withdrawal of estrogen secretion following ovulation causes petechial hemorrhages in the endometrium (metestrous bleeding) and the presence of blood in the vulval discharge. Most cows and heifers show

TABLE 14–1. Methods of Estrus Detection in Cattle

Principle	Method of detection	Comments
Sexual behavior (standing to be mounted)		Twice daily observations
	Observations	Night time (limited value)
	Visual	
	Videotape	
	Teasers fitted with marking devices	Teasers are (a) bulls surgically prepared to prevent release of sperm or copulation; (b) steers treated with testosterone, and (c) cows with cystic ovaries or those treated with androstenedione
	Chin-ball mating device	A halter fitted with a reservoir of dye that is released by a ball-type mechanism and marks a line on the back of the cow
	Grease	Smeared on brisket
	Collar	A pad soaked in dye or grease
	Detectors on cows	Applied on point of maximum pressure during mounting—sacral spine (detection is continuous)
	Heat mount detector (KaMaR)	Release of dye on pressure (unsuitable in wet weather)
	Tail paint	Removes hair at site when mounted
Physiologic changes related to estrus	Progesterone	Basal levels in milk or plasma; retrospective confirmation of estrus
	Cervical mucus	Alterations in physiochemical properties
	Ferning	Maximum on mucus dried on a glass slide
	Viscosity	Decreased
	Electrical resistance	Decreased as measured by a vaginal probe
	Vaginal pH	Decreased
	Uterine tone	Maximum on rectal palpation
	Estrus-related odors	Dogs trained to detect odors in vaginal mucus, milk, or urine
	Body temperature	A rise of 0.5 to 0.8°C during estrus but drops of ovulation; radio telemetric measurement of vaginal temperature
	Physical activity	Increased as measured by electronic pedometers

(Adapted from Foote (1975). J. Dairy Sci. *58*, 248; Britt (1977). J. Dairy Sci. *60*, 1345; Kiddy et al. (1983). J. Dairy Sci. *67*, 388; Vasquez et al. (1984). Proc. 10th Int. Congr. Anim Reprod & AI, III, 298; Zartman et al. (1983). Theriogenology *19*, 541).

bleeding on the second or third day after estrus. Apparently, metestrous bleeding bears no relationship to conception; it is only an indication that a cow has been in estrus. Cows showing blood-stained mucus at the time of insemination are less likely to conceive.

The actions of progesterone, secreted by the corpus luteum (CL), on the uterus and cervix are opposite to those of estrogen. During the luteal phase, cervical mucus is thick and tenacious, the cervical canal is tightly closed, and the myometrium relaxes. Progesterone levels in plasma are closely correlated with the growth, maintenance, and regression of the CL.

Most estrous periods can be detected by careful observation of cattle at least twice daily (Table 14–1). During checks for estrus, any distractions to cattle, such as feeding, should be avoided. Detection of estrus is improved by the use of bulls; they may be vasectomized or their penises may be surgically deflected or locked mechanically in the sheath. Other aids to detecting estrus include pressure-sensitive indicators placed on the rump of females and chinball markers or marking harnesses on bulls. When bulls equipped with chin-ball markers or harnesses mount an estrous female, an easily visible mark of dye or pigmented grease is left on the rump and tailhead of the female. Although nonestrous cows will occasionally be marked, the marking aids identify cows that should be observed closely for confirmation of estrus.

Ovulation

Cattle are unique among farm animals in that they ovulate 10 to 12 hours after the end of standing estrus or on the average 30 hours after the onset of estrus (Table 14–2). Except for the first postpartum estrous cycle, ovulations are preceded by behavioral signs of estrus. Cattle are spontaneous ovulators, but ovulation can be advanced by about 2 hours by service with a vasectomized bull. Similarly, manual massage of the clitoris for 10 seconds following artificial insemination of beef cows shortened the interval from beginning of estrus until the ovulatory surge of LH by more than 4 hours, shortened the time from beginning of estrus until ovulation by 4 hours, and increased the conception rate by 6%.

Normally, one follicle ovulates per estrous cycle in cattle. Two follicles ovulate approximately 10% of the time, and three follicles ovulate infrequently.

Follicles ovulate on the right ovary about 60% of the time and on the left ovary about 40% of the time. The first ovulation after parturition occurs more frequently on the ovary opposite to the uterine horn that previously carried the fetus.

Sperm Production and Release

The duration of one cycle of the seminiferous epithelium is 13.5 days for bulls, irrespective of the breed. Approximately 61 days (4.5 cycles seminiferous epithelium) are required for completion of spermatogenesis. Thus, an injury to the testes of a bull resulting from fever, heat stress, or transport stress could interfere with spermatogenesis and sperm production; it

TABLE 14–2. Female Reproductive Characteristics of Cattle and Buffalo

Parameter	Cattle Mean (range)	Buffalo Mean (range)
Sexual season	Polyestrous	Polyestrous
Age at puberty (months)	15 (10 to 24)	21 (15 to 36)
Estrous cycle		
Length (days)	21 (14 to 29)	21 (18 to 22)
Estrus (hours)	18 (12 to 30)	21 (17 to 24)
Ovulation		
Type	Spontaneous	Spontaneous
Time from onset (hours)	30 (18 to 48)	32 (18 to 45)
Number of eggs shed	1	1
Life span of corpus luteum (days)	16	16
Fertilizable life of ova (hours)	(20 to 24)	?
Entry of ova into uterus (hours after ovulation)	90 (64 to 96)	?
Gestation length (days)	280 (278 to 293)	315 (305 to 330)
Age at first calving (months)	30 (24 to 36)	42 (36 to 56)
Postpartum intervals (days)		
Uterine involution	45 (32 to 50)	35 (16 to 60)
First ovulation	30 (10 to 110)	75 (35 to 180)
Calving intervals (months)	13 (12 to 14)	18 (15 to 21)

would take at least 2 months before sperm quality returns to normal.

Daily sperm production, the number of potentially fertile sperm produced per day by the testes, is highly correlated with testicular size, which can be estimated by length and width measurements or scrotal circumference (Foote, 1984). Both testis size and scrotal circumference, however, are influenced by genotype and age. Thus, it is not possible to have standard measurements for all ages and breeds. Sperm production also varies widely among individual bulls with some variation among breeds.

The bull ejaculates 4 to 10 ml of semen containing 0.8 to 2.0 billion sperm per milliliter. Semen output is influenced by the age of bull, season of the year, and frequency of ejaculation. Normally, total sperm per ejaculate increases with the age of bull up to about 7 years and then declines. Large differences exist in semen output characteristics between bulls, between first and second ejaculates, and between intervals between collections.

Breeding

The bull's penis is of the fibroelastic type, relatively small in diameter and rigid when nonerect. Although the penis is more rigid during erection, it undergoes little enlargement. Protrusion is effected by straightening of the S-shaped sigmoid flexure. Vision appears more important than smell in sexual stimulation of a bull. The bull identifies the estrous cow by licking or smelling around her external genitalia and curling his upper lip in a characteristic manner—"Flehmen." Before mounting, the bull orientates himself behind the cow and rests his chin and throat over the cow's rump. Estrous cows respond to chin-resting pressure by standing.

Mating in cattle is brief (less than 5 seconds) when compared to that in horses and swine. As the partially erect penis protrudes from the sheath and accessory fluid dribbles, the bull mounts and straddles the cow. After the penis penetrates the vagina (intromission), sudden contractions of the abdominal muscles of the bull lead to maximum intromission and ejaculation. The force of the muscular contraction lifts the bull's hind legs off the ground as an active leap forward. This ejaculatory thrust deposits the semen in the anterior vagina near the external os of the cervix.

Most dairy herds in the United States use an artificial insemination service, but over 90% of beef cattle are bred by natural service. Usually, one bull is assigned to about 30 to 60 cows in either single or multiple-sire mating pastures. Under range conditions, the number of females mated per unit time depends on many interrelated factors such as male≠female ratio and the aggressive interactions among bulls.

Social ranking of bulls, largely controlled by age and seniority within groups, can influence their sexual activity. Calves born to cows exposed as a herd to three or four bulls showed that the oldest or the second oldest bull in the group sired over 60% of the calves while the youngest bull sired less than 15% of the calves (Chenoweth, 1981). Breed differences exist in the libido of bulls. Holsteins react more quickly to stimulation at semen collection than most other breeds; Zebu bulls have a slower reaction time than European breeds.

Most beef herds have restricted breeding seasons of 9 to 12 weeks so that cows calve in spring when abundant feed is available. Heifers are bred at an optimum target weight that varies with breed (Table 14–3). Matings should be planned to avoid disproportionately large calves in dams with small pelvic areas.

Gestation and Parturition

Gestation lengths vary from 276 to 295 days, and lengths are longest in Brown Swiss and Brahman. Differences in gestation length are associated with twinning, sex of calf, and parity of cow.

TABLE 14–3. Optimum Body Weight (and Age) to Breed Heifers

Breed	Body Weight (kg)	Age (Months)
Holsteins	340	15
Brown Swiss	340	15
Jerseys	225	13
Jerseys	225	13
Guernseys	250	13
Ayrshire	275	13
Hereford	270	15
Angus	250	13
Charolais	330	14

Several clinical changes in the pregnant female indicate approaching parturition. The muscles and ligaments of the rump and tailhead soften and relax, the tailhead is elevated 24 to 48 hours before calving, and the vulva swells. As calving nears, the vulva discharges thick, stringy mucus, the udder enlarges, and the teats appear to be distended with milk. A day or two before calving, the cow may become restless and keep to a small isolated area, which she defends against other cows. Confinement and interference at this time can result in prolonged parturition.

During the first stage of labor (dilation of the cervix), heifers, but not cows, may be restless and show signs of abdominal pain. As the calf enters the birth canal, abdominal straining commences and the animal lies down in a lateral or sternal position. The amnion or the "second water bag" appears at the vulva. With further straining the calf is delivered; most calves take at least 45 minutes to stand and may take a few hours to suckle for the first time. Cows take about 4 to 6 hours to expel the placenta. They tend to eat the afterbirth more frequently than do sheep.

Puerperium

The postpartum period is the time following parturition during which lactation is initiated and reproductive cycles are established.

Involution of the Uterus

Between parturition and the first estrus, the uterus must involute if conception is to occur. Immediately after calving, the uterine horn that carried the fetus (gravid horn) is considerably larger than the opposite nongravid horn. Both horns lack firm muscle tone. The weight and size of the uterus soon decrease, the number and size of myometrial cells decrease, and the muscle tone of the uterus gradually improves. The uterus involutes most quickly in primiparous cows and cows that are suckling calves (Table 14–2).

Ovarian Function

The interval from parturition to first ovulation shows considerable variability (Table 14–2). Multiparous cows ovulate earlier than primiparous cows. Suckling and the plane of nutrition delay the time of the first postpartum ovulation in beef cows. The incidence of first postpartum ovulation without estrous behavior is relatively high. Thus, the first estrus may not reflect the resumption of ovarian cyclicity. Usually, estrus is observed for the first time at about 35 days postpartum in dairy cows. The conception rate is lower at first postpartum estrus than at subsequent estrous periods. Dairy cows are bred after 50 days postpartum and should conceive by 80 days to maintain a calving interval of 12 months.

Reproductive Performance

Measures of Reproductive Efficiency

The reproductive efficiency of both dairy and beef cattle can be evaluated by several methods (Table 14–4). The 60- to 90-day nonreturn rates evaluate fertility of bulls and efficiency of inseminators in artificial insemination (AI) centers. First service conception rates are based on a rectal diagnosis of pregnancy conducted 6 to 8 weeks after insemination. Although both nonreturn rates and conception rates estimate the proportion of cows estimated to be pregnant, differences between them have long been recognized. The nonreturn rate overestimates the conception rate by about 10 to 15%. Much of this difference is related to failure of estrous de-

TABLE 14–4.   Measures of Reproductive Efficiency

Trait	Definition
First calving	Age (months)
Days open	Days calving to conception
First-service conception rate (%)	$\dfrac{\text{No. pregnant first service}}{\text{No. bred first service}} \times 100$
Calving interval (days)	$\dfrac{\text{Days between successive calving}}{\text{Total cows}}$
Services per conception	$\dfrac{\text{No. of services in all cows}}{\text{Total conceptions}}$
Pregnancy rate (%)	$\dfrac{\text{No. of cows pregnant}}{\text{Total cows in herd}} \times 100$
Calving rate (%)	$\dfrac{\text{No. of calves born}}{\text{Total cows in herd}} \times 100$
Net calf crop (%)	$\dfrac{\text{Total calves weaned}}{\text{Total cows in herd}} \times 100$

tection, anestrus, some early embryonic deaths, sale or death of cows, and the presentation of cows for return insemination beyond a 60- to 90-day period.

The calving to conception interval or "days open" is a valuable index reflecting efficiency of estrus detection and the fertility of both females and males in a herd. Since gestation length is a fixed interval, both calving intervals and days open are usually influenced by similar factors; the latter has the advantage of early detection of problem cows.

The percentage of cows pregnant, the index widely adopted in beef herds, has greater significance when the breeding season is short. A breeding season of about three estrous cycle lengths provides a cow at least two or three matings. Calf crop measures pregnancy losses and calf mortality at calving, whereas the percentage of calves weaned reflects the reproductive efficiency of the breeding season, ease of calving, mothering ability, and calf survival.

General Fertility

The optimal calving interval for both beef and dairy cattle is 12 months, but 12-month intervals are seldom achieved. Fertility is often measured as the net calf crop for naturally bred beef cattle and as the calving rate to first service for artificially inseminated dairy cattle. The net calf crop for beef cattle, or the percentage of cows that wean calves each year, is estimated at 70 to 75%. For dairy cattle the percentage of cows calving to first service is only about 50%.

Improving Reproductive Performance

Because 95% of the beef females in the United States are bred by natural service, the bull must produce semen of high potential fertility and possess sufficient libido and physical stamina to detect estrus and mate repeatedly (Chenoweth, 1981). Reproductive performance of beef cattle can often be improved considerably by thorough evaluation of bulls for breeding soundness (Fig. 14–2).

Failure of the beef female to express either a pubertal or postpartum estrus early in the breeding season is a serious problem. Conception early in the breeding season for both heifers and cows permits early calving and the weaning of older, heavier calves. Beef cattle must receive adequate nutrition so that heifers attain puberty and maximal pelvic growth at an early age and postpartum females express estrus and have acceptable fertility early in the breeding season.

To maintain a 12-month calving interval in a dairy herd, at least 90% of cows should show standing estrus by day 60 postpartum and conceive by 85 days postpartum (Fig. 14–3). Conception rates were lower when cows were bred earlier than a 60-day postpartum interval than at later intervals (Berger et al., 1981). In herds where the incidence of uterine infections, acyclicity, and cystic ovarian disease were reduced by reproductive herd health programs, conception rates were higher and

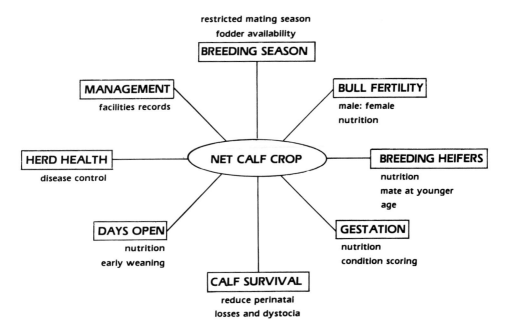

FIG. 14–2.   Methods of increasing the net calf crop in beef cattle.

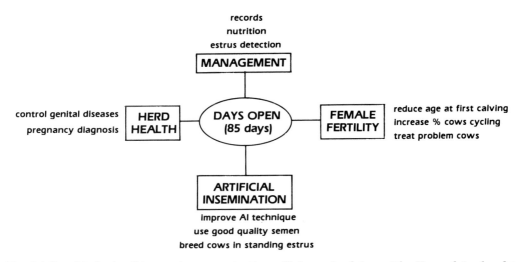

FIG. 14–3.   Methods of improving reproductive efficiency in dairy cattle. For a dairy herd to achieve a 12-month calving interval, at least 90% of cows should be cycling by 60 days postpartum and conceive within 85 days (days open).

days open were shorter for cows bred at 50 days postpartum than those bred at later postpartum intervals (Heider et al., 1980; Stevenson et al., 1983).

Days open can be reduced by increasing efficiency of estrus detection. Thus, a greater number of cows would be submitted for AI between 55 and 85 days postpartum. Most cows in estrus can be detected by careful observation at least twice daily and by using detection aids (Table 14–1) and prediction charts and by monitoring ovarian activity by milk progesterone or rectal palpation. These methods have increased the efficiency of estrus detection in some herds from 50 to about 90%. Also, contact with a bull results in an increased incidence of estrus and may stimulate ovarian activity in beef cattle early in the postpartum period (Alberio et al., 1987).

Several hormones have been employed to increase the incidence of estrus and ovulation during the second month after calving. Gonadotropin-releasing hormone (GnRH) injections early in the postpartum period or estrus induction techniques have given variable results.

Fertility to AI could be increased by inseminating only cows in estrus, proper semen thawing procedures, placement of semen in the uterus rather than the cervix or vagina, uterine and clitoral massage following insemination, and housing inseminated cows at temperatures below 23°C on the day after insemination (Gwazdauskas et al., 1980).

Treatment with human chorionic gonadotropin (hCG) did not improve the conception rate at the first insemination, but it may be beneficial for cows that require a repeat service (Helmer and Britt, 1986). The administration of GnRH or its analogs 0 to 6 hour before AI has little beneficial effects on first-service conception rates in dairy cattle. It may even have an antifertility effect and should not be recommended at first services in dairy cattle (Mee et al., 1990). GnRH, however, may improve the fertility of repeat breeders when administered at time of AI (Stevenson et al., 1990).

The effects of nutrition on ovarian function, particularly in lactating dairy cows, have been extensively studied. The problem in feeding high-producing cows is to stimulate their appetite to increase intake to minimize the severity and length of negative energy balance. During the post-partum period, fertility becomes confounded with milk production. Nutritional intake did not influence behavioral estrous traits provided that dietary restriction did not result in body weight loss (Knutson and Allrich, 1988). High-producing cows that were anestrous or cyclic between day 40 and 60 postpartum obtained more energy from body reserves for milk production during the first 2 weeks of lactation than cows cycling before day 40 postpartum (Staples and Thatcher, 1990). In post-partum beef cows, lipid metabolic status could influence luteal activity with a hyperlipidemia-enhancing luteal activity (Williams, 1989). Reduced luteal activity that is associated with a negative energy balance during the early postpartum dairy cow may be related to the reduced levels of insulin-like growth factor I in serum (Spicer et al., 1990). Recombinant bovine growth hormone (rbSt) used to stimulate lactation may adversely affect reproductive function in the dairy cow if administered before the first postpartum ovulation (Schemm et al., 1990).

BUFFALO

The world population of 130 million domestic buffaloes, *Bubalus bubalis,* has been broadly classified into the swamp or river type. The swamp buffalo (2n = 48 chromosomes) is the draft animal in the rice fields of the eastern half of Asia and is managed under range conditions similar to beef cattle. The river buffalo (2n = 50 chromosomes) is the dairy animal in countries extending from India and Pakistan to the Mediterranean countries and Egypt.

Puberty

The buffalo attains puberty at a later age than cattle (Table 14–2). The river type exhibits first estrus earlier (15 to 18 months) than the swamp type (21 to 24 months). First conception occurs at an average bodyweight of 250 to 275 kg, which is usually attained at 24 to 36 months of age.

The testes of the buffalo descend into the scrotum at 2 to 4 months of age, although they may be present at birth in some animals. Buffalo testicular quiescence extends from 0 to 7 months of age, followed by a period of rapid testicular growth and considerable androgenic activity (Ahmad et al., 1989). Spermatogenesis commences at 12 to 15 months, but the ejaculate contains viable spermatozoa only when animals are about 24 months old.

Estrous Cycles

Breeding Season

Buffaloes, like cattle, are polyestrous and breed throughout the year. Seasonal calving patterns reported in many countries have been attributed to ambient temperature, photoperiod, and feed supply. Apparently, the photoperiodic effect on estrous cyclicity is similar in both buffalo and cattle. Buffaloes calving in summer or fall resume ovarian cyclicity earlier than those in winter or spring (Ahmad et al., 1981). Probably decreasing day length and cooler ambient temperatures favor cyclicity. During summer, when ambient temperature and photoperiod are at their maximum, prolactin levels are highest (Kaker et al., 1982) and plasma progesterone levels are lowest (Rao and Pandey, 1982). High ambient temperatures may also contribute to this seasonality by depressing the male libido.

Cyclic Changes

Many cyclic changes in the ovaries, tubular genitalia, and hormonal secretions in the buffalo are comparable to those of cattle. Assessment of ovarian activity is based on combinations of daily estrus detection with a vasectomized male, rectal palpation, or laparoscopic observation of the ovaries and plasma progesterone assay. Progesterone levels in plasma and milk, as in cattle, reflect the endocrine activity of the CL, but levels are lower. Exogenous prostaglandin ($PGF_{2\alpha}$) will cause regression of the cyclic CL; $PGF_{2\alpha}$ of uterine origin, as in cattle, is probably the luteolysin in the buffalo.

Estrus and Ovulation

The length of the estrous cycle is about 21 days, and estrus lasts about 12 to 30 hours (Table 14–2). Overt signs of estrus are less intense than in cattle. Acceptance of the male is the most reliable sign of estrus in the buffalo. Less than a third of buffaloes in estrus is detected by homosexual behavior. A discharge of clear mucus rom the vulva, restlessness, increased frequency of urination, vocalization, and a drop in milk production are not reliable signs of estrus. Maximum ferning of mucus occurs during estrus but is not a substitute for standing estrus. Sexual receptivity toward the male can be determined as in cattle (Table 14–1) by a vasectomized male or an androgenized female buffalo fitted with a chin-ball mating device or the use of heat-mount detectors. The efficiency of these estrus detection aids, however, may be reduced because of the wallowing habits of buffaloes.

Estrus commences toward late evening with peak sexual activity between 6:00 P.M. and 6:00 A.M. Matings continue until late morning in the river buffalo but usually cease during daylight hours in the swamp buffalo. Ovulation, as in cattle, occurs 15 to 18 hours after the end of estrus or about 35 to 45 hours after the onset of estrus (Table 14–2). Ovulation is preceded by a surge of LH at the onset of estrus. A single egg is shed during one cycle.

Sperm Production and Release

The testes, accessory sex glands, and the penis of the buffalo are smaller than those of cattle. The sheath of the penis adheres close to the body in the swamp type, whereas it is more pendulous in the river type.

The buffalo, among farm animals except the boar, has one of the shortest spermatogenic cycles. The durations of the seminiferous epithelial cycle and spermatogenesis are 8.6 days and 38 days, respectively

(Sharma and Gupta, 1980). In general, the frequency of cell stages in the buffalo and cattle are similar. The short duration of spermatogenesis, the small testicular size, and low rate of daily sperm production as compared with cattle perhaps reflect species differences in length of the sexual season and mating behavior.

The normal ejaculate is grayish to milky white, rarely exceeds 5 ml, and has a sperm concentration between 300 to 1500 million cells per milliliter. Sperm motility is lower than in cattle.

Breeding

Male sexual behavior is similar but less intense than in the bull. Libido is suppressed during the hotter part of the day, particularly in the swamp buffalo. Sniffing of the vulva or female urine and the "Flehmen" reaction precedes mounting of the estrous female. Mating is brief and lasts only a few seconds, and the ejaculatory thrust is less marked than in the bull. After ejaculation, the buffalo dismounts slowly and the penis retracts gradually into the sheath.

Artificial insemination in buffalo is similar to that of cattle but is not commonly practiced because of the difficulty of detecting estrus. In countries such as Egypt, India, and Pakistan, however, artificial insemination centers provide a breeding service with either chilled or frozen semen for dairy buffaloes. Deep-frozen semen is now exported from India and Pakistan to upgrade or crossbreed indigenous buffaloes in several countries.

The numerical differences in chromosome numbers in the two types of buffaloes result in crossbreeds having an intermediate karyotype of $2n = 49$. Although both male and female crosses produce unbalanced gametes ($n = 24$ or 25), they are fertile, unlike other hybrids possessing chromosome complements differing from their parents.

Gestation and Parturition

The CL is maintained throughout gestation, but its role in the maintenance of pregnancy has not been established. Plasma progesterone levels remain elevated during pregnancy but decline to basal levels on the day of parturition. Estrus is generally suspended, but a few pregnant animals may exhibit one or more periods of anovulatory estrus.

The epitheliochorial placenta of the buffalo is of the cotyledonary type. Convex maternal caruncles fuse with fetal cotyledons to form placentomes that are distributed throughout both gravid and nongravid uterine horns.

Buffaloes have a longer gestation period than cattle (Table 14–2). The gestation length ranges from 305 to 320 days for the river buffalo and from 320 to 340 days for the swamp buffalo. A swamp female carrying a fetus sired by a river type has a gestation length that is intermediate (315 to 325 days). Buffaloes producing calves weighing about 35 kg had the shortest (about 308 days) gestation period, and buffaloes producing calves weighing either more or less than 35 kg had longer gestation periods. Calves were heavier at birth than were heifer calves (Usmani et al, 1987).

The endocrine mechanism initiating parturition in the buffalo is not fully understood; but about 15 days before parturition, plasma and levels of both estrone and $PGF_{2\alpha}$ metabolite increase and reach peak values at 3 to 5 days before parturition. The elevated levels of plasma progesterone during gestation drop sharply to basal levels on the day of parturition, whereas estrone and $PGF_{2\alpha}$ metabolite levels decline gradually to basal levels at 7 to 14 days postpartum. A marked rise in plasma cortisol occurs on the day of parturition; but its source, whether fetal or maternal, and role in the initiation of parturition in the buffalo is not known.

The signs of approaching parturition, the birth process, and the duration of the various stages of labor are similar to those of cattle. The first stage of labor lasts 1 to 2 hours, being longer in primiparous than in pluriparous buffaloes. During the second stage of labor, lasting 30 to 60 minutes, strong abdominal contractions cause rupture of the amnion and delivery of the fetus in anterior presentation with fully extended limbs. Fetal membranes are expelled 4 to 5 hours after delivery of the fetus. Twins are rare, and their occurrence is less than 1 per 1000 births.

Puerperium

Uterine involution is completed by 28 days for the suckled swamp buffalo as compared to 45 days for the hand-milked river buffalo (Table 14–5). Several factors influence the rate of postpartum uterine involution in the buffalo. Involution occurs earlier in normal than in abnormal parturitions, sooner in suckled than in nonsuckled or milked buffaloes, and earlier in low than in high milk producers, with increasing parity during winter and spring (Jainudeen, 1984).

The optimum time to breed in relation to uterine involution has not been established for the buffalo. The opportunity for matings or inseminations before completion of uterine involution is limited because the first postpartum ovulation occurs much later than uterine involution in the buffalo.

Ovarian Activity

An increase in follicular activity occurs particularly on the ovary opposite the previously gravid side, between days 30 to 60 postpartum, but only a few animals ovulate.

Progesterone remains at basal levels in the plasma between parturition and the resumption of ovarian cyclicity. Following the first postpartum ovulation, plasma progesterone levels are closely correlated with the morphologic and functional activity of the CL.

The postpartum interval to first ovulation is longer in buffalo than in cattle (Table 14–2). The interval is longer in the suckled swamp buffalo than in the milked river buffalo (Table 14–5). Most first postpartum ovulations are not preceded by estrus. First estrus is observed at 2 to 3 months after parturition (Jainudeen et al., 1983).

Among the physiologic factors, body condition, lactation, suckling, and age adversely affect ovarian function. Buffaloes in poor body condition and young females in their first lactation possess inactive ovaries and have extended periods of postpartum anestrus. Suckling significantly increases the interval from parturition to first estrus and ovulation in the buffalo. Ovarian cyclicity is restored earlier in nonsuckled than suckled river and swamp buffaloes (Jainudeen, 1984).

Reproductive Performance

Reproductive Efficiency

Reproductive efficiency of the buffalo can be measured by similar criteria as for cattle, particularly in dairy buffalo herds using AI or hand matings. Conception rates are 50 to 60% with chilled semen, 25 to 45% with frozen semen, and over 60%

TABLE 14–5. Uterine Involution and Ovarian Activity in the Buffalo*

Postpartum Interval (Days)	River Buffalo		Swamp Buffalo	
	Mean	Range	Mean	Range
Uterine involution	45	15–60	28	16–39
First detected estrus	75	35–185	90	40–275
First ovulation	59	35–87	96	52–140
Conception	125	85–150	180	40–400

* River buffalo: Chauhan et al. (1977). Ind. J. Dairy Sci. *4*, 286; El-Sheikh and Mohamed (1977). Ind. J. Anim. Sci. *47*, 165; El-Fadaly (1980). Vet. Med. J. Egypt. *28*, 399; swamp buffalo: Jainudeen et al. (1983). Anim. Reprod. Sci. *5*, 181.

with natural service. The pregnancy rates following a restricted breeding season of 2 to 3 months in swamp buffalo herds vary from 30 to 75% depending on the nutritional and lactational status of the females at joining. Calf crops as high as 80% have been reported in elite herds in many countries.

The calving interval is the fertility index widely used at the small farm level. Under range conditions, a buffalo usually produces two calves in 3 years. But in well-managed herds of dairy buffaloes, calving intervals of 14 to 15 months have been achieved. The calving interval is influenced by the individual cow, the year and season of conception, and parity. Conception during January to March led to the shortest calving interval, and during October to December, it led to the longest interval. The highest percentage of conceptions occurred 2 to 5 months after the peak rainfall (Lundstrom et al., 1982). Parity influences the calving interval, which is longer in primiparous than in pluriparous buffaloes.

Increasing Reproductive Performance

Delayed age at first calving, problems related to estrous detection and days open in the female, and loss of libido in the male are the major constraints to increasing reproductive rates in the water buffalo. Improvements in nutrition could increase growth rates and have hastened the onset of puberty. Similarly, management practices such as early weaning, induction of estrus with prostaglandins or intravaginal progesterone releasing devices, and better nutrition have hastened the resumption of early postpartum ovarian activity and reduced the days open in the water buffalo.

The seasonal nature of the breeding cycle and the long calving intervals under range conditions make it difficult for a buffalo to calve during the peak months of 2 successive years. The marked seasonal fluctuations in libido and semen quality may be overcome by providing cooling facilities for buffaloes during the hot season. Also, semen collected and frozen during the cooler months could be used to inseminate females during periods of high environmental temperatures. Induction of estrus with synthetic analogs of $PGF_{2\alpha}$ and fixed-time insemination with frozen semen may prove useful in restricting mating seasons so that calvings occur when water and green feed are abundant.

Reproductive management programs, as for dairy and beef cattle, have been adopted in large buffalo herds worldwide.

Females can be bred either naturally or by AI. Breeding males, as in cattle, should be tested for breeding soundness before assigning them to about 20 to 30 females in single-sire mating paddocks. If AI is planned, then estrus can be synchronized with $PGF_{2\alpha}$ or a progesterone-releasing intravaginal device, and animals can be inseminated at either a fixed time or on detection of estrus. Animals are examined for pregnancy at about 2 months after the end of the mating season or insemination and are separated into pregnant and nonpregnant groups. The adoption of these reproductive management programs combined with herd health service (as for cattle) and improved nutrition have virtually doubled the reproductive rates of the water buffalo.

REFERENCES

Ahmad, N., Chaudhry, R.A. and Khan, B.B. (1981). Effect of month of season of calving on the length of subsequent calving interval in Nili-Ravi buffaloes. Anim. Reprod. Sci. *3*, 301.

Ahmad, N., Shahab, M., Khurshid, S. and Arslan, M. (1989). Pubertal development in the male buffalo: Longitudinal analysis of body growth, testicular size and serum profiles of testosterone and oestradiol. Anim. Reprod. Sci. *19*, 61.

Alberio, E.H., Schiersmann, G., Carol, N. and Mestre, J. (1987). Effect of a teaser bull on ovarian and behavioural activity of suckling beef cows. Anim. Reprod. Sci. *14*, 263.

Berger, P.J., Shanks, R.D., Freeman, A.E. and Laben, R.C. (1981). Genetic aspects of milk yield and reproductive performance. J. Dairy Sci. *64*, 114.

Chenoweth, P.J. (1981). Libido and mating behavior in bulls, boars and rams. Theriogenology *16*, 155.

Foote, R.H. (1984). General evaluation of male reproductive capacity. Proc. 10th Congr. Anim. Reprod. & AI., X-1, Urbana–Champaign, IL.

Gwazdauskas, F.C., Lineweaver, J.A. and Vinson, W.E. (1980). Rates of conception by artificial insemination of dairy cattle. J. Dairy Sci. *64*, 358.

Heider, L.E., Galton, D.M. and Barr, H.L. (1980). Dairy herd reproductive health programs compared with traditional practices. J. Am. Vet. Med. Assoc. *176*, 743.

Helmer, S.D. and Britt, J.H. (1986). Fertility of dairy cattle treated with human chorionic gonadotropin (hCG) to stimulate progesterone secretion. Theriogenology *26*, 683.

Jainudeen, M.R. (1984). Reproduction in the water buffalo: postpartum female. Proc. 10th Int. Congr. Anim. Reprod. and AI, IV, XIV-43, Urbana—Champaign, Illinois, USA.

Jainudeen, M.R., Bongso, T.A. and Tan, H.S. (1983). Postpartum ovarian activity and uterine involution in the suckled swamp buffalo (*Bubalus bubalis*). Anim. Reprod. Sci. *5*, 181.

Kaker, M.L., Razdan, M.N. and Galhotra, M.M. (1982). Serum prolactin levels of non-cycling Murrah buffaloes (*Bubalus bubalis*). Theriogenology *17*, 469.

King, G.J. and Macleod, G.K. (1984). Reproductive function in beef cows calving in the spring or fall. Anim. Reprod. Sci. *6*, 255.

Knutson, R.J. and Allrich, R.D. (1988). Influence of nutrition on serum concentrations of progesterone, luteinizing hormone and estrous behavior in dairy heifers. J. Anim. Sci. *66*, 90.

Lundstrom, K., Abeygunawardena, H., de Silva, L.N.A. and Perera, B.M.O.A. (1982). Environmental influence on calving interval and estimates of its repeatability in the Murrah buffalo in Sri Lanka. Anim. Reprod. Sci. *5*, 99.

Matton, P., Adelakoun, V., Couture, Y. and Dufour, J.J. (1981). Growth and replacement of the ovarian follicles during the estrous cycle. J. Anim. Sci. *52*, 813.

Mee, M.O., Stevenson, J.S. and Scoby, R.K. (1990). Influence of gonadotropin-releasing hormone and timing of insemination relative to estrus on pregnancy rates of dairy cattle at first service. J. Dairy Sci. *73*, 1500.

Peters, A.R. and Riley, G.M. (1982). Is the cow a seasonal breeder? Br. Vet. J. *138*, 533.

Rao, L.V. and Pandey, R.S. (1982). Seasonal changes in plasma progesterone concentrations in buffalo cows (*Bubalus bubalis*). J. Reprod. Fertil. *66*, 57.

Schemm, S.R., Deaver, D.R., Griel, L.C., Jr. and Muller, L.D. (1990). Effects of recombinant bovine somatotropin on luteinizing hormone and ovarian function in lactating dairy cows. Biol. Reprod. *42*, 815.

Sharma, A.K. and Gupta, R.C. (1980). Duration of seminiferous epithelial cycle in buffalo bulls (*Bubalus bubalis*). Anim. Reprod. Sci. *3*, 217.

Spicer, L.J., Tucker, W.B. and Adams, G.D. (1990). Insulin-like growth factor-I in dairy cows: relationships among energy balance, body condition, ovarian activity, and estrous behavior. J. Dairy Sci. *73*, 929.

Staigmiller, R.B. and England, B.G. (1982). Folliculogenesis in the bovine. Theriogenology *17*, 43.

Staples, C.R. and Thatcher, W.W. (1990). Relationship between ovarian activity and energy status during the early postpartum period of high producing dairy cows. J. Dairy Sci. *73*, 938.

Stevenson, J.S., Call, E.P. and Scoby, R.K. (1990). Double insemination and gonadotropin-releasing hormone treatment of repeat-breeding dairy cattle. J. Dairy Sci. *73*, 1766.

Stevenson, J.S., Schmidt, M.K. and Call, E.P. (1983). Factors affecting reproductive performance of dairy cows first inseminated after five weeks postpartum. J. Dairy Sci. *66*, 1148.

Williams, G.L. (1989). Modulation of luteal activity in postpartum beef cows through changes in dietary lipid. J. Anim. Sci. *67*, 785.

Usmani, R.H., Lewis, G.S. and Naz, N.A. (1987). Factors affecting length of gestation and birth weight of Nili-Ravi buffaloes. Anim. Reprod. Sci. *14*, 195.

15
Sheep and Goats

M.R. JAINUDEEN AND E.S.E. HAFEZ

Domestic sheep (*Ovis aries*) and goats (*Capra hircus*) are two distinct species in the family Bovidae. They were among the first to be domesticated: sheep for wool and meat, and the goat for milk, meat, and fiber. The goat is important because it can be a major source of animal protein in the tropics. The world population of sheep is approximately 2.5 times that of goats. Each species possesses certain unique characteristics (Table 15–1). Reproduction in the ewe (female sheep) and the doe (female goat) are compared in this chapter.

SEXUAL SEASON

Female

Both sheep and goats are seasonally polyestrous so that the young are born during the most favorable time of the year,

the spring. The length of the sexual season varies with day length, breed, and nutrition. This seasonality is governed by photoperiodicity with estrus activity commencing during a period of decreasing day length. In temperate-zone latitudes, most breeds of sheep and goats are anovulatory and anestrous during spring and summer but start cycling as the length of daylight decreases during fall.

In the tropical zones, where there is less variation in day length, indigenous sheep and goats tend to breed throughout the year. Therefore, when temperate breeds are introduced into the tropics, they gradually lose their seasonality and follow the breeding patterns characteristic of the new environment. High environmental temperature and lack of feed may restrict

TABLE 15–1. Genetic and Physical Characteristics of Sheep and Goats

Characteristic	Sheep	Goat
Chromosome number	54	60
Taxonomy	*Ovis aries*	*Capra hircus*
Matings		
Buck × female	Sterile	Fertile
Ram × female	Fertile	Embryonic death
Habitat	Temperate zone	Arid tropical
World population	1.2 billion	500 million
Physical features		
Tail length	Short	Short
Tail carriage	Downward	Upward
Male scent glands	Absent	Present
Face and foot glands	Present	Absent
Lacrimal pits	Present	Absent
Beard	Absent	Present
Body coat	Wool	Hair

sexual activity during some months of the year in the tropics, but shortly after the onset of the rainy season, sexual activity increases, which is probably due to a change in feed availability. In Morocco, the D'Man breed has a very short seasonal anestrus allowing two lambings per year while all other breeds have a limited sexual season starting in June and ending in December.

Genotype influences the sexual season in the ewe and doe. With some ewes exhibiting estrus year-round, the Dorset, Merino, and Rambouillet sheep breeds, which originated near the equator, have longer sexual seasons than British breeds such as the Southdown, Shropshire, and Hampshire. Dairy goats such as the Toggenburg, Saanen, French Alpine, and the LaMancha have a restricted sexual season between August and February in most regions of North America. The Anglo-Nubian breed, developed in England by breeding English does with bucks from Nubia in Upper Egypt and Ethiopia, is less restricted to fall breeding, although sexual activity is highest during the fall. The sexual season of the Alpine dairy goat can also be extended under intense management but not beyond April. In the southern part of the United States (30° N latitude), meat-type of goats are anestrous between March and May while less than 40% of Rambouillet sheep are anestrous during the same period (Fig. 15–1).

During summer, the ovaries of anestrous ewes develop follicles and secrete estradiol when stimulated with LH. Follicular activity changes throughout the year in synchrony with the circannual patterns of prolactin secretion and day length, but apparently fluctuations in prolactin are not related to seasonality of mating in sheep.

The importance of day length in the seasonal control of reproductive activity in the ewe has long been recognized. Decreasing day length was thought to stimulate the endocrine changes associated with cyclicity, but later studies have shown that the sexual season reflects a loss of an active inhibition of tonic LH secretion. The frequency of LH discharges depends on the response to the negative feedback effect of estradiol; the response is low during the breeding season, rises during transition into anestrus, and remains elevated until the onset of the next breeding season, when it diminishes again (Fig. 15–2).

How photoperiodic signals are converted to neuroendocrine messages is not fully understood. Probably, sheep detect these changes in lighting by means of a built-in biologic clock located in the hypothalamus, and this information is transmitted to the hypothalamic–gonadal axis via the pineal gland. Melatonin, a pineal hormone, mediates the response to changes in the photoperiod in sheep. Melatonin levels are high during dark periods and low during light periods; probably these differences in the pattern of melatonin secretion act as a signal indicating day length to the neuroendocrine axis.

Probably, sheep detect these changes in lighting by means of a built-in 24-hour circadian clock located in the hypothalamus, and this information is transmitted to the hypothalamic-hypophyseal-gonadal axis via the pineal gland. Melatonin (N-acetyl, 5-methoxytryptamine), which is synthesized and released by the pineal gland exclusively at night, is believed to mediate the effects of photoperiod on the cyclic activity of the ewe. A long duration of melatonin secretion signals a short day, whereas a short duration of melatonin secretion signals a long day.

How melatonin codes for day length is not known. Two theories have been proposed: the duration of nocturnal melatonin secretion and the phase of melatonin release with respect to the light–dark cycle. According to the latter hypothesis, a photoperiodic response occurs when the period of melatonin secretion coincides with the rhythm of sensitivity to melatonin entrained by the light–dark cycle. In

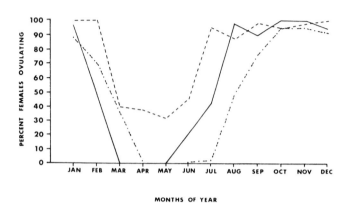

FIG. 15–1. Seasonal cycle of reproductive activity in goats and two types of sheep.

sheep, however, the evidence favors the first hypothesis. Under natural environmental conditions, a loss of response to the melatonin signal contributes to the cessation of the breeding season.

Male

The ram does not show a restricted mating season, but sexual activity is highest in the fall and declines in late winter, spring, and summer. Decreasing (or short) day lengths stimulate the secretion of FSH, LH, and testosterone in rams, while increasing (or long) day lengths inhibit these hormones.

Breeds differ in the magnitude of serum gonadotropin and testosterone secretion of mature rams in response to changes in day length. These differences are apparent during short days when the hypothalamo-pituitary-testis axis is most active.

The sexual activity of the buck (male goat) is also influenced by day length. Peak sexual activity occurs during the fall and coincides with the sharp rise in plasma testosterone level during the fall breeding season.

PUBERTY

Female

Puberty, the age at first ovulation, occurs at 5 to 7 months in does and 6 to 9 months in ewes (Table 15–2). Finewool or Merino sheep and the Angora goat fail to reach puberty during the first sexual season. Consequently, they may be 18 to 20 months old at first estrus. Early maturing breeds such as the pigmy goat or the Finn-sheep may reach puberty as early as 3 or 4 months.

The onset of puberty in sheep is influenced by genetic and environmental factors such as breed and strain differences, the nutritional planes and time of birth. First estrus occurs in ewe lambs at 30- to 50-kg body weight (50 to 70% of adult weight).

Many of the endocrine mechanisms leading to ovulation and first estrus are capable of operating long before they are called on to function. Ewe lambs born in the spring have tonic and surge modes of LH secretion and can attain puberty at 20 weeks of age, but the season delays pu-

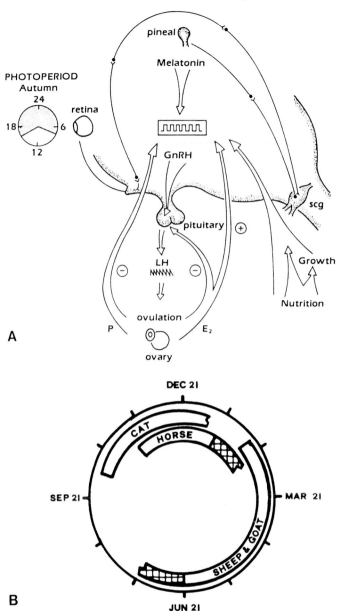

PHOTOPERIOD
Autumn

A

B

<figure>

FIG. 15–2. *A.* The events leading to first ovulation in ewe lambs at puberty or in adult ewes at the beginning of the sexual season. (From Foster et al. (1985). Neuroendocrine regulation of puberty by nutrition an photoperiod. *In* Adolescence in Females. S. Venturoli et al. (eds.). Chicago, Year Book Medical Publishers.)
B. Effects of photoperiod on ovarian activity in the sheep and goat at a latitude of 38.5° north (California). The open bars represent periods of ovarian inactivity (anestrus). The transition from anestrous to estrous (often erratic) is shown by the cross-hatched portion of the bars for the horse, sheep, and goat. (From Stabenfeldt, G.H. and Edqvist, L. (1984). Female reproductive processes. *In* Dukes' Physiology of Domestic Animals. 10th Ed. M.J. Swenson (ed.). Ithaca, NY, Cornell University Press.)
</figure>

berty in lambs born in spring until the fall when they are about 30 to 35 weeks of age. By contrast, lambs born in the fall are 30 weeks old during the adult anestrous season, but ovulations are delayed until shortly after the onset of the breeding season at which time they are 50 weeks old.

The physiologic events leading to puberty in the ewe lamb are analogous to those that regulate the onset of the sexual season in the adult ewe (Figs. 15–2 and 15–

3). Both internal and external cues time puberty, and diet affects the attainment of puberty through changes in LH secretion. Once growth requirements for sexual maturity have been satisfied, photoperiod cues are used to time the onset of puberty to the season of decreasing day length. Only ewe lambs that have been exposed to long hours of daylight, then to short hours of daylight, can accelerate their sexual development (Colas et al., 1987).

TABLE 15–2. Reproductive Parameters of Ewes and Does

Parameter	Ewe	Doe
Sexual season	Fall	Fall
Age at puberty (months)	6–9	5–7
Estrous cycle		
Length (days)	17	21
	(14–19)	(18–22)
Estrus (hours)	24–36	24–48
Ovulation		
Type	Spontaneous	Spontaneous
Time from onset (hours)	24–27	24–36
Number per cycle	1–3	2–3
Life span of corpus luteum (days)	14	16
Fertilizable life of ova (hours)	10–25	?
Entry of ova into uterus (hours after ovulation)	72	?
Gestation length (days)	149	149
Postpartum intervals (days)		
Uterine involution	27	?
First ovulation	<20	?

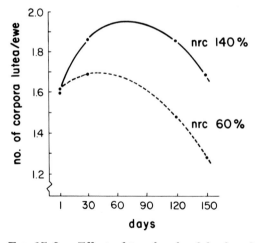

FIG. 15–3. Effect of two levels of feed and advance of breeding season on an average number of corpora lutea per ewe. (Feed levels were 60% and 140% of the National Research Council recommendations for maintenance; day 1 = September 9.)

Male

Puberty in the ram and buck is associated with a marked increase in testosterone secretion, spermatogenesis, and mating behavior. Testis size increases when ram lambs reach 8 to 10 weeks of age at body weights of 16 to 20 kg. This coincides with the appearance of primary spermatocytes and the enlargement of seminiferous tubules. In both species, copulation with ejaculation of viable spermatozoa occurs at about 4 to 6 months of age with live weights of 40 to 60% of mature weight.

As with the ewe lamb, the first exposure of ram lambs born in autumn to long hours of daylight, then to short hours of daylight accelerates their sexual development, depending on the breed (Colas et al., 1987). Serum testosterone rises at an earlier age in the goat (17 to 20 months) than in the ram lamb (25 to 28 months) (Chakraborty et al., 1989). As in cattle, sexual maturity is better correlated with body weight than age in both species.

In the ram, studies have addressed reproductive behavior (Hogg, 1984), hormonal profile (Hoaglund and Bolt, 1986), photoperiod control of LH secretion (Pelletier, 1986), functional arteriovenous anastomoses between the testicular artery and the pampiniform plexus of the spermatic cord (Noordhuizen-Stassen et al., 1985), the effects of photoperiod and nutrition on the testicular size of rams (Lindsay et al., 1984), semen characteristics after vasectomy (Thwaites, 1982), and retrograde flow of sperm in the urinary bladder (Pineda et al., 1987).

ESTROUS CYCLE

Length of Cycle

The length of the normal estrous cycle is 17 days for sheep and 21 days for goats, although considerable variation that is due to breed differences, stage of the breeding season, and environmental stress occurs in both species (Table 15–2). Abnormally short cycles observed in the ewe and the doe early in the breeding season may be associated with prematurely regressing corpus luteum (CL) or anovulation.

Duration of Estrus

Estrus lasts 24 to 36 hours in the ewe and 24 to 48 hours in the doe (Table 15–2). Duration of estrus is influenced by breed, age, season, and presence of the male. Wool breeds have longer estrous periods than meat breeds. Angora goats have a shorter duration of estrus (22 hours) than the dairy breeds. Estrus is of shorter duration in both species at the beginning and end of the breeding season, in the presence of the male, and in the first breeding season of young females.

Signs of Estrus

Signs of estrus are more conspicuous in does than ewes. A doe in estrus is restless, bleats frequently, and wags her tail constantly and rapidly; she may have a reduced appetite and a decreased milk production. Estrus in the ewe is relatively inconspicuous and is not evident in the absence of the ram. The vulva may be edematous, and a mucous discharge from the vagina may be evident in both species. A doe may occasionally exhibit homosexual behavior but not the ewe. Without the presence of the male, however, estrus is difficult to detect in both the ewe and the doe.

Male Influence on Estrus

The introduction of rams to ewes during the transition from the anestrous season to the breeding season stimulates them to ovulate within 3 to 6 days, and estrous activity occurs 17 to 24 days later. The CL of the first ovulation regresses prematurely in about half the ewes and is followed by a second ovulation associated with normal luteal activity. How this "ram effect" stimulates ewes to ovulate is not known, but ovulation is preceded by LH peaks that occur within 48 hours after ram introduction. The response of anovular ewes to the ram is due to an androgen-dependent pheromone secreted by the sebaceous glands of the ram.

The introduction of a buck into a group of seasonally anestrous dairy does not only may hasten the onset of the breeding season by several days but can also effectively synchronize them. Most seasonally anestrous does are detected in estrus within 6 days after introduction of the buck, and this is followed by ovulation and normal corpus luteum function. A period of sexual isolation is necessary to obtain a male effect in sheep, but brief contacts of the ewes with rams will not compromise a subsequent use of the male effect (Cohen-Tannoudji et al., 1987). Thus, ovulation induced by the "male effect" is more effective in the doe than the ewe.

OVULATION

Both the ewe and the doe are spontaneous ovulators (Table 15–2). The ewe normally ovulates near the end of estrus about 24 to 27 hours after the onset of estrus. Most goat breeds ovulate between 24 and 36 hours after onset of estrus, but the Nubian goat ovulates later, which is possibly due to a longer estrous cycle in this breed. Ovulation without estrus occurs before the onset of the breeding season in Nubian and other breeds of goats. The sequence of hormonal events during the estrous cycle is similar in both species, but the doe has a longer progesterone phase than the ewe.

Ovulation Rate

In many breeds of sheep and goat, two or more ova are shed during estrus. The ovulation rate is 1.2 for Merinos and 3 for the Finnish Landrace breed. In both species, the ovulation rate increases with age and reaches a maximum at 3 to 6 years, then declines gradually.

Among the environmental factors influencing ovulation rate, season and level of nutrition are important. Generally, ovulation rates are higher early in the breeding season than later (Fig. 15–4). "Flushing," or increasing the level of nutrition before mating, is commonly practiced in sheep to increase ovulation rate, but factors such as body size, weight, condition, and geno-

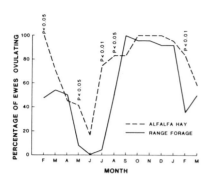

FIG. 15–4. The effects of two nutritional environments on the incidence of ovulation in sheep over 15 months. (From Hulet et al. (1986). Effects of nutritional environment and ram effect on breeding season in range sheep. *Theriogenology 25*, 317.)

type may also contribute to the increase in ovulation rate.

The highly fertile breeds of sheep include the Finnish Landrace, Romanov, Booroola Merino, and the D'Man breed. The high ovulation rate of the Booroola Merino is due to the action of a single gene, whereas in the Romanov, ovulation is under polygenic control. In all these high fecund breeds, a positive association exists between ovulation rate and plasma FSH in the periovulatory period (Bindon et al., 1986).

Driancourt et al. (1985) investigated ovarian follicular populations and preovulatory enlargement in Booroola and Merino ewes; Murdoch (1985) evaluated follicular determinants of ovulation. Various parameters in reproductive physiology of the ewe have been studied in depth: the role of retinal photoreceptors in the photoperiodic control of seasonal breeding (Legan and Karsch, 1983); ultrastructural changes in the epithelium of the oviduct (Hollis et al., 1984); sperm transport and release in the oviduct and preovulatory sequestering of cells in the caudal isthmus (Hunter et al., 1982; Hunter and Nichol, 1983); the time required for sperm to reside in the vagina to ensure conception (Tilbrook and Pearce, 1986); pregnancy di-

agnosis (Trapp and Slyter, 1983); and antiluteolytic activity of the conceptus during early pregnancy (Lacroix and Kann, 1986). Cummins et al. (1986) increased the ovulation rate by immunization of Merino sheep with a fraction of bovine follicular fluid containing inhibin activity.

BREEDING AND CONCEPTION

Most of the world population of sheep and goats is managed under free grazing conditions where natural mating is widely practiced. Unlike with cattle, artificial insemination (AI) of sheep and goats has been generally limited, owing to the high cost of labor, difficulty of accurately identifying superior sires, and low conception rates, especially with frozen semen.

Both the ram and the buck ejaculate a small volume of semen with a high concentration of spermatozoa (Table 15–3). Rams may copulate two or three times in a few minutes when first turned with ewes in estrus. They generally mate more frequently when more than one ewe is in estrus. The number of matings per day varies with individual males and with the climate and time when rams are introduced into breeding. Certain breeds copulate more frequently than other breeds. Normally, one adult ram is assigned to 30 ewes and one buck to 50 does.

Rams continuously bred produce volumes of semen and numbers of spermatozoa per ejaculate that are well below those considered adequate for AI. Ewes mated more than once are more likely to con-

TABLE 15–3. Reproductive Characteristics of the Ram and Buck

Characteristic	Ram	Buck
Age at puberty (months) (spermatogenesis)	4–6	4–6
Sexual season	None	None
Duration of seminiferous epithelial cycle (days)	10.3	?
Semen		
Volume (ml)	0.8–1.2	0.1–1.5
Concentration (billion/ml)	1.5	2–6
Mating (male:females)	1:30	1:50

ceive than those mated only once. Apparently, a ewe must accumulate adequate numbers of spermatozoa from several matings either with the same or with different rams before conception can occur.

The sudden introduction of the buck may induce estrus in many does in 1 day. This can result in many does not being mated. Breeding males may serve does as much as 20 times a day.

Copulation usually occurs before ovulation, and therefore spermatozoa are present in the oviduct by this time. Other spermatozoa are stored in the cervix (up to 3 days) and are continually released into the uterus, where they survive for about 30 hours. Eggs may remain viable for 10 to 25 hours, but abnormal development and lowered viability appear to increase with the age of either the sperm or ovum. In both species, eggs enter the uterus about 72 hours after ovulation.

GESTATION AND PARTURITION

Gestation

The normal gestation length for both species is about 149 days; the length varies between breeds and individuals (Table 15–4). In sheep, the early maturing breeds and the highly prolific breeds have shorter gestation periods than the slow-maturing wool breeds. Individual gestation periods within a breed vary up to 13 days. Gestation lengths for most breeds of goats are within 2 days of the species average, the exception being the Black Bengal breed, which averages 144 days (Table 15–4).

Heredity plays an important role in determining gestation length. The genotype of the fetus accounts for almost two thirds of the variation in gestation length of sheep. Male lambs are carried longer than female lambs, spring-born lambs longer than fall-born lambs, and singles longer than twins. Gestation length also increases with age of the dam.

The CL of pregnancy persists throughout gestation, but the two species differ in the source of progesterone for pregnancy maintenance. The sheep is a placenta-dependent species, whereas the goat is a CL-dependent species. During the first trimester, both species depend on the CL. Later, the placenta becomes the primary source of progesterone in the sheep, whereas the CL continues as the major source in the goat. Therefore, ovariectomy in the goat at any stage of pregnancy causes abortion.

Parturition

The fetus plays the key role in initiating parturition in both species, but parturition is preceded by regression of the CL in the goat.

Parturitions are spread throughout the day. Behavior of the ewe largely depends on the ease of parturition, but generally, the initial restlessness is broken by periods of lying, which are due to abdominal pain. Most lambs and kids are born head and forefeet foremost (anterior presentation). The duration of birth varies widely, particularly with a single oversized lamb or kid, with twins impacted in the birth canal, or with an abnormal presentation.

Twin births are usually more rapid than single births, but the interval between delivery of twins varies from a few minutes

TABLE 15–4. Gestation Lengths and Litter Sizes of Different Breeds of Sheep and Goats

Species	Breed	Gestation (days)	Litter size
Sheep	Wool breeds		
	Rambouilette	150	1.3
	Corriedale	150	1.5
	Merino	150	1.0
	Meat breeds		
	Dorset	144	1.4
	Suffolk	147	1.4
	Hampshire	145	1.4
	Prolific breeds		
	Finnsheep	144	2.7
	Romanov	145	2.3
Goats	Alpine	152	1.8
	Anglo-Nubian	148	2.1
	Angora	150	1.2
	Saanen	154	1.8
	Toggenburg	152	1.8
	Jamnapari	150	1.1
	Black Bengal	144	2.1

to an hour or more. Goats may be more efficient than sheep in recognizing that they have had twins.

Vigorous licking (grooming) and eating of any fetal membranes adhering to the neonate commence immediately after birth. Fetal fluids appear to play a critical role in attracting the ewe to her lamb. Ewes that have not yet lambed are attracted to the fluids and to the newborn lambs of other ewes, which leads to "lamb stealing."

Most lambs are standing within 15 minutes of birth, and within an hour or two, most ewes will allow the lamb to move toward the udder. The doe spends more time vigorously grooming and orienting the first-born, so that the second born, which is usually the weaker of the two, has a greater opportunity to suckle.

The "critical period" of attachment of the ewe to the lamb is short; if the lamb is removed at birth, it will be rejected by the ewe when presented to her 6 to 12 hours later. Some primiparous ewes display little interest and abandon their newborn lambs. Aberrant maternal behavior is more common with twin births, especially among Merinos.

The sheep is a classic example of a "follower species" as distinct from goats, a "hider species": that is, the young tend to follow their mothers from birth rather than lie hidden for several days while the dams are absent. Goats appear to be "hiders" for the first few days after birth, as judged by the behavior of feral goats in mountainous country, and there is a clear preference for maternal isolation at the time of birth.

Advancing the Breeding Season

A gestation length of about 150 days makes it possible for a ewe and doe to produce offspring more than once a year. But because of seasonal anestrus in ewes and does in the temperate zone latitudes, they do not cycle after parturition in the spring until the fall (autumn), with the result that only one lamb or kid crop per year is possible. If both species could be induced to breed during seasonal anestrus, they would give birth in the breeding season, thereby producing two crops annually.

Several methods can be used to induce breeding during seasonal anestrus in the ewe. They include a combination of progesterone and eCG, the "ram effect," altering day length by artificial lighting (8 hours light followed by 16 hours of darkness), and more recently with exogenous melatonin. The commercial availability of subcutaneous implants of melatonin provides a practical method of obtaining out of season breeding in seasonally anestrous breeds of sheep. The implant exposes the ewe to melatonin for 30 to 40 days, resulting in normal ovarian cyclicity in most ewes. Thus, melatonin will advance the normal breeding season so that ewes can be mated in spring or early summer, but it will not extend the breeding season if it is administered in the middle of the breeding season. In the seasonally anestrous goat breeds, the administration of melatonin to anestrous does will not significantly advance the breeding season.

PUERPERIUM

Changes occurring in the reproductive system during the puerperium include uterine involution and resumption of ovarian activity. Most of the data on the puerperium refer to sheep with a dearth of information for the goat.

In sheep, uterine involution is completed by 27 days and precedes the first estrus postpartum. No information is available for the doe. Since ewes and does are seasonal breeders, postpartum intervals to first estrus and ovulation are markedly affected by the season of parturition. The interval may be as short as 5 to 6 weeks in both sheep and goats or as long as 10 weeks in sheep and 27 weeks in some breeds of goats. If parturitions occur during the breeding season, both ewes and does will resume ovarian activity and conceive. The first postpartum ovulation in ewes that lamb during the breeding season occurs within 20 days and is not associated with overt estrus. Factors other than season that influence the resumption of ovarian activity include suckling, breed, nutrition and environmental temperature.

REPRODUCTIVE PERFORMANCE

Reproductive Efficiency

Reproductive efficiency depends on conception rate (fertility) or the proportion of ewes mated that conceive, the lambing rate (fecundity) or the number of lambs born of ewes lambing, and the lambing percentage or the number of lambs born per 100 ewes exposed. These rates depend on ovulation rate (number of eggs shed per estrus), which sets the upper limit for lambing percentage. Prolificacy is the relative number of live offspring produced in a given interval, such as a year. Similar methods are used to measure reproductive performance in the doe.

Conception rates are about 85% in mature sheep and goats in temperate zones during midbreeding season. The average lambing rate is about 150%. Marked differences occur in ovulation rate as a result of breed, age, year, season, and nutrition. Fertility is depressed near the equator near the beginning and the end of the breeding season. Fertility is also depressed during hot weather, in undernourished or overly fat females, in young and old females, when the estrogen content of forage is high, and when the females are parasitized or suffering from disease or other stress. Ovulation rate can be increased by changing the plane of nutrition ("flushing"). Ewes in normal body condition respond to flushing during the early part of the breeding season and during the late breeding season but not during midseason. Crossbreeding with breeds with a high ovulation rate (e.g., Booroola, Finn, and Romanov) may increase lamb crops by 250 to 400% and also may shorten lambing intervals.

Goals in the tropics maintain high fertility and twinning rates. Heat stress and insufficient nutrition depress the reproductive performance of temperate breeds of sheep and goats. This depression in the reproductive performance can be alleviated by crossing them with tropical breeds. Indigenous goat breeds in the tropics kid at intervals of 240 to 390 days, but some Indian breeds of goats such as the Jamnapari and Barbari have more than one kidding per year.

Artificial Regulation of Reproduction

Seasonality in reproduction limits reproductive rate of both the ewe and doe to one parturition per year. Manipulation of reproduction by genetic, physiologic, and environmental methods could increase the frequency of breeding per year and the litter size in these species.

Frequency of Breeding. A gestation length of approximately 150 days makes it possible for a ewe and doe to produce offspring more than once per year. Several methods have been investigated to reduce the lambing interval from once per year to three times in 2 years (8-month interval) or twice a year (6-month lambing interval).

Progestogen combined with equine chorionic gonadotropins (eCG/PMSG) was one of the earliest methods of inducing ovarian activity in anestrous ewes during the nonbreeding season; fertility rates averaged 30 to 60% at the induced estrus. Later, the "ram effect" mentioned previously was applied for out of season breeding. For example, Australian Merino, French Prealpes, and Ile de France, which have a restricted breeding season, could be made to breed in response to male stimulation at other times of the year.

Altering the day-length pattern by artificial lighting can increase the breeding frequency in sheep but has limited application. The discovery that melatonin can substitute for darkness may be used to mimic changes in reproductive activity of shortened day length. Feeding melatonin to seasonally anestrous ewes advanced the onset of the breeding season; this method may have future application in sheep breeding.

Litter Size. Practical methods are available for increasing ovulation rate which sets the upper limit for litter size. "Flushing" is widely used to increase ovulation rate. Ewes in normal body condition respond to flushing during the early part of the breeding season and during the late breeding season but not during mid-season.

Exogenous gonadotropins (eCG/PMSG) are employed to induce multiple ovulation in both species, but the response to the dose is highly variable and leads to embryonic losses. An alternative approach to gonadotropin therapy (twinning) is steroid immunization, which has a consistent response. Immunity to estrone or androstenedione leads to an increased frequency of LH pulses in anestrous ewes and to elevated levels of FSH in the case of estrone; the ovulation rate is increased by 0.6 ovulations per ewe. The technique involves two injections at 3- to 4-week intervals before ram introduction. The increase in ovulation rate was reflected by a 30 to 40% increase in the lambs reared; this technique may have future application in sheep breeding.

Although the heritability of fertility and fecundity appears to be low, prolificacy of sheep has been increased through selection. The most important traits of the Finn sheep and the Romanov ewe are their high prolificacy in lamb crops of 250 to 400% and their shorter lambing intervals. Therefore, systematic crossbreeding with these breeds could lengthen the natural breeding season and increase litter size of traditional breeds.

Extensive investigations were conducted on dairy and meat goats with emphasis on the following: seasonal breeding of dairy goats (Mohammad et al., 1984), estrus synchronization (Ott et al., 1980) reproductive efficiency (Erasmus et al., 1985; Thompson et al., 1983); hormonal profiles (Forsyth et al., 1985; Wathes et al.,

1986); semen-collection techniques (Memon et al, 1986); semen characteristics (Ali and Mustafa, 1986); sperm output, testicular sperm reserve, and epididymal storage capacity (Daudu, 1984); semen cryopreservation (Ritar and Salamon, 1983; Salamon et al., 1982); induction of luteolysis with prostaglandins (Bretzlaff et al., 1983); and removal of corpora lutea in pregnant goats and the effects of intrauterine indomethacin (Cooke and Knifton, 1980). Extensive investigations were also carried out on reproductive behavior, gonadal activity, testicular dimensions, and semen characteristics of the tropical creole meat goat (Chemineau, 1986a, 1986b; Chemineau and Xanda, 1982); embryo transfer (Armstrong and Evans, 1983); goat and sheep hybrids (Basrur, 1986); and intersex and freemartins (Basrur and McKinnon, 1986).

REFERENCES

Ali, B.H. and Mustafa, A.I. (1986). Semen characteristics of nubian goats in the Sudan. Anim. Reprod. Sci. *12*, 63.

Armstrong, D.T. and Evans, G. (1983). Factors influencing success of embryo transfer in sheep and goats. Theriogenology *19*, 31.

Basrur, P.K. (1986). Goat–sheep hybrids. *In* Current Therapy in Theriogenology, vol 2. D.A. Morrow (ed.). Philadelphia, W.B. Saunders.

Basrur, P.K. and McKinnon, A.O. (1986). Caprine intersexes and freemartins. *In* Current Therapy in Theriogenology, 2. D.A. Morrow (ed.). Philadelphia, W.B. Saunders.

Bindon, B.M., Piper, L.R., Cahill, L.P., Driancourt, M.A. and O'Shea, T. (1986). Genetic and hormonal factors affecting superovulation. Theriogenology *25*, 53.

Bretzlaff, K.N., Hill, A. and Ott, R.S. (1983). Induction of Luteolysis in goats with prostaglandin $F_{2\alpha}$. Am. J. Vet. Res. *44*, 1162.

Chemineau, P. (1986a). Sexual behaviour and gonadal activity during the year in the tropical creole meat goat. I. Female oestrous behaviour and ovarian activity. Reprod. Nutr. Dev. *26*, 441.

Chemineau, P. (1986b). Sexual behaviour and gonadal activity during the year in the tropical creole meat goat. II. Male mating behaviour, testis diameter, ejaculate characteristics and fertility. Reprod. Nutr. Dev. *26*, 453.

Chemineau, P. and Xande, A. (1982). Reproductive efficiency of creole meat goats permanently kept with males. Relationship to a tropical environment. Trop. Anim. Prod. *7*, 98.

Cooke, R.G. and Knifton, A. (1980). Removal of corpora lutea in pregnant goats: effects of intrauterine indomethacin. Res. Vet. Sci. *29*, 77.

Chakraborty, P.K., Stuart, L.D. and Brown, J.L. (1989). Puberty in the male Nubian goat: serum concentrations of LH, FSH and testosterone from birth through puberty and semen characteristics at sexual maturity. Anim. Reprod. Sci. *20*, 91.

Cohen-Tannoudji, J. and Signoret, J.P. (1987). Effect of short exposure to the ram on later reactivity of anoestrous ewes to the male effect. Anim. Reprod. Sci. *13*, 263.

Colas, G., Guerin, Y., Briois, M. and Ortavani, R. (1987). Photoperiodic control of testicular growth in the ram lamb. Anim. Reprod. Sci. *13*, 255.

Cognie, Y., (1988). Applications of immunological techniques to enhance reproductive performance in the ewe. Proc. 11th Int. Congr. Anim. Reprod and AI. Vol. 5, p. 192. University College, Dublin.

Cummins, L.J., O'Shea, T.O., Al-Obaidi, S.A.R. et al. (1986). Increase in ovulation rate after immunization of merino ewes with a fraction of bovine follicular fluid containing inhibin activity. J. Reprod. Fertil. *77*, 365.

Daudu, C.S. (1984). Spermatozoa output, testicular sperm reserve and epididymal storage capacity of the red sokoto goats indigenous to Northern Nigeria. Theriogenology *21*, 317.

Driancourt, M.A., Cahill, L.P. and Bindon, B.M. (1985). Ovarian follicular populations and preovulatory enlargement in booroola and control merino ewes. J. Reprod. Fertil. *73*, 93.

Erasmus J.A., Fourie A.J. and Venter, J.J. (1985). Influence of age on reproductive performance of the improved Boer goat doe. S. Afr. J. Anim. Sci. *15*, 5.

Forsyth, I.A., Byatt, J.C. and Iley, S. (1985). Hormone concentrations, mammary development and milk yield in goats given long-term bromocriptine treatment in pregnancy. J. Endocrinol. *104*, 77.

Hoaglund, T.A. and Bolt, D.J. (1986). Serum follicle stimulating hormone, luteinizing hormone, and testosterone in sexually stimulated intact and unilaterally castrated rams. Theriogenology *26*, 671.

Hogg, J.T. (1984). Mating in bighorn sheep: multiple creative male strategies. Science *225*, 526.

Hollis, D.E., Frith, P.A., Vaughan, J.D. et al. (1984). Ultrastructural changes in the oviductal epithelium of merino ewes during the estrous cycle. Am. J. Anat. *171*, 441.

Hunter, R.H.F., Barbwise, L. and King, R. (1982). Sperm transport, storage and release in the sheep oviduct in relation to the time of ovulation. Br. Vet. J. *138*, 225.

Hunter, R.H.F. and Nichol, R. (1983). Transport of spermatozoa in the sheep oviduct: preovulatory sequestering of cells in the caudal isthmus. J. Exp. Zool. *228*, 121.

Lacroix, M.C. and Kann, G. (1986). Aspects of the antiluteolytic activity of the conceptus during early pregnancy in ewes. J. Anim. Sci. *63*, 1449.

Legan, S.J. and Karsch, F.J. (1983). Importance of retinal photoreceptors to photoperiodic control of seasonal breeding in the ewe. Biol. Reprod. *29*, 316.

Lindsay, D.R., Pelletier, J., Pisselet, C. et. al. (1984). Changes in photoperiod and nutrition and their affect on testicular growth of rams. J. Reprod. Fertil. *71*, 351.

Memon, M.A., Bretzlaff, K.N. and Ott, R.S. (1986). Comparison of semen collection techniques in goats. Theriogenology *26*, 823.

Mohammad, W.A., Grossman, M. and Vatthauer, J.L. (1984). Seasonal breeding in United States dairy goats. J. Dairy Sci. *67*, 1813.

Murdoch, W.J. (1985). Follicular determinants of ovulation in the ewe. Domest. Anim. Endocrinol. *2*, 105.

Noordhuizen-Stassen, E.N., Charbon, G.A., deJong, F.H. et al (1985). Functional arteriovenous anastomoses between in testicular artery and the pampiniform plexus in the spermatic cord of rams. J. Reprod. Fertil. *75*, 193.

Ott, R.S., Nelson, D.R. and Hixon, J.E. (1980). Peripheral serum progesterone and luteinizing hormone concentrations of goats during synchronization of estrus and ovulation with prostaglandin $F_{2\alpha}$. Am. J. Vet. Res. *41*, 1432.

Pelletier, J. (1986). Contribution of increasing and decreasing daylength to the photoperiodic control of LH secretion in the Ile-de-France ram. J. Reprod. Fertil. *77*, 505.

Pineda, M.H., Dooley, M.P., Hembrough, F.B. et al. (1987). Retrograde flow of spermatozoa into the urinary bladder of rams. Am. J. Vet. Res. *48*, 562.

Ritar, A.J. and Salamon, S. (1983). Fertility of fresh and frozen-thawed semen of the angora goat. Aust. J. Biol. Sci. *36*, 49.

Salamon S. and Ritar, A.J. (1982). Deep freezing of angora goat semen: effects of diluent composition, method and rate of dilution on survival of spermatozoa. Aust. J. Biol. Sci. *35*, 295.

Thompson, F.N., Abrams, E. and Miller, D.M. (1983). Reproductive traits in Nubian dairy goats. Anim. Reprod. Sci. *6*, 59.

Thwaites, C.J. (1982). Semen quality after vasectomy in the ram. Livestock Prod. Sci. *8*, 529.

Tilbrook, A.J. and Pearce, D.T. (1986). Time required for spermatozoa to remain in the vagina of the ewe to ensure conception. Aust. J. Biol. Sci. *39,* 305.

Trapp, M.J. and Slyter, A.L. (1983). Pregnancy diagnosis in the ewe. J. Anim. Sci. *57,* 1.

Wathes, D.C., Swann, R.W., Porter, D.G. et al. (1986). Oxytocin as an ovarian hormone. Curr Top. Neuroendocrinol. *6,* 129.

16
Pigs

L.L. ANDERSON

SEXUAL DEVELOPMENT AND MATURATION

Genetic sex determines the development of gonadal sex, which in turn determines phenotypic and reproductive capacities. The Y chromosome and genes located on the autosomes are critical to the development of gonads, which are eventually capable of spermatogenesis. These are necessary indirectly for the development of the male reproductive system, body sex, and typical male behavioral characteristics. The porcine embryo has 38 ($2n$) chromosomes.

The gonadal anlage develops on the inner aspect of the mesonephros, which consists of coelomic epithelium, underlying mesenchyme, and primordial germ cells. The germ cells have an extraregional origin. Sex differentiation of the undifferentiated primordium begins when gonads differentiate into genetic males (Table 16–1). The Y-encoded testis-determining gene has been named *TDF* (*testis-determining factor*) in humans and *Tdy* (*testis-determining Y chromosome*) in mice. In eutherian mammals, evidence suggests that sex determination is equivalent to testis determination. A 35-kilobase region of the Y-specific sequence immediately adjacent to the pseudoautosomal boundary in which TDF must reside has been identified as a new gene in the human Y chromosome (Sinclair et al., 1990). This gene is conserved and Y-specific among a wide range of mammals (including the pig) and encodes a testis-specific transcript.

In testicular organogenesis, the germ cells are attracted to and encapsulated with somatic cells, initially in arrangements as seminiferous cords, which are delineated by connective tissue. The cords of cells eventually hollow into seminiferous tubules with connections to mesonephric tubules. Somatic cells within the seminiferous tubules differentiate into sustentacular cells (supporting or Sertoli cells). Between seminiferous tubules, mesenchymal cells differentiate into interstitial cells (Leydig cells). The testis then produces hormones that induce normal male phenotypic development.

In the genetic female, oogenesis occurs later with the obvious feature being the absence of testicular-inducing patterns of organogenesis. The surface epithelium of the presumptive ovary becomes separated from the central cellular mass. The ovarian cortex proliferates, and germ cells (oogonia) within this region transform into oocytes and enter early phases of premeiosis before they become separated from mesenchyme by a single layer of differentiating follicle cells. The follicles presumably prevent oocytes from entering meiotic processes beyond the diplotene phase. The primary follicles remain in this resting stage of development until puberty.

Mesonephric tubules stabilize in the male embryo as the wolffian ducts (e.g., epididymides, vas deferens, seminal vesicles, and prostate and bulbourethral glands); whereas in the female embryo, the paramesonephric tubules survive as

TABLE 16–1. Gonadal Development of Porcine Embryos

Day	Male	Female
21	Gonadal primordium	Gonadal primordium
22–24	Primitive cord cells Primordial germ cells	Primitive cord cells Primordial germ cells
26	Surface epithelium Mesenchyme Testicular cords Interstitium Testosterone production	Surface epithelium Mesenchyme Gonadal blastema
27	Sertoli cells	
29	AMH production	
30	Leydig cells	
31		Egg nests
35	3β-HSD production Testosterone maximal	
40		Meiosis of germ cells
60	Testicular descent	Primordial follicles
70		Primary follicles
90	Testes in scrotum	Secondary follicles

AMH = anti-Müllerian syndrome.

the müllerian ducts (e.g., oviducts, uterus, cervix, and the upper part of vagina). Both ducts are present in early embryonic development and are capable of developing as male or female internal and external genitalia. It seems that testes are body sex differentiators because they impose masculinity on the developing genital tract and on secondary sexual features and behavior. In their absence, or in the presence or absence of the ovaries, the genital tract and secondary sex characteristics develop as a normal female. Although the production of androgen from embryonic gonads influences development of internal and external genitalia, the secretion of anti-Müllerian hormone (AMH, or Müllerian-inhibiting substance [MIS]) by the testes seems essential for inducing the regression of the Müllerian ducts. MIS is composed of two subunits of 70,000 daltons each and is linked by disulfide bonds (Donahoe et al., 1987), and it is synthesized by Sertoli cells as early as day 27 and before the appearance of Leydig cells at day 30 of porcine fetal life. Bovine and human MISs share a high degree of homology (78%) in the primary amino acid sequences.

The gonadal primordium (ridge) in pig embryos at 21 and 22 days is composed of the surface epithelium, proliferating tissue of the primitive gonadal cords, and mesenchyme. The surface epithelium consists of columnar cells in a single layer and smaller cuboidal cells arranged in two or three layers. Primitive cord cells are derivatives of the epithelial cells. The cords are first found in the posterior part of the gonadal ridge, and by 22 days, their numbers have increased and they extend deeper into the mesenchyme. These cords are continuous with the surface epithelium. Primordial germ cells are round or elongated with diameters of 10 to 20 μm (Fig. 16–1c and e). These germ cells now undergo mitotic divisions in the gonadal ridge. The nucleus of these cells is round (i.e., 10 μm) and contains one or two nucleoli about 3 μm in diameter. The fine morphology of the germ cells is similar in both sexes at 21 and 24 days of embryonic life (Fig. 16–1e and f).

By 24 days, gonads of both sexes show further development of primitive cords in continuity with the surface epithelium (Fig. 16–1c and d). The gonadal blastema occupies space between the surface epithelium and the mesenchyme in the basal part of the gonad. In the central region, the gonadal blastema consists primarily of cells organized irregularly and is called the *blastema proper*.

At 26 and 27 days, the gonads protrude longitudinally along the medial mesonephric surface of both sexes (Fig. 16–1a and b). The testicular cords and interstitium are derived from gonadal blastema. Sustentacular cells of the testicular cords resemble primitive cord cells, and spermatogonia are similar to primordial germ cells. Interstitial cells have not yet differentiated into Leydig cells. Cells of the surface epithelium, primitive cords, mesenchyme, and primordial germ cells retain ultrastructural features that are similar in both sexes.

Gametogenesis and ovarian development in pig embryos from day 13 to birth and during the early neonatal period indicate mitotic and meiotic activities throughout these periods. The germ cells increase from approximately 5,000 at day 20 to a peak of 5,000,000 by day 50. Thereafter, germinal mitotic activity decreases and necrosis of germ cells increases. At birth, the population of germ cells is approximately 400,000. Throughout embryonic development, somatic mitotic activity follows a higher rate but a similar pattern to germinal mitotic activity. Premeiotic DNA synthesis and transformation of oogonia to oocytes continue at least to 35 days of postnatal life. Meiosis begins as early as day 40 of embryonic development. The premeiotic resting stage (diplotene) of porcine oocytes first appears by day 50 of embryonic life, and almost all germ cells are diplotene by 20 days after birth. The paucity of oogonia and absence of oogonial mitoses indicates completion of the process of oogenesis by day 100 of embryonic development.

Cellular and nuclear growth of germ cells increases greatly from the oogonial stage (13 μm in diameter) to the oocyte within a primordial follicle (27 μm in diameter). Cell sizes during early stages of meiotic prophase (leptotene, zygotene, and pachytene) are larger than those in oogonia. The oocyte remains in the diplotene stage to the time of ovulation, but it continues to increase in diameter during follicular maturation; growing follicles increase approximately threefold. The oocyte increases to a maximum diameter of 120 μm in graafian follicles near the time of ovulation, and the zona pellucida consists of a homogeneous matrix approximately 8.6 μm in thickness (Fig. 16–1h). Surface area of the cell membrane (vitelline membrane) is increased by irregularly spaced microvilli in contact with cell processes arising from coronal radiata banding the zona pellucida. Cortical granules about 0.20 μm diameter are numerous immediately beneath the oocyte membrane wall and near the Golgi complex. Other prominent features of the oocyte cytoplasm include homogeneous yolk globules, mitochondria often located near these globules, and both granular and agranular endoplasmic reticulum. The nucleus consists of an inner and outer nuclear membrane with numerous nuclear membrane pores. Within the nucleus, an eccentrically located nucleolus (about 7 μm in diameter) contains fibrils, granules, and spherical vacuoles.

Corona radiata cells are porcine granulosa cells on the outer aspect of the zona pellucida that are arranged in a radial pattern. These granulosa cells usually adhere to each other, and they project long-cell processes (microvilli) through the zona pellucida and perivitelline space, and these microvilli terminate as end bulbs in contact with the oocyte membrane wall. They are regarded as nurse cells for the growing oocyte during oogenesis; their nutritive material is conveyed by extensive cytoplasmic processes. These cells disappear soon after ovulation. Mitochondria

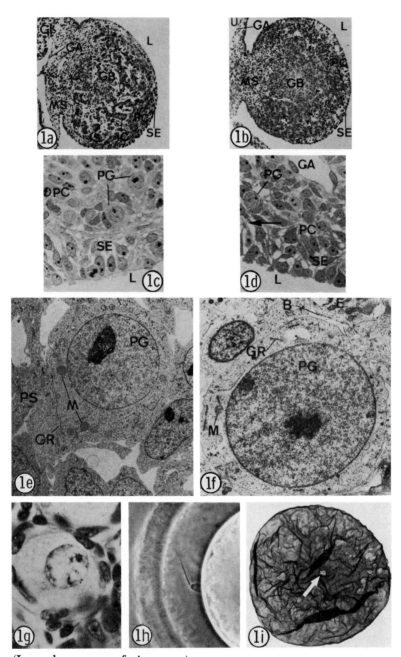

(Legend appears on facing page.)

formed in oocytes may include contributions of precursor materials from corona radiata cells, but these mechanisms are not clearly defined. The cortical granules are extruded through the vitelline membrane on contact with the fertilizing sperm.

Testicular development from the early fetal period to sexual maturity lags behind body growth from 7 to 14 weeks postcoitum. From 14 weeks postcoitum to 3 weeks postpartum, testicular growth exceeds body growth, primarily because of Leydig cell development. Although testicular weight increases in the prenatal period, a significant decrease in weight occurs 3 to 7 weeks postpartum as a result of Leydig cell regression. After 7 weeks postpartum, testicular growth again exceeds body growth, largely as a result of increases in the length and diameter of the seminiferous tubules. From 14 weeks postcoitum to 3 weeks after birth, the numbers of germ cells per testis show a constant doubling rate, but their numbers per tubule cross section decrease as a result of increasing tubular length. Morphogenesis is nearly complete by 25 weeks after birth.

HORMONE REGULATION IN THE BOAR

Porcine blastocysts are capable of synthesizing estrogens by day 12 (Fig. 16–1i). Fetal pig testes contain Δ^3-3β-hydroxysteroid dehydrogenase (3β-HSD) and thus contain steroidogenic capabilities before differentiation of Leydig cells. Histochemical evidence suggests the presence of 3β-HSD in Leydig cells by about day 35.

Testosterone concentrations in umbilical arterial serum are higher at day 35 (4 to 5 ng/ml) than concentrations either earlier or later (< 0.5 ng/ml) in fetal development. The fetal testes secrete testosterone during differentiation of the internal and external genitalia. Differentiation of the wolffian duct and development of the seminal vesicles, prostate, bulbourethral glands, and external genitalia occur between days 26 and 50. By day 29, pig testes produce sufficient AMH to induce regression of the müllerian ducts, and production of AMH by Sertoli cells lasts until after birth.

Serum testosterone concentrations are low during the later half of fetal development and increase to maximal levels by 2 weeks after birth. From 49 to 80 days postcoitum, serum LH, FSH, and prolactin remain low. These gonadotropins increase after day 90, reach peak levels during the first week after birth, and then gradually decrease by the seventh week. Testosterone production late in fetal life becomes gonadotropin dependent. Elongation of seminiferous tubules is probably increased

---

FIG. 16–1. *a.* Light micrograph of porcine fetal testis at day 26. *b.* Light micrograph of porcine fetal ovary at day 27. *c.* Light micrograph of male gonad in pig embryo at day 24. *d.* Light micrograph of female gonad in pig embryo at day 24. *e.* Electron micrograph of a cortical portion of a male gonad in pig embryo at day 24. *f.* Electron micrograph of a primordial germ cell with a prominent nucleolus of female gonad in pig embryo at day 21. *g.* Porcine oocyte in diplotene; note large eccentric nucleus. A single layer of flattened follicular cells surrounds the oocyte, thus forming a primordial follicle. *h.* Porcine spermatozoan in perivitelline space with head attached to vitelline membrane of ovum. *i.* Spherical porcine blastocyst (8.5-mm diameter with fluid-filled cavity) at day 12. Arrow indicates embryonic disc. *B,* surface epithelial basal lamina; *CA,* capillary; *E,* surface epithelial cell; *GB,* gonadal blastema; *GR,* granular endoplasmic reticulum; *IC,* interstitial cell; *IS,* interstitium; *L,* coelomic cavity; *M,* mitochondria; *MS,* mesenchyme; *PC,* primitive cords; *PG,* primordial germ cells; *PS,* pseudopod of cytoplasm; *SE,* surface epithelium. (*a* and *b.* From Pelliniemi, L.J. (1975). Am. J. Anat. *144,* 89. *c, d,* and *e.* From Pelliniemi, L.J. (1976). Cell Tissue *8,* 163. *f.* From Pelliniemi, L.J. (1975). Anat. Embryol. *147,* 19. *g.* From Black, J.L. and Erickson, B.H. (1968). Anat. Rec. *161,* 15. *h.* From Hunter, R.H.F. and Dziuk, P.J. (1968). J. Reprod. Fertil. *15,* 199. *i.* From Anderson, L.L. (1978). Anat. Rec. *190,* 143.)

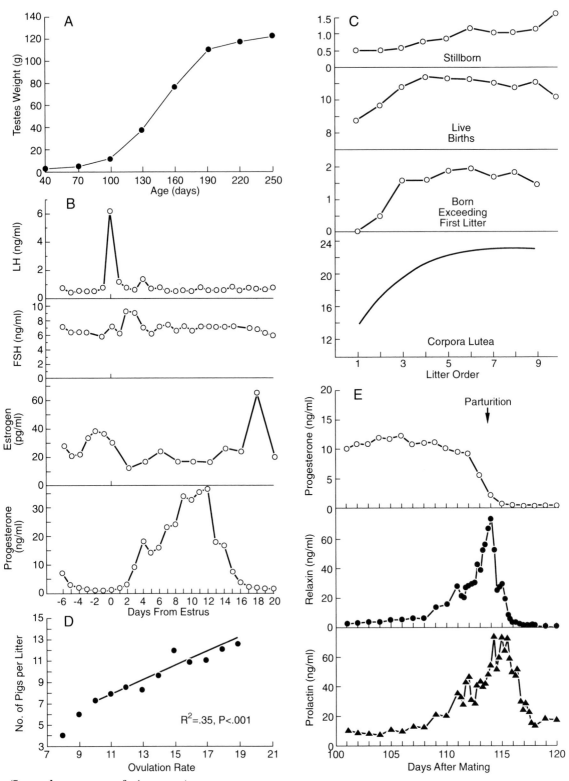

(Legend appears on facing page.)

at this time by FSH stimulation of Sertoli cells.

Testicular descent begins about day 60 postcoitum, with growth of the gubernaculum at a time when testosterone and gonadotropin blood levels are low. The testes traverse the inguinal canal in about 85 days and move to the base of the scrotum soon after birth. Patterns of LH and testosterone concentrations parallel testicular development during these prenatal and postnatal periods.

During prepubertal hypertrophy, the Leydig cells reach maximal diameters of 30 μm and show typical fine structural features that include an increase in numbers of mitochondria, development of agranular endoplasmic reticulum, and numerous cytoplasmic filaments. These and other cytoplasmic organelles resemble those in adult boars. Hypophysectomy in immature boars causes regression of the testes, epididymides, prostate, seminal vesicles, and bulbourethral glands. In mature boars, hypophysectomy results in testicular regression, decreased diameter of seminiferous tubules with ablation of spermatogenesis, reduced numbers of Leydig cells, and regression of accessory sex glands. Daily injections of human chorionic gonadotropin (hCG) re-establish the Leydig cells in these hypophysectomized animals, but the effect is transitory and essentially lost after 1 month.

From 40 to 250 days of age, the paired testes weight increases markedly (Fig. 16–2A). Testosterone concentrations in peripheral serum increase as pubertal development progresses, and concentrations decline near maturity. Estradiol-17β serum levels increase steadily throughout pubertal development, whereas LH remains relatively constant. Steroid sulfates such as dehydroepiandrosterone sulfate and the 16-androstenes may act as precursors to androgenic hormones in the boar. The estradiol-17β in the male may play a synergistic role with testosterone in sexual behavior and act on accessory sex glands as well as enhance testicular synthesis of testosterone.

In both pubertal and sexually mature boars, the intravenous injection of LH-releasing hormone (LH-RH) causes an immediate release of pituitary LH to peak values within 10 minutes. Pubertal and adult male pituitaries have similar sensitivities to LH-RH stimulation, and the circulating levels of testosterone in adult boars do not appreciably modify this response. In castrated males, plasma LH is sustained at higher basal levels, but the immediate release of LH in response to LH-RH follows a pattern similar to that in pubertal and mature boars. Testosterone and its metabolite, 5α-dihydrotestosterone (5α-DHT), provide both stimulatory and inhibitory effects on LH secretion in the boar. Direct intracerebral implantation of large amounts of 5α-DHT or testosterone into the mediobasal hypothalamus or amygdala inhibits release of LH from the pituitary gland, as reflected in lowered peripheral blood plasma levels of the gonadotropin, whereas implantation of lower amounts of these steroids in the

FIG. 16–2. *A.* Average paired testes weight in boars 40 to 240 days of age. *B.* Peripheral blood plasma concentrations of progesterone, estrogen, FSH, and LH during the estrous cycle in the pig. *C.* Reproductive performance in relation to parity in the pig. *D.* Litter size in relation to ovulation rate in primiparous gilts. *E.* Peripheral plasma concentrations of progesterone, relaxin, and prolactin during late pregnancy, parturition, and early lactation in Yorkshire gilts. (*A.* Adapted from Allrich, R.D. et al. (1982). J. Anim. Sci. *55*, 1139. *B.* Adapted from Parvizi, N. et al. (1976). J. Endocrinol. *69*, 193; Guthrie, H.D. et al. (1972). Endocrinology *91*, 675. *C.* Adapted from Lush, J.L. and Molln, A.E. (1942). Tech. Bull. U.S. Dept. Agric., 836; Rasbech, N.O. (1969). Br. Vet. J. *125*, 599. *D.* Adapted from Rhodes, M.T. et al. (1991). J. Anim. Sci. *69*, 34. *E.* Adapted from Li, Y. et al. (1991). Endocrinology *129*, 2907.)

brain elevates plasma LH levels. Thus, androgens modulate the secretion of hypothalamic hormones, which in turn control the release of LH from the adenohypophysis in the boar.

SPERM PRODUCTION

Behavior in pigs is sexually dimorphic as early as 1 month of age; mounting of penmates is observed more frequently for males than for females (Ford, 1990). Boars reach puberty at about 125 days of age. Spermatozoa are found in the testes, but there may be further delay before they are capable of fertilizing ova. Mounting activity occurs early (erection by 4 months), but sequential patterns of sexual behavior culminate after 5 months. First ejaculates occur at 5 to 8 months of age. The number of spermatozoa and the semen volume continue to increase during the first 18 months of life. The duration of one cycle of the seminiferous epithelium requires 8.6 days. On the basis of histologic features of the cells, eight stages can be described within this period, with the duration of stages one through eight being 0.9, 1.2, 0.3, 1.0, 0.8, 1.7, 1.6, and 1.0 days, respectively. The duration of the spermatogenic cycle (spermatogonia to mature spermatozoa) is approximately 34.4 days in the boar; thus, four cycles of the seminiferous epithelium occur during one spermatogenic cycle. The life span of primary spermatocytes is 12.3 days; secondary spermatocytes, 0.4 days; spermatids with round nuclei, 6.3 days; spermatids with elongated nuclei, 1.5 days, and spermatozoa, 6.2 days. The duration for transit of the spermatozoa through the epididymis is about 10.2 days. This period within the epididymides is necessary for spermatozoa to mature and acquire the ability to fertilize ova. Highest fertilization rates result with spermatozoa obtained from the proximal and distal caudal epididymidis. Testosterone sustains secretory activities of the accessory glands (e.g., seminal vesicles, prostate, bulbourethral glands), and these seminal fluids constitute a large proportion of the total ejaculate in the boar.

HORMONES AND PUBERTY IN GILTS

The fetal gonad differentiates to an ovary at about 35 days of gestation by the appearance of egg nests (Table 16–1). Primary and secondary follicles appear late in gestation. Steroidogenic activity of the fetal ovary occurs later than in the testis. FSH-secreting cells have been identified in fetuses 70 days old, and LH concentrations in the umbilical artery increase in response to LH-RH between 70 and 100 days. Serum levels of FSH, LH, and prolactin increase preceding birth. During the first 5 weeks after birth, LH and prolactin concentrations decrease, while FSH remains elevated to about 10 weeks of age. By 2 weeks after birth, the amplitude of LH pulses increases, and by 10 weeks, episodic LH release occurs spontaneously. Tertiary follicles develop at 8 weeks after birth and may indicate the period when follicular development becomes dependent on gonadotropins.

In pigs from 10 weeks of age until puberty (i.e., 25 weeks), the frequency and magnitude of serum LH peaks are greatest at 16 weeks, whereas FSH secretory spikes do not change. Spikes of FSH and prolactin occur with more than random synchrony throughout this period. The stimulatory estrogen feedback mechanism is essential to the onset of cyclic ovarian activity, but the negative feedback control of LH release by ovarian steroids is absent at birth and develops by 8 weeks of age. A negative influence by the ovary of prepubertal and postpubertal gilts is evident, but gilts respond differently to the removal of the ovaries. The LH serum levels increase within 2 days after ovariectomy of prepubertal (120 days old) and postpubertal (210 days old) gilts. The increase in LH secretion is delayed in prepubertal as compared to postpubertal gilts during the first 14 days after ovariectomy. Furthermore, the manner in which LH concentrations increase after ovariectomy is not influenced by chronologic age but rather reflects the pre- and postpubertal stage of development. The sensitivity of the hypothalamic-pituitary axis regulating LH secretion to the negative feedback action of estradiol-17β also decreases as gilts progress from the prepubertal to the postpubertal state. Infusion of LH-RH induces a significant increase in serum LH concentrations, leading to peak values (>6 ng/ml) 15 minutes later, which is followed by a decline of LH to basal levels.

During the prepubertal period, the ovaries contain numerous small follicles (2 to 4 mm diameter) and several (8 to 15) medium-sized follicles (6 to 8 mm). The uterus responds to increasing ovarian steroidogenic activity during the late stages of the prepubertal period; the uterus weighs 30 to 60 g during infantile stages as compared with 150 to 250 g in prepubertal gilts. As ovarian follicles develop in prepubertal gilts, there are corresponding increases in ovarian weights. Puberty is characterized by first estrus, ovulation of graafian follicles, and the release of ova capable of fertilization.

The age of puberty may be influenced by the level of nutrition, social environment, body weight, season of year, breed, disease or parasite infestation and management practices. Limiting energy intake to half that of the full-fed controls delays puberty more than 40 days. The presence of boars reduces age (191 vs 232 days) and body weight (105 vs 116 kg) to puberty. Puberty also is delayed in gilts penned individually as compared with those maintained in groups of 30 animals.

Progesterone concentrations in peripheral plasma during a prepubertal period of >20 days are low (e.g., 2 ng/ml) and remain low throughout the proestrous, estrous, and early metestrous periods of the first estrus. Since prepubertal gilts have no corpora lutea, the origin of the progesterone may be at least partly adrenal in origin. Profiles of progesterone during the luteal phase of the first estrous cycle follow a pattern typical of normal cycling gilts.

Maturation of ovarian follicles and ovulations can be induced by exogenous gonadotropins in prepubertal gilts after 60 days of age. For example, a single injection of pregnant mare serum gonadotropin (PMSG) followed by hCG induces ovulation in 90% of gilts 90 to 130 days of age, but few of them exhibit estrus or remain pregnant. In gilts 9 to 12 months old who have not exhibited a previous estrus, progesterone remains low (e.g., 2 ng/ml) throughout the proestrus; a similar gonadotropin regimen induces estrus, ovulation, recurrent estrous cycles, and normal fertility in a high percentage. Injection of LH-RH also induces ovulations in prepubertal gilts, and the corpora lutea from those ovulations sustain pregnancies.

ESTROUS CYCLE

Onset of estrus is characterized by gradual changes in behavioral patterns (e.g., restlessness, mounting of other animals, lordosis response), vulva responses (e.g., swelling, pink-red coloring), and occasionally a mucous discharge. Sexual receptivity lasts an average of 40 to 60 hours. The pubertal estrous period usually is shorter (47 hours) than later ones (56 hours), and gilts usually have a shorter period of estrus than sows. Breed, seasonal variation (e.g., longest estrus in summer and shortest in winter) and endocrine abnormalities affect the duration of heat.

Ova are released 38 to 42 hours after the onset of estrus, and the duration of this ovulatory process requires 3.8 hours. Ovulations occur about 4 hours earlier in mated than in unmated animals.

The length of the cycle is about 21 days (range: 19 to 23 days). The pig is polyestrous throughout the year; only pregnancy or endocrine dysfunction interrupts this cyclicity.

Ovarian Morphology and Hormone Secretion

There are about 50 small follicles (i.e., 2 to 5 mm in diameter) per animal, during the luteal and early follicular phases of the cycle. During the proestrous and estrous phases, about 10 to 20 follicles approach preovulatory size (8 to 11 mm), while the number of smaller follicles declines (those < 5 mm). During the luteal phase of the cycle, which occurs between days 5 and 16, the number of follicles 2 to 5 mm in diameter (with a few up to 7 mm) increases; whereas after day 18 (proestrous phase), an increase occurs primarily in the growth of preovulatory follicles (those ≥ 8 mm in diameter).

Soon after ovulation there is rapid proliferation of primarily granulosa and a few theca cells lining the follicle wall. These cells become luteinized to form luteal tissue thus the corpus luteum (CL). Initially, the corpus is considered a corpus hemorrhagicum because of the blood-filled central cavity, but within 6 to 8 days, the CL is a solid mass of luteal cells with an overall diameter of 8 to 11 mm. The relatively long luteal phase (about 16 days) is characterized by the rapid development of the CL to its maximal weight (i.e., 350 to 450 mg) by days 6 to 8, the maintenance of cellular integrity and secretory function to day 16, and then the rapid regression to a nonsecreting corpus albicans.

Characteristic cytologic features of a steroid-secreting cell include a large Golgi complex, few cisternal profiles of granular (rough) endoplasmic reticulum, and extensive agranular (smooth) endoplasmic reticulum, whereas a protein-secreting cell contains prominent granular endoplasmic reticulum with well-developed cisternae. Fine structural changes in the lutein cell indicate a close correlation between its morphology and steroid secretion during the estrous cycle.

During luteinization (day 1) granulosa cells at the periphery of the ruptured follicle are cuboidal to columnar and separated by irregular extracellular spaces that contain precipitated liquor folliculi. The cytoplasm in these peripheral cells contains granular endoplasmic reticulum and free polysomes. By day 4, luteinization is essentially complete; the cells are hyper-

trophied with masses of agranular endoplasmic reticulum. These cells typify the secretory phase (days 4 to 12) by their protein and steroid hormone production. During cell regression (days 14 to 18), there is an increase in cytoplasmic lipid droplets, in cytoplasmic disorganization, and in vacuolation of the agranular endoplasmic reticulum. At the terminal phase of the cycle, there is an increase in the number of lysosomes, in vacuolation of agranular endoplasmic reticulum and in invasion of connective tissue; these events result in formation of the corpus albicans.

Steroid-secreting activity of the corpora lutea is indicated by concentrations of progesterone and estrogen throughout the cycle (Fig. 16–2B). Progesterone levels are low at estrus (day 0), begin to increase abruptly after day 2, reach peak values by days 8 to 12, and then decline precipitously thereafter to day 18. These levels follow a pattern similar to the morphologic development and decline of the CL as well as ultrastructural changes in luteal cells. LH and dibutyryl cyclic adenosine monophosphate (c-AMP) stimulate *in vitro* production of progesterone by porcine luteal tissue (Felder et al., 1988; Huang et al., 1991). Insulin-like growth factors (i.e., IGF-I) promote differentiation and replication of cultured granulosa cells as well as increase FSH-stimulated production of progesterone, estrogen, cAMP, proteoglycans, and LH receptors (Adashi et al., 1985; Haseltine and Findlay, 1991). Gonadotropins, estrogen, and cAMP can stimulate IGF-I secretion by these cells (Hsu and Hammond, 1987). Epidermal growth factor (EGF) and transforming growth factor-β (TGF-β) can modulate steroidogenesis in porcine theca and granulosa cells (Caubo et al., 1989). For example, EGF inhibits production of estradiol by theca cells but has little effect on secretion of progesterone or androgens. These growth factors are produced by theca and granulosa cells and seem to modulate, in a paracrine or autocrine way, steroidogenesis and follicular differentiation. The life span and secretory function of this ephemeral structure in the pig can be prolonged by pregnancy or hysterectomy. Estrogen concentrations in peripheral plasma begin to increase coincident with the decline and disappearance of progesterone (Fig. 16–2B). Peak values occur 2 days preceding estrus and reflect rapid growth and maturation of Graafian follicles during the late proestrous phase of the cycle. Soon after estrus, estrogen declines and remains low during the luteal phase of the cycle. Increasing blood concentrations of estradiol secreted by the developing preovulatory follicles stimulate the preovulatory surge of gonadotropins (Kraeling and Barb, 1990).

Ovarian follicles depend on secretion of adenohypophyseal gonadotropins for their growth and maturation; hypophysectomy or hypophyseal stalk transection (Anderson et al., 1967) results in abrupt regression of these follicles. FSH in peripheral serum reaches peak levels on days 2 and 3, after the onset of behavioral estrus, and may reflect decreased use of FSH by the remaining, small ovarian follicles at this time (Fig. 16–2B). Ovarian follicular fluid of sows contains inhibin, a protein hormone, which can suppress the secretion of FSH. Concentrations of inhibin in serum increase during the late follicular phase, whereas FSH levels are inversely related to inhibin during this time. Inhibin concentrations decrease with the LH surge. Activin and activin-A are dimers of the β-subunits of inhibin ($\beta_A\beta_A$ and $\beta_A\beta_B$), and they are equipotent in their ability to stimulate FSH secretion without affecting LH secretion (Haseltine and Findlay, 1991). Follistatin is a single-peptide chain of 32,000 to 35,000 molecular weight distinct from inhibin and activin, which can inhibit the release of FSH but not LH from cultures of pituitary cells. Follicle-regulating protein (FRP) isolated from follicular fluid from the sow has a molecular weight of 15,000 and inhibits aromatase and 3β-HSD activities in granulosa cells. FRP inhibits secretion of progesterone and estradiol in porcine granulosa cells, as well as alters gonadotropin binding and adenylate cyclase activities by these cells. Although FRP has little effect on aromatase or 3β-HSD activities in porcine theca cells from medium follicles, it inhibits basal theca aromatase and 3β-HSD activities in large follicles, suggesting that the effects depend on the stage of follicular maturation.

Peripheral plasma levels of LH show one sharp peak at estrus and drop to low levels during the remainder of the cycle (Fig. 16–2B). There is no characteristic shift in LH secretion as related to the onset of luteal regression. Sequential bleeding from days 12 to 15 of the estrous cycle in gilts reveals an episodic pattern of secretion of FSH and LH as well as estradiol (Flowers et al., 1991). Prolactin concentrations in peripheral plasma peak during estrus and remain low during the luteal phase of the estrous cycle. Prolactin levels peak when estrogen is highest, and during estrus, prolactin profiles coincide better with the FSH peak than with the preovulatory LH peak. Sequential bleedings reveal an episodic pattern of LH secretion that is abolished after hypophyseal stalk transection, but injection of LH-RH in these stalk-transected gilts induces peak LH release within 15 minutes (Anderson et al., 1991). Deafferentation of the anterior hypothalamus and preoptic area abolishes episodic LH secretion, whereas LH-RH causes acute release of LH in such animals (Molina et al., 1986). In contrast, prolactin secretion remains consistently elevated after hypophyseal stalk transection of gilts as compared with sham operated controls (Anderson et al., 1982). Hypophyseal stalk transection dampens episodic secretion of growth hormone and results in elevated basal blood concentrations of the hormone as compared with controls (Klindt et al., 1983).

Thus, the hypothalamus is required for the tonic inhibition of prolactin secretion and for the regulation of both episodic release and tonic inhibition of basal secretion of growth hormone in the pig. Growth hormone-releasing factor (GRF) causes a greater peak release of growth hormone in hypophyseal stalk-transected gilts than in intact controls (Anderson et al., 1991).

Relaxin remains low in the luteal phase throughout the estrous cycle and shows no relationship to the high levels of progesterone secreted by these same cells during this brief period (Anderson, 1987).

Prostaglandin F (PGF) concentrations in utero-ovarian venous plasma increase during the estrous cycle to peak values between days 12 and 16, a period coinciding with onset of luteal regression. PGF and PGE_2 in uterine flushings increase from days 10 to 14 of the estrous cycle (Roberts and Bazer, 1988). Porcine endometrium also synthesizes *in vitro* the highest levels of $PGF_{2\alpha}$ during the mid- to late-luteal phase as compared with earlier stages of the cycle, and indomethacin blocks its production.

OVULATION RATE

Ovulation rate is associated with breed (lines or crosses), amount of inbreeding, age at breeding and weight at breeding. In inbred lines there is an average increase of 0.8 ova from the first to second estrous periods; ovulation continues to increase (1.1 more ova) at the third estrus, but little if any additional increase occurs beyond the fourth postpubertal estrus. Reproductive experience correlates with ovulation rate; ovulations increase with parity to seven or more litters (Fig. 16–2C). Inbreeding reduces ovulation rate, whereas crossing inbred lines increases the number of ovulations. The age at breeding in young gilts is positively correlated with ovulation rate. Weight at breeding is positively associated with ovulation rate when compared with weaning weight or weight at 154 days. Selection experiments based on a controlled gene pool over seven generations indicate that heritability of ovulation rate is 0.40 on weighted cumulative selection differential (Johnson et al., 1985).

Methods to Increase Ovulation Rates

Ovulations can be induced by single injection of PMSG or an injection of PMSG followed by an injection of hCG. The ovulatory response depends primarily on the dosage of PMSG. HCG induces ovulation in cycling gilts but causes little if any increase in ovulation rate. After an intramuscular injection of hCG (i.e., 500 IU) during the proestrous period, ovulations occur in most of the animals 44 to 46 hours later. The injection of PMSG induces superovulatory responses when given on days 15 or 16 of the cycle. The gonadotropins usually reduce the length of the cycle, increase the duration of estrus, and may increase the incidence of cystic follicles, but the ova shed are capable of acceptable fertilization rates.

Nutrition and Ovulation Rate

High-energy diets induce a higher ovulation rate in the pig when the diets are fed for a restricted duration. Although the number of ovulations is predominantly affected by genetic background, ovulation rate is usually affected positively, with increasing levels of energy intake. The levels of energy restriction before feeding the pigs a high-energy diet are an important factor influencing ovulation rate. A low level of energy intake (e.g., 3,000 to 5,000 kcal) is usually given before high-energy (e.g., 8,000 to 10,000 kcal) diets. The optimal duration of a high-energy regimen seems to be 11 to 14 days before expected estrus or mating. There is little evidence that increased protein intake during brief periods increases ovulation rate.

The administration of short- or long-acting insulin in combination with a high-energy diet consistently increased ovulation rate, reduced follicular atresia, and increased plasma estradiol concentrations (Cox et al., 1987). Altrenogest (17β-hydroxy-17-(2-propenyl) estra-4, 9, 11-triene-3-one) given orally for 14 days to gilts tended to increase ovulation rate, but its effect differed from those of flushing (Rhodes et al., 1991).

CONCEPTION RATE

The fertilization rate in pigs is usually high (> 90%). Low or high ovulation rates have little or no effect on fertilization rates. Loss of the whole litter may result from fertilization failure or death of all the embryos. Estimates indicate that approximately 5% of the litters are lost during the remainder of gestation. Early embryonic death results in resorption of the conceptus, whereas losses occurring after day 50 may result in abortion, fetal mummification, or delivery of stillborns at term.

EMBRYO SURVIVAL

Embryo loss is an important factor in the pig. At least 40% of the embryos are lost before parturition, and a major part of this loss occurs during the first half of gestation. Within the first 18 days, embryonic survival is reduced by 17%. By day 25, approximately 33% of the embryos die, and this increases to 40% by day 50. Although sows have greater fecundity than gilts, they also lose a greater proportion of their embryos during the first 40 days. With each 10% inbreeding in the dam, there results 0.55 to 0.76 fewer ova, loss of 0.53 more fertilized ova, and 0.8 fewer embryos by day 25. Crossing these inbred lines results in 0.55 more ova, 0.33 increase in number of fertilized ova, and 0.8 more embryos at day 25.

LITTER SIZE

Reproductive performance is measured primarily by the number of living pigs at birth or by the total farrowing or weaning weight of pigs produced by the dam within 1 year. Ovulation rates continue to increase with subsequent gestations, but litter size reaches maximal levels by the fourth or fifth parity (Fig. 16–2C). The number of pigs farrowed increases between the first and fourth litters, but by the eighth litter, the number of live births declines while the number of stillborn increases. When litter size is related to the age of the dam, reproductive performance

begins to decline after 4.5 years. The genetic contribution (heritability) to litter size is estimated as 0.17; most variation is attributed to environmental factors. Evaluation of several breed combinations provides estimates of heterosis and the average direct and maternal effects of the breeds. For example, pure lines of Duroc and Yorkshire animals average 13.8 corpora lutea, and when Duroc dams are bred to a boar of another breed, litter size increases by 1.44 pigs at farrowing. Survival rates at day 30, and farrowing and weaning of progeny from three-breed crosses exceed those progeny from two-breed crosses. Gilts of Yorkshire × Duroc breeding showed a direct relationship between ovulation rate and the total pigs (Fig. 16–2D). Neither covariate nor regression analysis provided evidence that prenatal survival was affected by ovulation rate (Rhodes et al., 1991).

PREGNANCY

Growth of Conceptuses

Ova are fertilized in the ampulla of the oviduct, and their arrival to this region may be aided by the rapid beat, in a downward direction, of cilia on the mucosal surface; in the isthmus region of the oviduct, there is an extensive upward ciliary current that may aid sperm ascent. Embryos are usually in the four-cell stage when they enter the uterus. Cleavage advances to morula stage by day 5 and then blastocyst formation by days 6 to 8. Hatching describes at least partial escape of the embryo from the zona pellucida, and it occurs on the sixth day; pig blastocysts may reach a size of 150 cells or more before hatching. Blastocysts are unevenly distributed throughout both uterine horns. Rapid development of conceptuses is indicated by intrauterine migration of the embryos, spacing of the embryos, and transition of blastocysts from spherical to extremely elongated forms and subsequent embryogenesis. By day 11, half the blastocysts rapidly elongate to filamentous forms, often exceeding 60 cm, and by day 13, embryos have completed this process (Anderson, 1978). These conceptuses become regularly spaced with no overlap of tubular membranes from other embryos in that horn. Protein content in individual conceptuses denotes exponential growth between days 9 and 18 and is independent of the developmental stage or potential loss of those neighbors nearest that conceptus.

Patterns of normal embryonic and fetal growth from days 20 to 100 of gestation increase exponentially from 0.06 to 1000 g. Fetal wet weight is highly correlated with placental length ($r = .64$), placental surface area ($r = .72$), and total areolae surface per placenta ($r = .65$). Specific uterine- and conceptus-derived proteins during endometrial differentiation and conceptus development include mitogens (IGF-I and -II and EGF); binding and transport proteins (uteroferrin, IGF- and retinol-binding proteins); protease inhibitors (plasmin and trypsin inhibitor); and interferon-related trophoblastic proteins (Simmen and Simmen, 1990). Their differential expression in early pregnancy may imply a functional importance during the period of maternal recognition of pregnancy and implantation. The synthesis of these proteins is related to progesterone-dependent differentiation of endometrial cells whose secretory activity may act as signals to initiate embryonic differentiation. Further, it is possible that secretory activity is initiated by factors implicated in activation of gene expression during initial cleavage stages of the embryos (Braude et al., 1988).

Hormones During Pregnancy

Corpora lutea are essential for maintenance of pregnancy to term in the pig. The CL develops to maximal weight by day 8 and is sustained to late pregnancy. Two porcine luteal cell populations of 30 to 50 μm in diameter and 15 to 20 μm in diameter occur during pregnancy. Production of progesterone seems associated with cell size and stage of pregnancy. After day 114, soon after delivery, there is a precipitous decline in luteal weight. Progesterone concentrations in peripheral blood increase to peak values by day 12, and gradually decrease to levels of 20 to 25 ng/ml by day 104. Relaxin gradually accumulates in luteal tissue to peak values during late pregnancy (days 105 to 110). Concentrations of unconjugated estradiol-17β in peripheral blood increase from 10 pg/ml at days 8 to 60 and rapidly increase to peak values (400 pg/ml) just before parturition (Anderson, 1987). Two peaks of estrone sulfate occur at days 30 and 112, respectively, and then drop at onset of parturition. The fetoplacental unit is the major source of estrogen production, as indicated by the finding of similar urinary excretory patterns in intact controls, as seen in sows after ovariectomy, hypophysectomy or adrenalectomy.

Immunocytochemical and ultrastructural evidence in the porcine pituitary indicate that most gonadotropic cells secrete both FSH and LH. In gilts hypophysectomized at day 4, pregnancy and luteal function are maintained to day 12, but pregnancy fails soon after hypophysectomy at days 70 to 90. Pregnancy is maintained at least 20 days; however, after hypophyseal stalk transection at day 70 or 90, the pig requires adenohypophyseal luteotropic support during a major part of gestation. Prolactin is luteotropic in the pig. In hypophysectomized and hysterectomized gilts given daily injections of purified porcine prolactin, both progesterone and relaxin plasma concentrations are maintained throughout a period of 10 days from days 110 to 120 (Li et al., 1989).

During early pregnancy (days 10 to 14), recoverable estrone, estradiol-17β, and estrone sulfate were greater in uterine flushings having tubular and filamentous blastocysts, whereas there was no change in these steroids in nongravid gilts (Bazer et al., 1984). From days 12 to 21, endogenous concentrations of prostaglandin F in utero-ovarian plasma remain lower in pregnant than nonpregnant gilts. There is also a greater frequency of PGF peaks in nonpregnant than pregnant pigs during this time. Furthermore, estradiol concentrations in utero-ovarian venous plasma are greater on days 12 to 17 of pregnancy as compared with nonpregnant animals. The blastocysts maintain luteal function during critical phases of early pregnancy by overcoming uterine luteolytic action, and they may contribute to the luteotropic effect by their production of estrogen (Ford and Stice, 1985). Uterine arterial blood flow increases two- to fourfold from days 11 to 13 of pregnancy. In pregnant pigs there is a temporal relationship between blastocyst elongation and increasing quantities of PGE_2 and $PGF_{2\alpha}$ as well as estrogens in uterine flushings (Geisert et al., 1982). Porcine blastocysts produce $PGF_{2\alpha}$ and PGE_2. In nonpregnant gilts, exogenous estrogen given on days 11 through 15 of the cycle maintains corpora lutea for prolonged periods, presumably by its action on the endometrium. When the uterus is removed (hysterectomy), the corpora lutea are maintained for a period exceeding that of pregnancy, and they produce progesterone and relaxin in a manner similar to that found in pregnant gilts (Anderson, 1987). Exogenous $PGF_{2\alpha}$ is luteolytic and induces abortion from day 23 of pregnancy onward.

During late pregnancy, corticosteroid concentrations increase within 24 hours of parturition and decrease during early lactation. Progesterone levels decline during the last days of pregnancy and drop abruptly to 0.5 ng/ml by day 1 postpartum (Fig. 16–2E). Estrone increases to peak concentrations until day 2 prepartum and then falls to basal levels after delivery of conceptuses. The rise in estrone as well as estradiol is associated with fetal maturity and is primarily of placental origin. The number of fetal adrenal cortical cells increases markedly from days 105 to 113 as well as the ability of these cells to secrete cortisol.

Relaxin is produced and accumulated in porcine corpora lutea throughout pregnancy and then released before parturition (Fig. 16–2E) (Huang et al., 1991; Li et al., 1991). The accumulation of cytoplasmic granules and relaxin activity in corpora lutea, beginning approximately on day 28, and their disappearance correlate with the rise and fall of relaxin in ovarian venous blood and peripheral blood just preceding delivery. Immunocytochemical localization of relaxin in granulosa lutein cells at the ultrastructural level is also correlated with changes in the numbers of granules and in the relaxin levels. Relaxin concentrations in peripheral serum remain consistently low (≤ 2 ng/ml) during the first 90 days of pregnancy, then increase to peak values 2 days before parturition and signal the discharge of accumulated relaxin from the corpora lutea (Fig. 16–2E). Relaxin abruptly declines just before delivery. The surge in relaxin levels that occurs in pigs experiencing progesterone-delayed parturition is not a sufficient stimulus to initiate parturition. Although the luteal cells produce both progesterone and relaxin, their secretion profiles differ during the last days of pregnancy (Fig. 16–2E). Relaxin mRNA using Northern analysis and *in situ* hybridization reveal relaxin gene expression in luteal tissue not only in pregnancy but also in the cycle and early lactation (Bagnell et al., 1990). Relaxin and estrogen are required for remodeling collagen and dilation of the cervix and for the growth of mammary parenchymal tissue of late pregnant gilts (Eldridge-White et al., 1989; Hurley et al., 1991).

Infusion of porcine relaxin during late gestation in the sow inhibits uterine myometrial contractions. Premature parturition in intact gilts or sows can be induced by the administration of exogenous $PGF_{2\alpha}$. Dexamethasone injections induce premature delivery, whereas feeding the dams methallibure delays onset of parturition. The role of the fetal pituitary and adrenal glands in initiating processes of parturition is implicated by the effects of fetal hypophysectomy or fetal decapitation on the prolongation of gestation beyond term. The antiprogesterone RU 486 given orally on days 111 and 112 induces parturition within 31 hours (Li et al., 1991). RU 486 abruptly decreases circulating concentrations of progesterone and causes an earlier peak release of relaxin in these gilts. The luteolytic effect of RU 486 likely results from preferential binding to progesterone receptor in the uterus.

Postpartum Estrus

Immediately after delivery, peripheral blood levels of progesterone, estrone, estradiol, and relaxin decline to basal levels during early lactation (Fig. 16–2E). Estrus frequently occurs within 1 to 3 days after parturition. If mated, the sow fails to conceive at this estrus because the ovarian follicles are immature and ovulation usually does not occur. The postpartum estrus is observed in sows with low concentrations of estrogen in peripheral plasma and may result from peak levels of fetoplacental estrogens just preceding parturition. Restricting the diet of primiparous sows during lactation had no effect on plasma LH or estradiol concentrations or subsequent reproductive performance (Armstrong et al., 1986).

LACTATION

With the exception of the postpartum estrus, sows rarely exhibit estrus during lactation. Ovarian morphology during the anestrous period indicates an absence of gonadotropic stimulation. The average diameter of the ovarian follicle decreases (i.e., from 4.6 to 2.7 mm) during the first week after parturition and then gradually increases (i.e., ≥ 5 mm) by the fifth week of lactation. Uterine weight and length decline rapidly for 21 to 28 days following parturition; thereafter, both remain constant. The endometrium is thinner and the uterine glands are less numerous, particularly in the basal region near the myometrium.

The lactational anestrus may be a period of depressed FSH release and reduced LH synthesis. Prolactin concentrations in peripheral plasma are high at parturition, increase in response to suckling by the piglets, and decline soon after weaning (Fig. 16–2E). After an ovariectomy performed during lactation, LH serum concentrations remain low, whereas FSH increases. Prolactin levels, but not LH, increase acutely with suckling or weaning. Estrogen, whether of endogenous or exogenous origin, causes surges in LH, FSH, and prolactin in the postpartum sow.

Sow at Weaning

Removal of the litter from the sow after 3 to 5 weeks of lactation results in follicular development, estrus, and ovulation within 4 to 8 days. At weaning, a transient increase occurs in plasma LH and hypothalamic LH-RH content. During the postweaning period, plasma concentrations of estradiol-17β increase gradually and are terminated by the preovulatory surge of LH at estrus. Increases in plasma FSH levels coincide with the LH surge, at least in some animals. Prolactin secretion is increased around estrus in weaned sows, and it may be associated more with estrus than the ovulation process (Fig. 16–2E).

REFERENCES

Adashi, E.Y., Resnick, C.E., D'Ercole, A.J., Svoboda, M.E. and Van-Wyk, J.J. (1985). Insulin-like growth factors as intraovarian regulators of granulosa cell growth and function. Endocr. Rev. *6*, 400.

Anderson, L.L. (1978). Growth, protein content and distribution of early pig embryos. Anat. Rec. *190*, 143.

Anderson, L.L. (1987). Regulation of relaxin secretion and its role in pregnancy. Adv. Exp. Med. Biol. *219*, 421.

Anderson, L.L., Berardinelli, J.G., Malven, P.V. and Ford, J.J. (1982). Prolactin secretion after hypophysial stalk transection in pigs. Endocrinology *111*, 380.

Anderson, L.L., Dyck, G.W., Mori, H., Henricks, D.M. and Melampy, R.M. (1967). Ovarian function in pigs following hypophysial stalk transection or hypophysectomy. Am. J. Physiol. *212*, 1188.

Anderson, L.L., Ford, J.J., Klindt, J., Molina, J.R., Vale, W.W. and Rivier, J. (1991). Growth hormone and prolactin secretion in hypophysial stalk-transected pigs as affected by growth hormone and prolactin releasing and inhibiting factors. Proc. Soc. Exp. Biol. Med. *196*, 194.

Armstrong, J.D., Britt, J.H. and Kraeling, R.R. (1986). Effect of restriction of energy during lactation on body condition, energy metabolism, endocrine changes and reproductive performance in primiparous sows. J. Anim. Sci. *63*, 1915.

Bagnell, C.A., Tashima, L., Tsark, W., Ali, S.M. and McMurty, J.P. (1990). Relaxin gene expression in the sow corpus luteum during the cycle, pregnancy, and lactation. Endocrinology *126*, 2514.

Bazer, F.W., Marengo, S.R., Geisert, R.D. and Thatcher, W.W. (1984). Exocrine versus endocrine secretion of prostaglandin $F_2\alpha$ in the control of pregnancy in swine. Anim. Reprod. Sci. *7*, 115.

Braude, P., Bolton, V. and Moore, S. (1988). Human gene expression first occurs between the four- and eight-cell stages of preimplantation development. Nature *332*, 459.

Caubo, B., DeVinna, R.S. and Tonetta, S.A. (1989). Regulation of steroidogenesis in theca cells from porcine follicles by growth factors. Endocrinology *125*, 321.

Cox, N.M., Stuart, M.J., Althen, T.G., Bennett, W.A. and Miller, H.W. (1987). Enhancement of ovulation rate in gilts by increasing dietary energy and administering insulin during follicular growth. J. Anim. Sci. *64*, 507.

Donahoe, P.K., Gate, R.L., MacLaughlin, D.T., Epstein, J., Fuller, A.F., Takahashi, M., Coughlin, J.P., Ninfa, E.G. and Taylor, L.A. (1987). Mullerian inhibiting substance: gene structure and mechanism of action of a fetal regressor. Recent Prog. Horm. Res. *43*, 431.

Eldridge-White, R., Easter, R.A., Heaton, D.M., O'Day, M.B., Petersen, G.C., Shanks, R.D., Tarbell, M.K. and Sherwood, O.D. (1989). Hormonal control of the cervix in pregnant gilts. I. Changes in the physical properties of the cervix correlate temporally with elevated serum levels of estrogens and relaxin. Endocrinology *125*, 2996.

Felder, K.J., Klindt, J., Bolt, D.J. and Anderson, L.L. (1988). Relaxin and progesterone secretion as affected by luteinizing hormone and prolactin after hysterectomy in the pig. Endocrinology *122*, 1751.

Flowers, B., Cantley, T.C., Martin, M.J. and Day, B.N. (1991). Episodic secretion of gonadotropins and ovarian steroids in jugular and utero-ovarian vein plasma during the follicular phase of the oestrous cycle in gilts. J. Reprod. Fertil. *91*, 101.

Ford, J.J. (1990). Differentiation of sexual behavior in pigs. J. Reprod. Fertil. Suppl. *40*, 311.

Ford, S.P. and Stice, S.L. (1985). Effects of the ovary and conceptus on controlling uterine blood flow in the pig. J. Reprod. Fertil. Suppl. *33*, 83.

Geisert, R.D., Renegar, R.H., Thatcher, W.W., Roberts, R.M. and Bazer, F.W. (1982). Establishment of pregnancy in the pig. I. Interrelationships between preimplantation development of the pig blastocyst and uterine endometrial secretions. Biol. Reprod. *27*, 925.

Haseltine, F.P. and Findlay, J.K. (eds.). Growth Factors in Fertility Regulation. Cambridge, England, Cambridge University Press, 1991.

Hsu, C.J. and Hammond, J.M. (1987). Gonadotropins and estradiol stimulate immunoreactive insulin-like growth factor-I production by porcine granulosa cells in vitro. Endocrinology *120*, 198.

Huang, C.J., Stromer, M.H. and Anderson, L.L. (1991). Abrupt shifts in relaxin and progesterone secretion by aging luteal cells: luteotropic response in hysterectomized and pregnant pigs. Endocrinology *128*, 165.

Hurley, W.L., Doane, R.M., O'Day-Bowman, M.B., Winn, R.J., Mojonnier, L.E. and Sherwood, O.D. (1991). Effect of relaxin on mammary gland development in ovariectomized pregnant gilts. Endocrinology *128*, 1285.

Johnson, R.K., Zimmerman, D.R., Lamberson, W.R. and Sasaki, S. (1985). Influencing prolificacy of sows by selection for physiological factors. J. Reprod. Fertil. Suppl. *33*, 139.

Klindt, J., Ford, J.J., Berardinelli, J.G. and Anderson, L.L. (1983). Growth hormone secretion after hypophysial stalk transection in pigs. Proc. Soc. Exp. Biol. Med. *172*, 508.

Kraeling, R.R. and Barb, C.R. (1990). Hypothalamic control of gonadotropin and prolactin secretion in pigs. J. Reprod. Fertil. Suppl. *40*, 3.

Li, Y., Huang, C.J., Klindt, J. and Anderson, L.L. (1991). Divergent effects of antiprogesterone, RU 486, on progesterone, relaxin and prolactin secretion in pregnant and hysterectomized pigs. Endocrinology *129*, 2907.

Li, Y., Molina, J.R., Klindt, J., Bolt, D.J. and Anderson, L.L. (1989). Prolactin maintains relaxin and progesterone secretion by aging corpora lutea after hypophysial stalk transection or hypophysectomy in the pig. Endocrinology *124*, 1294.

Molina, J.R., Hard, D.L. and Anderson, L.L. (1986). Hypothalamic deafferentation and LHRH on LH secretion in prepuberal gilts. Biol. Reprod. *35*, 439.

Rhodes, M.T., Davis, D.L. and Stevenson, J.S. (1991). Flushing and altrogenest affect litter traits in gilts. J. Anim. Sci. *69*, 34.

Roberts, R.M. and Bazer, F.W. (1988). The function of uterine secretions. J. Reprod. Fertil. *82*, 875.

Simmen, R.C.M. and Simmen, F.A. (1990). Regulation of uterine and conceptus secretory activity in the pig. J. Reprod. Fertil. Suppl. *40*, 279.

Sinclair, A.H., Berta, P., Palmer, M.S., Hawkins, J.R., Griffiths, B.L., Smith, M.J., Foster, J.W., Frischauf, A.-M., Lovell-Badge, R., and Goodfellow, P.N. (1990). A gene from the human sex-determining region encodes a protein with homology to a conserved DNA-binding motif. Nature *346,* 240.

17
Horses

E.S.E. HAFEZ

The various breeds of the domestic horse (*Equus caballus*) are members of the family *Equidae,* which belongs to the order *Perissodactyla.* The horse has several unique aspects of reproductive endocrinology and pregnancy. Whereas other large farm species such as the cattle, swine, and sheep have been highly selected for reproductive efficiency, as well as other productive traits, the only selection practiced with horses has been their ability to walk or run.

Race horses are usually aged from January 1 in the year that they are born, and it has been the practice to breed them as early in the year as possible so that, as 2-year-olds, the offspring have maximal physical advantage.

BREEDING SEASON

Stallion

The breeding season of stallions is not well marked, and semen can be collected throughout the year. However, remarkable seasonal variations are noted in reaction time, number of mounts per ejaculate, volume of gel-free semen, total number of spermatozoa per ejaculate, sperm agglutination, and motility in fresh and in diluted semen.

The effects of season on seminal plasma are greater than those on spermatozoa. Spermatozoa in first ejaculates are less affected by season than those in second ejaculates. This differential effect on first and second ejaculates is noted for most semen characteristics (Pickett et al., 1975).

Mare

The reproductive cycle of the mare is subject to the greatest variability of all the domestic animals. Some mares appear to be truly polyestrous; they can produce offspring at any time of the year. However, the great majority of the mare population are seasonally polyestrous. Although many mares in the northern hemisphere show behavioral estrus in February, March, and April, estrus during this time is often unaccompanied by ovulation, and conception rates in mares bred during the period are low. In the northern hemisphere, the best conception rates usually occur in mares bred from May to July. The same trends occur in mares in the southern hemisphere for the corresponding seasons. Although mares who feed primarily on grass normally breed only during summer and go into anestrus in winter, those that are well fed and stabled tend to cycle throughout the year. The onset of the fertile breeding season is closely associated with management.

Mares can be classified into three categories according to their breeding season:

1. Defined breeding season: The wild breeds of horses manifest several estrous cycles during a restricted breeding season that coincides with the longest days of the year; the foals are born during a restricted foaling season.
2. Transitory breeding season: Some domestic breeds and some individual mares manifest estrous cycles throughout the year, but ovulation

accompanies estrus only during the breeding season, and the foals are born during a limited foaling season.

3. Year-round breeding: Some domestic breeds and some individual mares exhibit estrous cycles accompanied by ovulation throughout the year.

Thus, it is evident that although some mares, at certain latitudes, may show estrous cycles throughout the year, they do not necessarily conceive during all estrous periods.

In localities where there is a breeding season, the two transitory periods preceding and following the breeding season are characterized by variability of ovarian activity and sexual behavior. At this time the ovarian follicles develop only to limited degrees and then undergo atresia. Also there is a high frequency of prolonged estrus or estrus of short duration as well as irregular estrous cycles during these periods.

Near the equator, there is little seasonal variation in the length of the estrous cycle. In temperate regions, mares are seasonally polyestrous, with the breeding and nonbreeding seasons occurring during the summer and winter months, respectively. Photoperiod is perhaps the most important environmental signal and entrains the pituitary–gonadal axis, since artificial photoperiod treatments hasten follicular development and onset of the breeding season. The mare exhibits a photoperiodically entrained seasonal pattern of LH secretion. The cyclic reproductive behavior during the breeding season is mediated by the stimulatory and inhibitory actions of estradiol and progesterone (Garcia and Ginther, 1978). The exposure of mares to additional hours of light during winter will induce estrus and hastens the onset of the breeding season.

The arbitrary assignment of January 1 as the birth date for all foals born in a given year has stimulated a demand in the equine industry for the administration of hormones to advance the onset of the natural breeding season in mares by 3 to 4 months; thus, foals would be born nearer to the first of the year. Several hormonal treatments were used with varying success such as: pregnant mare serum gonadotropin (PMSG), human chorionic gonadotropin (hCG), equine pituitary extracts, gonadotropin-releasing hormone (GnRH), progesterone, and prostaglandins.

Neural impulses are generated as a result of light incident on photoreceptors in the eye. The impulses are transmitted to the pineal gland where they regulate the synthesis and secretion of melatonin. The pineal gland and possibly melatonin seem to mediate changes in neuroendocrine-gonadal activity in response to changing photoperiod. In the mare, both superior cervical ganglionectomy and pinealectomy have altered the ability to respond to a stimulatory photoperiod.

REPRODUCTIVE PARAMETERS IN STALLIONS

Sexual Maturity

The testes of the stallion descend into the scrotum at 1 to 3 weeks of age. In a few cases, the testes are already in the scrotum at birth. Postnatal growth of the testes begins during the eleventh month, and the left testis develops earlier and grows faster than the right. At this time, there is also a gradual outward development of the seminiferous tubules around the right testis (Fig. 17–1). The age at which stallions are first used for natural or artificial breeding is determined primarily by managerial conditions.

Semen Production

The cycle of the seminiferous epithelium can be divided into eight stages on the basis of meiotic divisions, shape of the spermatid nuclei, and location of spermatids with elongated nuclei. The characteristics of semen and spermatogenesis are summarized in Tables 17–1 and 17–2 and Figure 17–2.

The ejaculate is composed of six to nine jets resulting from the contractions of the

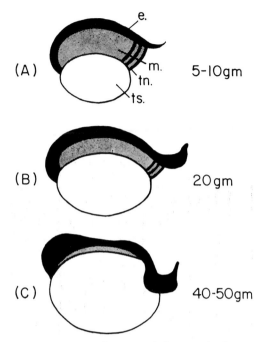

(A) e. m. tn. ts. 5-10gm

(B) 20gm

(C) 40-50gm

FIG. 17–1. Developmental changes in the attachment of epididymis with the testis in relation to sexual maturity. Figures on right indicate testis weight, *e.*, epididymis; *m.*, thin membrane; *tn.*, tendon; *ts.*, testis. *A.* Loose attachment between testis and epididymis: note tendon attachment at head of epididymis. *B.* Elongation of epididymis. *C.* Epididymis fully developed and completely attached to testis. (Adapted from Nishikawa (1959). Studies on Reproduction in Horses.)

urethra. The volume of each succeeding jet in the ejaculate reduces to about 50% of its initial value; 70% or more of the spermatozoa and the basic biochemical constituents are contained in the first three jets.

The gelatinous material in semen, secreted by the seminal vesicles, has no effect on the motility or the fertilizing ability of spermatozoa. The volume of gel, composing about one third of the ejaculate, varies considerably and is not characteristic of the individual stallion. This is in contrast to gel obtained from boar ejaculates, which is a constant feature of the ejaculates. Ejaculates containing gel seem to require fewer mounts and a shorter re-

action time and possess a slightly larger volume of gel-free semen than ejaculates without gel.

Fructose is present in negligible quantities in stallion semen, whereas relatively large quantities of ergothioneine and citric acid are present. Although the majority of the lipids of stallion spermatozoa are phospholipids, the percentage of phospholipid is much lower than that for the bull or the boar. The lower percentage of phospholipid may be related to the great sensitivity of stallion spermatozoa to stress as compared with spermatozoa of other species.

Semen characteristics are influenced by the degree of sexual stimulation, frequency of ejaculation, age, testicular size, and method of semen collection. Season of the year influences the physical and biochemical characteristics of semen as well as blood hormone levels, sexual behavior, and fertility of both sexes. Spermatozoal output and libido of stallions are greatest during spring and summer and least during fall and winter. These changes in reproductive capacity coincide with the natural breeding season of mares. The concentration of plasma testosterone of stallions is also influenced by season and may mediate the patterns of seminal and behavioral characteristics.

The minimal number of motile spermatozoa necessary for maximal conception rate has not been established, although 500×10^6 motile spermatozoa per insemination have been recommended.

Ejaculation

During ejaculation the urethral diverticulum of the penis is in close apposition to the external cervical orifice of the mare. Semen is ejaculated under high pressure directly into the uterus. The final seminal jets ejaculated when erection is ceasing and the penis is being withdrawn are probably deposited in the vagina. The patterns of ejaculation and emission have been carefully studied (Tischner et al., 1974).

TABLE 17–1.   **Some Reproductive Parameters in the Stallion**

	Reproductive Parameters or Characteristics	Values (Average)
Sexual maturity	Postnatal growth of testis	1 year
	Sperm appear in testis	1 year
	Sperm appear in ejaculate	13 months
	Sexual maturity	2 years
Testicular and Epididymal Morphology	Testicular weight (g)	150–170 gm
	Epididymal weight (g)	20–30 gm
	Volume of tubules and testis	55–70%
	Length of tubules and testis	2300–2600 m
	Weight (without tunica albuginea)	14–20 m
Spermatogenesis and Sperm Transport in Male Tract	Duration of seminiferous tubule cycle judged by ^{3}H-thymidine injection	13 days
	Life span of primary spermatocytes	19 days
	Life span of secondary spermatocytes	0.7 days
	Life span of spermatids with round nuclei	8.7 days
	Life span of spermatids with elongated nuclei	10 days
	Interval for labeled sperm to enter input of epididymis	35 days
	Interval from isotope injection until it appears in ejaculate	40 days
	Time of transport of sperm in excurrent ducts	8–11 days

(Data collected from Swierstra, E. E., Gebauer, M. R., and Pickett, B. W., 1974. Reproductive physiology of the stallion, I. Spermatogenesis and testis composition. J. Reprod. Fertil. *40*, 113.)

TABLE 17–2.   **Biochemical Characteristics of Semen Fractions of the Stallion**

Semen Fraction	Origin	Physical Characteristics	Biochemical Characteristics
Presperm	Urethral glands	Watery	High NaCl content, no ergothioneine, citric acid, or GPC
Sperm rich	Epididymal and ampullary glands	Milky, nonviscous	High sperm concentration, ergothioneine and GPC; little NaCl and citric acid
Postsperm	Seminal vesicle	Highly viscous	Low sperm concentration High content of citric acid Low ergothioneine and GPC
Penile drip	Tail-end sample	Watery	No spermatozoa; lacks any secretory products of epididymis, ampulla, and seminal vesicles (e.g., GPC, citric acid)

GPC = glyceryl phosphorylcholine diesterase.
(Adapted from Mann, T., Leone, E. and Polge, C. (1965). The composition of the stallion's semen. J. Endocrinol. *13*, 279; Mann, T., Short, R. V. and Walton, A. (1957). The tail-end sample of stallion semen. J. Agric. Sci. Camb. *49*, 301.)

The process of emission is variable because the number of jets per ejaculate varies from 5 to 10 with an average of 8. The early jets occur under high pressure in a stream with characteristic spatter. The later jets, accompanied by declining erection and withdrawal of the penis from the vagina, are associated with low pressure. Of the total time of ejaculation, 24% involves actual emission of semen; the rest comprises intervals between successive seminal jets. The first 3 jets contain 80% of the ejaculated spermatozoa. The total number of spermatozoa and the ergothioneine content gradually decrease in successive jets (Tischner et al., 1974). The terminal jets from 4 to 10, with low concentrations of sperm cells and ergothioneine, consist mostly of the so-called mucous fraction and correspond to fraction 3 described by Mann et al. (1957).

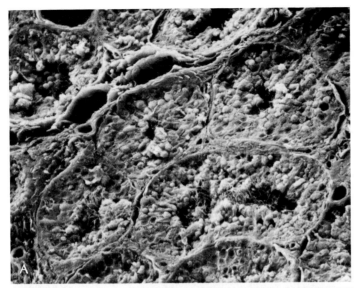

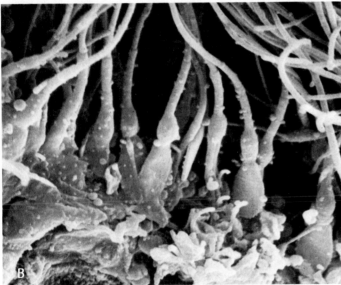

FIG. 17–2. Scanning electron micrograph of equine testis. *A.* Note irregular shape of seminiferous tubules and tails of spermatozoa protruding in the lumen. (440×) *B.* Spermiation: spermatozoa with cytoplasmic droplets are released from the Sertoli cells (5,280×). (Courtesy Dr. Larry Johnson (1978). Fertil. Steril. *17,* 21.)

ESTROUS CYCLES

Table 17–3 shows some of the unique and remarkable characteristics of reproduction in horses (Allen, 1984; Allen and Pashen, 1984).

Estrus

During estrus, the vulva becomes large and swollen; the labial folds are loose and readily open on examination. The vulva becomes scarlet or orange, wet, glossy, and covered with a film of transparent mucus. The vaginal mucosa is highly vascular, and thin watery mucus may accumulate in the vagina. The cellular components of the vaginal smear have no value for detecting estrus. During estrus, the cervix dilates enough to admit two to four fingers; during diestrus only one finger can be inserted.

During estrus, the mare assumes a stance characteristic of urination. The tail

TABLE 17–3. Unique Anatomic, Physiologic, and Endocrine Characteristics of Reproduction in the Horse

Parameters	Unique Reproductive Characteristics
Development of ovary	During fetal life, cortical tissue entirely surrounds the medullary portion. During neonatal life, cortical tissue becomes confined to one area and is nearly surrounded by medullary tissue.
Site of ovulation on the ovarian surface	Follicles can only ovulate through the surface of the ovary adjacent to cortical issue ("ovulation fossa").
Accessory ovulation during luteal phase of estrous cycle	Ovulation unaccompanied by estrus occurs.
Pattern of follicular growth	A small group of follicles develops during late diestrus, some of which enlarge differentially to ovulate during subsequent estrus; remaining follicles may ovulate during early luteal phase and others regress without ovulation.
Primary CL	Primary CL of pregnancy declines in secretory activity from 14 to 16 days after ovulation (similar to the time that complete luteolysis would normally occur in the cycling mare). This causes a slow and steady fall in peripheral plasma progesterone concentrations during the next 20–25 days until the initiation of the secondary rise, days 35–45. This coincides with the onset of secretion of equine chorionic gonadotropin (eCG), formerly known as pregnant mare serum gonadotropin (PMSG).
Accessory corpora lutea	A secondary progesterone rises from the formation of the first of what eventually becomes a whole crop of secondary corpora lutea that develop in the mare's ovaries between day 40 to 150. By day 120, 3 to 30 accessory luteal structures arise from both normal ovulation and luteinization of unruptured follicles. All primary and secondary corpora lutea regress and leave the ovaries small and completely inactive for the remainder of gestation.
Gonadotropins associated with ovulation	Prolonged rise of LH surge during estrus that continues after ovulation.
Life span of CL during nonpregnancy	Spontaneous prolongation of CL life span is common; corpora lutea that fail to regress at normal time persist for 2 months.
FSH content of pituitary	High
Ovarian response to FSH	Low
Egg transport in oviduct	Mare can discriminate between fertilized and unfertilized eggs, which may be retained in oviducts during pregnancy and nonpregnancy for up to 7 months.
Presence of placental hormone (PMSG)	PMSG found in large quantities; secreted by endometrial cups during early pregnancy.
Placental progesterone	Placental tissue contains appreciable quantities of progesterone, and the placenta is secreting sufficient progesterone to maintain pregnancy from about day 100.
Endometrial cups	Endometrial cups, a series of small, ulcer-like, endometrial outgrowths form in a circle around the conceptus in the gravid uterine horn. They first appear as pale, slightly raised plaques in the endometrium at day 38 to 40 after ovulation and enlarge steadily during the next 20 to 30 days. They become concave or saucer-shaped on the surface, and they regress in the central regions of the structure. After days 70 to 80, degenerating cups become pale and cheesy in appearance, and their concave surface becomes filled with a sticky, honey-colored exocrine secretion. Between days 100 to 140, each necrotic cup and its attached exocrine secretion is sloughed off the surface of the endometrium to lie free in the uterine lumen.
Interspecies breeding	Several equid species can interbreed, producing viable, but infertile, offspring. Fetal genotype exerts a profound influence on both the total amount of eCG secreted during pregnancy and its rate of disappearance from maternal blood after the peak concentration. In mares conceived by a jack donkey so that they are carrying interspecies mule conceptuses, the peak serum eCG concentrations of only 8 to 30 IU ml reached by day 45 to 55 are five- to tenfold lower than those in mares carrying normal intraspecies horse conceptuses. eCG activity disappears again from the blood as early as day 70 to 80, and hence much sooner in gestation than the 120- to 140-day period that is usual for normal horse pregnancy. Successful transfer of a horse embryo into the donkey and vice versa.

(Adapted from Stabenfeldt, G.H., Hughes, J.P., Evans, J.W., and Geschwind, I.I. 1975). Unique aspects of the reproductive cycle of the mare. J. Reprod. Fertil. Suppl. *23*, 155.

is raised, urine is expelled in small amounts and the clitoris is exposed by prolonged rhythmic contractions.

The duration of estrus varies among individuals and also among estrous cycles of the same mare. Long duration of estrus in the mare may be due to the following factors: (1) The ovary is surrounded mostly by a serous coat, and some follicles have to migrate to reach the ovulation fossa to rupture. (2) The ovary is less sensitive to exogenous FSH than that of other species (e.g., cattle, sheep), so that the preovulatory follicle requires a longer time to reach maximal size. (3) The level of LH is low compared with FSH, and this delays ovulation. The intensity of behavioral estrus varies both throughout the estrous period and among individual mares at comparable stages of the period.

The duration of estrus is prolonged in old mares, in mares underfed during the early part of the breeding season, and during twin ovulations.

Corpus Luteum

Most ovulations occur on days 3, 4, or 5 of estrus, 24 to 48 hours before the end of behavioral estrus (i.e., the time of ovulation is more closely related to the end than to the onset of estrus). Follicular size and the day of ovulation are consistent in mares from one cycle to another. Ovulation takes place after the first meiotic division. The fertility of mating gradually rises to a peak about 2 days before the end of estrus and then falls sharply on the last day.

The ruptured follicle can be palpated up to 24 hours after ovulation as a soft fluctuant area. The developing CL, however, cannot be detected by rectal examination 48 hours after ovulation because it develops within the ovarian stroma.

The CL reaches only one half to three fourths the size of the follicle at the time of ovulation. The maximal size is attained at 14 days, when luteal cells enlarge and have a peripheral vacuolation (Figs. 17–3 and 17–4). Spontaneous prolongation of

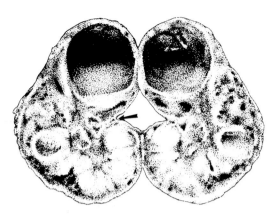

Fig. 17–3.   Ovary of the mare cut in halves. Note ovulation fossa (arrow).

the CL, accompanied by follicular activity and without any signs of estrus for periods of 2 to 3 months, is common (Hughes et al., 1975). Corpora lutea that fail to regress at the normal time persist for about 2 months and are characterized by having a white connective tissue core. Most of the granulosa cells that undergo luteinization 24 hours after ovulation become secretory.

Endocrine Control of Estrous Cycles

FSH. In normally cycling mares, two FSH surges occur at approximately 20 and 11 days before ovulation. Both FSH and LH concentrations surge around the time of ovulation. FSH and LH surges cause development of follicles from less than 2 mm in diameter through to ovulation. The late estrous–early diestrous surge of FSH appears to initiate development of up to 20 follicles. The mid-diestrous surge may be important for the subsequent development of follicles destined to ovulate 10 to 13 days later.

The ovary of the mare is less sensitive to FSH than is that of the cow, ewe, and goat. Injection of massive doses of PMSG during the nonbreeding season is ineffective for inducing ovulation of follicles. Injection of PMSG toward the end of the estrous cycle is also ineffective in promoting follicular

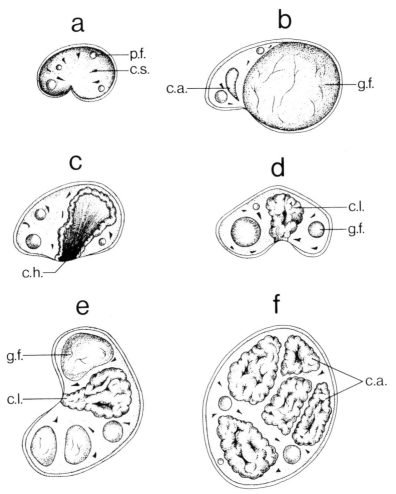

FIG. 17–4.   Cross section of ovaries (drawn to scale) of the mare at different stages of reproduction. *A.* Nonbreeding season. The ovary is small and contains primary follicles (*p.f.*) and scars (*c.s.*) from degenerating corpora lutea. *B.* Breeding season. During estrus, the ovary contains a mature graafian follicle (*g.f.*) and corpus albicans (*c.a.*) from previous ovulation. *C.* Three days after ovulation. The corpus haemorrhagica (*c.h.*) develops from the walls of ruptured graafian follicle. *D.* Ten days after ovulation. Fully developed corpus luteum (*c.l.*); graafian follicles (*g.f.*) start to develop for subsequent cycle. *E.* Pregnancy—60 days. The corpus luteum of pregnancy (*c.l.*) is maintained, and graafian follicles (*g.f.*) develop as a result of circulating PMS. *F.* Pregnancy—80 days. Accessory corpora lutea (*c.a.*) develop from the unruptured follicles.

development. The administration of hCG shortens estrus and hastens ovulation. Injection of hCG is frequently used in an attempt to decrease the number of inseminations or matings per cycle and to synchronize ovulation time more accurately with mating.

LH.   The regulation of LH secretion involves two mechanisms: (1) a central ner-

vous system pituitary component responsible for a basal circannual rhythm of LH release, entrained to an environmental parameter (most probably photoperiod) and independent of ovarian influences and (2) an ovarian (steroidal) component that modifies the primary LH rhythm during the breeding season (Garcia and Ginther, 1978). In ovariectomized mares, concentrations of LH follow a seasonal pattern (low basal concentrations in winter; high basal concentrations in summer). The cyclic changes in LH concentrations during the breeding season seem to result from the modulation of high basal LH concentrations by ovarian steroids.

Levels of LH increase by the onset of estrus, reaching a maximum 1 to 2 days after ovulation. This rise in LH may stimulate maturation of the follicle throughout estrus. An inverse relationship between progesterone and LH levels occurs, suggesting a negative feedback, but there is no such relationship between FSH and progesterone concentrations. LH levels show a prolonged rise during estrus that continues after ovulation. A significant decrease from peak levels is not observed until the third day after ovulation, from which time levels continue to decline toward diestrous values.

The pattern of plasma LH in the mare differs from that in other species, and it is possible that persistence of high concentrations of LH results from a long half-life of the endogenous LH. This in turn may be responsible for the relatively large number of second ovulations detected in many estrous cycles (Geschwind et al., 1975). It seems that LH may be sensitive to progesterone feedback control in that levels do not start to rise until after the CL has regressed completely. On the other hand, high circulating progesterone levels apparently do not constitute an effective negative-feedback control mechanism once LH release has begun.

The administration of 2000 IU of hCG shortens estrus and hastens ovulation. Injection of hCG is used to accurately synchronize ovulation time with mating in an effort to decrease the number of inseminations or matings per cycle. Repeated hCG injection does not cause refractoriness.

In the mare, the uterus exerts its luteolytic effect on the CL primarily through a systemic utero-ovarian pathway. This conclusion is supported by the following findings in mares: (1) hysterectomy prolonged the life of the CL, but unilateral hysterectomy failed to indicate that a local utero-ovarian relationship was involved; (2) local administration of prostaglandin $F_{2\alpha}$ ($PGF_{2\alpha}$), a postulated uterine luteolysin, into the uterus did not improve its luteolytic efficacy over systemic administration given intramuscularly; (3) the vascular anatomy of uterus and ovaries provides limited potential for the local transfer of a luteolysin between uterus and ovary through a veno-arterial pathway (Douglas et al., 1976).

Progesterone. In the absence of ovulation, with or without follicular growth, there are prolonged periods of low progesterone levels. The daily intramuscular injection of 100 mg or more of progesterone during the midcycle prevents estrus and ovulation, but a dose of 50 mg per day inhibits only estrus. The interval between termination of treatment and estrus appears to depend on dosage. To counteract habitual abortion in the mare, the usual dosage is 250 to 500 mg every 10 to 30 days.

Induction of Estrus and Ovulation

Saline Infusion. The technique of intrauterine saline infusion has been used routinely to induce estrus in anestrous mares. Anestrous mares are affected only near the beginning and end of the breeding season when anovulatory heats are induced. Diestrous mares infused between days 5 and 9 return to heat 4 days earlier than expected, and induced estrus is accompanied by ovulation. Mares in prolonged diestrus may show ovulatory heats within 3 to 9 days of infusion (Arthur, 1975). Repeated infusions are clinically harmless, but postinfusion bacteriologic swabs from the uterus are positive.

Synchronization of Estrus. Mares are usually mated or artificially inseminated after estrus has been detected with a teaser stallion and follicular development has been assessed by rectal palpation of the ovaries. Synchronization of estrus and ovulation would allow mares to be inseminated at predetermined times without the need to detect estrus or palpate the ovaries.

Two treatments effectively influence ovarian activity in the mare: (1) induction of luteolysis with prostaglandin $F_{2\alpha}$ ($PGF_{2\alpha}$) or analogues of $PGF_{2\alpha}$ and (2) induction of ovulation during the follicular phase by an injection of hCG.

Prostaglandins. Of the farm species studied, the mare is most sensitive, on a body-weight basis, to the luteolytic effects of systemically (intramuscular or subcutaneous) administered $PGF_{2\alpha}$. Systemically administered $PGF_{2\alpha}$ is as effective in causing luteolysis in hysterectomized as in intact mares, indicating that the principal site of action of exogenous $PGF_{2\alpha}$ is not at the uterine level.

Prostaglandin $F_{2\alpha}$ and its analogues have been used to control the estrous cycle of the mare. The treatment causes a prompt cessation of secretion by the CL as indicated by a rapid fall in plasma progesterone levels. The infusion of 10 mg of $PGF_{2\alpha}$ on days 7 to 9 after ovulation causes a sharp fall in plasma progesterone levels and induces estrus and ovulation. This induced estrus is longer than the natural cycle but the time of ovulation in relation to the end of estrus is normal. The time of return to estrus following luteolysis does not depend on the amount of $PGF_{2\alpha}$. Luteolysis can be induced as early as day 5 following natural ovulation (Oxender et al., 1975). Prostaglandin $F_{2\alpha}$ ($PGF_{2\alpha}$) and its synthetic analogues are luteolytic in mares and cause abortion.

Intramuscular administration is as effective as subcutaneous administration, and 1.25 mg $PGF_{2\alpha}$ is the minimal effective systemic dose for inducing luteolysis. Administration of $PGF_{2\alpha}$ into the uterus or directly into the CL does not improve the luteolytic efficacy of the intramuscular injection of $PGF_{2\alpha}$.

Ova and Ova Transport. At ovulation, the ovum is without corona radiata but is enclosed in a large irregular gelatinous mass of ovarian origin, which separates

from the egg within 2 days. Fertilized ova are transported in the uterus, whereas unfertilized ova are trapped for several months in the isthmus of the oviduct. The ovum undergoes degeneration and fragmentation during the ensuing months. If a mare has a succession of sterile estrous cycles followed by a fertile mating, the developing embryo may outrun the unfertilized eggs trapped in the oviduct and enter the uterus.

Nonfertilized eggs may be retained in the oviducts of pregnant and nonpregnant mares for up to 7 months (Fig. 17–5). This indicates that the mare can discriminate

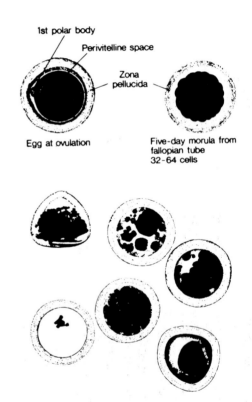

FIG. 17–5.   A normal horse egg before and after fertilization and degenerating oviductal eggs ranging in age from 1 to 7.5 months. The mechanisms by which the equine unfertilized ova are trapped in the oviduct are unknown. (From van Niekerk and Gerneke (1966). Onderstep. J. Vet. Res. *33*, 195; redrawn by Short (1972). *In* Reproduction in Mammals. Austin and Short (eds.). Cambridge, Cambridge University Press.)

between fertilized and nonfertilized eggs, allowing the fertilized egg to pass into the uterus while retaining nonfertilized eggs. Retained eggs are more common in heavy than in light breeds and are found more frequently in early than in late pregnancy.

Little is known about the function of the acellular capsule, which replaces the zona pellucida in the horse and then surrounds the embryo throughout its preattachment life in the uterus. The passage of a substance through the capsule to the embryo is influenced by the size and chemical nature of the substance's molecule.

The time when fertilized ova arrive in the uterus in the mare is much later (> 144 hours) than in the cow, and the cleavage stage of equine ova at arrival is more advanced than that in cattle. Transuterine migration of ova occurs in 50% of cases.

Extensive investigations conducted on equine reproduction physiology and management included the following: ovarian changes during ovulation and pregnancy (Genther, 1979; Squires et al., 1974); endocrine profile in pregnant and postpartum mares and cryptorchid stallions and following increased photoperiods (Ganjam et al., 1974, 1975; Oxender et al., 1979); energy undernutrition during weaning (Ellis and Lawrence, 1978); and manipulation of the estrous cycle and ovulation luteal function by prostaglandin $F_{2\alpha}$, by hCG and GnRH, and by intrauterine saline infusion (Kenney et al., 1975; Neely et al., 1974, 1979; Michel and Rossdale, 1986).

GESTATION

Gestation length in the mare ranges from 315 to 360 days and is influenced by maternal size, fetal genotype, and the stage of the breeding season when conception occurs. Development *in utero* can also be affected by degenerative wear and tear changes of the endometrium such as cystic fibrosis and glandular atrophy (Allen and Pashen, 1984). Fetal growth is retarded as a result of impaired placental function in mares exhibiting such changes, and gestation may be lengthened as a consequence.

Pregnancy Diagnosis and Developmental Horizons

Several methods are used for pregnancy diagnosis in the mare (Table 17–4). Diagnosis of pregnancy by rectal palpation of the ovaries and uterus is accurate 40 to 50 days after conception. A mouse biologic test that depends on PMSG to stimulate the ovaries of 21-day-old immature mice is accurate after 35 days of gestation of pregnancy. A qualitative hemagglutination-inhibition test for PMSG in serum is commercially available as a rapid test (MIP test, Diamond Labs). This test must await the serum rise in PMSG, because the test is not usable until 35 to 40 days after conception. Early pregnancy diagnosis can be done by ultrasound with 15% false-negative diagnosis.

The major developmental horizons of the equine fetus are summarized in Table 17–5.

Twinning

Twinning is rare. The natural occurrence of identical twins in the mare is virtually precluded by her general inability to carry twin conceptuses to term. This is primarily due to the competition of the placenta for contact with the maternal endometrium, which results in a net placental insufficiency for both conceptuses (Allen and Pashen, 1984). The usual outcome is for the more disadvantaged of the two fetuses to die during the second half of gestation and so initiate abortion. Monozygotic (identical) twins are valuable research tools in several types of biologic investigations. While monozygotic twins occur naturally in cattle, sheep, and women, albeit at a low frequency, they have not been reported to date in equids. In 2,673 thoroughbred mares, the spontaneous dizygotic twin conception rate was 2%.

Twin pregnancy is unwanted in the horse because of the high rate of abortion and a tendency to poor postnatal development in the few twin foals that survive to

TABLE 17–4.   Pregnancy Diagnosis in the Mare (Ginther, 1979)

Days After Ovulation	Criteria	Method	Comments
16–24	No behavioral, physical, or hormonal signs of estrus	Estrous detection	Few pregnant mares show estrus (nonpregnant mares may fail to show estrus due to pseudopregnancy or silent estrus) Mucous membranes and cervix are given for estrus and diestrus Tense tone is good presumptive indicator before bulge is detectable; does not differentiate from pseudopregnancy High values (1 ng/ml) are presumptive indicators but do not differentiate from pseudopregnancy or cycles of unusual length
16–17	Presence (nonpregnant) or absence (pregnant) of estrus in response to estrogen	Single injection of estrogen detection for estrus	False-positives in pseudopregnancy or early embryonic death
28–term	Changes in stained vaginal mucus	Mucin test	Positive results as early as day 20 effective after day 80; false-positives from pseudopregnancy
45–90	PMSG in blood	Immunologic and biologic tests	Special precautions to differentiate from anestrus Hemagglutination kits available in some countries Biologic tests involve injection of serum into rodents or frogs Accuracy of approximately 90%, but false-positives can result from maintenance of endometrial cups after abortion
60–term	Uterine content	Rectal palpation	Ballottment and palpation of fetus
90–term	Fetal heart beat	Ultrasonography	Transducer placed in rectum; fetal pulse occasionally detected as early as day 40, consistently between days 90 and 240
150–term	Estrogens in urine	Chemical (Cuboni) biologic tests	Adding chemicals to urine and observing fluorescence; reliable after day 150

PMSG = pregnant mare serum gonadotropin.

term. Thus, most twins that are conceived are deliberately aborted early in gestation, and the mare is remated in an attempt to produce a singleton pregnancy during the same breeding season. In most dizygotic twin pregnancies, there is invagination of the adjacent allantochorions. Identical blood groups are found in twin foals, indicating chimerism and macroscopic or microscopic anastomosis between both chorions. Stillbirth is frequent in twin pregnancies, and only one half of the foals born survive. Twin pregnancies are not desirable in view of the high peri- and

TABLE 17–5. Developmental Horizons of Equine Fetus

Days of Pregnancy	Head	Legs	Reproductive Organs	Hair	Conformation
40	Ears rudimentary Eyelids External nares	Elbows and stifles	Migration of genital tubercle begins	Nil	Head between forelegs
45	—	—	Sex determinable	Nil	
55	Ears-triangle fold cover opening eyelids closed except for 1 mm slit	Hocks and fetlocks	Prominent vulva or penis Mammary papillae (0.25- mm dots)	Nil	Prominent brain case
60	Eyelids closed or almost closed nares—1 × 0.5 mm slits	Soles and frogs	—	Nil	Unmistakably equine
80	—	Points of shoulders and hips	Mammary papillae are raised buds Scrotum; pale bulge, 2 cm behind umbilicus	Nil	Head and neck in normal position
100	Ears: 1 cm long and curled forward and down Eyes bulging	Hooves: pale yellow, raised coronary band	Clitoris recessed to postnatal position	On lips	Muscle groups easily recognized
120	—	—	Vulval lips meet at ventral commissure Prepuce pendulous	On chin, muzzle, eyelids	—
150	—	Ergots, 5 mm	Glandular shaped mammae in female Palpable gubernaculum in scrotum	Eyelashes	—
180	—	—	Suspension of mammary gland in female	Early mane and tail hairs	—
210	—	—	Suspension of mammary gland in female	Mane hair, 2.5 mm	—
240	—	—		On ears, poll, back of tail Vibrissae on throat, chin, muzzle	—
270	—	—	—	Body covered with fine hair Tail switch	—
300	—	Prominent pad covering soles	—	Full-term coat	—

(Data of Ginther, 1979, 1984.)

postnatal losses and the poor viability and racing performance of twins. Subsequent conception rate is not affected by twin birth if the mare foals at full term, but it decreases following abortion.

Ovarian Function

Four distinct stages of ovarian function are recognized.

1. During early pregnancy, a single CL verum is present; it was believed that this regressed at approximately day 40 of gestation, but according to subsequent observations (Squires et al., 1974), the primary CL persists beyond day 40.

2. Between day 40 and 150 of pregnancy, ovarian activity occurs. As many as 10 to 15 follicles (over 1 cm in diameter) undergo luteinization to form the accessory corpora lutea. The recovery of recently ovulated ova from the oviducts suggests that some of these follicles ovulate even though unfertilized ova are retained in the oviduct for several months. Usually, each ovary contains 3 to 5 accessory corpora lutea (Fig. 17-4).

3. From the fifth to the seventh month, though both primary and secondary corpora lutea and the large follicles regress completely, the mare does not show signs of estrus, which is due to placental secretion of progesterone until the end of gestation.

4. From the seventh month onward, only vestiges of the corpora lutea and small follicles are present, but during the last 2 weeks of gestation follicular activity commences in preparation for the postpartum estrus ("foaling heat").

The primary and secondary corpora lutea and the placenta all contribute to the total progesterone pool during pregnancy. The corpora lutea progesterone concentration in the peripheral plasma is closely correlated with morphologic changes in the corpora lutea. Similarities and differences in ovarian function observed between pregnant and hysterectomized mares suggest that, while PMSG does not appear to stimulate follicular develop-

ment, it does prolong the life span and stimulate the secretory activity of the primary CL and induced ovulation and/or luteinization of secondary follicles in pregnant mares (Squires and Ginther, 1975). Ovariectomy does not terminate pregnancy, if performed after day 70 of pregnancy.

Placenta

The placenta of the mare is classified as diffuse, microcotyledonary, and epitheliochorial (Fig. 17-6 and 17-7). The outer surface of the chorion is closely studded with tufts of branching villi that enter into corresponding invaginations in the endometrium to form small globular structures known as *microcotyledons*. Microcotyledons, which are a distinctive feature of the mature equine placenta, are fully formed by the fifth month of gestation. The primary folds of trophoblast become elaborately subdivided as gestation proceeds. These changes are reflected in the structure of the maternal crypts, which receive the fetal villi.

Within each microcotyledon, chorionic and uterine epithelia are in intimate contact, and a microvillous junction is formed at the fetal–maternal boundary.

Placental Barrier. The following mechanisms control the passage of gases, nutrients, ions, or hormones across the placental barrier: (1) those related to diffusion across the placental tissues, i.e., permeability, diffusion distances, total surface area, and concentration gradients between maternal and fetal blood vessels; (2) rates of supply and removal on either size of the placenta, the presence or absence of specialized exchange areas, the direction of blood flow in these areas, and the existence of shunts or unequal flows; and (3) specialized mechanisms that assist the passage of substances and, in the case of oxygen, differences in hemoglobin O_2 affinity and O_2 capacity between fetus and mother (Silver and Comline, 1975).

The primary CL that develops at the site of the fertile ovulation regresses about

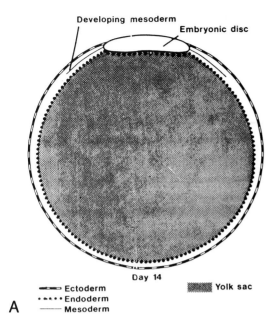

Day 14

■□■ Ectoderm
• ▲ • ▲ Endoderm
—— Mesoderm

▨ Yolk sac

A

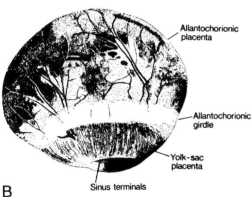

Allantochorionic placenta

Allantochorionic girdle

Yolk-sac placenta

B   Sinus terminals

FIG. 17–6. *A.* Equine conceptus of 2 weeks of gestation (diameter, 16 mm) is spherical, located in the uterine body, the conceptus not attached to its eventual location in the caudal portion of a uterine horn. Mesodermal tissue grows from the embryonic disc into the area between the trophoblast (ectodermal origin) and the endoderm of the yolk sac. The mesoderm gives origin to supportive mesenchyme or connective tissue blood vessels. Some islands of rudimentary vessels are already visible, histologically (From Ginther, 1979). *B.* Equine conceptus, 7 weeks of gestation, the size of an orange. Cells become detached around the allantochorionic girdle at this stage to invade the endometrium and form the endometrial cups. (From Short (1972). *In* Reproduction in Mammals. C.R. Austin and V. Short (eds.). Cambridge, Cambridge University Press).

day 160 of gestation and is replaced by secondary corpora lutea. The primary and secondary corpora lutea and the placenta all contribute to the total progesterone pool during pregnancy. The luteal progesterone concentration in the peripheral plasma is closely correlated with morphologic changes in the CL.

Similarities and differences in ovarian function observed between pregnant and hysterectomized mares suggest that, while PMSG does not appear to stimulate follicular development, it does prolong the life span and stimulate the secretory activity of the primary CL and induce ovulation and/or luteinization of secondary follicles in pregnant mares (Squires and Ginther, 1975).

Endocrine Profile

Steroids. Plasma progestogen levels decline in midpregnancy and remain low until a few days before parturition, when they increase again. During pregnancy there are two peaks of plasma progestogens. The first, which occurs during the third month, coincides with high levels of PMSG and is probably produced by the endometrial cups or the secondary CL. The second peak occurs in the eleventh month and probably represents the secretion of placental progestogens. Blood estrogen levels are highest at midgestation and decrease significantly before parturition. The pregnant mare, moreover, excretes some other estrogens that are peculiar to the mare and other equids.

During the fourth to eighth months, estrone levels exceed 100 ng/ml and then decline toward parturition. The high concentrations of estrone in midpregnancy are associated with gradually increasing concentrations of equilin, which tend to plateau after the sixth month at just under 100 ng/ml and decline only in the last month of pregnancy.

Gonadotropins (PMSG). The endometrial cups, which are present from the second to the fourth months of pregnancy, are the source of the gonadotropin PMSG,

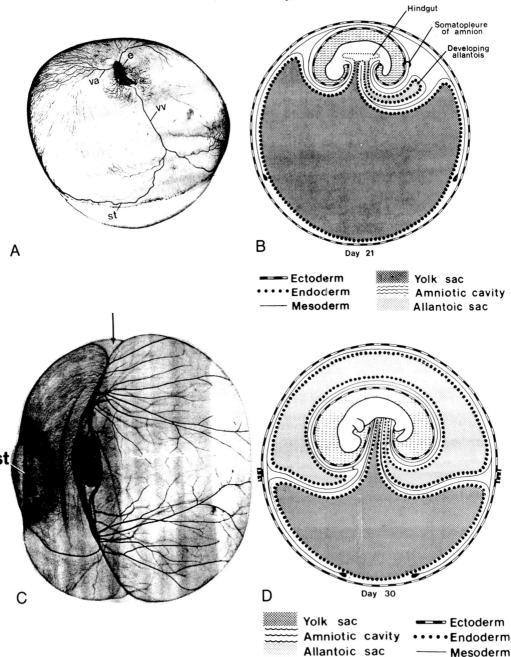

FIG. 17–7. *A and B.* Spherical conceptus from a pony mare: *e,* embryo; yolk sac vasculature (*vv,* vitelline vein; *va,* vitelline artery); *st,* sinus terminalis; the prominent collecting vein that encircles the vesicle. The vesicle is 2.6 cm in diameter when submerged and flattened slightly to a diameter of 3.5 cm on removal of the fluid in which it was submerged. Note completion of amniotic cavity and emergence of the allantois from the hind gut. The allantois grows into the exocoelom between the somatopleure and splanchnopleure. *C and D.* The exposed vesicle as viewed from embryonic pole. The dark spot in center of the vesicle is the embryo. Prominent vessels are in the allantochorion. Sinus terminalis is still prominent. Chorion (arrow) between allantois (right) and yolk sac (left) is the location of the chorionic girdle. The mesoderm remains avascular. The allantois continues to grow, and the yolk sac recedes. Because the yolk sac remains attached at the bilaminar omphalopleure, the embryo is pulled by the receding yolk sac (From Ginther, 1979).

which circulates in the maternal blood between 40 and 130 days of gestation. The maternal ovaries are thus stimulated, forming ovarian follicles, many of which ovulate and form accessory corpora lutea, while others luteinize without ovulating. The accessory corpora lutea persist until about 180 days of gestation and then degenerate. During the remainder of gestation, no lutein tissue is formed. If a mare aborts about the 35th day of gestation, when the fetal cells have already invaded the endometrium, the endometrial cups continue to develop normally and secrete PMSG, and the corpora lutea that are present may be maintained.

Several factors influence PMSG levels: season, maternal size, parity, and fetal genotype. A high level of PMSG occurs in the serum of a mare carrying twin fetuses if a set of endometrial cups develops in both uterine horns. The sudden fall in the blood level of this hormone in a mare that aborts compared to the maintenance of a high blood level in another in which resorption has taken place suggests that the conceptus may be necessary for the continued function of this hormone.

The fetal genotype has a pronounced effect on PMSG concentration in the mother. Blood serum of mares bred to a jack donkey contains only about 10% of the PMSG concentration in mares bred to a stallion. It appears that the allantochorion may provide a stimulus, possibly chemical in nature, that regulates the secretory activity of the endometrial cups.

PMSG disappears from the blood of mares carrying mule fetuses by the third month of gestation, which is much earlier than in mares carrying horse fetuses. PMSG concentration is high in a donkey mare carrying a hinny fetus. In surgical removal of the conceptus from the uterus on or after day 38 of gestation or fetal death occurring after day 40, PMSG production continues normally as though the mare is still pregnant (Hay and Allen, 1975). The endometrial cups, once functional, have a life span that is independent of the conceptus.

PMSG may play a major role in stimulating secondary follicular development and accessory CL development during the first half of gestation, but similarities in follicular development in hysterectomized and pregnant mares indicate that other factors may be responsible for follicular development in pregnant mares (Squires et al., 1974).

FOALING

The time of foaling, which usually takes place between nightfall and daybreak, seems to be influenced by photoperiods and quietness in the stable. In England, 86% of foalings occur between 1900 and 0700 hours (7:00 P.M. and 7:00 A.M.), with a maximal incidence between 2200 and 2300 hours (10:00 P.M. and 11:00 P.M.).

The imminence of foaling is suggested by the degree of mammary hypertrophy, waxing of the teats, and possibly the discharge of milk from the udder. The best indication that the first stage has begun is the onset of patchy sweating behind the elbows and about the flanks. This sweating commences about 4 hours before foaling and increases as the stage progresses. The tail is frequently raised or held to one side.

Induced Parturition

Parturition can be induced by various doses of estrogen, prostaglandins ($PGF_{2\alpha}$), and oxytocin. The time of appearance and degree of expression of the major clinical signs of parturition, and the time for completion of delivery and the passage of the placenta are influenced by increasing doses of oxytocin. Estrogen is useful in softening and relaxing the cervix when it is tight but is not essential to induction when the cervix is already soft and dilating.

Progesterone (500 mg/day) administered daily from day 318 of pregnancy shortened gestation, while estrogen (50 mg/day) administered on the same schedule as progesterone had no such effect. Parturition can be induced in the mares of large-sized breeds by daily treatment with 100 mg of dexamethasone for 4 days. However, parturition has not been successfully induced in pony mares. Single or low doses of dexamethasone do not induce parturition. The mode of action of dexamethasone in causing premature birth in the equine is unknown. Dexamethasone seems to induce a normal parturition, because all prepartum signs—including vulva dilatation, mammary development, and sinking in the flank area—are normal.

Indications for elective induction of parturition in the mare include delayed parturition resulting from uterine atony, prolonged gestation, prevention of injury at foaling, preparturient colic, injury to the mare and impending rupture of the prepubic tendon, and obtaining colostrum-deprived foals for research purposes. Fertility is not adversely affected by induced parturition.

Postpartum Estrus (Foal Heat)

Postpartum estrus usually occurs 5 to 15 days after foaling. Some mares, however, may show estrus as late as 45 days after parturition; such estrus may have been preceded by a quiet ovulation. The interval between postpartum estrus and the following estrus may be affected by the milk yield. Breeding at the postpartum estrus may cause an increased percentage of abortion, dystocia, stillbirth, and retained placenta. This may be due to the introduction of bacteria into the uterus before it is completely involved and while it still lacks contractility.

Involution of the uterus after normal foaling is rapid. Regression in size is almost complete by the first day of "foal heat." The relatively low conception rate from copulation during this period appears to indicate that involution of the endometrium is not complete in all mares.

EQUINE HYBRIDS

There are several equine hybrids:
Horse (stallion)×donkey (jenny)=hinny
Donkey (jack) × horse (mare) = mule
Zebra × donkey (jenny) = zebronkey
Zebra × horse (mare) = zebrorse
These hybrids of both sexes are infertile because horses, donkeys, and zebras have different chromosome numbers and the hybrids have a number intermediate between their parents. The germ cells of the hybrids proceed through mitosis, but there is a block to meiosis, because paring of homologous chromosomes is impossible as a result of uneven chromosome numbers (McDonald, 1989). Testosterone (Leydig cells) is produced in the male hybrid and libido exists, but the block to spermatogenesis causes infertility (see Fig. 17–5). Estrogen is not produced by the hybrid ovary, however, because meiosis must occur for the follicle to develop sufficiently to elaborate estrogen. Consequently, very few female mules produce enough sex steroids to exhibit estrus.

REPRODUCTIVE FAILURE IN MARES

Conception and foaling percentages differ widely. In a few pony studs, conception rate and foaling rates are 100%. In most studs, the foaling rate is much lower than the conception rate. In general, the conception rate is influenced by the breed, nutrition, and age of the dam and management practices. For example, the conception rate from first service is lower in Thoroughbred mares than in most other breeds. The conception rate of foaling mares served during foal heat is lower than the first-service pregnancy rate of foaling mares served after the foal heat.

Reproductive efficiency in horses is low compared to that in other farm animals. Reproductive failure in mares may be due to hormonal dysfunction, genital infection, inadequate management, and improper detection of estrus.

Estrous Irregularities

Irregularities in the estrous cycle are associated with seasonal changes in the photoperiod, nutrition, and climate. Variations in patterns of cyclic behavior include cycle length and estrous behavior, failure of ovulation and follicular development, and spontaneous prolongation of the corpora lutea. "Quiet ovulation," anovulatory estrus, "split estrus," and prolonged estrus are not uncommon.

Split estrus is commonly observed in healthy mares during the early spring. In such cases, behavioral estrus is interrupted by an interval of sexual nonreceptivity. Fairly frequently, the follicle that is present at the beginning of the first part of the split estrus continues its growth normally throughout the period and will ovulate. Prolonged estrus, lasting 10 to 40 days, may also occur in early spring and in mares used for heavy draft.

Intrauterine infusion of saline may induce estrus in some mares with irregular or no ovarian activity. The distention of the uterus by the infused saline acts as a stimulus to release pituitary gonadotropins. Intrauterine saline infusion in diestrus shortens the ovulatory interval by inducing premature luteolysis, but during estrus it has little effect on cycle length.

Anestrus

There are three forms of anestrus: (1) a winter anestrus that lasts 11 weeks in which follicles rarely reach 35 mm before regressing without ovulation and plasma levels of progestogen are 1 ng/ml; (2) a CL that persists for 5 to 13 weeks with elevated plasma progestogen levels, usually in November and December; and (3) cyclic ovulatory patterns unaccompanied by estrus (Hughes et al., 1975).

Evans and Irvine (1977) designed a regimen of exogenous GnRH to reproduce in acyclic (anestrous) mares the sequence of changes in plasma FSH and LH that occur in the normal cycle, in an attempt to induce follicular development culminating in ovulation. A single injection of GnRH in anestrous mares will cause an increase in serum FSH to 3.7 times baseline, which is comparable to the peak increases occurring during the estrous cycle; however, the induced increase in LH is much less than that of the cyclic peak. GnRH in com-

bination with appropriate progesterone treatment in the acyclic mare treated toward the end of the nonbreeding season can consistently induce normal cyclic pituitary and ovarian activity culminating in ovulation (Evans and Irvine, 1977).

Prenatal Mortality

Prenatal mortality is frequent in lactating mares mated early in the season or mated after foal heat. Prenatal death is also common in certain horse families. Higher prenatal mortality in yearlings compared to adult mares may be due to inadequate progestogen levels to maintain pregnancy, immaturity of the yearlings, their greater nutritional requirements for growth and maintenance, and the physical stresses imposed on them by the husbandry procedures. Infection of the fetus *in utero* is a significant cause of prenatal mortality in the later months of pregnancy.

Ovarian Neoplasms

Neoplasms of the equine reproductive organs are uncommon, whereas teratoma and granulosa cell tumors are not uncommon. Ovarian tumors have been classified according to their histogenetic origin: (1) stromal and derived from the mesenchymal core of the germinal ridge, with possible contributions from connective and vascular tissues of the hilus; (2) differentiated epithelial cells, such as the granulosa, theca, and lutein cells, a syndrome associated with hormonal imbalance; (3) dysgerminoma, a rare tumor similar to the seminoma of stallions; and (4) cystadenoma derived from the surface coelomic epithelium and of tubular ingrowths in the gonadal cortex.

Granulosa cell tumor is a common neoplasm that affects only one ovary. Its incidence increases with age, and it is usually associated with overproduction of steroid hormones leading to clinical signs of excessive estrogenization. The surface of the granulosa cell tumor is smooth, the cut surface may be either solid or cystic, and its white or yellow color depends on the amount of ovarian lipids. The teratoma, a true tumor composed of multiple tissues foreign to the part in which they arise, is noted in mares 1 to 5 years of age.

Endometrial Cysts and Related Pathologic Conditions

Focal enlargements of the uterus palpable through the rectal wall have various causes. Lymphatic lacunae seem to be common in older mares and may occasionally give rise to a large endometrial cyst or cause widespread change throughout the uterine horns. In cases of myometrial atony and endometrial atrophy, repeated uterine infusions of hot (40° to 45°C) saline with or without antibiotics may enhance myometrial tone. The response is rapid but transient.

Genital Infections

Uterine infections cause shortening of the estrous cycles. Experimental intrauterine inoculation of *Streptococcus zooepidemicus* into mares during diestrus may shorten the length of the estrous cycle. Chronic endometritis includes latent, purulent, hypertrophic, and atrophic types and pyometra. Several factors may cause endometritis in the mare: breeding at the wrong stage of the estrous cycle; too frequent matings during estrus; poor hygiene at mating or foaling; excessive work during the breeding season, especially at estrus; atony of the uterus as a result of dystocia, general debility or old age; the retention of part of the placenta at abortion or foaling. Prognosis and treatment of infertile mares are based on the breeding history, clinical data, and histopathologic findings of endometrial biopsy and cervical mucus.

The internal reproductive organs can be examined by endoscopy. A human rhinolaryngoscope can be used. The induction of artificial pneumoperitoneum and the installation of an endoscopic peritoneal fistula device are used to prolong the observation period. New concepts of endo-

scopic instrumentation and surgical techniques have enlarged the scope of medical endoscopy in clinical and basic research.

Excessive or prolonged intrauterine infusion of antibiotics in the treatment of chronic endometritis in mares is usually followed by the establishment of fungi and yeasts in the genital tract.

Intrauterine Growth Retardation. Virus infection of the fetus may lead to stunted development in some species, although viruses have not yet been implicated in the pathogenesis of fetal growth retardation in the horse. However, chronic placental infection may interfere with placental exchange and thereby impair fetal growth. For example, birth weight is greatly reduced in cases of rhinopneumonitis and fungal placentitis.

Excessive Length of Umbilical Cord

The length of the umbilical cord is not correlated with gestational age, foal's body weight, sex or viability, dam's age or parity, or surface area, width, or length of the allantochorion. However, cord length is correlated with weight of the allantochorion and allantoamnion and the length of the nonpregnant horn. Several pathologic conditions of unknown origin cause excessive elongation of the umbilical cord. Reproductive failures associated with these conditions include (1) strangulation by the cord around the fetus; (2) excessive twisting around the amniotic or allantoic portion of the fetus, causing vascular occlusion and/or urinary retention; or (3) necrosis of the chorioallantois at the cervix. Strangulation of the fetus may cause abortion, with deep grooves present around the head, neck, thorax, and back with apparent local edema.

Mild urachal obstruction is compatible with normal pregnancy. The umbilical cord may become twisted with multiple urachal dilations that prevent normal sealing of the bladder apex at birth. Excessive twisting of the umbilical cord threatens the integrity of the urachus and umbilical vessels; the effects depend on the completeness, duration, and site of the compression.

Abortion

The average abortion rate in mares is high (10%). This may be due to peculiarities in the hormonal balance of the mare during pregnancy. Abortion is lowest between 3 and 6 years of age, and most abortions that are due to infection occur during the later stages of pregnancy. During the fifth and tenth months of pregnancy, the mares are endocrinologically susceptible to abortion owing to hormonal deficiencies. It is recommended to avoid sudden changes in the diet or the amount of physical exercise at these times. Postabortum conception rate is low, especially in older mares.

Abortion in older mares may be due to uterine inadequacies. The normal endometrium is thrown into more or less longitudinal folds that vary in size with the estrous cycle. Implantation occurs at the junction of the body and horns of the uterus, and the folds in this region can undergo atrophy after several pregnancies. The atrophic areas appear to have a reduced number of endometrial glands and, in some cases, contain collagen and/or inflammatory cells.

Neonatal Abnormalities and Neonatal Mortality

Microphthalmos (button eye) and entropion are regular congenital abnormalities in Thoroughbreds. The degree of microphthalmos is variable and may be so severe that the globe is obscured behind a well-developed third eyelid. The cornea is often distorted and pigmented, and the palpebral aperture is usually smaller than normal; the condition can be bilateral or unilateral. Entropion is both congenital and hereditary and may lead to corneal opacity and ulceration.

Barker Syndrome (Convulsive Foal Syndrome, or Neonatal Maladjustment Syndrome). This syndrome affects Thoroughbred foals, often those that have experienced an easy birth, and occurs within minutes after birth to 24 hours later. Clinical symptoms include jerking movements of the head, limb, and body musculature; hyperexcitability; inability to stand; convulsions; opisthotonus; and erection of the tail. There may also be collapse of the external nares, deep inspiratory movement, and a barking sound. If able to stand, the foal may walk around aimlessly. Recovery occurs in about 50% of cases and is usually complete.

The syndrome is associated with necrosis of the cerebral cortex, diencephalon, and brain stem, and with severe hemorrhage in the white and gray matter of the cerebral cortex and in the cerebellum.

Ocular Changes. The eye of the foal, which is open at birth, has a clear cornea and ocular media. The fundus is differentiated into tapetum lucidum and tapetum nigrum and is similar to the fundus of the adult horse. Ocular changes in the convulsive foal syndrome include asymmetry of pupils, apparent blindness, variable pupil size, scleral splashing, and retinal petechiae. These clinical signs are not always present, even in severe cases. Small round retinal hemorrhages may occur, which are clearly visible as red dots against the background of the tapetal fundus. These hemorrhages occur at 1 and 2 days of age in convulsive foals and persist only a few days.

Neonatal Mortality. Neonatal mortality may be a result of weakness of the mother or the foal or bacterial infection through the umbilical cord of the young. Proper management, clean stables for foaling, and sanitary precautions at foaling are the common preventive methods of neonatal mortality.

Recommendations for Breeding Techniques

Careful testing for estrus with the stallion, routine examination of the vagina, and rectal palpation of the reproductive organs may help to improve conception rate. Whenever possible, the time of ovulation should be predicted, because the duration of estrus and the time of ovulation from the onset of estrus may differ between individuals. Conception rate depends primarily on the time and number of inseminations.

On occasion, the mare may strain (as in micturition and defecation) after mating and evacuate most of the semen from the uterus. This may be prevented by having the mare walk for a while after mating. The mare is susceptible to endometritis, especially after foaling, because the cervix of the mare is not a strong barrier to the introduction of bacteria. The mare is more prone to a deficiency in LH than other farm animals; such deficiency may be alleviated by the use of exogenous LH. The intravenous injection of 1500 to 3000 IU of hCG may cause ovulation during anovulatory estrus, provided the ovarian follicle is at least 3 cm in diameter.

REPRODUCTIVE FAILURE IN STALLIONS

Reproductive failure in stallions includes abnormal sexual behavior, ejaculatory disturbances, and poor semen characteristics.

Abnormal Sexual Behavior and Ejaculatory Disturbances

Abnormal sexual behavior of stallions includes (1) failure to attain or maintain an erection with poor or excellent libido; (2) incomplete intromission or lack of pelvic thrusts after intromission, poor libido or pain from injuries incurred during breeding; (3) dismounting at onset of ejaculation because of injury or pain; (4) failure to ejaculate in spite of a complete prolonged erection and repeated intromissions; (5) good ejaculation for a short time, but no further ejaculation without sexual rest, although libido remains high; and (6) masturbation (Pickett and Voss, 1975). Impotent stallions respond well to retraining, and recovery can be achieved without pharmacologic treatment. Masturbation in breeding stallions, an abnormal sexual behavior, may be treated by the use of a stallion ring, but this may cause hemospermia.

Ejaculatory disturbances are manifested differently in individual stallions, from normal copulation with or without occasional ejaculation. In most cases, penile erection is associated with several copulatory movements that terminate in complete or incomplete failure of ejaculation. Ejaculatory disturbances—transitory, intermittent or permanent—may occur during the first two or three breeding seasons or after several seasons of normal activity. To ensure that ejaculation has taken place after intromission, one holds the hand under the base of the penis. In the absence of ejaculation, a few weak urethral waves may be felt, but when ejaculation takes place it feels like the contents of a 10-ml syringe being transported along the urethra. In a stallion of good fertility, it is usual to feel about five of these waves; in the stallion with lower fertility, one sometimes feels only about one and a half waves.

Ejaculatory disturbance may arise from directed blocking of nerve impulses or from fatness, poor condition, or exhaustion resulting from frequent services. Stallions usually also react strongly to unfamiliar surroundings, and psychic factors of this nature may inhibit the normal stimulation from the supraspinal centers. Ejaculatory disturbance may be due to failure of contraction of smooth muscles in the reproductive tract as a result of refractoriness of these cells to norepinephrine, exhaustion of the norepinephrine depots, or failure to release norepinephrine from the sympathetic nerve endings.

Poor Semen Characteristics

This may include one of the following: azoospermia, absence of sperm in the ejaculate; oligozoospermia, decreased sperm concentration per milliliter of semen; teratospermia, increased percentage of morphologically abnormal spermatozoa; asthenospermia, decreased sperm motility; or hemospermia, hemorrhage in semen.

Hemospermia results from urethritis in the ejaculatory ducts. Hemospermia may occur occasionally, in isolated instances or in each ejaculate, irrespective of frequency of ejaculation. Affected stallions frequently require several mounts to ejaculate and often exhibit pain on ejaculation. Semen quality as determined by motility, sperm numbers, and morphology is usually unaffected, and the cause of the infertility is unknown. Urethroscopic examination, urethrography, bacterial and viral cultures, biopsy, surgery of the urethra, and histocytologic examination are used for diagnosis (Voss and Pickett, 1975). The exact cause and location of the hemorrhage should be known before treatment is initiated.

Several species of microflora have been found in the semen: *Pseudomonas* spp., *Escherichia coli, Klebsiella, Aerobacter (Enterobacter), Proteus* spp., *Staphylococcus* spp., *Streptococcus* spp., and other gram-positive and gram-negative rods. These microorganisms, however, do not seem to affect the fertility. Most *Streptococcus* spp. in the semen are contaminants from the prepuce.

Recommendations for Breeding Techniques

The detrimental effect of frequent ejaculations on the number of sperm per ejaculate is pronounced in the stallion. In natural breeding, where several mares may exhibit estrus simultaneously, a stallion may copulate several times on one day; this causes a decline in fertility. The use of artificial insemination during such periods of mating will improve the conception rate. The stallion ejaculates directly into the uterus, and in most cases there is little semen left in the vagina. The transfer of semen from the vagina to the uterus following insemination is seldom necessary, but this is recommended with wriggling mares or if a stallion is apt to dismount the mare with the penis still erect, as this pulls semen back into the vagina.

REFERENCES

Allen, W.R. (1984). Hormonal control of early pregnancy in the mare. Anim. Reprod. Sci. *7*, 283–304.

Allen, W.R. and Pashen, R.L. (1984). Production of monozygotic (identical) horse twins by embryo micromanipulation. J. Reprod. Fertil. *71*, 607–613.

Arthur, G.H. (1975). Influence of intrauterine saline infusion upon the estrous cycle of the mare. J. Reprod. Fertil. Suppl. *23*, 231.

Douglas, R.H., Del Campo, M.R. and Ginther, O.J. (1976). Luteolysis following carotid or ovarian arterial injection of prostaglandin $F_{2\alpha}$ in mares. Biol. Reprod. *14*, 473.

Ellis, R.N.W. and Lawrence, T.L.J. (1978). Energy undernutrition in the weanling filly foal. Br. Vet. J. *134*, 205.

Evans, M.J. and Irvine, C.H.G. (1977). Induction of follicular development, maturation and ovulation by gonadotropin in releasing hormone administration to acyclic mares. Biol. Reprod. *16*, 452.

Ganjam, V.K., Kenney, R.M. and Flickinger, G. (1975). Plasma progestagens in cyclic, pregnant and postpartum mares. J. Reprod. Fertil. Suppl. *23*, 441.

Ganjam, V.K., Kenney, R.M. and Gledhill, B.L. (1974). Increased concentration of androgens in cryptorchid stallion testes. 1. J. Steroid Biochem. *5*, 709.

Garcia, M.C. and Ginther, O.J. (1978). Regulation of plasma LH by estradiol and progesterone in ovariectomized mares. Biol. Reprod. *19*, 447.

Geschwind, I.I., Dewey, R., Hughes, J.P., Evans, J.W. and Stabenfeldt, G.H. (1975). Plasma LH levels in the mare during the estrus cycle. J. Reprod. Fertil. Suppl. *23*, 207.

Ginther, O.J. (1979). Reproductive Biology of the Mare. Cross Plains, WI, O.J. Ginther.

Ginther, O.J. (1984). Intrauterine movement of the early conceptus in barren and postpartum mares. Theriogenology *21*, 633.

Hay, M. and Allen, W.R. (1975). An ultrastructural and histochemical study of the interstitial cells in the gonads of the fetal horse. J. Reprod. Fertil. Suppl. *23*, 557.

Hughes, J.P., Stabenfeldt, G.H. and Evans, J.W. (1972). Clinical and endocrine aspects of the estrous cycle of the mare. Proc. A. Meeting, Am. Ass. Equine Pract.

Hughes, J.P., Stabenfeldt, G.H. and Evans, J.W. (1975). The estrous cycle of the mare. J. Reprod. Fertil. Suppl. *23*, 161.

Kenney, R.M., Ganjam, V.K., Cooper, W.L. et al. (1975). The use of prostaglandin $F_{2\alpha}$-THAM salt in mares in clinical anoestrus. J. Reprod. Fertil. *23*(Suppl.), 247.

Mann, T., Short, R.V. and Walton, A. (1957). The "tail-end sample" of stallion semen. F. Agric. Sci. Camb., *49,* 301.

McDonald, L.E. (1989). "Reproductive Patterns of Horses" *In* Veterinary Endocrinology and Reproduction, 4th Ed. L.E. McDonald (ed.). Philadelphia, Lea & Febiger.

Michel T.H. and Rossdale, P.D. (1986). Efficacy of hCG and GnRH for hastening ovulation in thoroughbred mares. Equine Vet. J. *6,* 150.

Neely, D., Hughes, J.P. and Stabenfeldt, G.H. (1974). The influence of intrauterine saline infusion on luteal function and cyclic ovarian activity in the mare. Equine Vet. J. *6,* 150.

Neely, D.P., Stabenfeldt, G.H., Kindahl, H. et al. (1979). Effect of intrauterine saline infusion during the late luteal phase on the estrous cycle and luteal function of the mare. Am. J. Vet. Res. *40,* 665.

Nishikawa, Y. (1959). Studies on Reproduction in Horses. Tokyo, Japan Racing Association.

Oxender, W.D., Noden, P.A. and Hafs, H.D. (1979). Estrus, ovulation and plasma hormones after prostaglandin $F_{2\alpha}$ in mares. J. Reprod. Fertil. Suppl. *23,* 251.

Oxender, W.D., Noden, P.A. and Hafs, H.D. (1977). Estrus, ovulation, and serum progesterone, estradiol, and LH concentrations in mares after an increased photoperiod during winter. Am. J. Vet. Res. *38,* 203.

Pickett, B.W. and Voss, J.L. (1975). Abnormalities of mating behavior in domestic stallions. *In* Equine Reproduction. I.W. Rowlands, W.R. Allen and D.P. Rossdale (eds.). Oxford, Blackwell Scientific Publications.

Pickett, B.W., Faulkner, L.C. and Voss, J.L. (1975). Effect of season on some characteristics of stallion semen. *In* Equine Reproduction. I.W. Rowlands, W.R. Allen and P.D. Rossdale (eds.). Oxford, Blackwell Scientific Publications.

Silver, M. and Comline, R.S. (1975). Transfer of gases and metabolites in the equine placenta: a comparison with other species. J. Reprod. Fertil. Suppl. *23,* 589.

Squires, E.L., Douglas, R.H., Steffenhagen, W.P. et al. (1974). Ovarian changes during the estrous cycle and pregnancy in mares. J. Anim. Sci. *38,* 330.

Squires, E.L., Garcia, M.C. and Ginther, O.J. (1974). Effects of pregnancy and hysterectomy on the ovaries of pony mares. J. Anim. Sci. *38,* 823.

Squires, E.L. and Ginther, O.J. (1975). Follicular and luteal development in pregnant mares. J. Reprod. Fertil. Suppl. *23,* 249.

Tischner, M., Kosiniak, K. and Bielanski, W. (1974). Analysis of the pattern of ejaculation in stallions. J. Reprod. Fertil. *41,* 329.

Voss, J.L. and Pickett, B.W. (1975). Diagnosis and treatment of haemospermia in the stallion. *In* Equine Reproduction. I.W. Rowlands, W.R. Allen and P.D. Rossdale (eds.). Oxford, Blackwell Scientific Publications.

18
Poultry

M.R. BAKST and J.M. BAHR

This chapter provides a brief overview of the reproductive processes in domestic poultry. Because of their economic importance, the chicken (*Gallus domesticus*) and turkey (*Meleagris gallopavo*) provide the focus of the discussion.

THE FEMALE

The Egg

The egg is a complex structure chemically and physically; its complexity is determined by the requirements to protect and to provide sustenance for the embryo. The egg is formed basically of three components: the "central yolk mass," which is equivalent to the mammalian egg, the "white," and the shell (Fig. 18–1), although no component is homogeneous either structurally or chemically (Table 18–1). Moreover, the physical characteristics of eggs are difficult to define precisely because they vary from species to species as well as within species (Gilbert, 1971a, 1979).

The "central yolk mass" is bounded by the perivitelline layer and weighs about 19 g in the chicken, although its mass is age dependent. Lower weights are associated with pullets. The living cytoplasmic part of the cell, the *blastodisc* (or the *blastoderm* if the egg is fertile), occupies a small fraction of the ovum. It is a grayish-white spot, 3 mm in diameter containing in the infertile egg the female haploid pronucleus. Unlike in the mammal, the female bird is the heterogametic sex.

The germinal disc floats on a cone of light-colored yolk ("white yolk") that extends downward to end in a ball, the *latebra* (Fig. 18–1). The chemical composition of white yolk differs from that of the yellow; it contains a greater proportion of protein and its structure has certain peculiarities. The major part of the "central yolk mass" is composed of the familiar orange-yellow viscid fluid (yellow yolk), which has been described as an oil–water emulsion with the continuous phase as aqueous protein. Scattered throughout this are various lipid droplets and yolk spheres.

The function of the yolk is to provide the material for embryogenesis. Chemically, it is a heterogeneous mass containing proteins, lipids, pigments, and a variety of minor organic and inorganic substances. The low-density fraction contains nearly all the lipid fraction as lipoproteins and much phosphorus. The water-soluble fraction (livetin), which comprises 10% of the mass, contains about 30% of the protein mainly as plasma albumin, one of the plasma glycoproteins, and plasma γ-globulin. The granular fraction is formed of phosvitin and includes most of the remaining phosphorus as well as the majority of the calcium and lipovitellins.

Surrounding the central yolk mass, and constituting about two thirds of the egg in weight, is a layer of albumen that has at least seven major regions, which are possibly produced by the rotation of the egg in the oviduct (Fig. 18–1). The albumen is almost pure aqueous protein and contains about 40 proteins (Table 18–1). Since the albumen surrounds the developing em-

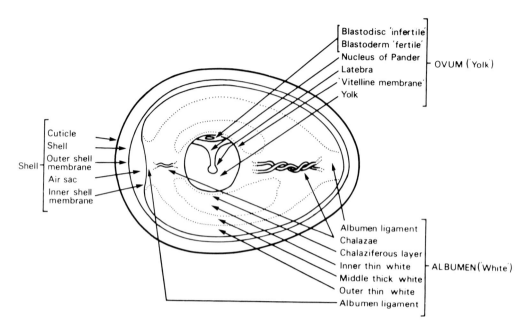

FIG. 18–1.   Diagram of the components of the egg. (Gilbert, A.B. (1971a). The egg: its physical and chemical aspects. *In* Physiology and Biochemistry of the Domestic Fowl. D.J. Bell and B.M. Freeman (eds.). New York, Academic Press.)

TABLE 18–1.   Some Characteristics of the Major Egg White Proteins from the Chicken Egg

Component	Percent	Molecular Weight	Biologic Properties
Ovalbumin	54.0	46,000	
Ovotransferrin	12–13	76,600–86,000	Binds iron, copper, manganese, zinc; may inhibit bacteria
Ovomucoid	11.0	28,000	Inhibits trypsin
Globulins	8.0	Between 36,000 and 45,000	
Lysozyme	3.4–3.5	14,300–17,000	Splits specific β- 1,4-D-glucosaminides; lyses bacteria
Ovomucin	1.5–2.9		Antiviral hemagglutination
Flavoprotein	0.8	32,000–36,000	Binds riboflavin
Ovomacroglobulin	0.5	760,000–900,000	
Ovoglycoprotein	0.5–1.0	24,400	
Ovoinibitor	0.1–1.5	44,000–49,000	Inhibits proteases, including trypsin and chymotrypsin
Avidin	0.05	68,300	Binds biotin
Papain inhibitor	0.1	12,700	Inhibits proteases, including papain and ficin

bryo, it forms an aqueous mantle preventing desiccation. It is also known to contribute material to the embryo during later development. Other functions have been ascribed to specific proteins, since many of the proteins *in vitro* have bactericidal properties, while others have enzymatic activity and some are enzyme inhibitors.

The shell is composed of three structures: the membranes, the mineralized part, and the cuticle. The two shell membranes are sheets of fibrous protein, together about 70 μm thick. At one end, the protein sheets separate to form the air sac. Functionally, the shell membranes provide the surface on which mineralization can occur; fibers from them penetrate outward to produce the organic matrix of the shell. They may reduce the speed of bacterial entry, allowing the bactericidal properties of egg white to act more effectively.

The egg shell is about 350 μm thick and is composed of radiating crystals of almost pure calcite (calcium carbonate). Running vertically through the shell are pores that allow gases to pass. The shell forms a physical barrier to substances that might adversely affect the microenvironment of the embryo. It also provides mechanical strength and a rigid support to maintain the orientation of the heterogeneous internal components. The shell's strength is determined mainly by its curvature and thickness, although other factors are involved. It also provides calcium for the developing embryo. The outer covering of the egg, the proteinaceous cuticle, reduces water loss and bacterial contamination.

Egg Formation

The formation of the egg involves the transport of large quantities of material across numerous biologic membranes, and the formation of many new substances, particularly specific proteins and lipids. The size and composition of the egg are affected by numerous genetic, environmental, and physiologic factors.

Ovary. In birds as in mammals, two ovaries and oviducts are formed during embryogenesis, but a characteristic feature of birds is the suppression of further development of these organs on the right side (Gilbert, 1979; Mittwoch, 1983). Production of the Müllerian-inhibiting substance by the ovary results in the regression of the right duct only (Hutson et al., 1983). Removal of the left ovary results in ovo–testis with both male and female tissue. The functional left ovary (Fig. 18–2) produces ova and acts as an endocrine organ secreting steroid hormones.

The ovary consists of a medulla, which contains connective tissue, blood vessels, and nerves, and a cortex. The cortex contains the oogonia, which give rise to the oocytes. The pear-shaped, immature ovary is about 15 mm long by 5 mm wide, lying in the body cavity, ventral to the aorta and cranial to the kidney and close to the two adrenal glands. The blood supply arises from the gonadorenal artery. Two veins drain blood from the ovary. It is extensively innervated from the sympathetic chain by way of the adrenal–ovarian plexus (Gilbert, 1979).

Follicular Development and Gametogenesis. At the onset of sexual maturity, ovarian weight increases. In the chicken this increase ranges from 0.5 g to between 40 and 60 g; most of this increase comes from the four to six developing follicles, the largest of which weighs about 20 g, with a diameter of about 40 mm.

Of the thousands of oocytes present, many enlarge in size to about 4 to 10 mm in diameter. The majority of the follicles in this size range, however, fail to develop further or become atretic. Every 25 to 27 hours, one of these small follicles enlarges and enters the follicular hierarchy. In the chicken, this follicle will continue to grow and will ovulate 5 to 7 days later. Growth of small follicles appears to be primarily regulated by FSH (Palmer, 1989). Maturation of the female pronucleus begins in the follicle and is completed in the oviduct. Completion of the first (reduction) division occurs 2 hours before ovulation, possibly under control of LH; the second (maturation) division occurs in the oviduct and may be initiated by the penetration of the sperm.

Development of the oocyte and yolk deposition can be considered in three phases, although others have separated the phases differently (Gilbert, 1979). The first, lasting for many months or years, is characterized by a slow deposition of material consisting mainly of neutral fat. During the second period, which may last several weeks, the size of the follicle increases

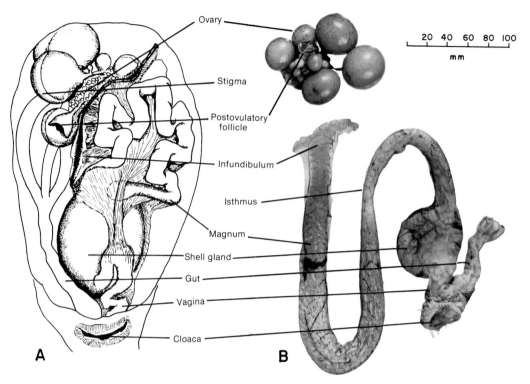

Ovary
Stigma
Postovulatory follicle
Infundibulum
Isthmus
Magnum
Shell gland
Gut
Vagina
Cloaca

20 40 60 80 100
mm

A   B

FIG. 18–2.   *A.* The ovary of the domestic hen *in situ*. *B.* The ovary and oviduct of the domestic hen.

from about 1 mm to 6 mm. During the last stage (the rapid-growth phase), lasting 7 to 8 days, the main mass of yolk material is laid down and follicular weight increases almost linearly. Production of yolk precursors in the liver is regulated by estrogen, whereas the uptake of yolk proteins by the follicle is controlled by gonadotropins.

The liver, not the ovary, is the major source of yolk proteins and phospholipids (Griffin et al., 1984). The structure of the follicle during the rapid-growth phase facilitates the transfer of yolk from the blood plasma to the oocyte. Thecal capillaries are fenestrated, and the cell layer adjacent to the oocyte, the granulosa layer, is characterized by wide intercellular channels. The oocyte surface is greatly increased by the highly convoluted oolema (also referred to as the vitelline membrane), which is actively engaged in pinocytosis.

The Oviduct: Structure and Function

The oviduct, about 700 mm long in the chicken, is suspended by the peritoneal dorsal ligament, which continues around it to form the ventral ligament. It is highly vascular, and the muscular layers are well supplied with nerves from the autonomic system (Gilbert, 1979).

The functions of the oviduct include deposition of albumen, membranes, and shell around the ovum; movement of the developing egg along the oviduct; and storage and transport of sperm (Fig. 18–6). The anterior end of the oviduct is also the site of fertilization. The oviductal wall consists of a highly folded luminal mucosa, an inner circular and outer longitudinal layer of smooth muscle, and an outer covering of peritoneal epithelium.

Infundibulum. The infundibulum actively engulfs the ovulated ovum and, if

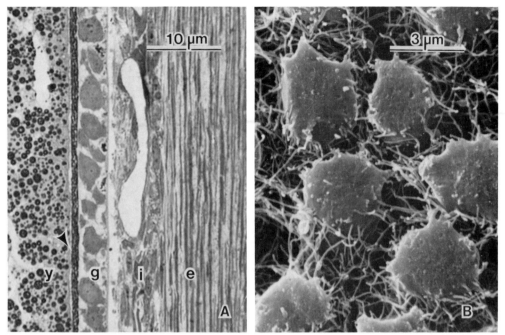

FIG. 18–3. *A.* Cross section of a maturing follicle (chicken) showing the theca externa (*e*), theca interna (*i*), the granulosa cell layer (*g*), the perivitelline layer (arrowheads) and yolk spheres (*y*). *B.* Scanning electron micrograph of the basal face of several granulosa cells. Numerous cytoplasmic processes traverse wide intercellular spaces and interconnect adjacent granulosa cells. (From Bakst, M.R. (1979). Scanning electron microscopy of hen granulosa cells before and after ovulation. Scan. Electron Microsc. III, 307.)

sperm are present, is the site of fertilization.

After passing through the more proximal funnel-shaped region of the infundibulum, the ovum reaches the "chalaziferous region," the narrower, glandular portion of this segment (Fig. 18–2). Secretions from this region form an "outer" perivitelline layer and probably contribute to the formation of the chalazae. The chalaziferous region is also one of two known sperm storage sites in the oviduct.

The magnum is the albumen-secreting region. It is the longest oviductal segment and is distinguishable from the infundibulum and isthmus by its greater external diameter, thicker walls, and more voluminous luminal folds (Figs. 18–2 and 18–6).

The majority of the 40 proteins found in albumen are formed in the oviductal mucosa; a possible exception is ovotransferrin (conalbumen), which appears to be similar to serum transferrin. The protein avidin is formed in the epithelial goblet cells, and the proteins ovalbumin and lysozyme are produced by the tubular glands. Ovotransferrin and ovomucoid may also be produced in the cells of the tubular glands.

Oviductal proteins are secreted as the developing egg mass passes down the magnum. Whereas the precise stimulus for secretion of these proteins is not known, three possibilities exist: (1) the developing egg causes release of the albumen by mechanical or other means, (2) hormonal mechanisms synchronize release, or (3) some neural coordinating mechanism is involved.

The isthmus, which forms the shell membrane around the developing egg, is characterized by narrower and thinner

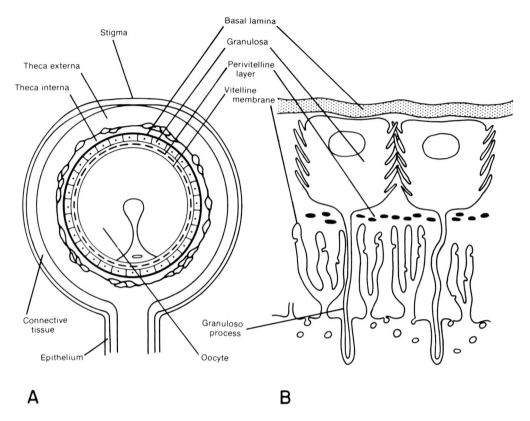

FIG. 18–4. *A.* Cross section of a maturing follicle. (Redrawn from Gilbert, A.B. (1979). Female genital organs. *In* Form and Function in Birds. A.S. King and J. McLelland (eds.). New York, Academic Press.)
B. Diagram of the oocyte surface and the granulosa layer.

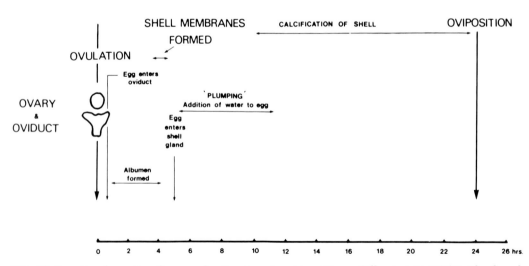

FIG. 18–5. Egg formation from evaluation to oviposition. (From Gilbert, A.B. (1971). The female reproductive effort. *In* Physiology and Biochemistry of the Domestic Fowl. D.J. Bell and D.M. Freeman (eds.). New York, Academic Press).

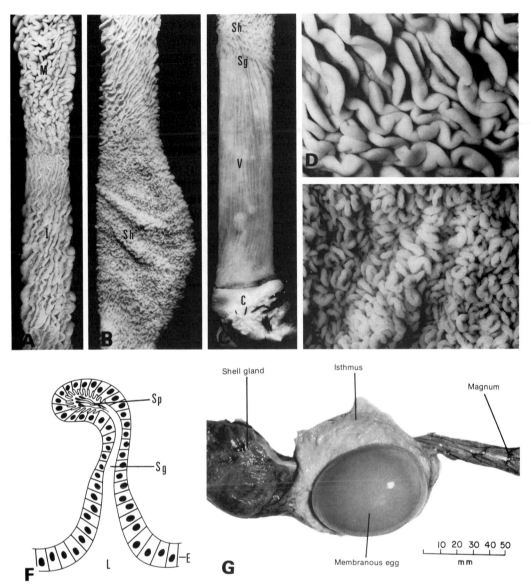

FIG. 18–6. *A*. The luminal surface of the magnum and isthmus. *B*. The luminal surface of the shell gland and its junction with the isthmus. *C*. The luminal surface of the vagina. *D*. Higher power view of the mucosal folds of the magnum. *E*. Higher power view of the mucosa folds of the shell gland. *F*. Sperm storage tubules located in the junction between the shell gland and the vagina. *G*. An egg *in situ* in the isthmus. Note the membranous covering only and the typical egg shape. *C*, cloaca; *E*, epithelium; *I*, isthmus; *L*, lumen of oviduct; *M*, magnum; *Sg*, sperm storage tubule; *Sh*, shell gland; *Sp*, spermatozoa; *V*, vagina.

walls, and by luminal folds less voluminous than those found in the magnum. Little is known of the mechanisms involved in the formation of the shell membrane proteins or their release and deposition on the egg.

It has been observed, however, that while the albumenous egg is entering the isthmus, a membrane is deposited on those parts in contact with the glandular tissue. In the chicken, the typical shape of the egg is produced by the membranes and not by the calcified shell, which is laid down on an already formed shape. At this stage, the membranes are loosely applied to the egg, which has about 50% of its final mass.

The shell gland, also referred to as the *uterus,* is characterized by a pouch-like section joined to the isthmus by a short "neck" and by extensive muscularization (Fig. 18–2). The egg remains in the shell gland for approximately 20 hours. During the first 6 hours or so, a watery fluid produced from the neck region passes into the egg, resulting in a twofold increase in the mass of egg white. However, this "plumping" may continue throughout the time the egg stays in the shell gland. Thereafter, the main process is calcification. During its stay in the shell gland, rotation of the egg around the polar axis leads to the completion of the formation of the chalazae, which started in the infundibulum, and the stratification of the albumen (see. Fig. 18–1).

Shell calcification probably starts in the isthmus where small projections from the membrane, the mammillary cores, are formed. In the uterus, growth of the calcite crystals continues at a constant rate of mineralization (about 300 mg calcium per hour). The oviduct does not store calcium, and about 20% of the calcium in the blood is removed as it passes through the uterus. The specific cells responsible for transferring calcium into the lumen appear to be the surface epithelial cells and not the tubular gland epithelial cells. The final task of the uterus is the formation of the cuticle and pigmentation; the latter consists of porphyrins deposited shortly before laying.

The vagina appears to be relatively short, primarily because its cranial half is tightly folded and bound together by connective tissue (Fig. 18–2). The muscular layer is well developed, and the luminal folds are high and narrow. The vagina serves as a passage for the formed egg from the uterus to the cloaca at oviposition. It also serves an important function in the selection, transport and storage of sperm.

Egg Transport and Oviposition. The transport of the egg along the oviduct is similar in all domestic poultry. The developing egg spends about 15 minutes in the infundibulum. In the magnum, its speed averages about 2 mm/minute and hence it takes about 2 or 3 hours to traverse this region (Fig. 18–5). The egg takes about 1 to 1½ hours to pass through the isthmus. About 20 hours of its total time in the oviduct (about 26 hours) is spent in the uterus. Passage through the vagina takes a few seconds. Although the mechanism for transport of the egg along the oviduct is not fully understood, egg-induced distention of the oviduct has been shown to excite the smooth musculature and to increase the rate of egg transport in quail.

It is not known precisely how oviposition is initiated, but both hormonal and neural mechanisms are involved (Shimada and Saito, 1989). Contraction of the shell gland musculature forces the formed egg through the vagina at oviposition. This may be under neural control, for stimulation of the central nervous system can affect it, but hormones are also involved.

Arginine vasotocin, which is released from the posterior pituitary, and prostaglandins, which originate from the postovulatory follicle formed 26 hours earlier, also contribute to the contraction of and egg expulsion from the shell gland.

With the contraction of the uterine musculature, relaxation of the uterovaginal "sphincter" occurs, possibly analogous to the cervix of mammals. The egg is then pushed further into the vagina, and the general distention of the vaginal wall brings into operation the bearing-down reflex. This involves changes in respiration and stance, and contraction of the abdominal body muscles.

Sperm Storage, Transport, and Fertilization. Unlike most mammals in which sperm spend a considerable amount of time in the male tract and a relatively short time in the female tract, chicken and turkey sperm are probably stored no longer than 4 to 5 days in the ductus deferens. After copulation or artificial insemination, however, sperm spend prolonged periods of time (up to 32 days in the chicken, 70 days in the turkey) housed within the oviduct sperm storage tubules located at the uterovaginal junction (Fig. 18–6). How sperm enter, survive, and exit these sperm storage tubules is not known.

Transport of sperm to the uterovaginal junction is rapid, less than an hour; however, only viable sperm enter the sperm storage tubules. Although first thought to be associated with oviposition, current evidence suggests that the release of stored sperm is continuous or episodic (Bakst, 1981). These sperm ascend the oviduct by way of smooth muscle contractions and/ or ciliary activity and accumulate in the mucosal folds and short tubular glands at the distal infundibulum. At ovulation, sperm are released (probably by distention of the infundibulum) to fertilize the ovum. Sperm that make contact with the perivitelline layer undergo an acrosome reaction and, presumably by the action of the trypsin-like enzyme acrosin, hydrolyze the perivitelline layer. The sperm then pass through this investment, contact, and subsequently fuse with the oolema (Howarth, 1984).

Polyspermy is observed in the hen ovum, yet only one male pronucleus fuses with the female pronucleus. *In vitro* studies indicate that chicken and presumably turkey sperm do not require a period of "capacitation" before penetrating an ovum (Howarth, 1970). Whether sperm released from the oviductal sperm storage tubules require a period of capacitation before penetrating the ovum *in vivo* is not known.

THE MALE

Semen: Physical and Chemical Properties

Morphology of Chicken and Turkey Spermatozoa. Ejaculated chicken and turkey sperm are filiform in shape and are nearly indistinguishable by light and scanning electron microscopy.

Compared to the mammalian sperm head, the chicken and turkey sperm heads are morphologically simple (Bakst, 1980; Lake, 1981). The cone-shaped acrosome contains homogeneous material and is enveloped by a continuous acrosomal membrane. There is no equatorial segment or postacrosomal dense lamina typically seen in mammalian sperm. Separating the acrosome from the nucleus is the subacrosomal space, which is occupied by the perforatorium. The nucleus consists of condensed chromatin granules and is enveloped by a double nuclear membrane. The neck region, which joins the head with the tail segment, is formed by a centriolar complex. The axoneme, the motor component of the tail, originates from the distal centriole. Surrounding the centriolar complex are about 30 mitochondria, which form the midpiece. The annulus, a dense ring, marks the distal boundary of the midpiece and the proximal boundary of the principal piece. The principal piece of chicken and turkey sperm lacks the fibrous sheath and outer dense fibers observed in mammalian sperm. The axoneme, however, is enveloped by an amorphous sheath.

Composition of Seminal Plasma and Sperm. The chemical composition of seminal plasma is known to contain between 50 and 60 constituents (Lake, 1971, 1981). Seminal plasma is essentially an aqueous solution of salts, proteins, and some amino acids. In the absence of "transparent fluid" (a cloacal transudate), chicken seminal plasma differs considerably from that of the mammal. It is low in chloride and almost completely lacking in fructose, citrate, ergothioneine, inositol, phosphoryl choline, and glycerophosphoryl choline. Glutamate is the chief anion.

Testis and Duct System

In the avian male, the testes together weigh between 14 and 60 g, depending on the species. They are suspended from the dorsal body wall just posterior to the lung and ventral to the kidney. Blood is supplied by way of the anterior renal artery and the testicular artery, and there is no pampiniform plexus as seen in mammals (Lake, 1981).

In contrast to the arrangement in mammals, the seminiferous tubules are not grouped into evident lobules surrounded by connective tissue but instead branch and anastomose freely within the tunica albuginea. In the mature cock, extensions of the tunica penetrate between the tubules to act as a supporting framework. Interstitial tissue is negligible, but it contains the androgen-secreting Leydig cells. The seminiferous tubules of immature males are lined by a single-cell layer of Sertoli cells and stem spermatogonia, while mature males have irregularly shaped tubules lined by a multilayered germinal epithelium. The spermatogonia give rise to the primary spermatocytes, secondary spermatocytes, and spermatids. The latter progressively transform into spermatozoa (spermiogenesis).

The time required for maturation of the sperm in the testis depends on the avian species. Usually, spermatogonia multiply about the fifth week after hatching, and primary spermatocytes appear about the sixth week. About the tenth week, these cells multiply rapidly, secondary spermatocytes appear, and tubules increase in size. Spermatids first appear soon afterward, and continued development occurs in the tubules until the twentieth week. Thereafter, the testis appears capable of producing spermatozoa in large quantities.

Chicken and turkey males lack the characteristic coiled and subdivided epididymis present in most mammals. Testicular sperm pass from the seminiferous tubules through the rete testis to the ductuli efferentes. From the ductuli efferentes, sperm pass through a series of connecting ductules and are then transported to the ductus epididymis. Together these ducts are termed the *epididymal region*. The ductus epididymis opens into the ductus deferens, which is the primary sperm storage site in the male. The ductus deferens is a highly convoluted tube, which at its distal end, straightens and dilates slightly, passes through the cloacal wall, and terminates as a wart-like extension projecting into the cloaca (Fig. 18–7). There are no accessory reproductive organs such as the seminal vesicles, prostate, Cowper's gland, and urethral glands associated with the ductus deferens. In nonejaculated chickens, sperm traverse the ductus deferens in about 84 hours, while in ejaculated males, sperm require 24 to 48 hours.

The male has no intromittent organ (e.g., penis), but a phallus makes contact with the everted vagina during copulation. Erection of the phallus is a result of its engorgement with a lymph-like fluid derived from the *corpus vascularis paracloacalis* (vascular body), a craniolateral extension of the phallus located in the wall of the cloaca.

Testicular sperm recovered from chickens are fertile but only when surgically introduced into the anterior half of the oviduct (Howarth, 1984). Semen removed from the proximal portion of the ductus deferens is highly fertile after vaginal insemination (Bakst and Cecil, 1981).

CONTROL OF GAMETE PRODUCTION

The Female

Initiation of Egg Production

The female chicken reaches sexual maturity at 18 to 20 weeks of age. She will start to lay eggs at this time and reach peak production rates of 90% within several weeks. The young chicken will lay many eggs on sequential days before skipping a day. This pattern of daily egg laying followed by a skip day is called a *sequence,* or *clutch.* As the chicken ages, the clutch length shortens; e.g., she will drop from 10 to 20 eggs in a clutch to 4 to 5 eggs in a clutch, and the production rate will decrease to 60 to 70%. This gradual decrease

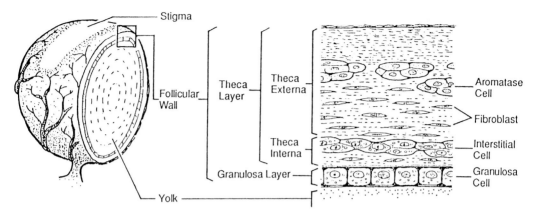

FIG. 18–7.   Anatomic structure of the preovulatory follicle. The thin follicular wall consists of the theca and granulosa layers. The theca layer is divided into the theca externa and theca interna. The theca externa consists of aromatase cells (estrogen-producing cells), fibroblasts, and extracellular matrix. The theca interna consists primarily of interstitial cells (sites of progestin and androgen synthesis). The granulosa layer, separated from the theca layer by the basal membrane, is a single cell layer and is the primary site of progesterone synthesis in the preovulatory follicles.

in the number of eggs laid in a clutch is the result of increase in the time required for the largest follicle to become competent to ovulate and of a greater interval between ovulations. For a more extensive review of this topic, see Bahr and Palmer (1989).

Anatomy and Function of the Ovary

The ovary of the laying chicken contains numerous small follicles (1 to 10 mm in diameter), five to six larger preovulatory follicles arranged in a hierarchy, and several postovulatory follicles. The preovulatory follicles are numbered according to size, with the F1 being the largest follicle and the next follicle to ovulate; F2, the second largest follicle, will ovulate the day after the F1 follicle ovulates, and so on. The follicle consists of the oocyte and several layers of tissue, namely, the vitelline membrane and zona radiata (the innermost layers); the perivitelline layer; granulosa layer; theca layer (interna and externa); loose connective tissue; and the superficial epithelium (the outermost layer) (see Figs. 18–3, 18–4, and 8–7). The granulosa layer is a single-cell layer, whereas interstitial cells, fibroblasts, and

aromatase cells are present in the theca interna and externa layers. The granulosa layer produces primarily progesterone with low amounts of androgens. The interstitial cells of the theca interna layer produce some progesterone and principally androgens, whereas the aromatase cells of the theca externa layer are the site of estrogen production (Nitta et al., 1991). As the preovulatory follicles grow (F5→F1), there is a significant increase in progesterone production by the granulosa layer and a gradual decrease in androgen and estrogen secretion by the theca layer (Bahr et al., 1983; Etches and Duke, 1984). These dramatic changes in steroid production are the result of a change in responsiveness to gonadotropins (i.e., the granulosa layer becomes more responsive to LH as the F1 follicle approaches ovulation) and of the removal of an inhibition of the theca layer (specifically, androgens and estrogen) on progesterone production by the granulosa layer (Johnson et al., 1987).

Steroid production by the ovary is essential for reproduction and egg laying in the chicken (Fig. 18–8). Progesterone induces the preovulatory LH surge in a positive feedback manner and is required for the

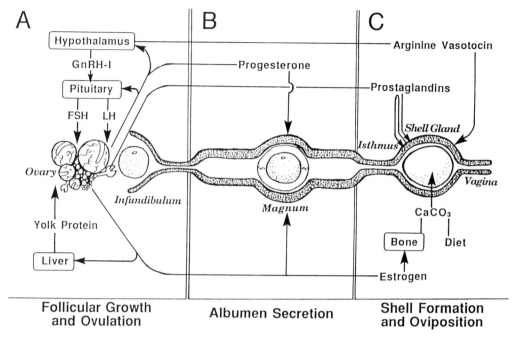

FIG. 18–8. Summary of the endocrine regulation of, *A,* follicular growth and ovulation; *B,* albumen secretion; and *C,* shell formulation and oviposition in the chicken. Note: *A, B,* and *C* represent separate stages of the ovulatory cycle. (From Nitta, H., Osawa, Y. and Bahr, J.M. (1991). Multiple steroidogenic cell populations in the thecal layer of preovulatory follicles of the chicken ovary. Endocrinology *129,* 2033.)

function of the reproductive tract, specifically, the production of albumen. Androgens are necessary for the expression of secondary sex characters and are precursors for estrogen production. Estrogens, produced primarily by the small follicles (1 to 10 mm in diameter) induce the synthesis of yolk proteins by the liver, interact (synergize) with progesterone to cause albumen secretion, mobilize calcium from medullary bones, and promote the secretion of calcium by the shell gland to form the egg shell.

Other hormones, besides steroids, are required for egg production. Catecholamines, specifically, norepinephrine, may have a role in ovulation. Arginine vasotocin of posterior pituitary origin and prostaglandins produced by the largest preovulatory and postovulatory follicles

promote contractions of the shell gland and oviposition of the egg.

Ovulatory Cycle

The chicken, unlike the mammal, has only a follicular phase. Because the chicken does not get pregnant, there is no need for a corpus luteum. Therefore, the cycle of follicular growth and hormonal changes that culminates in ovulation is called the *ovulatory cycle.* Approximately every 25 to 27 hours, an egg is laid (Fig. 18–5). During this cycle, there is a small increase in blood LH at the time of lights off ("crepuscular" meaning at dusk) and a preovulatory surge 4 to 6 hours before ovulation (Johnson and van Tienhoven, 1980a, 1980b; Wilson and Sharp, 1973). In contrast to the changes in LH, blood levels of FSH are relatively constant throughout the cycle, with the exception of lower levels 9 to 3 hours before ovulation.

The chicken lays an egg at a later time each day until the egg is laid late in the afternoon (Fig. 18–9). This egg will be the last egg laid in the sequence. In contrast to previous eggs laid in sequences during which oviposition is followed by ovulation of the next egg 10 to 30 minutes later, no ovulation occurs. As a result, no egg is laid the next day. This day is called "pause day." The chicken will reset her endocrine clock and will lay the first egg of the next sequence early the next day. Thus, the chicken begins a new sequence with each egg laid at a later time each day.

Molting

Once a year, a chicken will molt, or lose feathers, if exposed to natural daylight.

Molting can be artificially induced through stress or by blocking release of pituitary LH. A molt is preceded by a gradual decrease in egg production. It is hypothesized that the development of a gradual insensitivity of the hypothalamus to stimulatory daylight and the positive feedback action of progesterone on the release of LH may cause this decrease in the number of ovulations and, ultimately, of egg production (Williams and Sharp, 1978). Molting is characterized by cessation of ovulations and egg laying, regression of the reproductive tract, decreased blood levels of LH and progesterone, and an increase in thyroxine. Generally, a molt will last 4 to 6 weeks, after which the chicken will return to lay. Egg production and quality will be improved compared to the premolt performance. In commercial

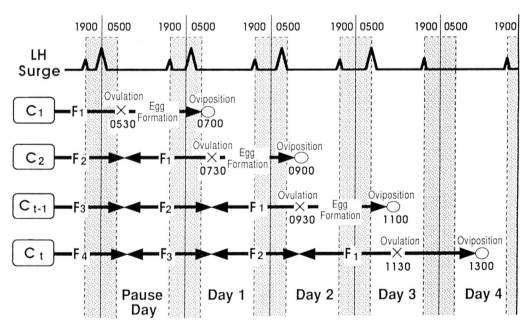

FIG. 18–9. Diagrammatic description of events during the ovulatory cycle of a chicken laying a sequence of four eggs. The shaded area indicates the time of lights off. C_1 (first egg laid), C_2 (second egg laid), C_{t-1} (third egg laid) and C_t (terminal egg laid) refer to the position of the egg in the sequence. LH concentrations in the blood are elevated slightly at the time of lights off (crepuscular) followed by the LH surge. The F_1 follicle ovulates 6 hours later and is oviposited approximately 26.5 hours later. The LH surge occurs at a later time each night until eventually no LH surge occurs. Consequently, ovulation and oviposition do not occur. The day no egg is laid is called *pause day*. (From Nitta, H., Osawa, Y. and Bahr, J.M. (1991). Multiple steroidogenic cell populations in the thecal layer of preovulatory follicles of the chicken ovary. Endocrinology *129*, 2033.)

production units, chickens are molted when egg production decreases to 50 to 60%. Molt can also be effectively and humanely induced by giving chickens a gonadotropin-releasing hormone (GnRH) agonist that blocks LH release and causes regression of the reproductive tract (Dickerman and Bahr, 1989). A more complete review of the reproductive endocrinology of the chicken is presented by Bahr and Johnson (1991).

The Male

It is generally believed that FSH controls seminiferous tubule growth and differentiation and that LH affects the interstitial Leydig cells, which produce the steroid hormones. Increased levels of testosterone and androstenedione accompany the latter stages of spermatogenesis and the onset of semen production in chickens (Culbert et al., 1977; Sharp et al., 1977). The rise in plasma testosterone continues after the onset of semen production (about 20 weeks) and finally stabilizes after 35 to 36 weeks (Culbert et al., 1977). The survival of ductus deferens sperm is not androgen dependent, but the phallus and vascular bodies, structures associated with the transparent fluid formation, appear to be androgen dependent. Little is known about the role of hormones in the maintenance of the ductus deferens.

BREEDING PRACTICES AND THE APPLICATION OF ARTIFICIAL INSEMINATION

The advantages of breeding by artificial insemination (AI) include: reducing the relative number of breeder males to females; accelerating genetic progress by allowing greater selection pressures; reducing the spread of reproductive pathogens (particularly the mycoplasmas); overcoming periods of low semen production that are due to disease or environmental stress; and overcoming problems associated with natural matings, e.g., physical incompatibility, low libido, and leg and foot problems. The disadvantages of AI are due to economics and include: the associated high cost of labor; the need to use caged as opposed to floor-reared breeders; the need for skilled labor; and the lack of documentation illustrating potential savings derived from an AI program.

NATURAL MATING

In birds, the introduction of semen into the female is associated with complex courtship behavior. A diurnal rhythm in mating frequency exists in males and is correlated with semen production. Libido in the male, however, is not necessarily correlated with high fertility, and there is a tendency for the most frequent copulators to produce many aspermic ejaculates. In addition, the dominant male because of his size may not be the most sexually active, but he may prevent other males from mating successfully.

Libido in the female is affected by her rearing environment (whether or not males were present) and by her social ranking. Receptivity (crouching) varies from hen to hen, and this affects the chance of successful mating because the female probably determines whether or not the sexual advances of the male will lead to copulation.

ARTIFICIAL INSEMINATION

Artificial insemination is basically a two-step procedure. First, semen is collected from the male; and second, semen is deposited within the female's reproductive tract. Preparation of semen for short-term (liquid state; 24 hours or less) or long-term (frozen state; indefinitely) storage is reflective of the needs and preference of the breeder. Although some turkey breeders may inseminate "neat" semen (undiluted), the vast majority dilute semen with an extender (diluent). An extender is a buffered salt solution containing various substrates for the purposes of diluting the semen and supporting the viability of the spermatozoa. Refer to Bakst (1990) for detailed explanations of semen extenders and semen storage techniques (liquid storage and cryopreservation).

As a result of successful short-term storage of turkey semen, centralized "stud farms" have been established by many turkey breeders. In a central facility, males are subject to management protocols intended to both optimize semen production and lower production costs. Economic benefits include savings in feed because breeder males require less protein (10 vs. 17%) and a savings in energy because males require lower light intensity than hens (20 lux or more vs. 50 lux or more) to stay in semen production. The total number of males can be reduced to 1 male to 20 hens, which lowers production costs and also permits greater selection pressure for improving the performance of the market bird. Finally, labor costs are lower because the same crew often collects semen early in the day and inseminates later in the day.

Long-term storage of semen at −196 °C (liquid nitrogen) is accomplished by freezing semen in an extender containing a suitable cryoprotectant. Subsequent fertility in the chicken following AI of thawed spermatozoa is about 60 to 70%, while that of the turkey is generally less than 50%. Although the potential for worldwide distribution of genetic material exists, the commercial application of frozen semen technology has been limited primarily to the freezing of semen from selected genetic lines of birds for subsequent pedigree breeding. However, cryopreservation techniques are being used to preserve semen obtained from nondomesticated, endangered species of birds. Maintenance of a diverse genetic pool through the use of cryopreservation of semen would help alleviate problems associated with repeated inbreeding caused by dwindling numbers within the species.

Semen Collection, Evaluation, and Insemination. The abdominal massage technique of semen collection involves a gentle massaging of the abdomen while the opposite hand simultaneously strokes the lower back and tail feathers of a restrained male. When phallic tumescence is achieved, the collector's hands are placed around the cloaca and the thumb and forefinger of the upper hand gently squeeze the cloaca with a downward pressure while the lower hand exerts slight upward pressure. To minimize the spread of pathogens, care must be taken by the collector not to touch the cloacal structures. The semen, which pools on the phallus after each squeeze of the cloaca, is collected into a clean, dry tube. Generally, males can be ejaculated twice weekly without affecting semen volume and sperm concentration.

Semen evaluation begins at the time of semen collection. Good-quality semen should be viscous (chicken semen less viscous than turkey) and cream-white. The use of semen that is discolored, watery, or contaminated by fecal material, urates, or blood will lead to lowered fertility, particularly if the semen is subjected to short- or long-term storage. If possible, a critical evaluation of the semen should be performed on an individual basis, particularly when selecting male breeders. The parameters listed previously—as well as semen volume, sperm concentration, motility, morphology, and percentage of live sperm—should all be used to evaluate a semen sample.

Insemination involves the placement of a predetermined volume (generally less than 0.1 ml) of semen with a minimum of 100 to 200 million viable spermatozoa within the hen's vagina. Semen is placed within narrow (about 5 mm outside diameter) inseminating straws, either manually or with a mechanical semen dispenser, and the straw is then mounted on a dosing syringe or gun. The vaginal orifice is exteriorized for insemination by a procedure referred to as "breaking" or "venting." Venting involves the application of hand pressure around the hen's cloaca region. As with semen collection, the hands should not touch the cloaca. When the vagina is exteriorized, the inseminating straw is quickly and gently inserted until resistance is felt (about 4 to 6 cm). The hand pressure is released around the cloaca, and the inseminator ejects the semen as the vagina returns to its normal position.

Fertility and Hatchability. All eggs fertilized by sperm do not develop during incubation. Eggs are candled (an intense beam of light is transmitted through the egg that highlights vascular development of the embryo) within the first 5 to 10 days of incubation to establish candling fertility. To determine true fertility, those eggs showing no sign of embryonic development by candling are opened and their blastodiscs are examined for evidence of early embryonic development. These procedures distinguish between fertility and hatchability problems.

Hatchability is expressed as the number of offspring hatched divided by the number of fertile eggs at candling. Factors that depress hatchability include farm management (improper handling, holding, transport, and storage of eggs before incubation and the improper management of the hatchery), diseases transmitted within the egg, and the genetics, nutritional status, and age of the hen. Peak embryonic mortality in the chicken and turkey occurs during the first 5 days and the last 3 days (days 18 to 21 in the chicken and 24 to 27 in the turkey) of incubation. Table 18–2 shows reproductive traits of some birds of domestic importance.

Semen Production

Many factors influence semen production by male breeders. There are wide differences in the onset of semen production and in semen quality between species, strains within species, and individuals within strains. Generally, chicken and turkey ejaculates average about 0.25 ml in volume and about 5 billion sperm per ml and 9 billion sperm per ml, respectively. Genetic improvement with such important parameters as semen volume and sperm concentration appears to be feasible with the turkey but less likely with the chicken (Sexton, 1983). Unfortunately, using semen-quality traits such as the preceding to predict semen fertility has produced contradictory observations (Wilson et al., 1979).

An important step for a successful AI program is the selection of breeder males. With the turkey, lighting and feeding programs should begin early enough to ensure full expression of their growth poten-

TABLE 18–2. Comparative Reproductive Performance* of Some Birds of Commercial Importance

Species	Incubation Period (Days)	Age of Sexual Maturity (Months)	Egg Weight (g)	No. Eggs in First Laying Year	Fertility (%)	Hatchability of Fertile Eggs (%)
Chicken *(Gallus gallus)*						
Layer	21	5–6	58	300	97	90
Broiler	21	6	65	180	92	90
Turkey *(Meleagris gallopavo)*	28	7–8	85	90	90	84
Duck *(Anas platyrhynchos)*						
Layer	27–28	6–7	60	300	95	75–80
Meat type	28	6–7	65			
Goose *(Anser anser)*						
Small type	30	9–10	135	30–70	70	70
Large type	33	10–12	215			
Pheasant *(Phasianus colchicus)*	24–26	10–12	30	50–75	95	85
Guinea fowl *(Numida meleagris)*	27–28	10–12	40	80–200	90	95
Quail *(Coturnix coturnix)*	15–16	1.5–2	10	300	90	75–85

* Only general figures are given since values are greatly affected by breed, location, and nutrition. In particular the values given in the last three columns depend greatly on management practices, and it is unlikely that fertility and hatchability will be the same for all species.

tial by market age (about 18 weeks). After selection for size, conformation, leg fitness, and other economically important traits, males should be maintained on a restricted diet, which results in a body weight about 30% less than full-fed males at 30 weeks of age. At this time, 10 to 12 males per 100 hens can be selected as breeders based primarily on semen quantity and quality.

REFERENCES

Bahr, J.M. and Johnson, P.A. (1991). Reproduction in poultry. *In* Reproduction in Domestic Animals, 4th Ed. P.T. Cupps (ed.). New York, Academic Press.

Bahr, J.M. and Palmer, S.S. (1989). The influence of aging on ovarian function. Poult. Biol. *2*, 103.

Bahr, J.M., Wang, S.C., Huang, M.Y. and Calvo, F.O. (1983). Steroid concentrations in isolated theca and granulosa layers of preovulatory follicles during the ovulatory cycle of the domestic hen. Biol. Reprod. *29*, 326.

Bakst, M.R. (1980). Ultrastructure of chicken and turkey gametes, fertilization, and oviductal sperm transport: a review. Eighth Int. Congr. Anim. Reprod. A.I., Madrid, Vol. 2, pp. 511–517.

Bakst, M.R. (1981). Sperm recovery from oviducts of turkeys at known intervals after insemination and oviposition. J. Reprod. Fertil. *62*, 159.

Bakst, M.R. (1990). Preservation of avian cells. *In* Poultry Breeding and Genetics. R.D. Crawford (ed.). Amsterdam, Elsevier Science Publishers.

Bakst, M.R. and Cecil, H.C. (1981). Changes in the characteristics of turkey ejaculation semen and ductus deferens semen with repeated ejaculation. Reprod. Nutr. Dev. *21*, 1095.

Culbert, J., Sharp, P.J. and Wells, J.W. (1977). Concentrations of androstenedione, testosterone, and LH in the blood before and after the onset of spermatogenesis in the cockerel. J. Reprod. Fertil. *51*, 153.

Dickerman, R.W. and Bahr, J.M. (1989). Molt induced by gonadotropin-releasing hormone agonist as a model for studying endocrine mechanisms of molting in laying hens. Poult. Sci. *868*, 1402.

Etches, R.J. and Duke, C.E. (1984). Progesterone, androstenedione and oestradiol content of theca and granulosa tissue of the four largest ovarian follicles during the ovulatory cycle of the hen (*Gallus domesticus*). J. Endocrinol. *103*, 71.

Gilbert, A.B. (1971a). The egg: its physical and chemical aspects. *In* Physiology and Biochemistry of the Domestic Fowl. D.J. Bell and B.M. Freeman (eds.). New York, Academic Press.

Gilbert, A.B. (1971b). The ovary. *In* Physiology and Biochemistry of the Domestic Fowl. D.J. Bell and B.M. Freeman (eds.). New York, Academic Press.

Gilbert, A.B. (1979). Female genital organs. *In* Form and Function in Birds. A.S. King and J. McLelland (eds.). New York, Academic Press.

Griffin, H.D., Perry, M.M. and Gilbert, A.B. (1984). Yolk formation. *In* Physiology and Biochemistry of the Domestic Fowl. B.M. Freeman (ed.). London, Academic Press.

Howarth, B. (1970). An examination for sperm capacitation in the fowl. Biol. Reprod. *3*, 338.

Howarth, B. (1984). Maturation of spermatozoa and mechanism of fertilisation. *In* Reproductive Biology of Poultry. F.J. Cunningham, P.E. Lake and D. Hewitt (eds.). British Poultry Science, Ltd. Oxford, The Aden Press, Ltd.

Hutson, J.M., MacLaughlin, D.T., Ikawa, H., Budzik, G.P. and Donahoe, P.K. (1983). Reproductive Physiology IV. R.O. Greep (ed.). New York, University Press.

Johnson, A.L. and van Tienhoven, A. (1980a). Plasma concentrations of six steroids and LH during the ovulatory cycle of the hen, *Gallus domesticus*. Biol. Reprod. *23*, 386.

Johnson, A.L. and van Tienhoven, A. (1980b). Hypothalamic-hypophyseal sensitivity to hormones in the hen. I. Plasma concentrations of LH, progesterone, and testosterone in response to central injections of progesterone and R5020. Biol. Reprod. *23*, 910.

Johnson, P.A., Stoklosowa, S. and Bahr, J.M. (1987). Interaction of granulosa and theca layers in the control of progesterone secretion in the domestic hen. Biol. Reprod. *37*, 1149.

Lake, P.E. (1971). The male in reproduction. *In* Physiology and Biochemistry of the Domestic Fowl. D.J. Bell and B.M. Freeman (eds.). New York, Academic Press.

Mittwoch, U. (1983). Heterogametic sex chromosomes and the development of the dominant gonad in vertebrates. Am. Nat. *122*, 159.

Nitta, H., Osawa, Y. and Bahr, J.M. (1991). Multiple steroidogenic cell populations in the theca layer of preovulatory follicles of the chicken ovary. Endocrinology *129*, 2033.

Palmer, S.S. (1989). Follicle stimulating hormone and steroidogenesis in ovarian granulosa cells during aging in the domestic hen. Doctoral thesis, University of Illinois, Urbana.

Shimada, K. and Saito, N. (1989). Control of oviposition in poultry. Poult. Biol. *2*, 235.

Sexton, T.J. (1983). Maximizing the utilization of the male breeder: a review. Poult. Sci. *62*, 1700.

Sharp, P.J., Culbert, J. and Wells, J.W. (1977). Variations in stored and plasma concentrations of androgens and luteinizing hormone during sexual development in the cockerel. J. Endocrinol. *74*, 467.

Williams, J.B. and Sharp, P.J. (1978). Age-dependent changes in the hypothalamo–pituitary–ovarian axis of the laying hen. J. Reprod. Fertil. *53*, 141.

Wilson, S.C. and Sharp, P.J. (1973). Variations in plasma LH levels during ovulatory cycle of the hen (*Gallus domesticus*). J. Reprod. Fertil. *35*, 561.

Wilson, H.R., Piesco, N.P., Miller, E.R. and Nesbeht, W.G. (1979). Prediction of the fertility potential of broiler breeder males. Wlds. Poult. Sci. J. *35*, 95.

V. techniques for improving reproductive efficiency

19
Semen Evaluation

E.S.E. HAFEZ

The spermatozoon is unique in its form, function and density. The mature sperm cell is a terminal cell, the end product of a complex developmental process, and it cannot undergo further cell division or differentiation. The ideal method of evaluating the fertility of a breeding male, other than his ability to produce pregnancy, is by the examination of his semen.

The evaluation of the ejaculate is an important part of the physical examination of an infertile male. A semen analysis is simple to perform, and important conclusions can be obtained from the results (Table 19–1). The standards for a species can be established, and any deviations from these "normal standards" can be recognized and correlated with fertility. Certain terms are used to express deviations in semen characteristics (Table 19–2).

EVALUATION AND FERTILITY

Semen evaluation in relation to fertility is conducted more often in bulls than in other species. In general, the minimal standards for a classification of a "probably fertile" specimen of bull semen are as follows: over 500 million spermatozoa per milliliter are present, more than 50% of motile sperm make forward progression, and more than 80% of the spermatozoa conform to normal morphology. If any of these criteria is not met, particularly with samples of three or more ejaculates, the bull is suspected of being infertile. However, only when motile spermatozoa are totally absent and the reproductive system

has been carefully examined for disease can it be stated that the bull is sterile.

Semen evaluation should be rapid and effective so that carefully collected samples can be processed to preserve initial quality and fertility. No single test has been developed that is an accurate predictor of the fertility of individual ejaculates, but when several tests are carefully combined, ejaculates can be selected for use that have a higher fertility potential. Semen samples are tested for various physical characteristics including (Figs. 19–1, to 19–3; Table 19–3) color; odor (sample is noted for any unusual odor); viscosity (sample is drawn up by pipetting and extruded twice along the side of the test tube, and if the sample is not runny, it is marked as viscous); and pH (pH paper is used to determine the pH of the sample).

A wet mount of the sample is placed on a clean glass slide and observed for the following: white blood cells, red blood cells, spermatogenic cells, crystals, debris, and agglutination (Fig. 19–3). A standardized scheme of semen analysis has been established (Table 19–2).

Appearance and Volume

Semen should have a relatively uniform, opaque appearance indicative of high sperm cell concentration. Translucent samples contain few sperm. The sample should be free from hair, dirt, and other contaminants. Semen with a curdy appearance, containing chunks of material (other than the gel in boar and stallion semen), should not be used; this indicates

405

TABLE 19–1.   Evaluation of the Ejaculate

Parameter	Data Collection	
Semen collection	Date and time of collection Place of collection	Method of collection Frequency of ejaculations within last 4 weeks
Macroscopic evaluation	Volume (mL) Color Viscosity pH Cellular debris Crystals	Odor Spermatozoa count per milliliter Centrifugation results if sperm count is low
Duration (% motile)	4.6 hrs after collection	24 hrs after collection
Rating (% sperm)	Very rapid progressive movement Motility without progression	Slow progressive movement Nonmotile
Patterns	1. Progressively motile 2. Vibratory circular 3. Darting 4. Rotating 5. Asymmetric head and or flagella 6. Sperm and cytoplasmic droplet	7. Agglutinated sperm 8. Pathologic movement (circular, oscillating, shivering) 9. Rolling movements 10. Whiplash motility within a small radius
CellSoft-CASA Calculates	Sperm cell concentration Concentration of motile cells Average linearity of forward progression Motility index Histogram of velocity distribution Objective quantitative evaluation of motility-enhancing and inhibiting agents and technique	Percentage of motile cells Average velocity of the sperm sample Average velocity of cells with and without linear forward progression Percentages of morphologic types Histogram of forward progression distribution Printed report of complete semen analysis results Data storage files on patients and referring physicians
Programs for sperm banks	Storage and reporting on donor characteristics and history Specimen inventory and consumption updating system tracks each straw and specific location in tank or freezer	Data storage system for physician list and donor test results
Computer-assisted cell counter program	Computer-assisted counting of standard or user-selected morphologic types and nonsperm cell constituents makes the clicker counter obsolete Printed report of morphology data	Automatic ongoing percentage calculation of morphologic types Tone sounds for every 100 cells counted Distinctive alarm to signal mistaken hits of counter keys "Erase" key to erase mistaken hits

TABLE 19–2.   Semen Analysis Nomenclature

Parameter	Evaluation Criterion	Nomenclature
Volume	None Reduced Increased	Aspermia Hypospermia Hyperspermia
Sperm concentration	Zero Reduced Normal Increased	Azoospermia Oligozoospermia Normozoospermia Polyzoospermia
Sperm motility	Decreased	Asthenozoospermia
Sperm viability	All dead	Necrozoospermia
Abnormal spermatozoa	High percentage	Teratozoospermia

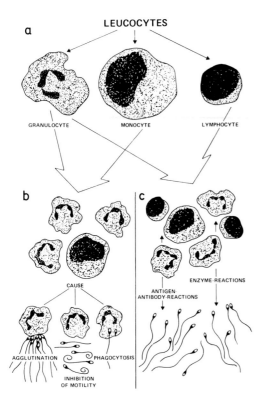

a

LEUCOCYTES

GRANULOCYTE   MONOCYTE   LYMPHOCYTE

b   c

CAUSE   ANTIGEN-ANTIBODY-REACTIONS   ENZYME-REACTIONS

AGGLUTINATION   PHAGOCYTOSIS

INHIBITION OF MOTILITY

FIG. 19–1. Cellular interactions among granulocytes, monocytes, lymphocytes, and spermatozoa. These interactions cause sperm agglutination, arrested motility, phagocytosis, antigen–antibody interactions, and enzyme reactions. (Courtesy of Professor A. Riedel).

Sperm Concentration

Accurate determination of the number of spermatozoa per milliliter of semen is extremely important because it is a highly variable semen characteristic. When combined with the volume of the ejaculate, this quantity of spermatozoa determines how many females can be inseminated, each with the optimal number of sperm cells. A sperm count is taken using a hemocytometer.

Sperm Count

1. A 20-fold dilution is made by mixing the semen with a spermicidal solution in one of the following ways: (a) one drop of semen is added to 19 drops of spermicide, or (b) 0.1 ml of semen is added to 1.9 ml of spermicide, or (c) using a white blood cell pipette, semen is drawn to the 0.5 mark halfway up the stem and the spermicide solution subsequently to the II mark at the top of the bubble chamber. Common spermicidal solutions include 5% triphenyltetrazolium chloride in physiologic saline, 5% chlorazene (chloramine-T) in physiologic saline, 5g $NaHCO_3$ and 1 ml of 35% concentrated formaldehyde made up to 100 ml in physiologic saline.

2. The preparations are thoroughly mixed using standardized pipette shakers, and one drop is added to both sides of a standard blood cell hemocytometer.

3. Spermatozoa are allowed to settle by keeping the hemocytometer in a humid (wet) chamber for 1 hour. A humid chamber may be constructed by placing a wet sponge inside a fairly airtight, plastic box. The 1-hour incubation is not essential but increases the accuracy of the count because all spermatozoa will have precipitated onto the hemocytometer rather than floated.

4. The spermatozoa in the appropriate squares of the hemocytometer are counted by light microscopy at ×100 or ×400, using a manual counter for convenience. Only the outside and middle squares are counted, and only those lying

infection of the reproductive system. Some bulls consistently produce yellow semen, owing to the presence of a harmless pigment riboflavin. This should not be confused with urine, which has its own distinctive odor.

In general, young animals and those of smaller size within a species produce smaller volumes of semen. Frequent ejaculation results in lower average volume, and when two ejaculates are obtained consecutively, the second usually has the lower volume. Small volume is not harmful, but if accompanied by a low sperm concentration, the number of sperm available is limited.

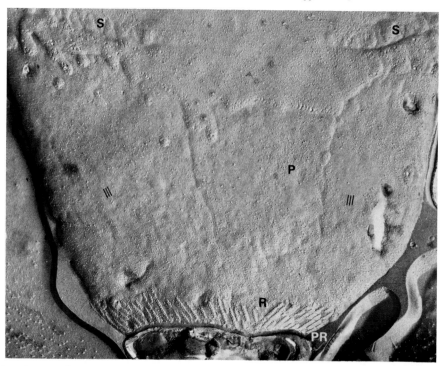

FIG. 19–2.   Sperm ultrastructure after freeze-etching techniques. General view of postacrosomal region. The plasma membrane is split by the fracture and shows numerous particles (*P*). Underlying differentiations of the postacrosomal lamina are visible: anterior serrations (*S*), striations (*III*) and posterior parallel rows of particles oriented in various directions (*R*). Caudally the postacrosomal lamina is limited by the posterior ring (*PR*) (37,000×). (Photograph courtesy of Dr. J. Flechon.)

in the square itself and on the top and right sides are counted (Fig. 19–4). Both sides of the hemocytometer are counted and the average computed.

5. *Sperm concentration* refers to the number of spermatozoa per milliliter of semen. The sperm count is the total number of spermatozoa in the ejaculate. Both are important and should be calculated. The hemocytometer has a grid containing five major squares: A, B, C, D, and E. The central square "E" is subdivided into 25 smaller squares. The four small squares in the corners are labeled E_1, E_2, E_3, and E_4, and the central small square is E_5. Normally, either all the spermatozoa in the major square E are counted or only the ones in small squares E_1 through E_5. When counting, include all the spermatozoa within the designated squares and those that cross the lines at the top and righthand sides.

Major square E is 1 mm long, 1 mm wide, and the thickness of the fluid between the coverslip and the hemocytometer is 0.1 mm. The total volume represented by major square E is thus 0.1 mm^3 or 10^4 ml. The multiplication factor of major square E is therefore 10^4 or 10,000. If all the spermatozoa in major square E are counted and the number is multiplied with the multiplication factor (10,000), the number of spermatozoa per milliliter of the solution applied to the hemocytometer is obtained. When this is multiplied with the sperm dilution factor, normally 20, the concentration of spermatozoa in the original semen sample is obtained. From this information, the total number of spermatozoa in the semen (sperm count) is calculated by multiplying the sperm concentration by the volume of the ejaculate.

If only the spermatozoa in small squares (E_1, E_2, E_3, E_4, and E_5) are counted, the

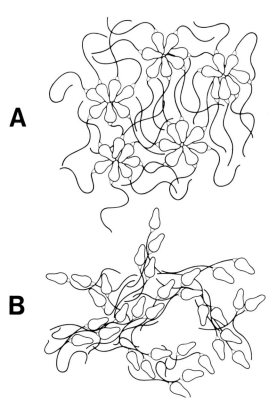

A

B

FIG. 19–3. *A* and *B* show different patterns and intensities of sperm agglutination.

multiplication factor is five times greater than if the entire major square E is counted and is thus 50,000. If all major squares are counted, as in the cases of very low sperm concentrations, the multiplication factor is five times smaller, i.e., 2,000.

When the spermatozoa number more than 200 per high-power field, a 1:100 dilution should be made. This is done by taking 0.1 ml of semen and mixing it with 9.9 ml of the spermicide using a graduated pipette. Some clinicians routinely use a 1:100 or a 1:200 dilution because they feel that it gives more accurate results. The dilution factor for undiluted semen is 1; for semen diluted 100 times, it is 100; and for semen diluted 200 times, it is 200.

The Makler counting chamber is now used extensively in various research and *in vitro* fertilization (IVF) centers (Fig. 19–5).

SPERM MORPHOLOGY

Semen from most males contains some abnormally formed spermatozoa. Usually, this is not associated with lower fertility rates until the proportion of abnormal sperm exceeds about 20%; even then, cer-

TABLE 19–3. **Motility Pattern of Spermatozoa from Fertile Males and Males Suspected of Infertility**

Patterns of Motility and Morphology	Sperm Tail	Sperm Head	Sperm Movements and Progression
Vibratory circular	Slow or rapid quivering from side to side; vibrations of various types and frequency bent in a curved shape; immotile	Immotile or vibrating in one place	Motility without progression; perpendicular, oblique, or horizontal clockwise or counterclockwise motion
Darting	Vibration with high velocity	Irregular; propelling; no rotation	Minimal and erratic; wandering path
Rotating	Undulations of small amplitude pass down tail	Whole sperm rotates around its axis; periodic "flashing" effect	Rapid forward progress in a straight line
Asymmetric head and/or flagella	Amplitude of tail wave is asymmetric at both sides	Irregular; propelling; usually no rotation	Circular orbits if rotation is absent
Sperm with cytoplasmic droplet	Amplitude of tail waves is unequal; rapid vibrations	Irregular, often rocking; seldom rotational	Perpendicular, oblique, seldom progressive
Agglutinated sperm	Decreasing, vibrating motion; slow, vibrating motion	Slow; irregular propelling; rocking	Depends on type of agglutination

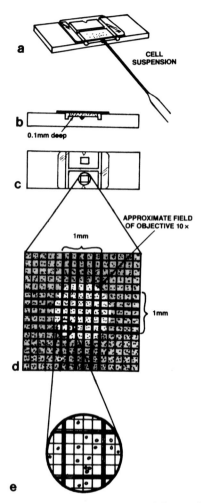

FIG. 19–4. *a,* Hemocytometer slide used for estimating the concentration of spermatozoa in a semen sample, and thereby its dilution potential for use in artificial insemination. *b, c, d,* Each square is of known area and the depth between coverslip and slide is also known, enabling cells per unit volume to be calculated (*e*).

tain types of abnormalities may not be associated with infertility. Large numbers of abnormal sperm can be detected in samples when estimating the percentage of motile cells. A semen film is carefully made (Fig. 19–6). Phase-contrast and particularly Normarski interference optics are helpful. A more precise estimate of the types of abnormal sperm and their incidence can be gained from slides prepared with an india-ink background or with the supravital stain.

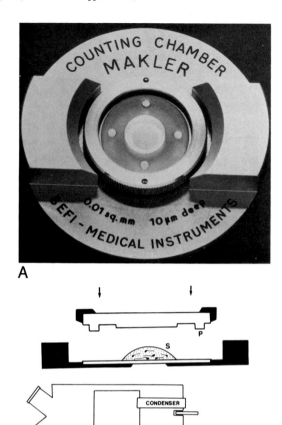

FIG. 19–5. (*Top*) The chamber after the cover has been placed on the lower base. (*Bottom*) Cross section of counting chamber. C = cover glass; L = lower part; P = elevated quartz pin. Dark area indicates the metal portion of the chamber. *A.* Before a drop of the specimen applied on the lower part is covered. *B.* After placement of the cover glass. The drop has been spread with the 10 μm space of the chamber.

Several stain mixtures have been used to estimate the percentage of live spermatozoa. These methods are subject to variations between stain batches and are influenced by the pH of the stain and the temperature and duration of staining. Dif-

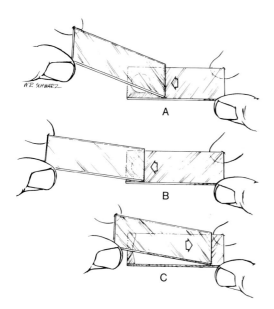

FIG. 19–6. Preparation of semen smear. *A.* A drop of semen is placed on a glass slide. *B, C.* Another glass slide is used to prepare the smear without damage to the sample. Estimation of sperm motility when placed against bovine cervical mucus.

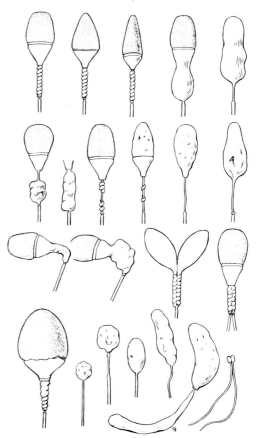

FIG. 19–7. Drawings of major morphologic abnormalities in mammalian spermatozoa (Fujita, 1975).

ferential and morphologic stains reveal structural abnormalities of spermatozoa (Fig. 19–7). A Papanicolaou stain is placed on an air-dried smear of the sample for 2 minutes. The slide is rinsed to remove excess stain and allowed to air dry. Observation of normal and abnormal forms are made, and the percentage of each type is noted (Fig. 19–8).

Special attention should be given to the acrosome, as this plays an important role in fertilization. The apical ridge of the acrosome of bull or boar sperm deteriorates with aging or injury of the cell, and the acrosin enzyme may be lost. Eventually, the acrosome may loosen and be lost. This can be seen only with appropriate phase or interference microscopes or with specially stained preparations.

Morphologic abnormalities of spermatozoa can be primary, secondary, or tertiary. Primary abnormalities are due to the failure of spermatogenesis, whereas secondary abnormalities occur during the passage of spermatozoa through the epididymis. Damage to spermatozoa resulting during or after ejaculation or from the improper handling for the artificial insemination (AI) is designated as a tertiary abnormality.

For routine examination in AI centers, the abnormal spermatozoa are classified as follows: abnormal or detached heads; cytoplasmic droplets attached to the anterior, middle, or distal part of the midpiece; coiled or bent tails, and other abnormalities (Fig. 19–8).

Inherited Sperm Defects

A variety of structural defects of spermatozoa can cause sterility or subfertility

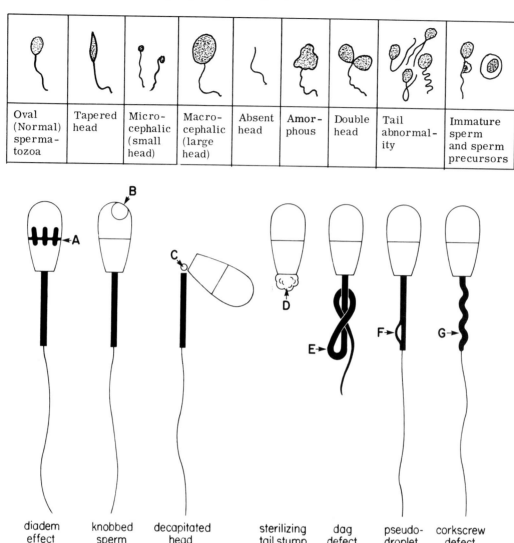

Oval (Normal) spermatozoa	Tapered head	Microcephalic (small head)	Macrocephalic (large head)	Absent head	Amorphous	Double head	Tail abnormality	Immature sperm and sperm precursors

diadem effect   knobbed sperm   decapitated head   sterilizing tail stump   dag defect   pseudo-droplet   corkscrew defect

FIG. 19–8.   Morphological anomalies of spermatozoa. (*Top*) Chart for recording of sperm abnormalities. This chart could be drawn on one tally while doing microscopic evaluation of semen samples. (*Bottom*) Some inherited sperm abnormalities associated with reproductive failure in bulls. *A*, Diadem effect; *B*, knobbed sperm; *C*, decapitated head; *D*, sterilizing tail stump; *E*, dag defect; *F*, pseudodroplet; *G*, corkscrew defect.

in bulls and boars by interfering with fertilization. Some of these sperm defects are inherited; however, the mode of inheritance is not clear because of the small number of animals that have been investigated. The defect, confined to the anterior border of the postnuclear cap, results from invaginations of the nuclear membrane and is a sign of disturbed spermatogenesis. The knobbed-sperm defect, found mostly in Friesian bulls, takes the form of an acrosome; it affects all spermatozoa in the ejaculate and affected bulls are sterile. It is an inherited characteristic and is due to an autosomal recessive gene. A similar knobbed-sperm defect was noted in the semen of large White boars. After insemination, affected spermatozoa failed to fertilize eggs.

The decapitate defect is an abnormality of the sperm tail in the semen of sterile Guernsey bulls (Fig. 19–8). It is associated with an ultrastructural abnormality in the neck or implantation region of the spermatozoon. These defective spermatozoa disintegrate into isolated heads and tails in the caput epididymis. In the dag defect noted in the semen of three infertile Danish Jersey bulls, the main piece is strongly coiled and folded over the midpiece, giving the impression of a short tail. It is due to elevated levels of zinc in spermatozoa as well as in the seminal plasma. Over 60% of the sperm heads had short tail stumps, 2 to 3 μm long. Another sperm defect found in sterile Friesian bulls is the pseudodroplet defect that is characterized by a rounding or elongated thickening of the midpiece. A rare sperm-tail defect noted in aging bulls, especially in the Red Dane breed, is a midpiece shaped like a corkscrew in 15 to 50% of spermatozoa; these sperm were dead.

Live/Dead Sperm

The proportion of live to dead cells can be estimated by supravital staining with a stain mixture such as nigrosin-eosin. The cells that were alive when the stain was applied exclude the stain, and the dead cells stain red with eosin against the dark nigrosin background. The results are highly correlated with visual estimates of progressively motile cells, but the latter averages are lower than the percentage of unstained spermatozoa.

Supravital Triple-Staining Technique

Routine semen analysis usually includes rating of sperm morphology since a low percentage of normal head forms is correlated with decreased fertility potential. Sperm morphology is generally determined using staining methods that do not distinguish between live and dead sper-

matozoa. However, the morphology of live spermatozoa correlates better with the fertility potential than with the overall sperm morphology of an ejaculate. In staining techniques, it is important that normal acrosomal reactions be clearly distinguished from the degenerative reaction of dead sperm. A triple-staining technique permitting direct assessment of normal acrosome reaction of fixed sperm could be used for scoring reacted spermatozoa in fresh and capacitated, normal and abnormal semen (Plachot et al., 1984, Jager et al., 1985) (Fig. 19–9).

Semen fractions of 200 μl are incubated at 37°C for 15 minutes with an equal volume of 2% trypan blue in phosphate-buffered saline, pH 7.4 (PBS). In trypan blue mixtures, the supravital staining percentage is determined directly after the incubation. Prior to fixation, the semen-supravital stain mixtures are pretreated at room temperature as follows:

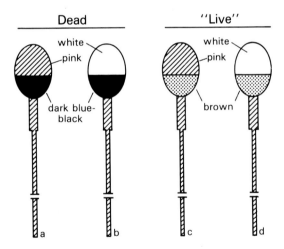

FIG. 19–9. Schematic illustration of staining patterns of spermatozoa stained with the triple-stain technique. *a.* Dead spermatozoon with intact acrosome. *b.* Dead spermatozoon without intact acrosome. *c.* "Live" spermatozoon with intact acrosome. *d.* "Live" spermatozoon without intact acrosome. (From Jager, S., Kuiken, J. and Kremer, J. (1985). Triple staining of spermatozoa for routine investigation of human semen. Technical aspects. Arch. Androl. *13,*)

A. A smear is made from undiluted or from 5 to 10 times diluted mixture (10 mixtures).

B. The mixture is diluted with 2 ml PBS, and the suspension is allowed to sediment for 4 hours.

C. The mixture is centrifuged at 400 to 1800 g for 10 minutes. The pellets are resuspended in 2 ml PBS and again centrifuged at the same speed (12 mixtures).

The triple-stained slides are examined at 1000× to 1250× magnification with a bright field microscope. From each semen sample, two preparations are investigated, and in each preparation, 100 spermatozoa are counted and classified according to presence or absence of acrosome, vital or nonvital sperm, and normal or abnormal head form (Fig. 19–9). In triple-stained preparations, particular attention is paid to tail abnormalities and the presence or absence of cytoplasmic droplets and round cells.

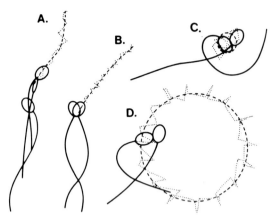

FIG. 19–10. Various patterns of sperm motility from the ampula and the ejaculate: *A.* Rolling ejaculated sperm; *B.* Ejaculated sperm that did not roll; *C.* Ampullary sperm a small circle, whiplash motility; *D.* Ampullary sperm a circle of moderate radius, about 20 μm. (From Suarez, D.S., Katz, D.F. and Overstreet, J.W. (1983). Movement characteristics and acrosomal status of rabbit spermatozoa recovered at the site and time of fertilization. Biol. Reprod. *29,* 1277–1287.)

SPERM MOTILITY

Spermatozoa are highly specialized cells that are well designed to accomplish a single objective: fertilization of an ovum. To achieve fertilization, however, the sperm must first gain access to the egg. During their transport in the male and female reproductive tracts, spermatozoa encounter different environments in which they must survive. The capacity of progressive motility develops as the morphology and metabolic machinery of the spermatozoa mature (Fig. 19–10).

Factors Affecting Sperm Motility

Motility is essential for fertility. However, motility, while an essential feature of healthy spermatozoa, is not necessarily indicative of fertilizing capacity. Normal spermatozoa lose fertilizing ability before they lose motility. Furthermore, abnormal spermatozoa may exhibit normal movement and yet be incapable of fertilizing an egg. While motility may assist in the transport of spermatozoa from the site of

deposition to the site of fertilization, it is probably secondary to other transport mechanisms such as muscular contractility and ciliary motion of the female reproductive tract. Sperm motility per se becomes crucial in facilitating passage through the cervix and uterotubal junction; even more important, it makes possible the actual penetration of the cumulus cells and zona pellucida of the ovum. Several endogenous and exogenous factors influence sperm motility (Fig. 19–11).

Patterns of Sperm Motility

Spermatozoa are driven by a propulsive apparatus, the flagellum, equipped with contractile proteins strategically arranged in longitudinal organelles, the coarse fibers, and with associated subfilaments, and microtubules, to provide the propulsive force necessary to overcome internal structural resistance and external viscous drag of extracellular fluids. The flagellum propagates repetitive sinusoidal (or nearly

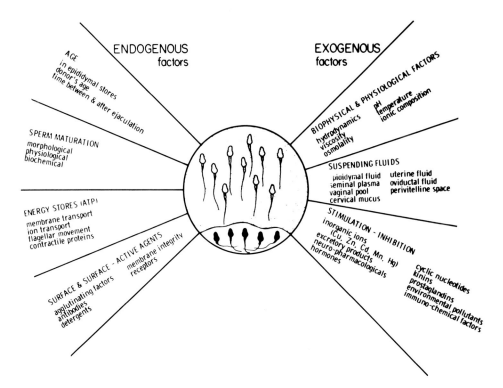

FIG. 19–11. Some endogenous and exogenous factors known to influence sperm motility.

so) waves in a coordinated sequence down the coarse fibers by alternating contraction–relaxation cycles. For the sperm cell to achieve effective progressive motion, the coordination of the waves must be attained and maintained as a consequence of developmental processes effected by programmed changes in the medium.

Spermatozoa are sensitive to environmental conditions, and as in other excitable tissues and cells, the cell membrane at the environmental interface may be adaptively equipped with specific receptor sites.

Spermatozoa exhibit a vast spectrum of diversity even within a single ejaculate, not the least evident variables being the shape and speed of the individual spermatozoon (Figs. 19–12 and 19–13). This diversity has both physiologic and morphologic significance and therefore probably plays a crucial role in the selection process during the development, maturation, and transport of spermatozoa (Table 19–3).

Techniques to Measure Sperm Motility

Among the features of spermatozoa that have long held the attention of investigators is that of motility. Several techniques have been devised to study, describe, and quantitate sperm motility. The simplest of these involves a visual appraisal of the percentage of motile sperm and the quality of the motility of individual spermatozoa.

Sperm motility in the ejaculate or dilute suspension is estimated visually under several fields using light microscopy. The percentage of progressively motile cells should be estimated using a high-power (400×) microscope with a preheated stage at 37°C to 40°C. The fresh semen should be prepared as a thin film on a microscope slide, diluted with sufficient physiologic solution (such as saline) so that individual cells are visible. At 400×, the percentage of motile sperm, their rate of motility, and their gross morphology can be scrutinized. Despite the subjective nature of such eval-

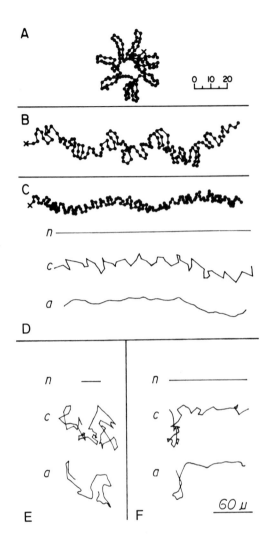

FIG. 19–12. *A, B,* and *C.* Traces of head–neck junction of motile epididymal spermatozoa. The sperm head–neck junction was marked on 150 consecutive frames (1 sec. total). *A.* The motility of a typical caput sperm incubated for 15 min at 37°C in assay buffer with theophylline without forward motility pattern (FMP). *B.* Shows the trace of a caput spermatozoon incubated identically, but with the addition of a saturating concentration of crude FMP. *C.* Shows the trace of a typical caudal sperm incubated similarly with neither theophylline nor FMP added. The scale in *A* is in micrometers, and the *X's* mark the points at which the traces begin. (From Acott et al. (1983). Movement characteristics of bovine epididymal spermatozoa: effects of forward motility protein and epididymal maturation. Biol. Reprod. *29,* 389–399.) *D, E,* and *F.* The net, curvilinear, and average paths for three typical 2-second tracks of sperm movement (61 points at 30 frames per second). *n,* The net displacement path connecting the first and last points; *c,* the curvilinear path of the sperm head–midpiece junction; *a,* the five-point moving average of the curvilinear path. Paths were redrawn from computer generated images. (From Tessler, S. and Olds-Clarke, P. (1985). Linear and nonlinear mouse sperm motility patterns: A quantitative classification. J. Androl. *6,* 37.)

uations, the percentage of motile sperm is positively correlated with fertility. The low correlations between sperm motility and fertility may result from the low accuracy and precision of the visual method to evaluate spermatozoal motility, the influence of other attributes of sperm quality on fertility, the imprecision in measuring fertility of individual ejaculates, and the influence of many factors unrelated to semen such as parity of the females, season of year, month the semen is used, and herd management.

Motility in Seminal Plasma and Biologic Fluids

The motility and survival of spermatozoa depend on an optimal ratio between the prostatic and vesicular fluids. The secretions of the seminal vesicles contain one or more factors that exert a deleterious effect on sperm motility and survival. The prostatic fluid, on the other hand, stimulates motility. On contact with the prostatic fluid, spermatozoa are protected against the negative influences exerted by the vesicular fluid.

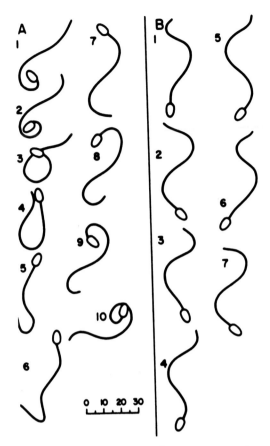

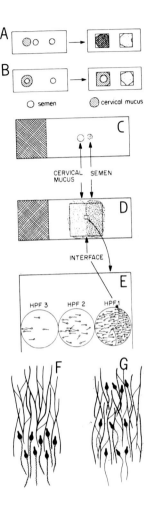

FIG. 19–13. Traces of motile caput spermatozoa showing typical wave propagation. Sperm tails were traced from sequentially selected frames taken of caput sperm incubated for 15 min at 37°C in assay buffer plus theophylline in, *A*, the absence and, *B*, the presence of crude FMP. The scale is in micrometers. (From Acott et al. (1983) Movement characteristics of bovine epididymal spermatozoa: effects of forward motility protein and epididymal maturation. Biol. Reprod. *29*, 389–399.)

As spermatozoa move from the seminal plasma to cervical mucus, the pattern of tail movement alters. During penetration of mucus at midcycle, there is little if any change in the rate of progressive motility; however, the rate of flagellar beating and rotation of the head are greatly reduced. In highly viscous mucus, the speed of forward motion is reduced or stopped entirely and the flagellum generates a wider arc.

FIG. 19–14. *A, B.* Sperm–cervical mucus contact test. The slide test for *in vitro* sperm penetration in cervical mucus. *C.* A drop of semen and a drop of cervical mucus are placed on a glass slide. *D.* A coverslip is placed on the slide and pressed slightly. *E.* Quantitative (number of sperm per high-power microscopic field, 400×) assessment of sperm penetration in cervical mucus, HPF$_1$; HPF$_2$; HPF$_3$ consecutive high-power microscopic fields from the interface. Change in motility pattern of spermatozoa as a result of sperm agglutination in sperm–cervical mucus contact test. *F.* Spermatozoa loaded with spermagglutinins stick to glycoprotein filaments as soon as they contact cervical mucus. *G.* Cervical mucus containing spermagglutinins provides the penetrating spermatozoa with the spermagglutinins causing the spermatozoa to stick to glycoprotein filaments.

Once through the cervical canal, spermatozoa encounter the intrauterine environment. Little is known concerning what influence, if any, uterine fluid exerts on sperm motility. However, the pattern of motility appears to be responsive to metabolites in the various fluids of the female reproductive tract. For example, the velocity of sperm movement increases in the presence of oviductal or peritoneal fluid. The patterns and rate of sperm motility can be evaluated when a drop of semen is

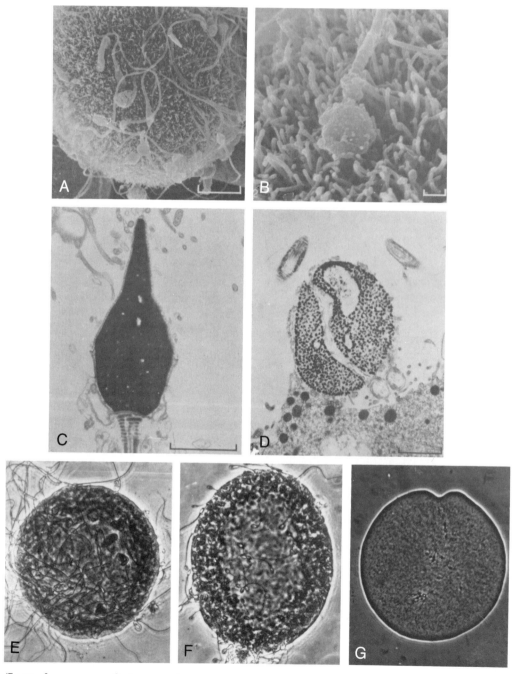

(**Legend appears on facing page.**)

mixed on a glass slide with a drop of cervical mucus or a drop of vaginal fluids (Fig. 19–14).

To improve the quality of semen for use in *in vitro* fertilization programs, and to separate sperm bearing X and Y chromosomes, sperm penetration patterns in cervical mucus and other biologic fluids are being studied.

Photoelectric and Electronic Methods

Photoelectric and electronic methods of observing sperm cell velocity, swimming patterns and the proportion of moving spermatozoa as they pass a phototube have been developed. However, the instrumentation is expensive and not available for general use. Other objective methods to evaluate sperm motility include cinematography and videotape, scattering of a light beam, and image analysis by computers.

Two-dimensional "tracking" techniques (e.g., multiple-exposure photography, cinematography, and videomicrography) that follow the position of the sperm head–midpiece junction reveal differences among sperm motility patterns. A quantitative method is used to distinguish types of sperm motility using a new parameter, the linear index. Using this method, spermatozoa are tracked by videomicrography, and the following are calculated: net displacement velocity; curvilinear velocity of the sperm head; "average" velocity (a five-point moving average of the track); the progressiveness ratio; the curvilinear progressiveness ratio; and a linear index (Tessler and Olds-Clarke, 1985).

With the increased use of multiple-exposure photography, cinematography, and videomicrography techniques, attention has been focused on the shape of sperm swimming patterns. A change in the movement characteristics of mammalian spermatozoa appears to be important, if not necessary, between the time of insemination and the time of arrival at the site of fertilization. Typically, the majority of motile spermatozoa in the ejaculate swim in linear trajectories ("progressive" or "straight-swimming" spermatozoa), while those spermatozoa examined from the oviduct swim in erratic, nonprogressive patterns.

Motion picture films of sperm suspensions are prepared to evaluate sperm motility. A drop of semen is mixed with a drop of 99-mm sodium citrate on a glass slide; a glass coverslip is used. When extended semen is evaluated, semen from several straws is transferred to a vial and mixed. A 10-μl aliquot is placed on a glass slide, covered, and evaluated (O'Conner et al., 1982). Evaluation of the tracks left by motile sperm on negatives prepared with a short-time exposure provides precise information but is very tedious.

FIG. 19–15. Reaction of human sperm (*A,B,C,D*) and monkey sperm (*E,F,G*) with zona-free hamster eggs. *A.* Scanning electron micrograph of a zona-free hamster oocyte with morphologically abnormal spermatozoa associated to the oocyte microvilli. *B.* Scanning electron micrograph of a round head spermatozoon attached to the oocyte microvilli. *C.* Transmission electron micrograph of a human sperm with a cytoplasmic drop (arrows) that has already undergone the acrosome reaction. This spermatozoon is associated with the oocyte microvilli of the hamster oocyte as preliminary to the membrane fusion process. *D.* Section through a grossly abnormal sperm head associated with the zona-free hamster oocyte. Note that this sperm head has two nuclear components and the chromatin appears abnormally condensed. (From Barros et al. (1985). Selection of morphologically abnormal spermatozoa by human cervical mucus. *Arch. Androl. 16*) *E,F,G.* Zona-free hamster eggs (fixed and stained with Lacmoid) after incubation with hamster sperm (*E*) or monkey sperm (*F,G,*). Swollen sperm head, indicating initial steps of fertilization, are visible in *A*. No sign of penetration was observed with monkey sperm. (From Kreitmann et al (1982). Ovum collection transfer in primates. *In* In Vitro Fertilization and Embryo Transfer. E.S.E. Hafez and K. Senin (eds.). Lancaster, UK, MTP Press.)

The rate of movement can be estimated on an arbitrary scale by microscopic observation. Circular or reverse motion is often a sign of cold shock or of a medium that is not isotonic with semen. Oscillatory motion frequently occurs in aged and dying spermatozoa.

FERTILIZING ABILITY OF SPERM

The standard procedures for semen analysis (sperm count, sperm morphology, and sperm motility) are relatively poor indicators of the fertilizing capacity of spermatozoa. A few laboratory techniques have been developed to evaluate the physiologic integrity of sperm such as survival, transport, and fertilizing ability. An ideal test is simple, rapid, and objective with a high correlation with fertility. Numerous tests have been proposed, and many have significant correlations with fertility. Unfortunately, with most of these biophysical procedures, there is a percentage of "false-positive" and "false-negative" results. This is mainly due to the lack of proper controls, to possible interaction with microbiologic contaminants of the semen, and to the variability in the technical details that are often not adequately described in the literature.

The method most commonly used is the Hamster test. The evaluation of sperm fertilizability is based on the penetrability of the sperm into zona-free hamster ova. This technique has been widely used to evaluate the fertilizability of human sperm for *in vitro* fertilization centers. Another test recently described is the hypoosmotic swelling test (HOS), which is based on the evaluation of functional integrity of sperm membranes (Jeyendran et al., 1985), but future research is needed to apply both of these techniques to the evaluation of bovine and ovine sperm.

Hamster Test (Zona-Free Hamster Ova Test)

This test involves a number of steps including the preparation and *in vitro* capacitation of sperm to be tested, superovu-

TABLE 19–4. *In Vitro* Penetration of Zona-Free Mammalian Oocytes by Heterologous Spermatozoa

Spermatozoon	Oocyte	Percentage of Penetration
Guinea pig	Hamster	100
P. Maniculatus	Hamster	100
P. Ceocopus	Hamster	2
Gerbil	Hamster	8
Mouse	Hamster	100
Rat	Hamster	83
Human	Hamster	95
Pig	Hamster	36
Rabbit	Hamster	63
Rat	Mouse	9
Hamster	Mouse	2
Hamster	Rat	14
Mouse	Rat	100
Mouse	Rabbit	81
Rat	Rabbit	37
Bovine	Hamster	90

Compiled by Barros and Leal, 1982)

lation of golden hamsters with the subsequent removal of the zona pellucida of eggs by using trypsin, incubation of sperm with zona-free hamster ova, and the evaluation of sperm penetration in the ova.

Zona-free hamster ova thus prepared are added to 0.2 to 0.3 ml of capacitated spermatozoa suspended under silicone oil in a sterile petri dish. Zona-free ova are incubated at 37° to 38°C under 5% $CO_2 : 95\%$ air in atmospheric pressure for a few hours. The cultured ova are washed with fresh BWW medium to remove spermatozoa. Ova are then transferred to a glass slide and fixed in a mixture of ethanol and acetic acid for 2 to 3 hours and then stained with 0.3% acetolacmoid stain. Stained ova are examined by phase-contrast microscopy ($400\times$ to $1000\times$) for the occurrence of sperm penetration (presence of swollen sperm heads with attached or closely associated tail within the vitellus). Ova are considered penetrated when a swollen sperm head (or heads) or male pronucleus or pronuclei and corresponding sperm tail(s) are found within the vitellus (Fig. 19–15).

TABLE 19–5. Reproductive Cycle of Female Golden Hamsters

Time	Day 1	Day 2	Day 3	Day 4
Midnight				
1 A.M.				
2	Late diestrus	Estrus	Mid-diestrus	Late diestrus
3		Ovulation		
4, 5, 6				
7	Vaginal discharge is a clear, thin fluid;	Postovulatory discharge has copious quantity of a thick, creamy white opaque material with a pungent cheesy odor	Vaginal discharge is yellowish; sometimes a waxy plug	
8	only a small amount			
9				
10	Vaginal smear not distinctive			
11		Animals rarely breed after this time		
Noon		Metestrus (4 hrs) Vaginal smear with oval nucleated cells		
1 P.M.	Proestrus (3 hrs) Vaginal smear shows		Vaginal smear shows very few cells	Vaginal smear with cells quite sparse
2	non-nucleated squamous cells			
3		Early diestrus (total time for diestrus is more than 70 hours)		
4				
5		Leukocytes are quite characteristic on the vaginal smear		
6				
7	Estrus (12 hrs) Animals may be	Animals do not breed	Animals do not breed	Animals do not breed
8	bred during this			
9	stage			
10	Vaginal smear shows no leukocytes; nucleated cells,			
11	epithelial type			
Midnight				

(H. Magalhaes, 1970)

Hypo-osmotic Swelling Test

This is a simple and economic test used as an additional tool in evaluating the fertilizing ability of human spermatozoa (Jeyendran et al., 1985) and the functional integrity of the sperm membrane. To perform this test, 0.1 ml of undiluted ejaculate is mixed with 1 ml of solution consisting of equal parts of fructose and sodium citrate at 150 mOsm in water. After incubation for 30 to 60 minutes at 37°C, the spermatozoa are observed with phase-contrast microscopy and the proportion of sperm exhibiting tail swelling is determined.

The HOS test correlates highly with the ability of human spermatozoa to become

TABLE 19–6. Chemical Indicators of Secretory Activity

Secretions of Organs	Biochemical Markers to Evaluate Functional Activity of Organs
Prostate	Citric acid, acid phosphatase, zinc
Epididymis	Glycerylphosphorylcholine
Seminal vesicle	Fructose, proteins, prostaglandins

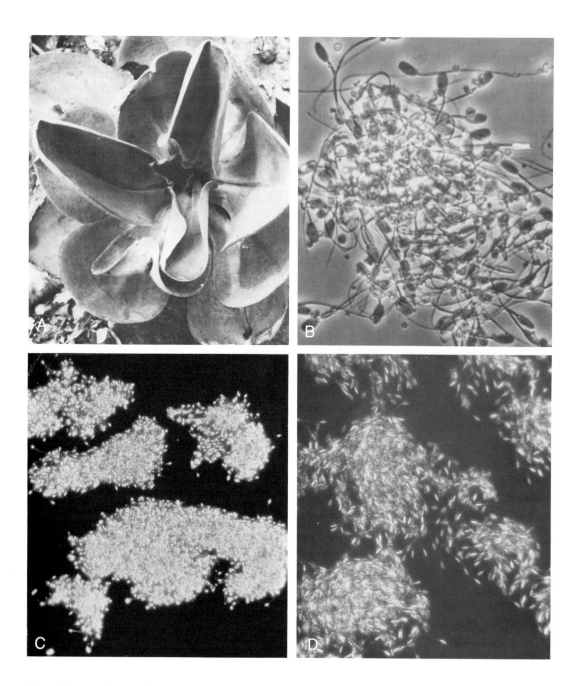

FIG. 19–16.   Immobilization and agglutination of spermatozoa as induced by *Echeveria gibbiflora*, commomly known as "Oreja de Burro" (OBACE), a Mexican plant used for contraception in women. *A.* Photograph of the leaves from *Echeveria gibbiflora* in rosette arrangement. *B.* Magnification of a clot of washed agglutinated spermatozoa from a rabbit using phase-contrast microscopy (830×). *C.* Agglutination pattern of washed spermatozoa from a human treated with OBACE (350×). *D.* Phase-contrast micrograph of the agglutination pattern of pig or bull spermatozoa induced by OBACE (350×). (From Huacuja et al. (1985). Immobilization and agglutination effect of Echeveria gibbiflora aqueous crude extract on human spermatozoa. Arch. Androl., *40,* 71–79.)

capacitated and penetrate denuded hamster oocytes (hamster test), whereas there is less correlation between the hamster test and the standard semen parameters. HOS tests the standard semen parameters in regard to the capacity of spermatozoa to fertilize human oocytes *in vitro*. If the results of the HOS test are used in combination with the standard semen parameters, false-negatives can be avoided and false-positives can be further minimized. Several methods are applied to evaluate the viability and fertilizability of sperm (Tables 19–4, to 19–6; Figs. 19–2, 19–16).

Induced Agglutination of Sperm

There are some 200 species of plants whose extracts or infusions have been used as contraceptives. One of these plants is the "Oreja de Burro" (OBACE), the common name for *Echeveria gibbiflora* of the family *Crassulaceae* (33 genera and 1300 species) (Huacuja et al., 1985). This plant is found growing profusely in the Valley of Mexico and surroundings and is popularly used as a diluted aqueous extract of ground leaves for a vaginal postcoital rinse (Fig. 19–2).

REFERENCES

Acott, T.S., Katz, D.F. and Hoskins, D.D. (1983). Movement characteristics of bovine epididymal spermatozoa: effects of forward motility protein and epididymal maturation. Biol. Reprod. *29,* 389–399.

Barros, C. and Leal, J. (1982). *In vitro* fertilization and its use to study gamete interactions. *In In Vitro* Fertilization and Embryo Transfer. E.S.E. Hafez and K. Semm (eds.). Lancaster, England, MTP Press.

Barros, C., Vigil, P., Herrera, E., Arguello, B. and Walker, R. (1985). Selection of morphologically abnormal spermatozoa by human cervical mucus. Arch. Androl. *16,* 255–260.

Fujita, T. (1975). Abnormal spermatozoa and infertility (man). *In* Scanning Electron Microscopial Atlas of Mammalian Reproduction. E.S.E Hafez (ed.). Tokyo, Japan, Igaku Shoin.

Huacuja, L., Taboada, J., Ortega, A., Merchant, H., Reyes, R. and Delgado, N.M. (1985). Immobilization and agglutination effects of *Echeveria gibbiflora* aqueous crude extract on human spermatozoa. Arch. Androl. *40,* 71–79.

Jager, S., Kuiken, J. and Kremer, J. (1985). Triple staining of spermatozoa for routine investigation of human semen. Technical aspects. Arch. Androl. *13.*

Jeyendran, R.S., Van der Ven, H.H., Reid, D., Perez-Pelaez, P., Diedrich, K. and Zaneveld, L.J.D. (1985). The hypoosmotic swelling (HOS) test as an indicator of the fertilizing capacity of human spermatozoa, current clinical and basic investigations. *In* ACOG, 33rd Clinical Meeting. New York, Elsevier.

Kreitmann, O., Lynch, A., Nixon, W.E. and Hodgen, G.D. (1982). Ovum collection, induced luteal dysfunction, *in vitro* fertilization, embryo development and low tubal ovum transfer in primates. *In Vitro* Fertilization and Embryo Transfer. E.S.E. Hafez and K. Semm (eds.). Lancaster, UK, MTP Press.

Magalhaes, H. (1970). Hamsters. *In* Reproduction and Breeding Techniques for Laboratory Animals. E.S.E. Hafez (ed.). Philadelphia, Lea & Febiger.

O'Connor, M.T., Amann, R.P. and Saacke, R.G. (1982). Comparisons of computer evaluations of spermatozoal motility with standard laboratory tests and their use for predicting fertility. J. Anim. Sci. *53,* 1368–1376.

Plachot, M., Mandelbaum, J. and Junca, A. (1984). Acrosome reaction of human sperm used for *in vitro* fertilization. Fertil. Steril. *42,* 418–423.

Suarez, D.S., Katz, D.F. and Overstreet, J.W. (1983). Movement characteristics and acrosomal status of rabbit spermatozoa recovered at the site and time of fertilization. Biol. Reprod. *29,* 1277–1287.

Tessler, S. and Olds-Clarke, P. (1985). Linear and nonlinear mouse sperm motility patterns: a quantitative classification. J. Androl. *6,* 34–44.

Zaneveld, L.J.D. and Polakoski, K.L. (1977). Collection and physical examination of the ejaculate. *In* Techniques of Human Andrology. E.S.E. Hafez (ed.) Amsterdam, North Holland, Elsevier.

20
Artificial Insemination

E.S.E. HAFEZ

Artificial insemination (AI) is the most important single technique devised for the genetic improvement of animals. This is possible because a few highly selected males produce enough spermatozoa to inseminate thousands of females per year, whereas only relatively few progeny per selected female can be produced per year even by embryo transfer. Methods have been developed for inseminating cattle, sheep, goats, swine, horses, dogs, cats, poultry, and a variety of laboratory animals and insects. The earliest carefully documented use of AI was in 1780 when Spallanzani, an Italian physiologist, obtained pups by this method. Other scattered reports appeared in the 19th century, but it was not until 1900 that extensive studies with farm animals began in Russia and shortly thereafter in Japan.

Major advantages of AI are as follows: (1) genetic improvement, (2) control of venereal diseases, (3) availability of accurate breeding records necessary for good herd management, (4) economic service, and (5) safety through elimination of dangerous males on the farm. AI is practically essential in conjunction with synchronization of estrus programs, and it has been proposed as a means of sex control through separation of spermatozoa containing X- and Y-chromosomes.

When properly done, disadvantages are few. However, it is necessary to have sufficiently well-trained personnel to provide proper service, and to have appropriate arrangements for corralling females for detection of heat and insemination, particularly under range conditions.

Artificial insemination in farm animals offers several advantages for genetic improvement, disease control, and economical aspects:

1. Enables the widespread use of outstanding sires and dissemination of valuable genetic material even to small farms.
2. Facilitates progeny testing under a range of environmental and managerial conditions, thereby further improving the rate and efficiency of genetic selection.
3. Leads to improved performance and potential of the national herd, and permits coordination of a breeding policy on a national basis.
4. Permits crossbreeding to change the production emphasis, such as switching from milk to beef.
5. Accelerates the introduction of new genetic material through the export of semen and reduces international transport costs.
6. Enables the use of deep-frozen semen after the donor is dead, thus aiding preservation of selected lines.
7. Permits use of semen from incapacitated or oligospermic males.
8. Reduces the risk of spreading sexually transmitted diseases.
9. Is usually essential after synchronization of estrus in large groups of animals.

10. Provides a necessary research tool for investigating many aspects of male and female reproductive physiology (Hunter, 1982).

The genetic improvement achieved by AI of dairy cattle has resulted from the use of proven-tested sires. Obtaining semen at the earliest possible age from bulls being proven tested is desirable to hasten identification of superior sires. Ultimately, the genetic impact of a superior sire is limited by the number of sperm produced, which is a direct function of testicular size.

Carefully selected young dairy bulls should be sampled as soon as possible and rigidly culled after the progeny test. Only a few outstanding sires need be selected to breed a large cow population, provided proper procedures of sexual preparation, semen collection, and processing are used to harvest and preserve the maximal number of viable sperm from each sire. Similar types of performance and progeny test programs are important to make maximal genetic progress with meat-type farm animals. AI facilitates cross-breeding, requiring that only one breed be maintained on the farm.

Development of AI in beef cattle has been slower in the United States and many other countries because of the difficulty of heat detection and insemination under range conditions, restrictive regulations of the breed associations, and the considerable genetic improvement that can be made for highly heritable traits, using performance-tested bulls, without AI.

MANAGEMENT OF MALES AND SEMEN COLLECTION

The production of high-quality semen depends on males that have been kept under good conditions. When young males are properly fed and managed, semen can be collected successfully at the following approximate ages: bulls, 12 months; rams, goats, and boars, 7 to 8 months; stallions, 24 months. (Tables 20–1 to 20–3)

Physical Condition of Males

Feeding has a notable effect on rate of sexual development in all farm animals. When energy intake is restricted, the rate of growth is decreased, testis growth is retarded, age of puberty is increased, and sperm output may be reduced. Prolonged deficiencies of essential nutrients can cause infertility. On the other hand, excessive feeding is wasteful and may produce fat, sluggish males.

Testis size is important because of the high correlation between testis size and sperm-producing potential. Testis size increases rapidly as puberty approaches, and by 1 year of age, bulls have reached approximately 50% of their mature potential. Testis size also is a highly heritable trait that is easily monitored by measuring scrotal circumference.

Semen Collection

Of major importance to an AI program is the correct collection of semen. This involves scheduling males for semen collection at optimal intervals, sexual preparation, and correct techniques of semen collection.

Mounts and Teasing Procedures. Live mounts—such as a teaser female, another male, or a castrated male—have proven to be the most successful techniques for routine semen collection. Some males, especially boars, can be trained to mount dummies equally well (Fig. 20–1). An estrogen-treated female may provide added incentive during the training period. Dummies may be constructed to hold the artificial vagina. Dummies have an advantage over live mounts in providing stability, and over teaser females particularly in permitting disease control. In either case, a strong mount providing adequate support should be provided. Live mounts should be restrained to minimize lateral as well as forward movement and still provide easy access for semen collection. Good footing is necessary. Convenient

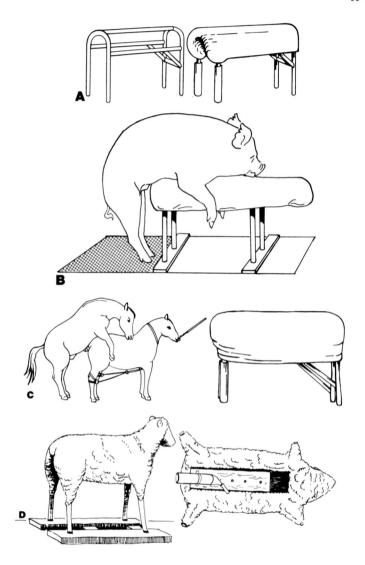

FIG. 20–1. Dummies and mounts used for collecting semen from farm animals. *A, Left to right.* Dummy cow constructed from steel pipe. Completed dummy covered and well padded. *B.* Boar mounting padded dummy. A mat to give secure footing is provided. *C, Left to right.* Mare hobbled, restrained, and tail-bandaged before using as a mount; padded dummy. *D, Left to right.* Side view of a portable dummy for rams. Bottom view showing artificial vagina secured for semen collection.

posts should be included for restraining bulls during sexual preparation.

Sexual preparation before semen collection from bulls increases the number of sperm cells obtained by as much as 100%. False mounting a bull several times and/or intensive teasing for 5 or 10 minutes without false mounting is effective. Fluids from the accessory sex glands secreted during this preparatory period may flush out contaminating material from the urethra. Stimuli that are effective in increasing the sexual response of bulls include changing the teaser, changing the location of the teaser, bringing a new bull into the collection area, and false mounting. Various combinations should be tried with sluggish males to keep the intensity of the sexual stimuli high. Beef bulls generally exhibit less libido than dairy bulls and require more ingenuity to provide proper sexual stimuli before semen collection.

Frequency of Semen Collection. Increasing the frequency of semen collection decreases the number of sperm per collection but increases the number of sperm obtained per unit of time. Thus, frequent ejaculation of superior sires provides more spermatozoa to inseminate more females. Billions of sperm can be obtained per normal male per week from any farm animal if properly managed at the time of semen collection (Table 20–1).

Bulls. Under practical conditions, artificial breeding organizations often prefer to collect semen from bulls twice a day 2 days per week to harvest more sperm to freeze at one time. With this procedure, a majority of the sperm produced can be collected. With liquid semen programs, bulls can be ejaculated three times per week and semen made continuously available from each bull by using it over a period of 2 to 3 days. Bulls can be ejaculated

TABLE 20–1. Frequency of Semen Collection and Preparation of Artificial Vagina

Species	Frequency of Collection	Preparation of Artificial Vagina
Cattle	Collect semen twice a day 2 days/week to harvest more sperm to freeze at one time. With liquid semen, bulls can be ejaculated three times per week and semen made continuously available from each bull by using it over a peiod of 2–3 days. Bulls are ejaculated daily without reducing fertility, but the number of sperm per ejaculate is reduced and more stimuli often are required for proper sexual preparation.	The temperature of the AV is more important than the pressure it exerts on the penis. Water is used to control both, but final pressure may be adjusted by pumping in air. Temperature inside AV is near 45°C, but 38°C–55°C has been employed. Place assembled AV in incubator at 45°C or slightly higher if cooling will occur prior to semen collection. Semen collection tube is maintained near body temperature to prevent sperm damage on ejaculation that is due either to overheating or to cold shock.
Sheep	Rams are ejaculated many times a day for several weeks before severely depleting epididymal reserves of sperm. This is due to small epididymal reserves. Rams often mate or are ejaculated many times per day during the season. Bucks are ejaculated less frequently than rams.	AV temperature and technique of collection is similar to cattle. Forward thrust of the ram is less vigorous but rapid. Semen collector must coordinate movements swiftly with those of the ram. AV may be attached to a dummy.
Boar	Males expel large numbers of sperm in each ejaculate and deplete their epididymal reserves more quickly. Regular semen collections not more than every other day are recommended. If daily ejaculates are required for several days, a short sexual rest for 2–3 days is recommended.	Pressure is especially important for collecting semen. The boar ejaculates when curled tip of penis is firmly engaged in the sow's cervix, the AV or the operator's hand. When using the AV or the gloved hand, pressure is exerted on the coiled distal end of the penis throughout ejaculation. Once ejaculation has started, the boar remains quiet for the few minutes required for ejaculation. Ejaculate consists of three fractions: (1) presperm fraction, (2) the sperm-rich fraction, and (3) postsperm fraction. Both pre- and postsperm fractions contain mostly seminal fluids with gelatinous, pellet-like material from Cowper's glands. This material tends to seal the cervix of sow during mating, preventing loss of semen. Presperm fraction is discarded before sperm-rich fraction is collected or gel can be filtered in horses.
Horse	Males expel large numbers of sperm in each ejaculate and deplete their epididymal reserves quickly. Regular semen collections not more than every other day are recommended. If daily ejaculations are required for several days, a short sexual rest for 2–3 days is recommended.	Before ejaculation wash the penis with warm soapy water and rinse with clean water to remove smegma and other debris on the surface of the penis. The mare should be hobbled. AV is larger than it is for other animals to accommodate the stallion's erect vascular penis.

daily without reducing fertility, but the number of sperm per ejaculate is reduced and more stimuli often are required for proper sexual preparation.

Rams. Rams can be ejaculated many times a day for several weeks before severely depleting epididymal reserves of sperm. This is because of the small ejaculates (Table 20–2) and the large epididymal reserves. Rams often mate or are ejaculated many times per day during the breeding season. Bucks have similar semen characteristics but are not ejaculated as frequently as rams.

Boars and Stallions. These animals expel large numbers of sperm in each ejaculate and deplete their epididymal reserves more quickly. It is best not to attempt regular semen collections more often than every other day. If daily ejaculations are required for several days, a short sexual rest for 2 or 3 days is recommended.

Artificial Vagina. The best procedure for collecting semen is with the artificial vagina (AV). The AV is simple in construction and simulates natural copulation. The basic design is illustrated with an AV for bulls (Fig. 20–2). The unit provides suitable temperature, pressure, and lubrication to evoke ejaculation, and a calibrated tube is attached to collect the semen. Sanitation and the technical skill of both the semen collector and handler of the male are important. Such skill should lead to obtaining semen of high quality and minimizing the possibility of injury during collection. A separate sterile AV should be used for collecting each semen sample. The frequency of semen collection and the preparation of the AV are summarized (Table 20–1 and Figs. 20–1 and 20–2).

The AV should be lubricated carefully with sterile lubricant. During collection, the AV should be held parallel and close to the cow slanted in line with the expected path of the bull's penis. The penis should be guided into the AV by grasping the sheath with the hand immediately behind the preputial orifice (Fig. 20–3).

Insertion of the penis is usually best accomplished on the upward movement as soon as the bull mounts. Precise timing is required. As the bull thrusts forward for ejaculation, the operator allows the AV to move forward with the thrust and aligned with the penis. Then he gently tilts the artificial vagina down so the semen can run into the collecting tube. The experienced operator will alter the conditions of the AV and the semen collection procedure slightly according to the sexual behavior of individual males.

The AV for stallions must be larger than for other farm animals to accommodate the stallion's erect vascular-muscular penis. Many types of AVs have been developed (Fig. 20–4). A handle to maintain a firm grip on the AV is necessary because of its size and the vigorous thrusting of a stallion. The AV is partially filled with water to give an internal temperature of 45°C to 50°C. Air space connected to an expansion valve is provided to permit expansion of the liner when the penis engages the AV and increases the pressure. This pressure and friction stimulates the stallion to ejaculate. When pulsations begin at the base of the penis, which is characteristic of ejaculation, the end of the AV with the collection bottle should be lowered sufficiently to allow semen to flow into the collection vessel. Ejaculation is completed in about 25 seconds. Artificial vaginas for semen collection in rabbits are used extensively for research purposes (Fig. 20–5).

Electroejaculation. Electrical stimulation is the preferred method, only when males cannot be trained or refuse to serve the AV (often under range conditions); also, injuries and infirmities may make mounting impossible. This method can be used successfully in the bull, ram, and buck, and it is possible to obtain a semen sample of reduced volume from the boar. It is not desirable to collect and use semen from males unable to serve because of a probable genetic defect. Portable electroejaculators that run on 110 volts as well as on the 12-volt car ignition system are

TABLE 20–2. Detection of Estrus and Procedures of Insemination

Species	Detection of Estrus	Procedures for Insemination
Cattle	Cows in loose housing are observed early in morning and evening every day for standing when mounted by other cows. Nonpregnant cows are turned morning and evening and watched for 20 to 30 minutes each time for standing heat.	Insemination while standing in a stanchion or stall is recommended. Beef cows in estrus are penned and a squeeze chute provided to restrain the animal during insemination. Stress should be avoided. Semen is deposited in the cervix with the aid of a speculum. The rectovaginal technique is more effective and more widely used. By manipulation of the cervix with the hand in the rectum, the inseminating catheter is passed just through the annular rings of the cervix. Part of the semen is deposited through the cervix into the uterus and the remainder in the cervix catheter is withdrawn. With the straw inseminating gun, most spermatozoa are transferred to the cow. Semen is expelled slowly to avoid sperm losses in the catheter. A common error is to penetrate beyond the body of the uterus into the uterine horns.
Sheep	Difficult to detect. Vasectomized rams with marking crayons or colored grease paint applied to brisket of ram or contained in a harness. Changing ram and/or color.	Ewe is held by putting hind legs over a rail or placing her in an elevated crate during insemination. A rotating platform arrangement with the inseminator in a pit can inseminate more than 100 ewes per hour. This permits one person to put a ewe on platform, another to inseminate and a third to release the ewe. Insemination with aid of a speculum and light permits semen to be deposited into or through the cervix rather than the vagina.
Pigs	Sound, sight, and smell of a vasectomized or intact boar in an adjacent pen are helpful. Sows in heat seek the boar and assume a rigid stance (lordosis) and their ears become erect when mounted, or similarly when hands are placed firmly on their back. The vulva swells and reddens as blood flow increases. Sows come into estrus 3–8 days after weaning their litter. Weaning time is used as a method of synchronizing estrus.	Insemination can occur without restraining the sow to avoid semen loss. With some rubbing and pressure on back, the sow stands calmly during AI. The insemination tube is guided into the cervix because the vagina tapers directly into the cervix, which itself tapers. It is not possible to pass the catheter into the uterus, but with inflated cuff, most of 50 ml is forced into the uterus. Large semen volume and high sperm numbers are required.
Horses	Mares are teased daily with a stallion in special teaser paddocks. Indications of acceptance of stallion are elevation of tail, spreading of legs, standing, frequent urination, and contractions of the vulva "winking."	The mare is restrained by hobbles, backed against baled hay or a board wall, or put in a breeding chute to protect the inseminator. The area around vulva is scrubbed before insemination to minimize contamination. Arm placed in a plastic sleeve, lightly lubricated, is inserted into vagina and index finger inserted into cervix. Inseminating catheter is guided into the uterus to deposit 20 to 50 ml of raw or extended semen.

available with different probe sizes for different species.

Bull. A rectal probe with either ring or straight electrodes or finger electrodes can be produced to provide the electrical stimulation. The penis usually erects, and the semen is collected without the possibility of contamination in the prepuce. Sine waves are equal to or better than pulse waves for stimulation.

Excess fecal material is removed from the rectum, and the lubricated probe or

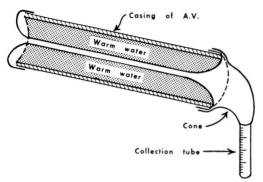

FIG. 20–2. Artificial vagina for bulls shown in longitudinal section to illustrate construction.

gloved hand is inserted into the rectum. Voltage is gradually increased, with repeated rhythmic stimulation periods alternated with short rest periods. Experience is necessary to achieve the proper combination for erection followed by ejaculation. Secretion from the accessory sex glands takes place at lower voltages and ejaculation at higher voltages. Semen samples obtained with an electroejaculator are usually of larger volume with a lower concentration of sperm, but the fertility and total sperm numbers are equivalent to samples obtained with an AV.

Bulls have been ejaculated by this method for a period of several years with no apparent ill effect. However, there usually occurs some stimulation of motor nerves with limb extension, so a restraining rack with good footing should be used.

Rams. The ram responds exceptionally well to electrical stimulation, and the response is more rapid than in the bull. It is recommended that stimuli be applied every 7 seconds with increments of 1 volt. Ejaculation usually occurs with four to seven stimuli. Semen can be collected with the ram in a standing or recumbent position on a table. The glans penis should be lightly secured with sterile gauze so that the filiform appendage and urethra are directed into the collection tube prior to ejaculation to minimize loss of semen.

Ejaculate volume is slightly larger than for samples collected with the AV, and sperm concentration is correspondingly lower. Male goats can be ejaculated in a similar fashion.

Boar. An electrostimulator designed for use in the ram also can be used in the boar. Because of the fat insulation it may be necessary to apply 10 volts or more to initiate ejaculation. This results in discomfort and causes the animal to strain; therefore, an anesthetic or analgesic is recommended to immobilize the boar. A small volume of semen usually is obtained. The procedure cannot be recommended for use in the boar. Electroejaculation is used in nonhuman primates (Fig. 20–6).

Massage Method. If an electroejaculator is not available, massage by way of the rectum of the vesicular glands and ampullae of the vas deferens can induce semen flow in the bull. Massage of the sigmoid flexure also may be desirable to cause protrusion of the penis so that an assistant can collect the semen with a minimum of bacterial contamination. Semen so collected usually has a lower sperm concentration than ejaculates obtained with the AV.

INSEMINATION OF THE FEMALE

High fertility with AI depends on (1) high-quality semen, (2) proper technique of thawing and inseminating the semen, (3) healthy females in sound breeding condition, and (4) insemination at the proper time of the estrous cycle. The latter is extremely important. Viable sperm must be in the vicinity of the egg and capacitated (in most species at least) shortly after ovulation. Because ovulation is difficult to detect, insemination should be timed relative to estrus (Fig. 20–7).

Detection of Estrus

The best indication of estrus is when the female stands when mounted by the male or other females. However, this test often is not practical for AI. Cows, does, sows, and mares cycle about every 20 to 21 days, and ewes, about every 16 to 17 days. Sev-

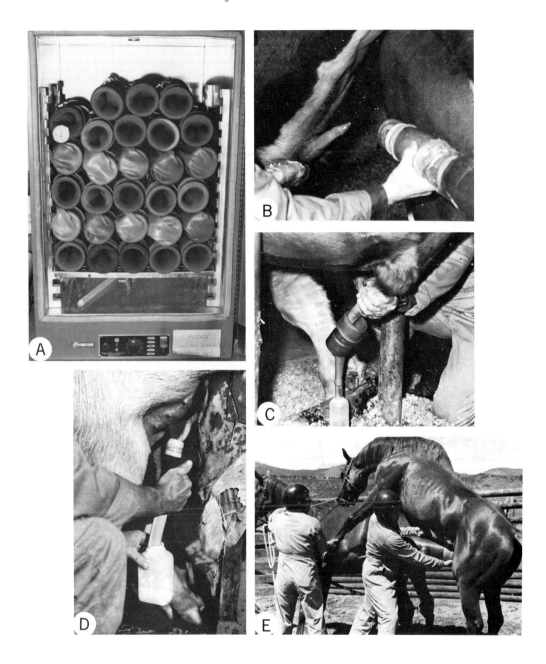

FIG. 20–3.   *A,* Assembled artificial vaginas (AVs) for bulls in an incubator. *B.* Proper technique of collecting bull semen with the AV. *C.* Achieving an erection and semen collection by electroejaculation in the bull. The semen collection tube is protected by a jacket of warm water. *D.* Collecting boar semen by applying manual pressure to a short AV. *E.* Collecting stallion semen. The handler of the stallion is holding the foreleg to prevent possible striking of the collector. (Courtesy of B.W. Pickett.)

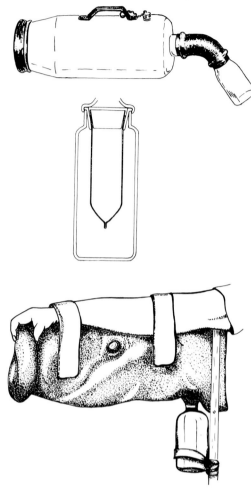

FIG. 20–4. (*Top*) Artificial vagina (modified Japanese model) for stallions. (*Middle*) Enlarged collection bottle fitted with a filter to remove the gel. (Adapted from Komarek et al. (1965). J. Reprod. Fertil. *10,* 337). (*Bottom*) Another type of artificial vagina for horses.

eral procedures have been used to detect estrus (Table 20–2).

Restlessness, bawling, and attempting to mount may be signs of coming into estrus in dairy and beef cattle. There are many aids for detecting estrus. These include pressure-sensitive devices placed on the backs of animals that change color when an animal stands for mounting, the use of surgically sterilized bulls carrying devices for marking females that stand, electronic

probes, and the discharge of clear mucus from the vagina. Reddish mucus on the tail is an indication that estrus occurred 1 or 2 days previously. Also, cows in estrus are more active, and this activity can be monitored by pedometers placed on the legs. Odors can be detected by specially trained dogs.

Because of the difficulty of detecting estrus in large herds, particularly in cold climates, a program of estrous cycle regulation could be advantageous. Several techniques that produce a highly synchronized and fertile estrus have been developed; however, not all drugs used in these techniques have been approved by the Food and Drug Administration for use in cattle in the United States.

Optimal Insemination Time

Animals should not be inseminated after parturition until the uterus is fully involuted and the females are cycling normally. Then, insemination near the time of ovulation is important. Because the length of estrus and time of ovulation are variable, it is necessary to give a range of insemination times that yield "optimal" results. Cows should not be inseminated before 50 days after calving for best conception rates; otherwise, more inseminations per conception are required. Conception rate also is lower when cows are inseminated during the first part of estrus. A practical procedure is to check for estrus twice daily and inseminate on the same day all cows first seen at the morning check. Cows first seen in estrus in the evening should be inseminated the next morning. There is no precisely defined "best" time.

In cattle, ovulation occurs some 24 hours after peak LH concentrations. Thus, the optimal time for insemination is about 14 hours before ovulation. Ovulation follows the LH surge by 24 hours in heifers given daily progesterone injections for 9 or 18 days. Ideally, the LH surge precedes insemination by about 10 hours (Kazmer et al., 1981). Variation in timing among

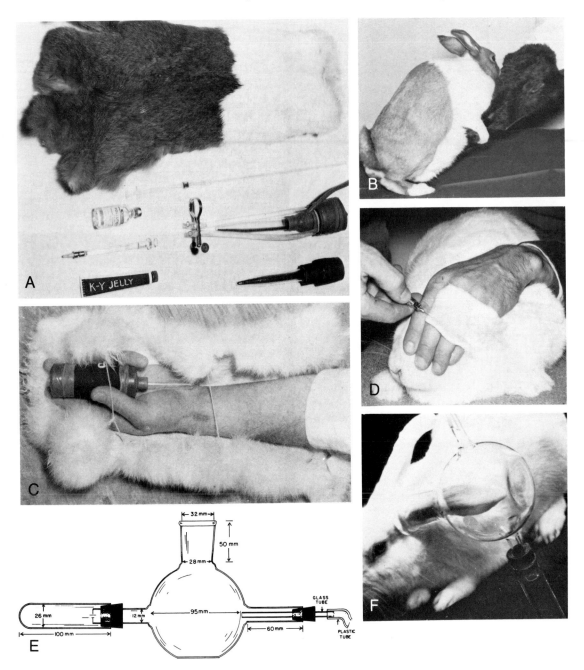

FIG. 20–5. *A*, Fur, artificial vaginas, K-Y Jelly, and other equipment used for semen collection and artificial insemination of the rabbit. *B*, One method of collecting semen with an artificial vagina employs a rabbit's pelt, which the buck mounts. *C*, Holding the artificial vagina within the rabbit's belt. *D*, Positioning the rabbit for an intravenous injection by means of the ear vein: the rabbit's rump is against a firm object and its eyes are covered. A simple technique for collecting blood from the ear vein. *E*, A 500-ml flat-bottomed boiling flask modified into a vacuum reservoir for collection of blood. *F*, The vacuum reservoir is placed against the rabbit's head; a centrifuge tube is attached to it. (*E, F*, From Hoppe et al. (1970). Lab. Anim. Care.)

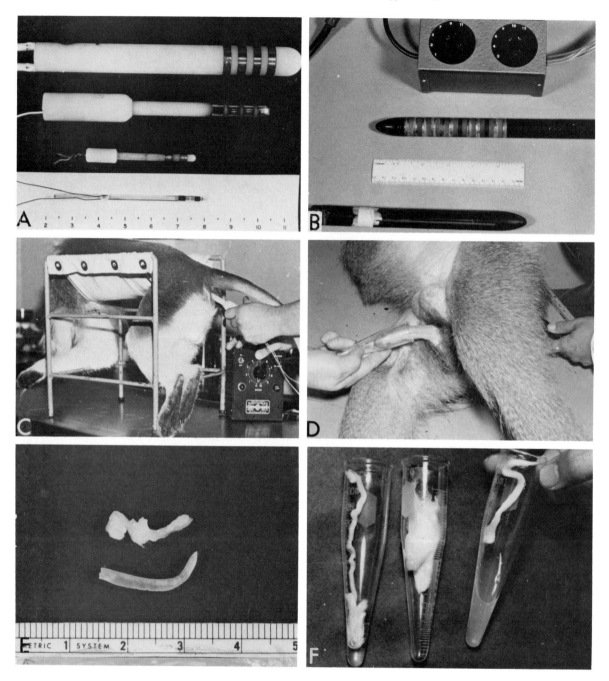

FIG. 20–6. *A*. Rectal probes used for electroejaculation of various species of primates. *B*. Rectal probes showing horizontal ring electrodes used for electroejaculation of baboons. These can be selected in any combination of two using the switch box shown in the top of the picture, and longitudinal electrodes. *C*. Electroejaculation of a patas monkey using a sling to support the animal in a convenient position. *D*. Electroejaculation of a baboon lying on its side in an extended position. *E*. Seminal coagulum from a rhesus monkey showing an amorphous mass characteristic of coagulation after ejaculation and a mass conforming to the urethra that is formed during ejaculation. *F*. Semen collected from baboons showing a liquid fraction and two types of coagulum. The amorphous mass coagulated after ejaculation and the strings of coagulum formed during ejaculation. (*A* from Fussel et al. (1967). Lab. Anim. Care *17*, 528; *C* and *E* from Roussel and Austin (1968). J. Inst. Anim. Tech. *19*, 22.)

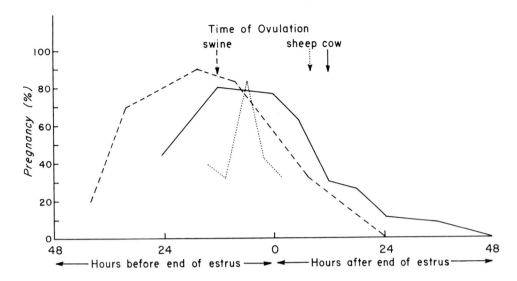

FIG. 20–7.   Relationship between time of insemination and fertility in the cow, sheep, and swine. ___ Cow; ------ swine; ..... sheep.

the occurrence of the LH peak, time of insemination, and the moment of ovulation occurs in untreated as well as synchronized animals (Table 20–1 and Fig. 20–7).

In the ewe, insemination should take place at the middle or during the second half of estrus. Double inseminations during estrus, particularly with frozen semen, increase fertility. Goats can best be inseminated about 12 hours after the onset of estrus and should be inseminated again the next day if they are still in estrus. Sows come into estrus about 3 to 5 days after farrowing, but they do not ovulate at this time and should not be bred. They come into heat 3 to 8 days after weaning their pigs and may be inseminated at this time. Since sows ovulate about 30 to 36 hours after the beginning of estrus, with rapid loss of fertility after ovulation, it is best to inseminate either late on the first day or early on the second day of estrus. An advantage of about 10% is gained by inseminating on both the first and second days of estrus.

Inseminating a mare during the first heat (foal heat), about 9 days after foaling, is not advised because the uterus is not fully involuted and the conception rate is lower. Mares may be inseminated at the next estrus about 30 days after foaling. Because mares have a long and variable estrus, it is best to inseminate at least every second day during estrus, starting on the second day. When mares are palpated daily, insemination can be done to coincide with ovulation, which precedes the end of estrus by 1 or 2 days.

Insemination Procedures

Several procedures are applied for insemination of various species (Fig. 20–8). Identification of the female is the first step. The breeding record should be checked for date of parturition; previous breedings are noted, and the current insemination is recorded. Basic breeding records are important for all species.

The number of sperm cells required for optimal conception rate for frozen semen is higher than that for liquid semen. Pellets require the same insemination equipment as ampules.

Pregnancy is a possibility in a previously inseminated cow, and the catheter should not be forced into the uterus; approxi-

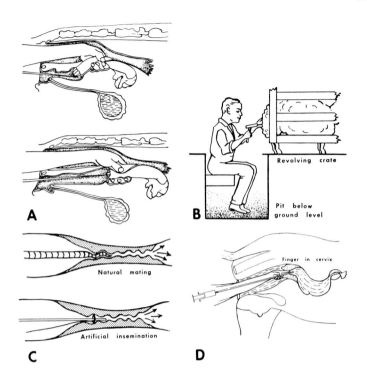

FIG. 20–8. Artificial insemination procedures. *A, Top.* Wrong way of holding cervix for rectovaginal technique of inseminating cows. *Bottom.* By using correct procedure, it is relatively easy to deposit semen through the cervix. (Redrawn from Bonadonna (1957). Nozioni di Fisiopathologia della Reproduzione e di Fecondazione Artificiale degli Animali Domestici. Milan, courtesy of T. Bonadonna). *B.* Pit and restraining crate facilitating ewe insemination. *C.* Comparison of cervical semen deposition in natural mating and artificial insemination in swine. Arrows indicate flow of semen into the uterus. *D.* For insemination of mares, the index finger in the cervix assists in guiding the catheter held by the other hand into the uterus.

mately 3 to 5% of pregnant cows show signs of estrus. The use of dye in extender when training technicians to inseminate reproductive tracts and intact cows at the specified location appears to be an extremely useful method to improve the accuracy of semen placement and the efficiency of technicians.

In sheep, frozen extended semen should be reconcentrated so that about 200 million motile sperm cells are inseminated. With unfrozen semen, 50 million motile sperm are sufficient. With progestogen treatment of ewes to induce estrus at a synchronized time, sperm number requirements may be as great as 1500 million cells. Double inseminations 12 hours apart increase fertility.

An insemination procedure for AI in pigs is shown in Figure 20–9.

FACTORS AFFECTING CONCEPTION RATE IN AI

Accurate measurement of fertility is an important part of any organized AI program. The major factors determining fer-

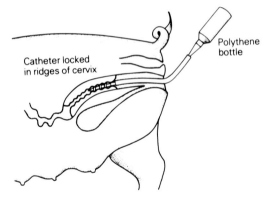

FIG. 20–9. General procedure for artificial insemination in pigs using a flexible rubber catheter and polythene bottle. The spiral-tipped catheter is introduced along the vagina and into the cervical ridges by an anticlockwise movement, after which the inseminate is delivered gently into the uterus by squeezing the bottle. (From Hunter, R.H.F. (1982). Reproduction of Farm Animals. New York, Longman.)

tility in artificial breeding are (1) the fertility of males used to produce the semen; (2) the care with which the semen is collected, processed, and stored; (3) the skill of the inseminating technician; and (4) management of the females. Males should be carefully selected, isolated, and tested before joining a stud. They should have completely normal testes, should produce high-quality semen, and should be free from disease. Those failing to meet standards should be culled. Regular health checks should be repeated periodically and all health codes followed.

The underline of males, particularly around the prepuce, should be clean at the time of semen collection. All equipment used for collecting, processing, and inseminating semen should be clean and sterile. Traces of washing solutions should be removed by proper rinsing. Thorough rinsing of liners with boiling distilled water, followed by isopropyl alcohol, should produce clean, sterile liners that dry readily before they are used. All glassware should be washed carefully, rinsed thoroughly in distilled water, and sterilized in an oven at 150°C for at least 1 hour. Special sanitary precautions are needed for semen collection. The collector should wear disposable plastic gloves. The mount should be covered or disinfected between collections.

Only high-quality semen should be processed for insemination. Antibiotics should be added to the semen. Frozen semen should be examined after freezing and inferior samples discarded. Semen can be stored successfully for a long time if stored continuously under liquid nitrogen at −196°C. However, lack of liquid nitrogen for even a few hours may result in complete destruction of a sperm bank.

Improper handling of semen during storage also decreases fertility. Placing sperm through the cervix or flushing cells through it (swine) is important. Skill and experience are required. Penetrating the cervix is particularly difficult in sheep and goats. The female should be in optimal breeding condition, and proper estrus detection is of extreme importance. More than one insemination per estrus increases conception rates. This is due to the diffi-

culty of predicting ovulation and appropriately timing each insemination.

Commercial AI organizations should monitor fertility and evaluate all contributing components possible. Ideally, this would be to gather complete information on young born, but this is not practical. A useful report, when all services are reported, is the 60- to 90-day report tabulated on a monthly basis. Two months after each month when the inseminations were performed (which is also about 90 days after the beginning of that month), the records of all inseminated cows are checked to determine what proportion were reported for reinsemination. With computers, it would be feasible to introduce a more precise time, such as a 60- to 75-day interval.

Pregnancy information may be obtained by palpation of the reproductive organs per rectum in cattle and horses, by milk progesterone assays in cattle and goats, by running an immunologic blood test for mares, and by ultrasonic measurements in sheep and swine. Information on litter size in swine also is important.

ARTIFICIAL INSEMINATION IN POULTRY

The male is held on some supporting surface by an operator, who restrains the bird by the legs, pinning its wings down to prevent flapping. The ejaculator then stimulates the male with the right hand by rhythmically massaging the extreme caudal portion of the bird's body just under the pubic bones. The purpose is to induce an ejaculatory reflex. A suitable container for the semen, a beaker, or a graduate cylinder is held in the palm of the right hand, leaving the fingers free to carry on the stimulation. Simultaneously, the left hand bends the tail feathers cephalad and presses gently on the urophygial region. When the ejaculatory reflex occurs, the thumb and index finger of both hands "milk" the male until the reflex disappears. The fingers of the left hand are also used to trap the semen in the lower end of the vasa deferentia to ensure complete

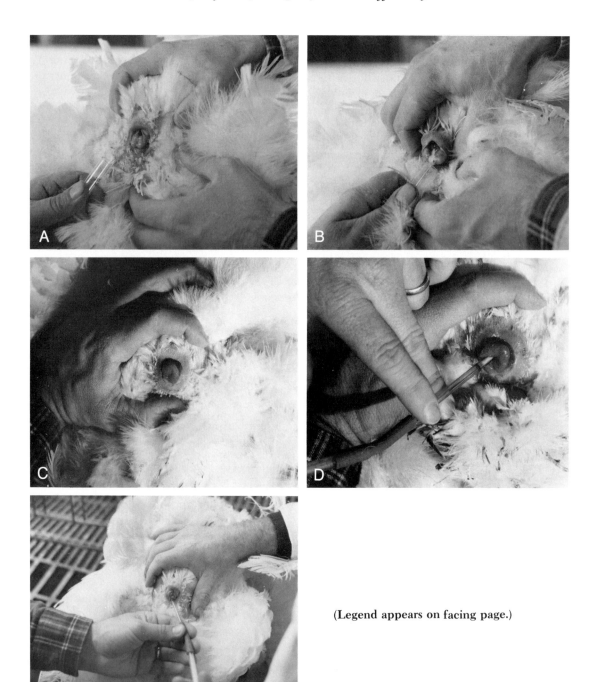

(Legend appears on facing page.)

ejaculation. A specially designed suction apparatus is frequently used to collect the semen directly from the male's copulatory organ into a thermos bottle kept at 10 to 15°C.

The interval between ejaculation and insemination should not exceed 30 minutes. The sperm remain immotile while in the male's excurrent ducts, but on contact with air, they immediately become extremely agitated. The later activity involves both oxidative and glycolytic processes leading to rapid chemical exhaustion of the substratum in which the sperm exist. If diluents are used, they are generally added just before insemination. The practical diluent is 1.025% physiologic saline solution buffered at pH 7.0 to 8.0. It gives best results when used 1 : 1 with the semen.

The dosages for insemination vary according to species. There is an inverse relationship between the concentration of the sperm in the semen and the required dosage. Dosages for insemination with undiluted semen are for the chicken—0.1 ml; for the turkey—0.05 ml; for the duck—0.3 ml; for the goose—0.05 ml.

The bird, resting on the left hand of an operator, is induced to evert its oviduct through a gentle pressure with the palms of both hands on the cloacal and visceral regions. Only a laying bird will respond easily to this treatment. When the lower end of the vagina is thus exposed, a syringe containing the semen is quickly inserted to the depth of about 3 cm and the semen is deposited. Before the syringe is withdrawn, the pressure on the abdomen is relaxed to permit the retraction of the oviduct. This is to prevent semen from being squeezed out by the retracting vagina.

Once started, AI should be repeated at weekly intervals in the chicken, and every 2 to 3 weeks in the turkey. When hens that are laying at an intense rate are inseminated artificially with highly functional sperm, they will lay their first fertile egg 48 hours after the insemination. Some of the technical details of AI in turkeys are shown in Figure 20–10.

REFERENCES

Hunter, R.H.F. (1982). Reproduction of Farm Animals. London, Longman.

Kazmer, G.W., Barnes, M.A. and Halman, R.D. (1981). Endogenous hormone response and fertility in dairy heifers treated with norgestomet and estradiol valerate. J. Anim. Sci. *53*, 1333–1340.

FIG. 20–10. *A.* Phallic tumescence has been achieved by a gentle massaging of the abdomen with one hand while simultaneously stroking the lower back and tail feathers with the other hand. The semen collector's hands are positioned for a "cloacal stroke." *B.* During a "cloacal stroke," the thumb and forefinger of the upper hand gently squeeze the cloaca with downward and inward pressure while the lower hand exerts slight upward pressure. Semen, which pools in the groove in the medial aspect of the phallus, is collected into a clean vial. To minimize the chance of spreading venereal disease, the semen collection crew must avoid contact with the phallus. *C.* The vaginal orifice is exteriorized for insemination by a procedure referred to as "breaking" or "venting." Hand pressure around (but not touching) the cloaca causes the vagina to evert. *D, E.* A predetermined number of sperm is contained in the insemination straw, which is then inserted gently into the vagina until resistance is felt (2 to 4 cm). The hand pressure around the cloaca is released as the inseminator ejects the semen into the vagina. (Photographs courtesy of Dr. M.R. Bakst.) These procedures are used when relatively few hens are to be inseminated. Commercial artificial insemination crews using mechanized equipment can inseminate 1000 turkey hens per man hour, and fertility is maintained above 90% during a 22-week egg production season.

21

X- and Y-Chromosome–Bearing Spermatozoa

E.S.E. HAFEZ

Female animals have two similar sex chromosomes (X and X), whereas males have two different sex chromosomes (one X chromosome and one smaller Y chromosome). The gametes (egg and sperm) are haploid cells containing either the X or the Y chromosome. Diploid somatic cells of females (homogametic sex) contain a pair of X chromosomes, but somatic cells of males (heterogametic sex) have XY sex chromosomes. The genetic sex is determined in the oviduct at the time of fertilization, and the sex of the offspring is determined by the sex chromosome within the spermatozoa.

Extensive investigations have been carried out for preselection and complete separation of X and Y sperm before artificial insemination (AI). Sex of the offspring can also be predetermined in embryos arising from diploid or haploid nuclear transplantation into recipient ova, parthenogenetic activation of ova, or fusion of two oocytes. Different cytogenetic and cytologic techniques are used to examine the diploid cells at an appropriate stage of fertilization to diagnose the genetic sex of the embryo. For example, fluorescence microscopy is used to detect the presence of a Y chromosome. Chromosome analysis is performed by culturing leukocytes or fetal cells to study the individual chromosomes using karyotyping procedures (Forsling, 1984).

This chapter addresses four concepts:

1. Morphologic, physiologic, biophysical, and immunologic differences between X and Y spermatozoa
2. Factors affecting primary and secondary sex ration
3. Techniques for separation of X and Y spermatozoa based on valid statistical evaluation of the results
4. Attempts to alter the sex ration by the use of "sexed" spermatozoa

BIOLOGY OF SPERMATOZOA

When spermatozoa are transported through the female reproductive tract, they undergo capacitation to acquire their fertilizing potential. Spermatozoa release and/or acquire various micromolecules and macromolecules on their plasmalemma as they migrate through the vaginal secretions, cervical mucus, endometrial secretions, oviductal fluid, and peritoneal fluid.

The degree of maturation and age of sperm in an ejaculate can influence density. Packed cell volume of bovine sperm is markedly affected by the osmolality of the medium. Live bull sperm placed in a hypo-osmotic saline solution swell to three times their normal size. Dead sperm do not swell or react osmotically. Live sperm placed in hyper-osmotic media shrank from a volume of about 25 μm^3 to 20 μm^3.

Cytogenetics of X and Y Spermatozoa

There are many potential differences between spermatozoa containing an X or a Y chromosome (Table 21–1). Sex chromosomes are responsible for any differences in DNA content. The presence of an X or a Y chromosome (Fig. 21–1) could cause a difference in size and shape of sperm, weight, density, motility (type and velocity), surface charge, and surface biochemistry or internal biochemistry (Foote, 1982a,b). The degree of difference may also be affected by other factors such as age of semen, repeat breeding (possible differential embryo mortality), and use of bulls that had been born co-twin with heifers (and have circulating XX leukocytes).

There are species variations in the mass differential of the X and Y chromosomes. The presence of large X chromosomes could result in greater weight and density of the X-containing sperm if size and other constituents are the same.

Sperm Plasmalemma

The external plasmalemma has different characteristics in different parts of the sperm. X and Y sperm have different surface characteristics at spermiation from the germinal epithelium. If ejaculated sperm are examined, such differences would be masked by components absorbed from the seminal plasma.

Karyotyping of Spermatozoa

The distinction of X and Y spermatozoa based on the fluorescence of the Y chromosome is facilitated by (a) quinacrine staining of sperm, which causes fluorescence of the long arm of the Y chromosome, and (b) a fluorescent spot (F body), which appears in 39 to 47% of the sperm in smears stained with quinacrine. Banding techniques are recommended: G-band and Q-band methods. Such procedures permit the accurate identification of individual chromosomes. The staining of chromosomes is carried out using a Giemsa dye mixture.

TECHNIQUES OF SPERM SEPARATION

Techniques used to separate sperm are discussed in Table 21–2. Experimental attempts have been hampered by the lack of laboratory tests to evaluate the degree of sperm separation. The presence of the F-body appears to be associated with the Y chromosome (Fig. 21–1).

Most of the techniques employed for sperm separation are based on nonequilibrium sedimentation (based on velocity of fall) or on equilibrium sedimentation on a density gradient (sedimentation to the level where specific gravities of sperm and the medium are equal). These techniques use simple gravity or centrifugation and are based on Stoke's law of sedimentation of a rigid sphere through an incompressible, viscous fluid at a low Reynolds' number (nonturbulent conditions). Aggregation of cells in the buffer is evaluated, and a concentration chosen at which aggregation is negligible.

Only two laboratory methods for separation of animal and human X and Y sperm

TABLE 21–1. Some Differences Between X and Y Sperm

Parameter	Difference	Evaluation
DNA	Less in Y sperm	Measurable and accepted
Size	X sperm is larger	Y sperm measured may or may not be representative of random sperm population
Identify	Y chromosome fluoresces	Species specific
Motility	Y sperm faster	Evidence primarily dependent on accuracy of F-body staining technique
Surface charge	X sperm migrate to cathode	No charge difference between X and Y sperm

(From Ericsson, R.J., and Glass, R.H. (1982). Functional differences between sperm bearing the X- or Y-chromosome. *In* Prospects for Sexing Mammalian Sperm. R.P. Amann and G.E. Seidel, Jr. (eds.). Boulder, Colorado University Associated Press.)

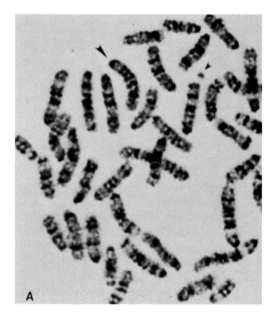

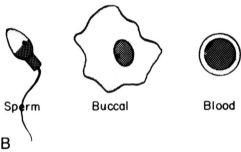

FIG. 21-1. *A.* Mitotic metaphase chromosome spreads stained to reveal G-banding. *A.* Chromosomes from a female XY^X. The large arrowhead designates the X; and small arrowhead, the Y^X chromosome (From Eicher, E.M., 1982, Primary sex determining genes in mice. *In* Prospects for Sexing Mammalian Sperm. R.P. Amann and G.E. Seidel, Jr. (eds). Boulder, Colorado, University Associate Press.) *B.* Localization of Y body in these cell types. Buccal cells: Y body usually found anywhere within the nucleus. Blood cells: lymphocyte Y body usually found near periphery of nucleus, appears crescent shaped. Spermatozoon: Y body usually found equatorially within sperm head (Lueck and Zaneveld, 1977).

appear valid, reproducible, and clinically applicable: albumin separation, which yields 75 to 80% Y sperm, and Sephadex filtration, which yields 70 to 75% X sperm (Beernink, 1986). The separation of X and Y sperm is based on the following:

1. Differences in the weight, density, or size of the X and Y chromosomes as a result of differences in the size of different components of the sperm.
2. Differences in haploid expression of X and Y chromosomes as a result of differences in the nature of sperm components: Defective allocation (nondisjunction) of sex chromosomes, to either the gametes or, after fertilization, to early cleavage products, will result in individuals with somatic cells containing only a single X chromosome (XO) (YO is lethal) or an extra X or Y chromosome (XXX, XXY or XYY).

Layered Separation over Albumin Columns

When semen is layered over columns of serum albumin, increased numbers of Y sperm are recovered from the albumin layers. Semen aliquots of 0.5 ml (diluted 1:1 with Tyrode's solution) are layered for 1 hour over a 7.5% solution of serum albumin in a glass column (8 × 75 mm). The initial sperm layer is then removed by pipette, the albumin centrifuged at 2800 to 3200 rpm for 10 minutes, and the sperm disc is resuspended in Tyrode's solution. The resuspended sperm is then layered over a two-layer serum albumin column. At 1 hour, the sperm layer is removed, and after another half hour, the 13% layer is removed. The 20% serum albumin is then centrifuged for 10 minutes, and the sperm disc is resuspended in 0.25 ml of Tyrode's solution, which is then inseminated into the uterus (Beernink and Ericsson, 1982).

Flow Cytometry and Sorting

With flow cytometry, high-speed measurements of components and properties of individual cells are made in a liquid suspension. Laser is used for monochromatic illumination of cells stained with fluorescent dyes. Light detectors sample the fluorescence produced by the interaction of light with dye and produce electrical signals proportionate to the intensity of fluo-

TABLE 21–2. Techniques Employed to Separate X- and Y-Chromosome–Bearing Spermatozoa

Techniques	Results
Sedimentation of immobilized sperm on media	Insemination with sperm that had sedimented the greatest distance produced 70% females
Skim-milk powder, glycine, sodium citrate, glycerol	Increase in number of male offspring when sperm from the top layers was used.
Albumin column	Successful results with frozen bull sperm preselected on albumin column before cryopreservation.
Velocity sedimentation	Sedimentation rates depend on size, density, and shape of sperm. Cell size difference is predominant factor in separation of types. Shape is usually the least important factor. Sperm heads have extremely aspherical shapes.
Centrifugation through density gradients	Sperm separated according to their sedimentation rates by centrifugation through density gradients, provided the density of the gradient material is less than that of the sperm. The advantage is that the time required for separation is much shorter. Shorter time does not improve theoretical resolution of separation, because diffusion is insignificant.
Motility and electrophoretic separation	Immotile sperm electrophoretically attracted to the anode at neutral pH. When electrophoretic separation is under conditions consistent with sperm motility, sperm migrate to the cathode. Sperm are oriented by electric field and swim in direction the head is facing. If negatively charged, sperm can be oriented so that the tail is facing the anode by virtue of its greater negative charge density and their intrinsic motility is greater than the electrophoretic mobility.
Isoelectric focusing	Separation performed in columns with the fluid stabilized using density gradients. Sperm layered on, or suspended in, this solution migrate electrophoretically until reaching an isoelectric point.
H-Y antigens	Sperm treated with H–Y antisera. Insemination with mouse sperm treated with antisera to a Y-linked histocompatibility antigen produced 45.4% males compared with 53% for controls.
Flow sorting by DNA content	Y-sorting is 72–80% successful. Disadvantages: low sorting rate and lack of sperm viability after sorting.
Sephadex column	Some 70% of X sperm found in certain fractions of the filtrate when sperm was placed on top of a column of Sephadex. 65–85% X sperm were found in certain fractions of filtrate.

(Data from Beernink, 1984; Bennett and Boyce, 1973; Bhatacharya et al., 1966; Corson et al., 1984; Ericsson and Glass, 1982; Hafs and Boyd, 1971; James, 1980; Meistrick, 1982; Moore and Hibbitt, 1975; Pinkel and Gledhill, 1982; Sherbet et al., 1972.)

rescent light from each object. This technique is useful in the evaluation of the degree of separation needed to produce populations enriched in X or Y sperm (Foote, 1982a,b).

Practical Application

Gender selection in farm animals is used for several purposes:

1. Produce more female progeny from superior females for herd and flock replacements and increased milk, meat, and pelt production
2. Produce more males for meat production from culled females and cross-breeding schemes, e.g., dairy–beef crosses
3. Ensure male progeny as herd sires from top dam–sire crosses

4. Ensure appropriate progeny when progeny testing young bulls
5. Avoid intersexes in multiple births

Gender selection in horses will provide more progeny for sale or for brood mare replacements. Good fertility of sexed sperm is important for commercial purposes. The fertility level also must be considered when determining how many breedings are needed to produce the desired number of sexed progeny. The number of inseminations needed to obtain an accurate assessment of reproductive ability of cattle is not precisely known (Foote and Oltenacu, 1980). Several thousand inseminations are required to evaluate true reproductive efficiency within a few percentage points.

FUTURE RESEARCH

Additional research is needed in the following areas:
1. Sperm motility: Sperm isolate themselves based on different progressive motility.
2. Sperm dimensions or density: Cells sorted through a device sensitive enough to detect minute differences.
3. Sperm cytogenetics: Chemical or immunologic reaction capable of selecting on sex chromosome content.
4. Sperm environment: Hormone or chemical condition resulting in penetration of the egg by an X or Y sperm (Ericsson and Glass, 1982).
5. Search for Robersonian chromosome rearrangements that include a sex chromosome: The availability of such chromosomes could facilitate specific breeding schemes suitable for selection for or against a female or male.
6. Detection of a t-like system associated with a Robertsonian translocation.
7. Cytogenetic sexing of cells isolated from an embryo and transfer of the selected embryo after short *in vitro* culture.
8. Selection of late fetuses after prenatal diagnosis on amniotic cells.
9. Immunoselection of embryos.

REFERENCES

Beernink, F.J. (1984). Factors influencing the human sex ratio. Presented at the Annual Meeting of the American Fertility Society, New Orleans.

Beernink, F.J. (1986). Techniques for separating X- and Y-spermatozoa. *In* Foundations of *In Vitro* Fertilization. C.M. Fredericks et al. (eds.). New York, Hemisphere.

Beernink, F.J. and Ericsson, R.J. (1982). Male sex preselection through sperm isolation. Fertil. Steril. *38*, 493.

Bennet, D. and Boyce, E.A. (1973). Sex ratio in progeny of mice inseminated with sperm treated with H-Y antiserum. Nature *246*, 308.

Bhattacharya, B.C., Bangham, A.D., Cro, R.J., Keynes, R.D. and Rowson, L. (1966). An attempt to determine the sex of calves by artificial insemination with spermatozoa separated by sedimentation. Nature *211*, 863.

Corson, S.L., Batzer, F.R., Alexander N.H., Shlaff, S. and Otis, C. (1984). Sex selection by sperm separation and insemination. Fertil. Steril. *42*, 756.

Eicher, E.M. (1982). Primary sex determining genes in mice. *In* Prospects for Sexing Mammalian Sperm. R.P. Amann and G.E. Seidel, Jr. (eds.). Boulder, Colorado University Associated Press.

Ericsson, R.J. and Glass, R.H. (1982). Functional differences between sperm bearing the X- or Y-chromosome. *In* Prospects for Sexing Mammalian Sperm. R.P. Amann and G. E. Seidel, Jr. (eds.). Boulder, Colorado University Associated Press.

Foote, R.H. (1982a). Functional differences between sperm bearing the X- or Y-chromosome. *In* Prospects for Sexing Mammalian Sperm. R.P. Amann and G.E. Seidel, Jr. (eds.). Boulder, Colorado University Associated Press.

Foote, R.H. (1982b). Prospects for sexing: present status, future prospects and overall conclusions. *In* Prospects for Sexing Mammalian Sperm. R.P. Amann and G.E. Seidel, Jr. (eds.). Boulder, Colorado University Associated Press.

Foote, R.H., and Oltenacu, E.A.B. (1980). Increasing fertility in artificial insemination by culling bulls or ejaculates within bulls. Proc. 8th Tech. Conf. Artif. Insem. Reprod. National Association of Animal Breeders, Columbia, pp. 6–12.

Forsling, M.L. (1984). Pocket Examiner in Endocrinology. London, Pitman Publishing.

Hafs, H.D. and Boyd, L.J. (1971). Galvanic separation of X- and Y-chromosome-bearing sperm. *In* Sex Ratio at Birth Prospects for Control. C.A. Kiddy and H.D. Hafs (eds.). American Society for Animal Science.

James, W.H. (1980). Gonadotrophin and the human secondary sex ratio. Br. Med. J. *281*, 711.

Lueck, J. and Zanaveld, L.J.D. (1977). Cytogenetics of spermatozoa: Y-chromosome staining. *In* Techniques in Human Andrology. E.S.E. Hafez (ed.). Amsterdam, Elsevier.

Meistrich, M.L. (1982). Potential and limitations of physical methods for separation of sperm bearing an X- and Y-chromosome. *In* Prospects for Sexing Mammalian Sperm. R.P. Amann and G.E. Seidel, Jr. (eds.). Boulder, Colorado University Associated Press.

Moore, H.D.M. and Hibbitt, K.G. (1975). Isoelectric focusing of boar spermatozoa. J. Reprod. Fertil. *44*, 329–332.

Pinkel, D. and Gledhill, B.L. (1982). Sex preselection in mammals: separation of sperm bearing Y and "O" chromosomes in the vole *(Microtus oregoni)*. Science *218*, 904.

Sherbet, G.V., Lakshmi, M.S. and Rao, K.V. (1972). Characterization of ionogenic groups and estimation of the net negative electric charge on the surface of cells using natural pH gradients. Exp. Cell Res. *70*, 113–123.

22
Pregnancy Diagnosis

M.R. JAINUDEEN AND E.S.E. HAFEZ

Knowing whether an animal is pregnant or not is of considerable economic value. In general, an early diagnosis of pregnancy is required soon after mating or insemination for the early identification of non-pregnant animals so that production time lost as the result of infertility may be reduced by appropriate treatment or culling. A diagnosis of pregnancy is also required to certify animals for sale or insurance purposes, to reduce waste in breeding programs using expensive hormonal techniques, and to help in the economic management of animal production.

During pregnancy, the conceptus inhibits the regression of the corpus luteum (CL) and prevents the animal from returning to estrus. Therefore, an animal not returning to estrus after service is assumed to be pregnant. This knowledge is widely used by farmers and artificial insemination (AI) centers as an indicator of pregnancy; but the reliability of the method depends on the accuracy of estrus detection in the herd. Both anestrus and estrus during pregnancy may also affect the reliability of this method.

Clinical and laboratory methods are available for the diagnosis of pregnancy (Fig. 22–1). The choice of method depends on the species, stage of gestation, cost, accuracy, and speed of diagnosis.

CLINICAL METHODS OF PREGNANCY DIAGNOSIS

Clinical methods depend on the detection of the conceptus—fetus, fetal membranes, and fetal fluids. The methods include rectal examination, radiography, and ultrasonic techniques.

Rectal Examination

Rectal examination is the accepted method of pregnancy diagnosis in the mare, buffalo, and cow. In this procedure, the uterus is palpated through the rectal wall to detect the uterine enlargement occurring during pregnancy, and the fetus or fetal membranes (Fig. 22–2, Table 22–1). This technique, which can be performed at an early stage of gestation, is accurate, and the result is known immediately.

Because of the small pelvic cavity, the ewe and sow are not suited for the rectal exploration of uterine contents. The middle uterine arteries, particularly in parous sows, however, are readily accessible for palpation through the rectal wall. The detection of a fremitus in one or both uterine arteries is a rapid and simple test for pregnancy in the sow from 28 days onward. A rectal-abdominal palpation technique has been used in sheep.

Radiography

Radiography can be used in determining pregnancy in sheep, goats, and swine. It is based on the identification of the fetal skeleton on an x-ray plate. Among the disadvantages of this method is that it can be applied only during the last third of gestation, it is costly, it necessitates restraint, and it poses a radiation hazard to the operator.

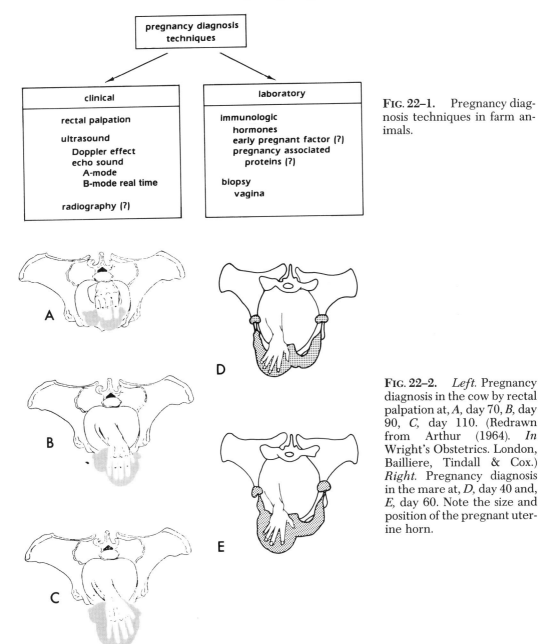

FIG. 22–1. Pregnancy diagnosis techniques in farm animals.

FIG. 22–2. *Left.* Pregnancy diagnosis in the cow by rectal palpation at, *A*, day 70, *B*, day 90, *C*, day 110. (Redrawn from Arthur (1964). *In* Wright's Obstetrics. London, Bailliere, Tindall & Cox.) *Right.* Pregnancy diagnosis in the mare at, *D*, day 40 and, *E*, day 60. Note the size and position of the pregnant uterine horn.

Ultrasonography

Ultrasound waves are inaudible to the human ear and operate at frequencies of 1 to 10 megahertz (MHz). Two types of ultrasound are employed in human and veterinary medicine: the Doppler phenomenon and the pulse–echo principle.

Doppler Phenomenon. In the Doppler phenomenon, sound waves striking a moving object are reflected to the transmitting source at a slightly altered frequency. The ultrasonic fetal pulse detector that is based on the Doppler phenomenon consists of a transducer and amplifier. The transducer (probe), when applied to the animal's abdominal wall or inserted into the rectum, emits a narrow beam of high-frequency waves (ultrasonic). Movements of the fetal heart or blood flow in the fetal (umbilical vessels) or maternal (uterine artery) circulation alter the frequency of these waves, which are reflected back to the probe, where they are converted into audible sound and amplified (earphones or speaker) or illuminated (oscilloscope).

Pulse–Echo Ultrasound. Pulses of ultrasound, generated by piezoelectric crystals in a transducer, on contacting tissues of varying acoustic impedance (resistance to the transmission), are reflected (echoed) to the transducer, then converted into electrical energy and displayed on a cathode ray oscilloscope in various ways. A- and B-mode are the basic forms currently in use (Fig. 22–3). A-mode (amplitude) is a one-dimensional display of echo amplitude versus distance, whereas B-mode (brightness) produces an accurate two-dimensional image of soft tissue cross sec-

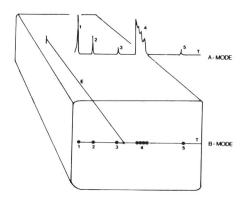

Fig. 22–3. A-mode and B-mode displays. An A-mode (amplitude) is formed by moving the electron beam (E) along the y-axis proportional to signal strength, and distance or time (T) along the x-axis. A B-mode display modulates the beam intensity in proportion to signal strength but maintains distance on the x-axis. The numbers show corresponding A-mode and B-mode signals. (From Powis, R.L. (1986). Ultrasound science for the veterinarian. *In* Vet. Clin. North Am. Equine Pract. *2*, 3–27.)

TABLE 22–1. **Diagnosis of Pregnancy in the Cow, Buffalo, and Mare by Rectal Palpation**

Animal	Month of Gestation	Major Findings
Cow Buffalo†	First	Quiescent uterus and a fully developed corpus luteum in one ovary.
	Second*	Enlargement and dorsal bulging of pregnant horn due to fetal fluids; on application of digital pressure, gives a resilient sensation. "Fetal membrane slip" or palpation of allantochorion; amnionic vesicle present anterior to the intercornual ligament.
	Third*	Descent of uterus commences; fetus is palpable.
	Fourth to Seventh	Uterus on abdominal floor, fetus difficult to palpate; cotyledons, 2–5 cm in diameter, are palpated as circumscribed areas in uterine wall; middle uterine arteries hypertrophy and pulse changes to a distinct fremitus.
	Seventh to term	Cotyledons, fremitus, and fetal parts are palpable.
Mare	First	Contracted and firm cervix; turgid uterine horns.
	Second*	Chorioallantoic sac (size of an orange) bulges ventrally in lower third of uterine horn; uterine horns are turgid.
	Third	Chorioallantoic sac grows rapidly and descends into uterine body, changes from spherical to oval, and tenseness is gradually lost. Uterus begins to descend.
	Fourth	Dorsal surface of the uterus is felt as a distended dome between the stretched broad ligaments. Fetus and/or fetal parts palpable.
	Fifth to Seventh	Uterus lies deep in abdominal cavity. Usually possible to palpate fetus, except in large pluriparous mares.
	Seventh to term	Fetus easier to palpate. Uterus begins to ascend.

* Period when pregnancy can be accurately diagnosed.
† Findings occur later than in cattle as a result of the longer gestation length.

tion. The brightness of the dots on the oscilloscope is projected in various shades of gray, comparable to a black and white photograph. If these images are produced and erased in rapid succession, they will reveal any motion in the tissue being imaged. This is the basis of B-mode "real-time" scanning.

B-Mode Real-Time Ultrasound. B-mode real-time ultrasound, developed in the 1970s for the diagnosis of pregnancy and fetal abnormalities in human medicine, was successfully applied to diagnose very early pregnancy in the horse about 10 years later. Since then, the technique has been used extensively in horse studs and the sheep industry and to a limited extent in goats, pigs, and cattle. Diagnostic ultrasound technology provides a noninvasive and rapid means of diagnosing pregnancy as well as estimating fetal numbers, viability, and their ages in sheep and other farm species.

The basic physical and diagnostic principles of ultrasonography have been reviewed elsewhere (Pierson et al., 1988; Powis, 1986; Taverne and Willemse, 1989). This discussion briefly outlines the basic equipment, procedures, and real-time images of ultrasonographs for pregnancy diagnosis in farm animals.

The major components of an ultrasound machine are an electrical pulse generator, a transducer, a scan converter, and video display (Fig. 22–4). A high-voltage electrical pulse of a few microseconds causes the piezoelectric transducer to vibrate and convert electrical to mechanical energy (ultrasound). The reflection of these waves (echoes) from tissue surfaces on reaching the transducer produces an electrical signal that is processed by a scan converter and displayed on a video monitor.

Depending on the display patterns they produce, transducers are of two types. A linear transducer produces a rectangular image, whereas the sector transducer produces a sector image similar to that of a "slice of a pie." The commonly used transducers in domestic animals are of the lin-

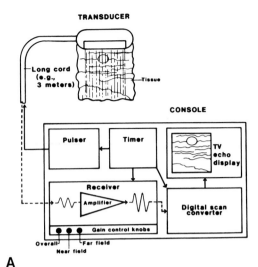

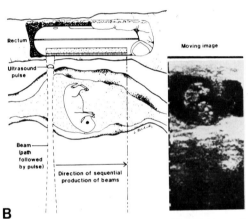

FIG. 22–4. *A.* Basic components of ultrasound scanner: a pulse generator, transducer, a scan converter, and a video display. *B.* The development of a moving image of a 48-day bovine fetus by transrectal ultrasonography. (From Pierson et al. (1988). Theriogenology *29,* 3–20.)

ear array type and have a frequency range of 3.5 to 7.5 MHz. Transducers with low frequencies (3.0 to 3.5 MHz) penetrate deeper and image deeper tissues than higher frequencies (5.0 to 7.5 MHz) that image closer to the surface. The images produced by low- and high-frequency transducers are comparable to the view of a tissue as seen under a microscope at low and high magnifications, respectively.

For scanning the uterus, the transducer is placed on the ventrolateral abdominal wall (transabdominal) or in the rectum (transrectal) of the test animal. The 3.5-MHz transducer is used for the transabdominal approach (goat, sheep, pig) and the 5.0- to 7.5-MHz transducers for the transrectal route (horse, cattle, sheep). Contact between transducer and the skin or the rectal wall is made with coupling gel or vegetable oil. Images of tissues seen on the screen are either black (nonechogenic) or various shades of gray (echogenic). The urinary bladder, embryonic vesicle, and fetal fluids appear black; the fetal skeleton, white; and the fetal membranes and maternal tissues, various shades of grey.

Horse. The B-mode real-time ultrasound technique offers an earlier diagnosis of pregnancy than with any of the current methods available for farm animals (Table 22–2). In the mare, it not only provides an early diagnosis of pregnancy (day 10 to 15) almost 100% accurate (Fig. 22–5A), but it also can detect twins, which are undesirable and usually aborted.

Cattle. The bovine conceptus is elongated and filamentous in contrast to the vesicular form of the equine conceptus, making the former difficult to visualize with the 3.5-MHz transducer used in the horse. However, with higher frequency transrectal probes (5.0 to 7.5 MHz), the embryonic vesicle can be detected as early as day 9 to 10, which expands in a localized area within the ipsilateral horn by day 18 to 20 (Curran et al., 1986; Boyd et al., 1990). The embryo, embryonic heart beat, and fetal membranes could be visualized by day 30 (Fig. 22–5B). The rate of correct diagnosis is low (33%) up to 16 days after insemination but improves significantly to reach almost 100% by day 20 with the 7.5-MHz rectal probe. The ability to assess the viability of the early conceptus opens up new frontiers in our understanding of early embryonic mortality in cattle. Detection of the genital tubercle between day 54 and 58 (Curran et al., 1989) or scrotal swellings and mammary teats by day 90 (Muller and Wittkowski, 1986) with a high degree of accuracy (85 to 95%) offers renewed hope for the dairy farmer wanting only female calves. The technique of ultrasonography in the buffalo is similar to that of cattle (Fig. 22–5C).

Sheep. The Doppler fetal pulse detector diagnoses pregnancy in ewes by day 60 of pregnancy with an accuracy of over 90% (Thwaites, 1981; Trapp and Slyter, 1983) but not accurate for counting fetal numbers. On the contrary, real-time ultrasonic scanning by the transabdominal approach offers an accurate, safe, and practical method of diagnosing pregnancy and determining fetal numbers in sheep (Fig. 22–5D) after day 40 of gestation (Gearhart et al., 1988; Taverne and Willemse, 1985). Although pregnancy can be diagnosed by

TABLE 22–2. Ultrasound Techniques of Pregnancy Diagnosis in Farm Animals

Species	Technique	Placement of Transducer	Earliest Day after Mating	Diagnostic Criteria	Accuracy (%)
Horse	B-mode RT	Transrectal	9	Embryonic vesicle	100
Cattle	B-mode RT	Transrectal	12	Embryonic vesicle	33
			20	Embryo, heart beat	100
Buffalo	B-mode RT	Transrectal	30	Embryo, fetal fluids	?
Sheep and goats	Doppler	Transabdominal	60	Fetal heart sounds	90
	A-mode	Transabdominal		Fetal fluids	70–90
	B-mode RT	Transabdominal	45–50	Fetus(es), placentomes	100
		Transrectal	20–22	Fetal fluids	<20
Pig	Doppler	Transabdominal	60	Fetal heart sounds	90
	A-mode	Same	60	Fetal fluids	70–90
	B-mode RT	Same	22	Allantoic fluid	

RT = real-time.
Transducer, 3.5 MHz (transabdominal); 5.0–7.5 MHz (transrectal).
Adapted from the literature cited in text.

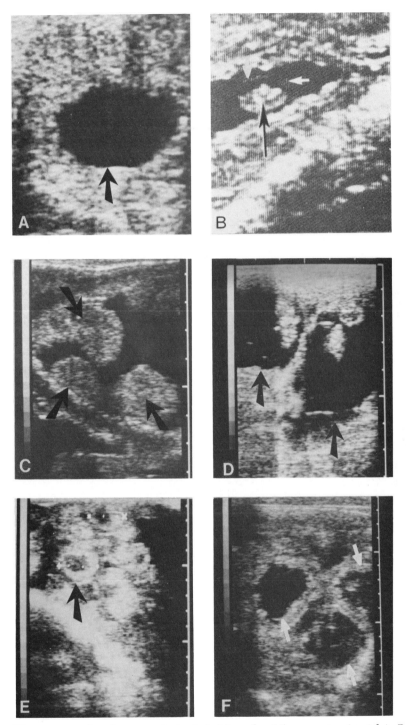

FIG. 22–5. Ultrasonographs of pregnant uteri. *A.* Mare day 17 conceptus (vesicle). *B.* Cow, day 31, embryo (black arrow), amnion (white arrow) encircling the fetus. *C.* Buffalo, day 50, placentomes. *D.* Ewe day 37, twins (arrows). *E.* Doe, day 45, placentomes. *F.* Sow at day 37, allantoic fluid within the uterus. (*A,* from Squires et al. (1988). Theriogenology *29,* 55–70; *B,* from Kastellic et al. (1988). Theriogenology *29,* 39–54.)

day 20 of gestation and fetal numbers by day 31 with a 5.0-MHz intrarectal probe (Buckrell et al., 1986; Gearhart et al., 1988), more false-negative diagnoses of pregnancy and lower probability of correctly identifying fetal numbers are associated with the transrectal than the transabdominal approach of scanning.

Goats. Pregnancy may be diagnosed, as in sheep (Fig. 22–5E), with the Doppler and A-mode techniques at midgestation but much earlier with real-time ultrasonography. The techniques of ultrasonography are similar to those in sheep. One advantage of real-time ultrasonography is in the diagnosis of pseudopregnancy (hydrometra) where fluid accumulates in the uterus but neither fetuses nor placentomes are detected. The age of the fetus between day 40 and day 105 could be determined by real-time ultrasonography by measuring the biparietal diameter (BPD) width of the head with the built-in electronic linear distance calipers (Haibel, 1988).

Pig. A-mode ultrasonography is probably the most frequently employed technique of pregnancy diagnosis by swine farmers after the absence of returns to service. The A-mode amplitude-depth ultrasonic analyzer in conjunction with a 2-MHz transducer has been used for pregnancy diagnosis in the pig (Fig. 22–6). A band of echoes is obtained from a depth of 15 to 20 cm in pregnant animals, as compared with only about 5 cm in nonpregnant animals. A 95% accuracy in pregnancy diagnosis can be achieved in sows and gilts between 30 and 90 days of gestation.

Real-time ultrasonography can also be used to diagnose pregnancy in the sow as early as day 18 but is more accurate after day 22 of gestation (Fig. 22–5F). Most errors in diagnosis between 18 and 21 days occur in sows that eventually give birth to less than five piglets.

LABORATORY METHODS

Laboratory diagnosis of pregnancy relies on detecting changes occurring in maternal tissues bearing a conceptus or substances produced by the conceptus and detected by immunologic assays in maternal blood, urine, or milk.

Vaginal Biopsy

The vaginal mucosa responds to the endocrine changes occurring during gestation by a reduction in the number of layers of the stratified squamous epithelium. This forms the basis for a pregnancy test in the ewe and sow (Fig. 22–7). A small sample of the vaginal mucosa is obtained with a biopsy instrument and is subjected to routine histologic procedures, such as formalin fixation, paraffin-wax embedding and hematoxylin and eosin staining, and microscopic examination.

Because the method involves sampling, processing, and microscopic examination, which are time consuming and costly, the vaginal biopsy technique has limited practical applicability.

Immunologic Diagnosis

The immunologic techniques for diagnosis of pregnancy rely on detecting or measuring the level of substances originating in the conceptus, the uterus, or ovaries that enter the maternal blood, urine, or milk. Immunologic tests are of two types. The first measures substances that are pregnancy specific and appear in maternal blood (equine chorionic gonadotropin [eCG]) or urine (human chorionic gonadotropin [hCG]) early in pregnancy. The second type of substances is not specific, but their levels in maternal blood, urine, or milk change during pregnancy, e.g., progesterone (Table 22–3).

Pregnancy-Associated Substances

Several protein-like substances have been identified in maternal blood during pregnancy. Some of these substances are products originating in the conceptus,

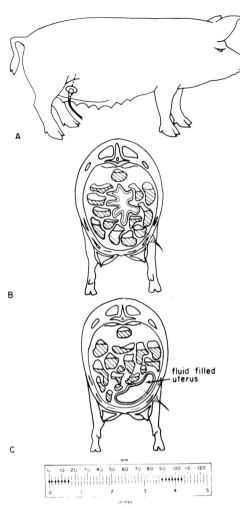

FIG. 22–6. Pregnancy diagnosis in swine by ultrasonic amplitude-depth analysis. *A.* Placement of transducer on the lower flank of the standing sow about 5 cm posterior to the umbilicus and just lateral to the nipple line. *B.* Display pattern of a sow or gilt that is not bred or is less than 30 days pregnant. *C.* Display pattern of a sow or gilt between 30 and 90 days of pregnancy. The first set of lights (0–15) represents the different layers of the abdominal wall, the gap in light pattern is due to fetal fluids, and the second set of lights (90–105) are the echoes from the distal wall of the uterus and adjacent intestines. Note that the gap in light pattern and the second set of lights are absent in a nonpregnant animal (Scanoprobe, Ithaco, Inc., Ithaca, N.Y.).

whereas others may be secreted at higher levels during gestation; thus, they can be used as indicators of pregnancy.

Early Pregnancy Factor. An early pregnancy factor (EPF) was first reported in the circulation of pregnant women (pre-implantation stage) and subsequently in the sow, ewe, and cow. EPF, which has immunosuppressive properties, can be detected in serum in reducing the number of rosettes formed in the rosette-inhibition test (Fig. 22–8) (Smart et al., 1981). EPF, identified by its immunosuppressive activity, is detected within a few days after conception in pig, sheep, and cattle. Besides diagnosing conception, a potential application for the EPF test could be for the early detection of fertilization failure or early embryonic mortality. However, the

EPF is a bioassay based on the inhibition of rosette formation (Fig. 22–8), which is time-consuming and has limited use in routine pregnancy testing in farm animals.

Pregnancy-Associated Antigens. Antigens specific to pregnancy have been reported in maternal tissues of various species including that of sheep, cattle, and horses (Findlay, 1980). These antigens are detected in maternal blood during the latter half of pregnancy and are of limited value in pregnancy tests.

A partially purified pregnancy-specific protein B (bPSPB) has been isolated from bovine placental tissue (Butler et al., 1982). A radioimmunoassay (RIA) has been developed that detects bPSPB in pregnant cow serum from day 24 of pregnancy until parturition (Sasser et al., 1986). This RIA

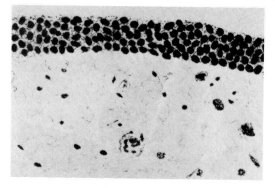

Pregnant

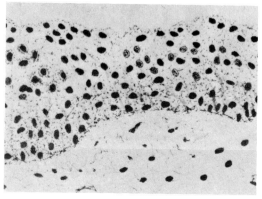

Non-pregnant

FIG. 22–7.   Pregnancy diagnosis in pigs by means of a vaginal biopsy and examination of the state of the epithelium. This is multilayered in cyclic animals compared with the two or three cell layers of the vaginal epithelium in pregnancy. (From Hunter, R.H.F. (1982). Reproduction of Farm Animals. New York, Longman.)

was more accurate than the progesterone RIA in detecting pregnancy and nonpregnant dairy cows 30 days after AI because bPSPB is pregnancy specific, whereas the progesterone assay (see next section) is not. Additionally, unlike the progesterone assay, the timing of bPSPB test is independent of the breeding date. The disadvantages are that it is not detectable in cow's milk or urine and also persists in the blood for several months after parturition, which could interfere with early diagnosis of the subsequent pregnancy.

Chorionic somatomammotropin is a placental lactogen (PL) found in the placental tissue of several mammalian species. It is first detected at day 16 in the ewe and between day 17 and 25 in the cow. It has not been used as a pregnancy test in cattle because it cannot be detected in maternal blood until the latter half of gestation. Pregnancy, however, can be diagnosed during midgestation in the ewe on PL levels with an accuracy of 97 to 100% for pregnancy and nonpregnancy, respectively (Robertson et al., 1980).

Hormones

Sensitive radioimmunoassays and enzyme immunoassays are available for the measurement of pregnancy-dependent hormones in body fluids. For example, pregnancy can be diagnosed in farm animals at a much earlier stage using the plasma or milk progesterone than was possible using clinical methods.

Progesterone. The measurement of progesterone has so far been the most widely used method of pregnancy detection in farm species. Although not pregnancy specific, progesterone can be used as a pregnancy test because the CL persists during early pregnancy in all farm animals. Progesterone levels are measured in biologic fluids such as blood and milk when progesterone is declining in nonpregnant animals. Normally, the sample is collected one estrous cycle length after an insemination or mating, e.g., 22 to 23 days in cows, 17 to 18 days in sheep, and 21 days in pigs. At this sampling time, the progesterone is low in a nonpregnant animal, whereas it is elevated in a pregnant animal (Fig. 22–9).

Milk is preferred to blood, particularly because progesterone levels are considerably higher in milk than in plasma and samples can be collected at milking time without inflicting much discomfort or pain on the animal. Commercial pregnancy testing services based on milk progesterone are available for dairy herds in several countries.

For pregnancy diagnosis in dairy cows, a sample of milk is collected between days

TABLE 22–3. Immunologic Methods of Pregnancy Diagnosis in Farm Animals

Pregnancy Test	Principle	Stage of Pregnancy	Sample	Technique	Species
Early pregnancy factor (EPF)	Detects immunosuppressive factor resulting from fertilization	Preimplantation	Serum	RIT	Cattle, sheep, pig
Progesterone	Predicts luteal activity	Implantation	Serum/milk	RIA/EIA	Cattle, sheep, horse, goat, pig, buffalo
Estrone sulphate	Determines fetoplacental function	Postimplantation	Serum/milk	RIA/EIA	Cattle, pig, horse, sheep, goat
Placental lactogen	Determines fetoplacental function	Postimplantation	Serum	RIA	Cattle, sheep
eCG (PMSG)	Determines placental activity	Postimplantation	Serum	HI	Horse
Pregnancy associated antigens	Identifies antigens specific to pregnancy	Postimplantation	Serum	HI	Cattle, sheep, horse

EIA = enzymoimmunoassay; HI = hemagglutination inhibition; RIA = radioimmunoassay; RIT = rosette inhibition test.

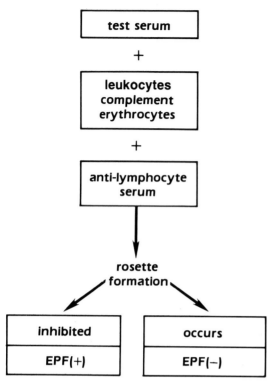

FIG. 22–8. Principle of the rosette-inhibition test for the detection of the early pregnancy factor (EPF). (From Smart et al. (1981). Early pregnancy factor. Its role in mammalian reproduction. Fertil. Steril. *35*, 397.)

22 and 24 after insemination. The progesterone concentration is correlated with the fat content of milk; the level will be higher in the afternoon than in the morning milk and higher in strippings than in bulk milk or foremilk. The sampling technique will vary from one laboratory to another, but most prefer the afternoon milk sample. A preservative, e.g., potassium dichromate or mercuric chloride, is added to prevent spoilage of milk during transport to the laboratory.

The progesterone concentration on which a positive diagnosis is based depends on whether the level was measured in whole milk, fat, or fat-free milk. Milk samples are tested for progesterone using automated radioimmunoassays, and results reach the farmer within 2 to 3 days. These methods are accurate but are relatively expensive, require laboratory facilities and results are available only after several days. One-step qualitative "cow-side" milk progesterone "kits" being developed should overcome some of these problems. Enzyme-linked immunoabsorbant assay (ELISA) and latex agglutination assay "kits" are available for testing on the farm

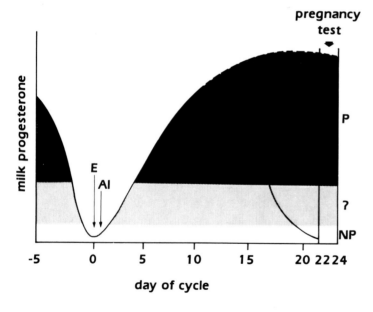

FIG. 22–9. The progesterone in milk as a method of pregnancy diagnosis in the lactating cow. The test is conducted at 22 to 24 days after estrus (*E*) and insemination (*AI*). The progesterone level in the milk sample declines in a nonpregnant cow (*NP*), whereas it remains elevated in a pregnant cow (*P*). The "?" is progesterone level in a cow 2 to 3 days before or after estrus and in doubtful pregnancy.

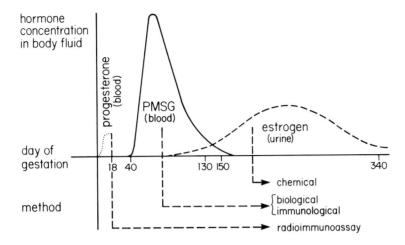

FIG. 22–10.   The laboratory methods of pregnancy diagnosis at various stages of gestation in the mare. (Redrawn from Walker, D. (1977). Laboratory methods of equine pregnancy diagnosis. Vet. Rec. *100*, 396.)

and take only a few minutes. The use of these qualitative tests for the early detection of nonpregnancy not only improves the reproductive performance of the herd but is economically feasible.

An elevated level of progesterone does not necessarily signify pregnancy. If a cow has a longer than normal estrous cycle length (e.g., 28 days) after insemination, a CL would be present on the day of sampling (22 days) and progesterone levels would be high. Another possibility is the occurrence of early embryonic mortality between sampling and confirmation of pregnancy by rectal palpation. Thus, a cow would be incorrectly diagnosed as pregnant (false-positive). For these reasons, the accuracy of predicting pregnancy has ranged from 75 to 90%. On the contrary, the accuracy for nonpregnancy will be 100% because cows with low progesterone in milk will not be pregnant (Table 22–4). Therefore, the milk progesterone test is more reliable for diagnosing nonpregnancy than pregnancy and can identify nonpregnant animals at a much earlier time than is possible by rectal palpation.

In herds where breeding dates are not available, e.g., in beef herds, a herd test for pregnancy may be based on the progesterone levels in three milk samples collected at 8-day intervals (Laing et al., 1980). For a positive test for pregnancy, the progesterone level must remain elevated at least in the last two samples.

The same basic principle of using the progesterone test for early diagnosis of pregnancy in cattle is also applicable to other farm species. The test is more reliable for nonpregnancy than pregnancy, as in cattle (Table 22–4). In some Asian countries, progesterone levels in milk or blood are used on an experimental basis as an early pregnancy test in the buffalo (Perera et al., 1980; Singh and Puthiyandy, 1980). The limitations of the test are similar to those in cattle.

The milk progesterone test has found limited application in other species. Sheep are not lactating at breeding time, and the test has to be conducted on blood samples. The inability to differentiate pregnancy from pseudopregnancy is a serious drawback in the goat. The accuracy of the test is low in the pig and horse as a result of the persistence of CL in the nonpregnant animal.

Estrone Sulphate.   Estrone sulphate is the major estrogen produced by the conceptus and can be measured in maternal plasma, milk, or urine in all farm species.

TABLE 22–4. **Progesterone Assay for Pregnancy Diagnosis in Farm Animals**

Species	Sample	Earliest Day after Mating	Accuracy of Diagnosis (%) Pregnancy	Nonpregnancy
Cattle	Milk/plasma	21–24	85	100
Goat	Milk/plasma	20–21	98	100
Buffalo	Milk/plasma	21–24	67	97
Horse	Milk/plasma	24	85	100
Sheep	Plasma	17–19	87	98
Pig	Plasma	19–24	86	100

Estrone sulphate is detectable in the plasma earlier in the sow (day 20) and mare (day 40) than in the goat and sheep (day 40 to 50) or cow (day 72) (Table 22–3).

Estrone sulphate can be detected in maternal plasma in the pig as early as day 17 postmating, rising to a peak by day 26 to 29 and declining thereafter.

Estrone sulphate test has the advantage over current methods of pregnancy diagnosis in the pig. It is more accurate earlier in gestation and is a better detector of nonpregnant sows than Doppler ultrasound (Atkinson et al., 1986). Although a relationship exists between litter size at birth and the levels of estrone sulphate in serum and urine on day 28, quantitative predictions of litter size using serum or urinary levels of estrone sulphate are relatively imprecise (Frank et al., 1987). The main disadvantage of the procedure is the difficulty of collecting blood or urine, but this could be circumvented by measuring estrone sulphate in feces (Choi et al., 1987).

Pregnancy can be confirmed in the dairy cow by measuring the level of estrone sulphate in a sample of milk after day 112 of pregnancy instead of confirmation by rectal examination (Booth and Chaplin, 1984). Pregnant goats can be identified by estrone levels in milk or plasma at 40 to 50 days of gestation (Holdsworth and Chaplin, 1982).

Both estrone sulphate and eCG levels (see the following section) may be used to diagnose pregnancy in the mare after day 40 of gestation. Because the developing fetus releases large quantities of estrone

sulphate into the maternal circulation between days 75 and 100 of gestation, estrone sulphate has the advantage over eCG for determining the viability of the fetus (Kindahl et al., 1982).

Gonadotropin. Equine chorionic gonadotropin (eCG or PMSG) appears in the blood of mares as early as 40 days following conception (see Fig. 22–9), and its detection has been regarded as evidence of pregnancy. Peak levels are found between 50 and 120 days (Walker, 1977), which gradually decline thereafter.

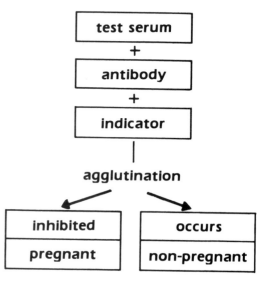

FIG. 22–11. The principle of the hemagglutination test for the detection of equine chorionic gonadotropin (eCG, PMSG). The antibody is raised against eCG and the indicator system is sensitized sheep erythrocytes. Note that inhibition of hemagglutination is positive for pregnancy and occurrence of hemagglutination is negative for pregnancy.

Immunologic diagnosis of pregnancy in mares is based on the principle that eCG, when present in the blood sample to be tested, prevents agglutination of sensitized sheep red cells by anti-eCG (hemagglutination-inhibition test, or HI). Agglutination of red cells means a negative result (i.e., no pregnancy), and inhibition of agglutination, a positive result (Fig. 22–11). This immunologic test is most accurate between 50 and 100 days of gestation. If the fetus dies during this period, however, plasma eCG levels remain elevated. Therefore, if eCG is measured after fetal death, false-positive results will be obtained.

REFERENCES

Atkinson, S., Buddle, J.R., Williamson, P., Hawkins, C.D. and Wilson, R.H. (1986). A comparison between plasma oestrone sulphate concentration and doppler ultrasound as methods for pregnancy diagnosis in sows. Theriogenology *26*, 483–490.

Booth, J.M. and Chaplin, V.M. (1984). Oestrone sulphate in milk as a test for pregnancy. Proc. 10th Int. Congr. Anim. Reprod. and AI. Vol. 11, 77. Urbana–Champaign, IL.

Boyd, J.S., Omran, S.N. and Ayliffe, T.R. (1990). Evaluation of real time B-mode ultrasound scanning for detecting early pregnancy in cows. Vet. Rec. *127*, 350–352.

Buckrell, B.C., Bonnett, B.N. and Johnson, W.H. (1986). The use of real-time ultrasound rectally for early pregnancy diagnosis in sheep. Theriogenology *25*, 665–673.

Butler, J.E., Hamilton, W.C., Sasser, R.G., Ruder, C.A., Hass, G.M. and Williams, R.J. (1982). Detection and partial characterization of two bovine pregnancy-specific proteins. Biol. Reprod. *26*, 925–933.

Choi, H.S., Kiesenhofer, E., Gantner, H., Hois, J. and Bamberg, E. (1987). Pregnancy diagnosis in sows by estimation of oestrogens in blood, urine or faeces. Anim. Reprod. Sci. *15*, 209–216.

Curran, S., Kastelic, J.P., and Ginther, O.J. (1989). Determining sex of the bovine fetus by ultrasonographic assessment of the relative location of the genital tubercule. Anim. Reprod. Sci. *19*, 217.

Curran, S., Pierson, R.A. and Ginther, O.J. (1986). Ultrasonographic appearance of the bovine conceptus from days 10 through 20. J.V.M.A. *189*, 1289–1294.

Findlay, J.K. (1980). Immunological diagnosis of early pregnancy. *In* Immunological Aspects of Reproduction and Fertility Control. J.P. Hearn (ed.). Lancaster, England, MTP Press.

Frank, G.R., Noble, R.C., Esch, M.W., Green, C. and Bahr, J.M. (1987). Direct estimation of estrone sulfate in serum and urine of pregnant swine as indicators of litter size at birth. Anim. Reprod. Sci. *15*, 121–129.

Gearhart, M.A., Wingfield, W.E., Knight, A.P., Smith, J.A., Dargatz, D.A., Boon, J.A. and Stokes, C.A. (1988). Real-time ultrasonography for determining pregnancy status and viable fetal numbers in ewes. Theriogenology *30*, 323–338.

Haibel, G.K. (1988). Real-time ultrasonic fetal head measurement and gestational age in dairy goats. Theriogenology *30*, 1053–1058.

Holdsworth, R. J. and Chaplin, V.M. (1982). A direct radioimmunoassay for oestrone sulphate in milk. Br. Vet. J. *138*, 455.

Humblot, H. et al. (1988). Diagnosis of pregnancy by radioimmunoassay of pregnancy-specific protein in the plasma of dairy cows. Theriogenology *39*, 257.

Kindahl, H. et al. (1982). Progesterone, prostaglandin $F_{2\alpha}$, PMSG and estrone sulphate during early pregnancy in mare. J. Reprod. Fertil. Suppl. *32*, 353.

Laing, J.A., Gibbs, H.A. and Eastman, S.A.K. (1980). A herd test for pregnancy in cattle based on progesterone levels in milk. Br. Vet. J. *136*, 413.

Muller, E. and Wittkowski, G. (1986). Visualization of male and female characteristics of bovine fetuses by real-time ultrasonics. Theriogenology *25*, 571–574.

Pierson, R.A., Kastelic, J.P. and Ginther, O.J. (1988). Basic principles and techniques for transrectal ultrasonography in cattle and horses. Theriogenology *29*, 3–20.

Perera, B.M.A.O. et al. (1980). Early pregnancy diagnosis in buffaloes from plasma progesterone concentration. Vet. Rec. *106*, 104.

Powis, R.L. (1986). Ultrasound science for the veterinarian. Vet. Clin. North Am. Equine Pract. *2*, 3–27.

Robertson, H.A. et al. (1980). Diagnosis of pregnancy in the ewe at mid-gestation. Anim. Reprod. Sci. *3*, 69.

Sasser, R.G., Ruder, C.A., Ivani, K.A., Butler, J.E. and Hamilton, W.C. (1986). Detection of pregnancy by radioimmunoassay of a novel pregnancy-specific protein in serum of cows and a profile of serum concentrations during gestation. Biol. Reprod. *35*, 936–942.

Singh, A. and Puthiyandy, R. (1980). Estimation of progesterone in buffalo milk and its application to pregnancy diagnosis. J. Reprod. Fertil. *59*, 89.

Smart, Y.C. et al. (1981). Early pregnancy factor. Its role in mammalian reproduction. Fertil. Steril. *35*, 397.

Taverne, M.A.M. and Willemse, A.A. (eds.). (1989). Diagnostic Ultrasound and Animal Reproduction. London, Kluwer Academic Publishers.

Thwaites, C.J. (1981). Development of ultrasound techniques for pregnancy diagnosis in the ewe. Anim. Breed. Abstr. *49*, 427.

Trapp, M.J. and Slyter, A.L. (1983). Pregnancy diagnosis in the ewe. J. Anim. Sci. *57*, 1.

Walker, D. (1977). Laboratory methods of equine pregnancy diagnosis. Vet. Rec. *100*, 396.

23

Assisted Reproductive Technology: Ovulation Manipulation, In Vitro Fertilization/Embryo Transfer (IVF/ET)

E.S.E. HAFEZ

The extensive investigations of mammalian embryos conducted during the last two decades have increased our depth of understanding of the normal biophysiologic events taking place during fertilization and early embryo development. The formulation of media that support these processes *in vitro* to the early blastocyst stage, and the refinement of procedures for routine embryo transfer into the genital tract of suitably prepared recipient females are the two fundamental achievements of the past two decades.

OVULATION INDUCTION AND SYNCHRONIZATION

Ovulation may occur spontaneously or as a reflex to a stimulus. Rabbits, ferrets, and some other mustelids, the cat, and the shrew do not ovulate spontaneously (Table 23–1). In the rabbit, ovulation occurs 10 to 13 hours after copulation or after some other stimulus, e.g., injection of LH, salts or copper and cadmium, electrical stimulation of the head or of the lumbar region of the spinal cord, or orgasm induced by contact with other females. However, ovulation usually cannot be provoked by mechanical stimulation of the cervix, as it can in the cat. Ovulation is usually induced in the rabbit by an intravenous injection of

20 to 25 IU of human chorionic gonadotropin (hCG) in about 0.25 ml of sterile physiologic saline. In the hamster, ovulation occurs regularly every 4 days. The time of ovulation is estimated in relation to the time of onset of estrus, i.e., the time when the female first permits breeding by the male, and in relation to the photoperiod in the room. Species differences are noted in characteristics of the estrous cycle, ovulatory mechanisms, time of ovulation, viability of the egg (Table 23–1), time of cleavage stages, and locations of the morulae and blastocysts in the female reproductive tract (Table 23–2).

Although the mammalian ovary contains hundreds of thousands of oocytes, the number of progeny a female produces is small. In farm animals, the number of times a female can become pregnant is severely limited by the extended duration of gestation. Furthermore, only one or two ova are usually shed per estrous cycle in nonlitter-bearing species. The number of offspring that a female can produce in her lifetime can be greatly increased by repeatedly allowing her to become temporarily pregnant, recovering the embryos in early pregnancy, and transferring them to the reproductive tracts of other females to complete gestation. The process can be

461

further amplified if the donor is superovulated.

The first successful embryo transfer was reported in rabbits. The first successful embryo transfers in farm animals were reported during the 1970s. Assisted reproductive technology/andrology (ARTA) is a new field of biomedical sciences in farm animals and man. A large body of literature on basic and clinical research is summarized in Tables 23–2 through 23–8.

There were several limitations of developing embryo transfer techniques to a practical scale comparable to artificial insemination. Previously, there were no reliable methods for superovulation and production of fertilized ova on a large scale, and there was no simple nonsurgical technique for collecting embryos. Some of these problems are being resolved, and embryo transfer, just as artificial insemination, could play a significant role in animal reproduction. Commercial companies for embryo transfer in farm animals have been established in Australia, Argentina, Canada, New Zealand, the United States and several countries in Europe (Church and Shea, 1977).

This chapter deals with basic concepts, physiologic mechanisms, and modern technology of superovulation, collection of ova, examination of ova for fertilization and normality, handling and storage of embryos, *in vitro* fertilization (IVF), embryo transfer, and genetic engineering.

Ovulation Induction During Anestrus

Several hormones are used to induce ovulation during estrus. A natural LH surge occurs as a result of positive feedback of estrogen secretion by the developing follicle. It may be appropriate to stimulate a surge of LH by the administration of gonadotropin-releasing hormone (GnRH), or an artificial LH-like surge can be caused by administration of hCG, an LH-like hormone.

The growth of ovarian follicles in anestrous females can be induced using various hormones; FSH with or without LH; and pregnant mare serum gonadotropin (PMSG) with or without hCG. FSH and LH have shorter biologic half-lives than the placental gonadotropins (PMSG and hCG). Thus, it is usually necessary to give multiple injections of FSH or FSH and LH to stimulate the same amount of follicular growth that would result from a single injection of PMSG or PMSG with hCG. One large dose of GnRH normally will cause a mature follicle to ovulate through release of endogenous LH and FSH. In cattle and sheep, estrus is not exhibited in response to gonadotropin injection alone. Estrus occurs only after previous exposure to elevated progesterone or synthetic progestogen.

In cattle, a preovulatory LH surge results from positive feedback of estrogen. A transient increase in progesterone and LH frequently follows the LH surge. The source of this transient increase in progesterone is LH or a small nonpalpable corpus luteum (CL). Estrus does not occur before this initial transient increase in progesterone. When the transient increase in progesterone decreases, estrus and ovulation occur within a few days. Ovulation can be induced in some anestrous postpartum cattle by administration of a single dose of GnRH (Tables 23–3 and 23–4). For cattle to respond to a single dose of GnRH, a mature follicle must be present on at least one ovary (Roche et al., 1981). The GnRH causes a preovulatory-like surge of LH, which then causes the mature follicle to ovulate (Table 23–5)

A combination of progestogen and estrogen is used successfully for ovulation induction in anestrous cattle. Estrogen conjugates (5 mg, estradiol valerate), is followed 7 to 12 days later with progestogen administered as an ear implant or as an intravaginal pessary. An enhanced response to this combination of estrogen

Sections of this chapter have been extracted from the fourth edition. Special and sincere thanks are due to Professors T. Sugie and G. Seidel, Jr.

TABLE 23–1. Species Differences in Type, Season, and Main Characteristics of Sexual Cycle in Laboratory Mammals

Ovulatory Mechanism	Species	Type and Season of Cycle	Length of Sexual Cycles (Days)	Duration of Heat	Time of Ovulation	Viability of Ova (Hours)
A. Spontaneous ovulation	Dog	In estrus at 4- to 8-month interval in spring and fall depending on breed; mono-estrous	Proestrus, 9 days; estrus, 7–9 days	7–13 days	2nd–3rd day of estrus	A few days
	Gerbil	Polyestrous	4–6	12–18 hrs		
	Guinea Pig	Polyestrous	16–19	6–15 hrs	10 hrs from onset of estrus	20
	Hamster	Polyestrous	4	4–23 hrs	Early estrus	10
	Mouse	Polyestrous (anytime)	4–5	9–20 hrs	2–3 hrs from onset of estrus	10–12
	Opossum	Polyestrous (seasonal)	22–38	1–2 days	Early in heat	
	Rat	Polyestrous (anytime)	4–6 (pseudo-pregnancy lasts 13 days)	9–20 hrs	8–11 hrs from onset of estrus	8–12
B. Reflex ovulation	Cat	Polyestrous (seasonal in spring and fall)	15–28 (pseu-dopregnancy lasts 36 days)	4–10 days	24–36 hrs post-copulation	
	Ferret	Polyestrous (April to Aug.)		In absence of male, 5 mo.	30 hrs post-copulation	30
	Mink	Polyestrous	8–9		42–50 hrs post-copulation	
	Rabbit	Polyestrous (anytime)	Pseudopreg-nancy lasts 14–16 days	No clearly defined period	10.5 hrs. post-copulation	8

(From Fox, R.R. and Laird, C.W. (1970). Sexual cycles. *In* Reproduction and Breeding Techniques for Laboratory Animals. E.S.E. Hafez (ed.). Philadelphia, Lea & Febiger.)

TABLE 23–2. Earliest Time when Cleavage Stages and Blastocysts Can Be Found with Some Regularity

Animal	Day Found				
	2-Cell Stage	4-Cell Stage	16-Cell Stage	Blastocyst	Implantation
Cat	Early 3	Late 3	4	5–6	13–14
Ferret	3	Late 3	4–5	6–7	11–12
Guinea pig	2	4	5	Late 5	6
Gerbil	2	3	Late 4	5	6
Hamster	2	3	Early 4	4	5
Mink	3	4	5–6	6–7	Delayed
Mouse	2	Early 3	Late 3	Early 4	Early 5
Opossum	3	3	4	Early 5	6
Rabbit	2	Late 2	Early 3	Late 3	7
Rat	2 and 3	Late 3	Late 4	5	Late 5

(From Enders, A.C., 1970. Fertilization, cleavage, and implantation. *In* Reproduction and Breeding Techniques for Laboratory Animals. E.S.E. Hafez (ed.). Philadelphia, Lea & Febiger)

TABLE 23–3. Hormones Used for Induction and Synchronization of Ovulation

Type of Hormone	Method of Administration	Biologic Activity
Gonadotropins		
Pregnant mares serum gonadotropin (PMSG)	Injection	Mimics FSH and stimulates follicular growth
Human chorionic gonadotropin (hCG)	Injection	Mimics LH and induces ovulation
PMSG + hCG	Injection	Combines action of FSH and LH
Gonadotropin releasing hormone (GnRH)	Injection	Induces release of LH and FSH from the anterior pituitary
Progestogens		
Progesterone	Injection, implant, pessary	Mimics action of corpus luteum (CL)
Synthetic progestogens*	Injection, implant, pessary, oral	Mimics action of CL
Estrogens		
Estradiol conjugates†	Injection, implant	Induces premature regression of CL and enhances response to progestogens
Prostaglandins		
Prostaglandin $F_{2\alpha}$ or analogues of $PGF_{2\alpha}$	Injection	Induces regression of CL during responsive phases

*Examples include Norgestomet, medroxyacetate progesterone (MAP), melengestrol acetate (MGA), fluorogestone acetate (FGA, Cronolone), and Altrenogest.
†Examples include estradiol valerate, estradiol benzoate, and estradiol cypionate. (Britt, 1986)

TABLE 23–4. Practical Methods for Inducing Estrus and Ovulation in Anestrous Farm Animals

Species Group	Treatment	Response
Cattle		
Prepubertal or postpartum suckled cows	Estrogen on day 1 followed by 7 to 12 days of progestogen, PMSG given on last day (optional)	Majority exhibit estrus within 5 days after treatment
Postpartum milked cows	GnRH on day 14 postpartum	Majority ovulate 1 day after treatment
Sheep and goats		
Prepubertal or seasonal anestrus	Progestogen for 12 to 21 days with PMSG given near the end of progestogen treatment	Majority exhibit estrus 2 to 4 days after treatment; PMSG required for good response
Swine		
Prepubertal or postpartum anestrus	PMSG alone PMSG on day 1 with hCG given 48–96 hours later PMSG + hCG given on day 1	Majority exhibit estrus 3 to 5 days after treatment
Horses		
Seasonal anestrus	Lengthen photoperiod by 4 hours per day	Majority cycle 4 to 6 weeks earlier than normal
Late anestrus	Progestogen for 15 days	Majority cycle within 1 week after treatment

GnRH = gonadotropin-releasing hormone; hCG = human chorionic gonadotropin; PMSG = pregnant mare serum gonadotropin. (Britt, 1986)

plus progestogen occurs when PMSG (400 to 800 IU) is given on the last day of progestogen treatment. Separating calves from their dams (2 to 3 days) after withdrawal of the progestogen also results in an increased response in terms of the percentage of cows that are induced to cycle (Wiltbank and Spitzer, 1978). The calf sep-

TABLE 23–5. Practical Methods for Synchronizing Estrus in Cyclic Farm Animals

Species	Method	Treatment Regimen	Response
Cattle	Prostaglandin	Detect estrus and AI for 5–6 days; give PGF to remaining animals on day 6–7 and AI at estrus.	Majority bred once in a 10- to 12-day period.
		Give PGF on day 1 and AI animals in estrus during next 5 days; give nonbred animals PGF on day 11 or 12 and AI at estrus or by fixed-time AI.	Majority bred once during the two 3- to 5-day periods.
		Give 2 injections of PGF 11 or 12 days apart and AI at estrus or by fixed time after second PGF.	Majority bred within a 3- to 5-day period; repeat cycles are synchronized.
	Estrogen plus progestogen	Estrogen plus progestogen injection on day 1 with progestogen implant for 9 days beginning on day 1, AI at estrus or by fixed time.	Majority bred within a 3- to 5-day period; repeat cycles are synchronized.
	Progestogen plus prostaglandin	Progestogen for 7 days with PGF given on day 6, AI at estrus or by fixed time.	Majority bred within a 2- to 3-day period; repeat cycles are synchronized.
Sheep	Progestogen plus PMSG	Progestogen for 12–14 days, PMSG given at progestogen withdrawal; breed at estrus or double AI.	Majority bred within a 2-day period.
	Prostaglandin	Give 2 injections of PGF 9 days apart, breed at estrus or double AI.	Majority bred within a 2- or 3-day period.
Goat	Progestogen plus PMSG	Progestogen for 18–21 days, PMSG at the time of progestogen withdrawal; breed at estrus or double AI.	Majority bred within a 2- to 3-day period.
	Prostaglandin	Give 2 injections 11–12 days apart; breed at estrus or double AI.	Majority bred within a 2- to 3-day period.
Swine	Progestogen	Progestogen for 14–18 days; breed at estrus.	Majority bred within a 4- to 7-day period.
Horse	Progestogen	Progestogen for 15 days; breed at estrus.	Majority bred within a 4- to 7-day period.
	Prostaglandin	One dose to mares in diestrus; breed at estrus.	Majority bred within a 3- to 5-day period.
	Prostaglandin plus hCG	PGF on day 1, hCG on day 7 or 8, PGF on day 15, hCG on day 21 or 22.	Majority bred within a 2- to 4-day period.

AI = artificial insemination; hCG = human chorionic gonadotropin; PGF = Prostaglandin F; PMSG = pregnant mare serum gonadotropin. (Britt, 1986)

aration temporarily removes the suckling-induced suppression of secretion of pituitary gonadotropins. This induction regimen will cause a majority of treated females to exhibit estrus within 5 days after progestogen withdrawal.

In sheep and goats, it is advantageous to advance the normal breeding season by 2 to 4 weeks. Anestrous sheep and goats can be induced to cycle by manipulating the photoperiod. This approach is practical only when females are confined indoors in intensive production facilities because it is

necessary to reduce the daily photoperiod (Ashbook, 1982; Corteel et al., 1982). The introduction of sexually active rams or bucks about 4 to 6 weeks before onset of the normal breeding season will stimulate about two thirds of the anestrous females to cycle earlier than normal. Hormonal induction of ovulation is based on use of progestogens to mimic a normal luteal phase. Progestogens (MAP, Cronolone, progesterone), administered for 12 to 21 days, is followed by gonadotropins (400 to 800 IU of PMSCG) given at progestogen withdrawal. If artificial insemination (AI) is to be used in induced females, two fixed-time inseminations are usually given at 48 and 60 hours, after the end of treatment. Several methods have been applied to detect and synchronize estrus. (Figs. 23–1 and 23–2).

SUPEROVULATION AND EMBRYO TRANSFER

Superovulation

Superovulatory treatments are widely used in embryo transfer programs to increase the supply of embryos from animals of superior genetic merit. The ovarian response and the yield of viable embryos following superovulation in these species remain highly variable, and when retarded

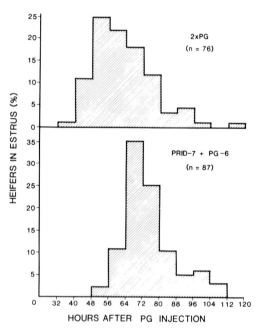

FIG. 23–1. Percentage of Holstein heifers detected in estrus after two different estrous synchronization treatments. Heifers were given two injections of prostaglandin F (PGF) 11 days apart (*top*) or a progesterone-releasing intravaginal device (PRID) for 7 days with PGF given on day 6 (*bottom*). (From Smith, R.D. et al. (1984). Insemination of Holstein heifers at a preset time after estrous cycle synchronization using progesterone and prostaglandin. J. Anim. Sci. *58*, 792.)

or abnormal embryos are recovered, it is difficult to determine whether the primary defect occurred before or after the time of ovulation (Miller and Armstrong, 1982).

The response to the superovulatory treatment can be predicted from milk progesterone pattern qualitatively but not quantitatively. A superovulatory treatment in terms of ovulation rate and number of embryos collected can be detected through measurement of milk progesterone concentrations prior to the collection of bovine embryo.

The proportion of superovulated ova capable of full development may vary between larger species, which are often monotocous, with longer cycle lengths, and polytocous species with much shorter cycles. Superovulation in the latter species, such as the hamster, produces a homogenous group of ova by drawing on a large pool of follicles that have already attained some degree of maturity. These follicles have already acquired the ability to respond to gonadotropic stimulation before exposure to exogenous gonadotropins. In contrast, in the species with longer cycles, relatively few follicles may be in each class of developing follicles, especially at later stages close to ovulation. Much of the maturation of follicle and ovum may occur during the more lengthy follicular phase of each ovulatory cycle. In these latter species, superovulatory treatment may either force less mature follicles, which lack the ability to respond fully to gonadotropic stimulation, to ovulate immature ova; or if initiated after the distinction of developing follicles into ovulatory and atretic subgroups, the treatment may induce ovulation of overly mature or degenerating ova (Fleming, 1982).

The following are effects of superovulatory treatment that might result in disturbances in the ova themselves or in the maternal environment on which the ova depend for their survival:

1. Genetic defects in the ova
2. Over- or undermaturity of the ova

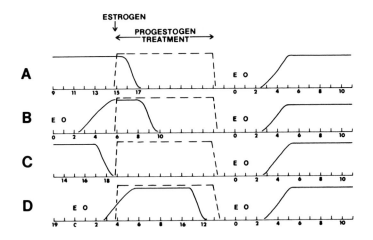

FIG. 23–2. Cattle can be synchronized with a combination of estrogen and progestogen. Letters *A, B, C, D* represent four cows on different days of their estrous cycle when treatment is started. The solid line represents progesterone secretion from the corpus luteum (CL). The broken line represents progestogen from an implant. Notice that treatment with estrogen causes the CL to regress early in cows B and D. Progestogen prevents estrus (E) and ovulation (DO) until it is withdrawn. (Britt, 1986.)

3. Maternal endocrine imbalance leading to altered oviductal transport and asynchrony between stages of embryonic development and endometrial sensitivity to implantation
4. Limitation in the capacity of the uterus to support an increased number of young (Fleming, 1982).

Methods of Superovulation

Usually, subcutaneous or intramuscular injections of PMSG or FSH are given to stimulate additional follicular growth. This treatment is often followed by intravenous administration of LH or hCG several days later to induce ovulation of the follicles, although exogenous LH or hCG is not required for adult cows, sheep, and goats. Methods of superovulation are summarized in Table 23–8. Some researchers inject 3 mg of estradiol-17β on day 19 and again on day 20, when cows are treated with PMSG on day 16 of the estrous cycle.

With current procedures, superovulation increases the yield of normal embryos about fivefold in the cow, goat, sheep, and rabbit but only slightly in pigs and horses (Fig. 23–4). With all species, there are tremendous individual variations in response. Many donors do not produce any normal embryos, while a few produce large numbers. For example, about half of the embryos recovered from a large group of superovulated donors are typically produced by one-fourth of the donors. Unfortunately, it is not possible to predict how a particular donor will respond; this is a major obstacle to successful application.

The single greatest advance in superovulation methodology in the last decade

TABLE 23–6. Percentages of Ewes in Estrus after Various Routes of Progestogen Administration

Route of Administration*	Hours Between End of Treatment and Onset of Estrus†					
	24	36	48	60	72	84
Oral FGA	—	—	29	54	4	4
Vaginal sponge (FGA)	9	40	41	8	2	—
Norgestomet implant	51	49	—	—	—	—

*All animals given pregnant mare serum gonadotropin on the last day of treatment.
†Oral FGA, 9 mg/day; vaginal sponge contained 40 mg FGA; Norgestomet implant contained 3 mg of steroid and was implanted subcutaneously.
(From Quinlivan, T.D. (1980). Estrous synchronization and control of the estrous cycle. *In* Current Therapy in Theriogenology. D.A. Morrow (ed.). Philadelphia, W.B. Saunders.

TABLE 23–7.   Summary of Historical Development of Embryo Transfer and Related Techniques

Author	Event	Species
Heape, 1890	First successful embryo transfer	Rabbit
Beidl et al., 1922	Successful embryo transfer	Rabbit
Nicholas, 1933	Successful embryo transfer	Rat
Warwick and Berry, 1949	Successful embryo transfer	Sheep and goats
Kvansnickii, 1951	Successful embryo transfer	Pig
Willett et al., 1951	Successful embryo transfer	Cattle
Marden and Chang, 1952	First intercontinental shipment of embryos stored at 10°C	Rabbit
Alberta Livestock Transplants, Ltd., 1971	First commercial company formed for embryo transfer in farm animals	Cattle
Whittingham et al., 1972	Offspring produced from long-term frozen embryos	Mouse
Wilmut and Rowson, 1973	Offspring produced from frozen embryos	Cattle
	International Embryo Transfer Society formed	—
Steptoe and Edwards, 1978	Baby girl born after embryo transfer	Man

TABLE 23–8.   Doses of Gonadotropins for Superovulation

Animal	Day of Estrous Cycle	Gonadotropin for Follicular Growth			Gonadotropin for Ovulation	
		PMSG (IU)	or	FSH (mg)	hCG (IU)	LH (mg)
Cow	15–16	1500–3000		20–50	1500–2000	75–100
Calf	—	1000–2000		20–50	1000–1500	50–75
Goat	16–17	1000–1500		12–20	1000–1500	50–75
Kid	—	1000–1200		10–15	1000–1500	50–75
Ewe	12–14	1000–2000		12–20	1000–1500	50–75
Lamb	—	1000–1200		10–15	1000–1500	50–75
Pig	15–16	750–1500		10–20	500–1000	25–50
Rabbit	—	25–75		2–3	25–75	2–3

hCG = human chorionic gonadotropin; PMSG = pregnant mare serum gonadotropin.

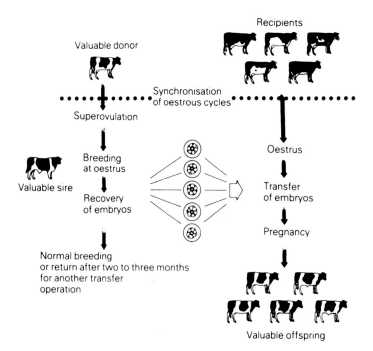

FIG. 23–3.   Advantages of embryo transfer. Embryos from a valuable donor mated to a valuable sire are transplanted to nonpedigree recipients that act as foster mothers for development of the pedigree calves. (From Hunter, R.H.F. (1982). Reproduction of Farm Animals. New York, Longman.)

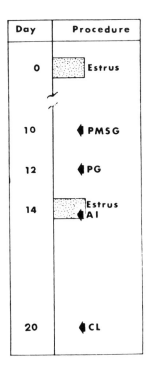

Day	Procedure
0	Estrus
10	⬥PMSG
12	⬥PG
14	Estrus ⬥AI
20	⬥CL

FIG. 23–4. The procedure of superovulation by gonadotropin and prostaglandin. *PMSG* = pregnant mare serum gonadotropin; *PG* = prostaglandin $F_{2\alpha}$; *AI* = artificial insemination; *CL* = observation of corpora lutea. (From Kanagawa et al. (1982). Ovulation rate in beef cattle after repeated treatments with gonatrophins and prostaglandin. *In* In-vitro Fertilization and Embryo Transfer. E.S.E. Hafez and K. Semm (eds.). Lancaster, England, MTP Press.)

has been the use of prostaglandin $F_{2\alpha}$ or $PGF_{2\alpha}$ analogues, such as cloprostenol, because superovulatory treatment can be initiated anytime between day 6 of the estrous cycle and natural CL regression. The optimal time for treatment, however, is between days 8 and 12 of the cycle in cattle (Betteridge, 1977). Not only does $PGF_{2\alpha}$ increase the flexibility of timing superovulation, but it is also an excellent treatment for producing large numbers of normal embryos. Most donors are in estrus 2 to 3 days after prostaglandin injection.

Sows are usually anestrous during the first 6 weeks of lactation. During the late summer and early autumn, the incidence of anestrus in weaned sows increases. Estrus and ovulation can be induced in anestrous sows and gilts by gonadotropin: PMSG is administered alone or in combination with hCG. A single injection of 400 to 1200 IU of PMSG will induce estrus in most anestrous sows and gilts. Injection of 500 to 1000 IU of hCG 48 to 96 hours after injection of PMSG will induce a well-synchronized ovulation. Ovulation can also be induced in anestrous swine by a single injection of a combination of PMSG (400 IU) and hCG (200 IU). The response to this combination treatment is similar to that which occurs when the gonadotropins are given separately. The advantage of the combination is that lower doses of each gonadotropin are needed. Induction of ovulation in gilts less than 160 days of age is not recommended, because these gilts often fail to maintain pregnancy. Pregnancy fails because CL in these young gilts regress during the third week after ovulation. Regression of the CL is due to the inability of the developing conceptuses to provide sufficient luteotropic support to overcome the luteolytic effect of prostaglandin from the uterus.

Insemination

Superovulated donors are usually inseminated more often and with more sperm per insemination than other donors. Even so, fertilization rates of ova from superovulated donors are usually considerably below those rates for ova from untreated donors (Elsden et al., 1976). This may be partly due to suboptimum sperm transport, ovulation over a period of time, defective oocytes, or other causes.

Repeated Superovulation

Experiments with repeated superovulation are sometimes difficult to interpret because they are often confounded by the sequelae of repeated surgery (Maurer and Foote, 1971). On the average, donors respond similarly to first, second, and third superovulatory treatments. The response to subsequent treatments, however, is less in some individuals, probably as a result of the production of antibodies against gonadotropins. This may be avoided to some extent by increasing the interval between hormone treatments. Antibody production may be minimized by using gonadotropins derived from the same species as the one being treated.

Egg Transport

Species differences are noted in egg transport in the oviduct and rate of cleavage (Table 23). In the mouse and rat, the ova move in a few minutes through the first coil of the ampulla of the oviduct to reach the dilated portion of the ampulla. In the mouse, in which transport of ova is relatively fast, the late morula or early blastocyst is transported to the uterus on the morning of the third day after fertilization, and by the afternoon of this day, all the blastocysts are in the uterus. In the rat transport of the ova takes a half-day longer than in the mouse. In the rabbit, a concentric coat of oviductal secretion is formed around the fertilized or unfertilized eggs while in the oviduct.

Collection and Manipulation of Oocytes

Embryos can be collected from the oviducts or uteri after the slaughter of the animal or excision of the reproductive tract, or they can be removed either surgically or nonsurgically from the intact animal (Table 23-9). Ova representing 40 to 80% of the corpora lutea can usually be recovered from superovulated, intact animals. Recovery rates are slightly higher from excised tracts. In some cases, the reason why the number of ova recovered is often considerably lower than the number of corpora lutea is unknown.

Some of the oocytes may not be picked up by the fimbria because of a greatly enlarged, superovulated ovary. Other possibilities include the loss of ova from the reproductive tract resulting from altered steroid levels, the formation of corpora lu-

tea without ovulation, and the failure to recover all ova present.

Surgical techniques have been used to collect ova from laboratory animals (Daniel, 1971) and farm animals (Dzuik, 1971; Murry, 1978). Ova reside in the oviduct for 3 to 4 days after estrus and then migrate to the uterus. Flushing the oviduct 1 to 3 days after estrus yields more ova than flushing the uterus 5 or more days after estrus. Uterine embryos, however, are often collected because they result in higher pregnancy rates (Newcomb and Rowson, 1975) and can be frozen more successfully with some species than younger embryos. Various methods and catheters have been used to collect ova surgically or nonsurgically (Fig. 23-5).

Surgical Methods

Oviductal ova can be flushed either from the fimbria toward the uterus or from the uterotubal junction toward the fimbria. In species other than the pig and horse, flushing toward the fimbria is the preferred method because a high percentage of ova can be recovered with little damage to the reproductive tract, although periovarian adhesions occur in some animals (Fig. 23-6).

As a result of the valve-like structure of the uterotubal junction in the sow and the mare, the flushing medium is introduced into the ampulla of the oviduct through the ostium of the fimbria with a small glass tube connected to a syringe. The medium is flushed toward the tip of the uterine horn and collected through a blunt needle or a fire-polished, fine glass tube punctured through the uterine wall. A disadvantage of this method is the frequent formation of postoperative adhesions of the uterus or oviduct.

Ova may be recovered from the uterine horns after they have left the oviducts, usually 5 days after estrus or later. The flushing medium is introduced into the base of the uterine horn and flushed toward the tip, where the medium is collected through a blunt syringe needle or a

TABLE 23-9. **Techniques of Ova Collection**

Techique	Species
Collection from Isolated Reproductive Tract:	
Remove reproductive organs and trim adjacent adipose tissue and ligaments.	All species
Flush each oviduct and uterine horn, avoiding contamination of flushings with blood.	All species
Surgical Methods:	
Flush 2–20 ml medium through the oviduct from the upper part of uterine horn toward the fimbria using a syringe and blunt needle; collect flushings through a small glass tube inserted into the infundibulum.	Cattle, sheep, goat, rabbit
Flush 15–20 ml medium through the oviduct from the infundibulum, through the uterotubal junction, and into the upper part of the uterine horn using a small glass tube attached to a syringe; collect flushings through a blunt needle or fine glass tube inserted into the uterine lumen through a puncture wound.	Pig, mare, some uses in other species
Flush the uterus from the base of the uterine horn toward the uterotubal junction or in the reverse direction; using 10–100 ml of medium, depending on the size of the uterus; collect flushings through a blunt needle or small glass tube inserted into the uterine lumen through a puncture wound.	All species
Nonsurgical Methods:	
Dilate cervix (heifers) with expander; insert Foley catheter, Sugie's instrument, or similar device into uterine horn by manual guidance per rectum; inflate ballon with air; irrigate uterine horn with 100–800 ml flushing medium; for mares, inflate balloon in cervix and flush both uterine horns simultaneously.	Cattle, horses

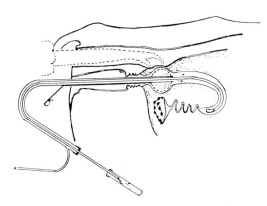

FIG. 23–5.   A nonsurgical technique for ova collection from the bovine uterus developed by T. Sugie.

small glass tube inserted into the lumen through a puncture wound in the uterine wall. The procedure may also be carried out in the reverse direction. Fewer ova are recovered with these procedures than by flushing the oviducts, and serious damage may result from the formation of uterine adhesions. A volume of 2 to 20 ml is used to flush the oviducts, whereas 10 ml

is used to flush the uterus, depending on its size (Fig. 23–7).

Nonsurgical Methods

For many applications, nonsurgical techniques for collection of ova are desirable because all surgical techniques may lead to the formation of adhesions and because there is less risk to the life and health of the donor with nonsurgical methods. There are two types of catheters for nonsurgical egg collection in cattle: a two-way flushing system and a three-way circulation system. The latter system minimizes flushing time and the fluid volume used and gives exceptional cervical penetration. It can also be used in maiden heifers (Fig. 23–8).

Nonsurgical methods have made repeated recovery from the same donor practical. One consequence is that ova are now often recovered from mares and cows without superovulation (Oguri and Tsutsumi, 1974; Elsden et al., 1976). Each uterine horn is filled with 30 to 60 ml of medium, which is then allowed to flow into the collection vessel while the uterus is

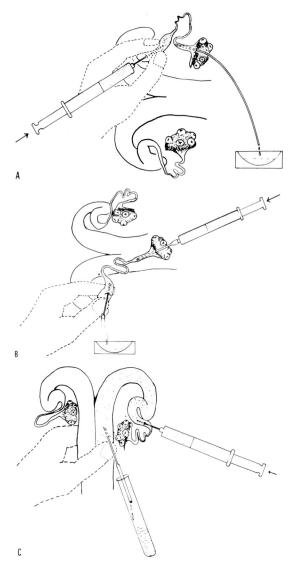

FIG. 23–6. Surgical techniques of ova recovery from slaughterhouse material. *A.* Flushing oviduct toward fimbria. *B.* Flushing oviduct toward uterotubal junction. *C.* Flushing uterus toward base of the uterine horn.

gently massaged through the rectum. This is repeated until 300 to 800 ml of medium have been used. The Foley catheter is then inserted into the other uterine horn and the process repeated. The same principle is used to recover ova from mares,

except that the balloon is inflated in the cervix and both horns are flushed simultaneously.

A syringe and needle can be used to aspirate follicular fluid with oocytes from slaughtered cows, mares, ewes, and gilts (Figs. 23–9, 23–10). Some 50% of the recovered oocytes are morphologically normal. The low recovery rate may be due to the difficulties in separating the cumulus cell-layer oocyte from the cumulus oophorus. Thus, it is possible that the best oocytes for *in vitro* culture are not recovered. Rupturing isolated follicles gives an almost 100% recovery rate and helps to distinguish atretic from nonatretic follicles.

Several techniques have been established for the perfusion of the ovary *in vitro* in an attempt to understand the physiologic mechanisms of ovulation (Koos et al., 1984). Various techniques were developed for perfusion of the isolated ovary developed recently for the study of ovulation. In these systems, ovulation occurs *in vitro* when the ovaries are stimulated by administration of either hCG *in vivo* or LH *in vitro* (Koos et al., 1984) (Fig. 23–11).

Preparation of Donors

1. The donor cow is placed in a squeeze chute, and its rear end is clipped before embryo collection.
2. The rear end of the donor is scrubbed. Local anesthetic and muscle relaxant are injected around the tail head for embryo collection.
3. A speculum is introduced into the donor guided by a rod with a round end to enable the operator to locate the cervix. An introducer is inserted through the cervix to enable accurate location. The introducer is then removed from the cervix and left within the uterus of the donor.
4. A three-way catheter is threaded through the introducer into the uterine horn. The catheter is made of

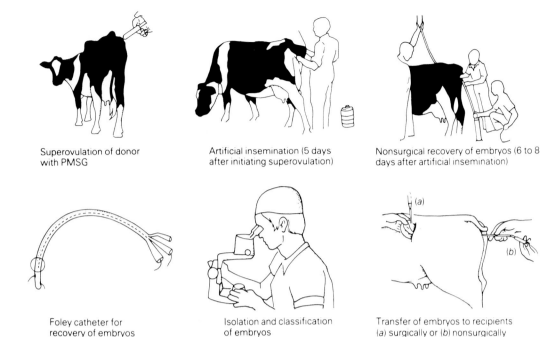

Superovulation of donor
with PMSG

Artificial insemination (5 days
after initiating superovulation)

Nonsurgical recovery of embryos (6 to 8
days after artificial insemination)

Foley catheter for
recovery of embryos

Isolation and classification
of embryos

Transfer of embryos to recipients
(a) surgically or (b) nonsurgically

FIG. 23–7.   Stages involved in nonsurgical recovery of embryos from a superovulated donor cow and their transfer to a recipient by surgical or nonsurgical techniques. (From Hunter, R.H.F. (1982). Reproduction of Farm Animals. New York, Longman.)

three separate tubes (placed in a plastic sheath), each with an external opening outside the donor that may be used either to introduce or collect liquids.

5. The plastic balloon at the other end is inflated to seal off the horn of the uterus into which the catheter is introduced. Using the catheter introduced into the uterine horn, embryos are flushed out with culture media and collected in dishes.

6. The collected embryos are examined with a microscope to evaluate their condition.

Selection of Ova for Transfer

After collection from the donor, ova are isolated under a microscope with a magnification of 10x to 15x. A fine pipette is used to move them into fresh culture medium for morphologic examination, usually with a compound microscope at 40x to 200x

magnification. Embryos should be kept in a container that prevents evaporation of the culture medium. Paraffin oil may be used frequently to cover the medium to prevent evaporation and contamination with microorganisms.

Usually, only morphologically normal ova are transferred; however, a few that appear morphologically abnormal may develop into normal young (Shea et al., 1976a, Elsden et al., 1978). Stages of embryonic development normally found at various times after ovulation are presented in Table 23–10 and Figure 23–12. Ova at any stage, from one cell to the hatched blastocyst, can develop to term following transfer to a suitable environment, but success rates may be lower with very early and very late stages. Under most conditions, embryos between the eight-cell (four-cell in pigs) and blastocyst stage result in the highest pregnancy rates. Older embryos may tolerate *in-vitro* han-

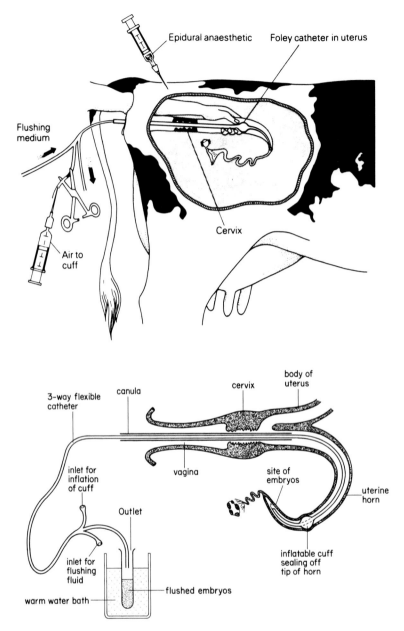

FIG. 23–8.   Use of a Foley rubber catheter with inflatable cuff for recovery of embryos from the uterus in cattle. A physiologic medium is introduced through the catheter, flushed around the uterine horn, and returns through the catheter to a collection dish (Hunter, 1982). The vulva is disinfected and a speculum passed into the vagina to the cervix. The central core of the speculum is removed and an introducer passed through it. The speculum is then withdrawn and the introducer passed through the cervix, using the rectal technique; it is inserted into the appropriate uterine horn as far as can easily be achieved without causing trauma. The introducer is held in position while the central insert is withdrawn, and the sterile three-lumen Bovine catheter is passed through it. If there is resistance to the free movement of the catheter, the assistant passing it should hold it in position while the operator releases his grasp on the introducer and corrects the cause of obstruction. The operator then relocates the introducer, and the catheter is passed as far as possible toward the uterotubal junction. (From Hunter, R.H.F. (1982). Reproduction of Farm Animals. New York, Longman.)

TABLE 23–10.   Stages of Embryonic Development at Various Times After Ovulation

Stage of Embryonic Development	Days after Ovulation, by Species					
	Cow	Mare	Ewe	Goat	Pig	Rabbit
1 Cell	0–1	0–1	0–1	0–1	0–1	0–1
2 Cell	0–2	0–2	0–1	0–1	0–1	0–1
4 Cell	1–2	1–2	1–2	1–2	2–3	1
8 Cell	2–4	2–3	2–3	2–3	3–4	1
Early morula	3–5	2–4	2–4	2–4	3–4	2
Compacted morula	4–6	4–5	4–5	4–5	3–5	2
Early blastocyst	6–7	5–6	5–6	5–6	4–5	3
Blastocyst	6–8	6–7	6–7	6–7	5–6	3
Expanded blastocyst	7–9	7–8	7–8	7–8	5–7	4–6
Hatching blastocyst	8–10	8–9	8–9	7–9	6–8	7

(Adapted from Betteridge, 1977)

dling better than younger embryos (Fig. 23–13).

Defective embryos showing any of the following morphologic anomalies should be discarded:

1. Blastomeres of variable, nonuniform size
2. Cellular debris in the morula
3. Collapse of the degenerated blastocyst within an oblong-shaped zona pellucida
4. Disintegrating mitotic figure
5. Indistinct foamy blastomeres
6. Fragmentation of cytoplasmic and nuclear material
7. Abnormal shape of morula or blastocyst (Fig. 23–14).

In Vitro *Maturation of Oocytes and Embryos*

Graafian follicles contain primary oocytes that normally complete morphologic development in the following sequence in response to the preovulatory LH surge:

1. The nuclear membrane (germinal vesicle) breaks down.
2. The secondary oocyte is formed by completion of the first meiotic division and extrusion of the first polar body. The metaphase plate for the second meiotic division is formed shortly thereafter.
3. Ovulation and rupture of the follicle occur.

In the horse and certain carnivores, ovulation probably occurs before formation of the secondary oocyte. In 1935, Pincus and Enzmann discovered that oocytes removed from the graafian follicles of rabbits before the LH surge and placed in suitable culture media would mature spontaneously. In recent years, this has been confirmed for several species; however, a high incidence of chromosomal abnormalities (McGaughey and Polge, 1971) and cytoplasmic deficiencies (Moor and Trounson, 1977) indicates that the process is not always normal.

Oocytes can be fully or partially matured *in vitro* and then fertilized, usually *in vivo.* In some of these studies, fertilization was clearly abnormal and may have been abnormal in most of them. Normal offspring, however, resulted from two of the studies. Best results were obtained when the entire follicle was cultured with the appropriate hormones (Moor and Trounson, 1977). This method apparently does not produce the abnormalities associated with *in vitro* maturation of isolated oocytes.

Embryo development occurs in several culture conditions, media and supplements, and gaseous atmospheres. Culture in sealed tubes yields results equal to those noted for microdrops of media under paraffin oil. A reduced oxygen atmosphere of 5% CO_2, 5% O_2, 90% N_2 is at least equal to, and, in some species, superior to, 5% CO_2 in air in promoting embryo development (Wright and Bondioli, 1981).

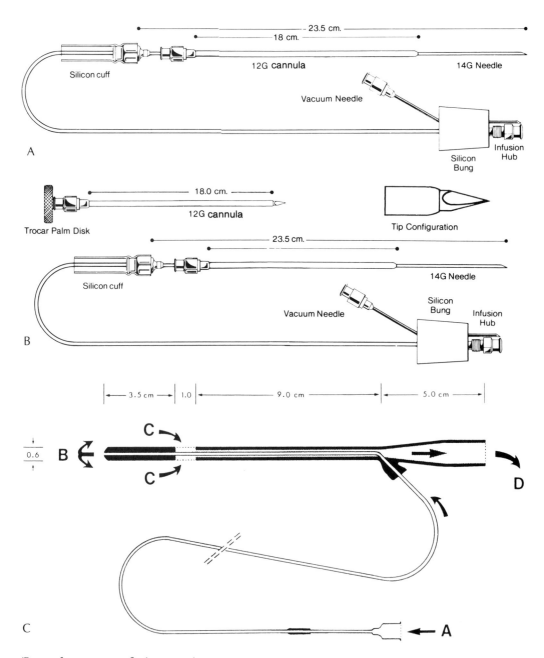

A

B

C

(**Legend appears on facing page.**)

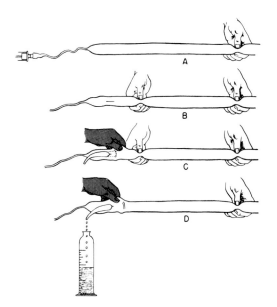

FIG. 23–10. Steps *A*, *B*, *C*, and *D* show the postmortem collection of porcine eggs and embryos.

The rates of fertilization, cleavage, and pregnancy in immature oocytes are lower than those in mature oocytes. Meiosis begins during early fetal period, then is arrested at the diplotene stage at birth until it is resumed by the preovulatory surge of gonadotropins. While meiosis is arrested, oocytes are continuously selected to grow from the pool of primordial oocytes. Resulting from the preovulatory surge of gonadotropins, full-grown oocytes in the follicles resume meiosis, complete the first meiotic division, and then enter a second period of arrest at metaphase II. The sequence of changes in the oocyte between the two periods of meiotic arrest are called *oocyte maturation,* which consist of nuclear, cytoplasmic, and membrane changes (Wassarman, 1988). The completion of these maturational changes leads to normal fertilization and embryonic development.

When full-grown oocytes are removed from the follicles before gonadotropin surge and cultured in medium, they resume meiosis and complete the first meiotic division *in vitro.* These oocytes, "spontaneously" matured *in vitro,* show very poor potential for normal fertilization and embryonic development. Removal of oocytes from the meiosis-inhibitory environment inside follicles is not sufficient for physiologic maturation of oocytes. Addition of gonadotropins and steroids into maturation medium promotes physiologic

FIG. 23–9. Ovum aspiration needle sets. *A.* Stainless steel, 14-gauge with special noncoring 60° bevel point. The useable length is 23.5 cm, allowing 4.5 cm to protrude from the cannula. Transparent Teflon lines the needle from 2 to 3 mm inside the tip to the flared end of the 75-cm extension that passes through the silicon bung. The bung is fitted with a vacuum needle for controlled aspiration and a Luer-Lok metal hub around the tubing outlet for infusion of culture medium. Lumen diameter of the Teflon lining is 1.2 mm ± 1 mm, equivalent to the lumen of an 18-gauge standard needle (Catalogue No. OPS-2). *B.* Polished stainless steel cannula 16.0 cm long with Luer-Lok hub, 12 gauge. Stainless steel trocar point extends 1 mm beyond the sheath, a knurled edge palm disk facilitates safe single-handed manipulation. (Needle Assembly) Stainless steel 14 gauge with special noncoring 60° bevel point. The useable length is 23.5 cm, allowing 4.5 cm to protrude from the sheath. Translucent Teflon lines the needle from 2 to 3 mm inside the tip to the flared end of the 75-cm extension that passes through a silicon bung. The bung is fitted with a vacuum needle for controlled aspiration and a Luer-Lok metal hub around the tubing outlet for infusion of culture medium. Lumen diameter of the Teflon lining the needle is 1.2 mm ± 1 mm, equivalent to the lumen of an 18-gauge standard needle (Catalogue No. OPS-3). *C.* Diagram of the apparatus used for nonsurgical collection of rabbit eggs from the vagina. Warmed flushing fluid is infused into a narrow tube injector: (*a*) the fluid flows through the catheter to the anterior part of the vaginal lumen; (*b*) then, the washings return to the catheter through the holes (*c*) and are recovered in the test tube; (*d*) arrows show the direction of the flow. (*A, B* from Tsutsumi et al. (1976). J. Reprod. Fertil. *48,* 393; *C* from Y. Tsutsumi (1980). Nonsurgical embryo recovery from rabbit vagina. Arch. Androl. *5,* 111–113.)

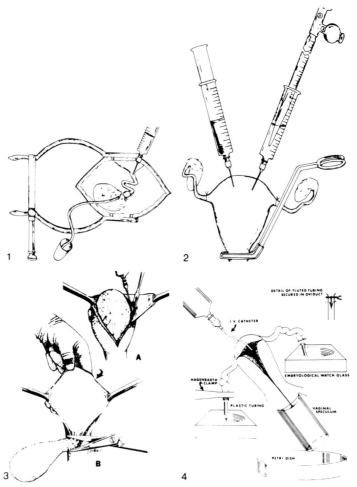

FIG. 23–11. Ova collection in monkeys. *I,* Retrograde flushing of the rhesus monkey oviduct for recovery of tubal ova. *II,* Uterine lavage in the rhesus monkey. *III,* Collection of preimplantation baboon embryos (*a* a spatula is used to separate the endometrium from the myometrium; (*b*) the uterus is inverted (arrow) and the endometrial sac containing the embryos is cut at the cervix uteri. *IV,* Collection of postimplantation baboon embryos. (I and II from Brackett et al. (1971) Cleavage of rabbit ova inseminated in vitro after removal of follicular cells and zonae pellucidae. Fertil. Steril. 22, 816–828; III and IV from Hendricks, A.G. (1971) Embryology of the baboon. Chicago, University of Chicago Press.)

maturation *in vitro* of extrafollicular oocytes and leads to an increase of the potential for fertilization and embryonic development. Also, culture of oocytes within intact isolated follicles (whole follicle culture) confer on the oocyte physiologic maturation *in vitro* (Xu et al., 1987) were able to induce pregnancy resulting from cattle oocytes matured and fertilized *in vitro.*

Transfer of Embryos
Nonsurgical Transfer

Results of nonsurgical embryo transfer have been summarized by Foote and Onuma (1970). With the technique developed by Sugie (1965), the cervix is bypassed. Currently, a more common method is to deposit ova in the uterus through the cervix with an AI straw gun

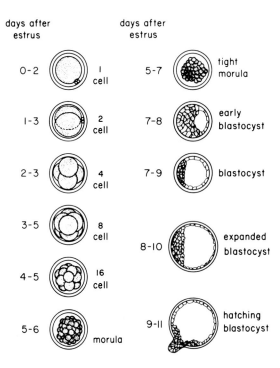

days after estrus

0-2 I cell

1-3 2 cell

2-3 4 cell

3-5 8 cell

4-5 16 cell

5-6 morula

days after estrus

5-7 tight morula

7-8 early blastocyst

7-9 blastocyst

8-10 expanded blastocyst

9-11 hatching blastocyst

FIG. 23–12. Morphologically normal bovine embryos recovered at various stages of development.

6 to 12 days after estrus (Sreenan, 1978; Trounson et al., 1978a).

Surgical Transfer

Embryos are usually transferred surgically. Midventral laparotomy under general anesthetic is the most common method, although flank and lumbar approaches are often used with cattle and rabbits. The reproductive tract is exposed as for ova collection. For transfer into the oviduct, the tip of a capillary pipette containing the embryos is inserted into the infundibulum and ampulla of the oviduct where embryos are then deposited in a drop or two of medium. When transfer is made to the uterus, the wall of the uterine horn is punctured with a blunt needle, and the embryos are expelled from the tip of the capillary pipette inserted into the uterine lumen.

For bovine embryo transfer, laparotomy may be performed under local anesthetic.

The tip of the uterine horn is exposed through an incision in the flank. The ovum is then deposited in the uterine lumen.

In sheep and goats, the recovery and transfer of embryos may be carried out by surgical procedures under general or local anesthetic with the animal restrained in a laparotomy cradle. The approach is invariably by midventral incision, and the genital tract is extracted out of the incision, and the oviduct or uterine horn is flushed to collect ova. Embryos are transferred with one or two drops of medium into the oviduct or the uterine horn extracted out of the incision (Sugie et al., 1982) (Fig. 23–15).

Selection and Preparation of Recipients

Pregnancy rate after embryo transfer is greatly influenced by the conditions and preparation of the recipients. An animal that is not fit for natural service cannot be used for embryo transfer. The females selected to be recipients must be good breeders, have an infection-free genital tract, and be 3 months past parturition (and not suckling). In addition, recipients must be sexually mature, cycling normally, in good condition, and not overweight. Several catheters have been used to transfer fertilized ova in the recipients.

Synchronization of Estrus Between Donor and Recipient

For successful embryo transfer, synchronization between the stage of ovum and the reproductive tract of the recipient is necessary (Fig. 23–16). This is usually accomplished by selecting recipients that were in estrus at the same time as the donor, either naturally or as a result of estrus synchronization (Sreenan et al., 1975). For optimum results, the recipient should be in estrus within 12 hours of the donor. Pregnancy rates decline drastically if the difference is greater than 24 hours in cows and 48 hours in sheep and goats. Recipients for embryos that have been frozen or stored at low temperature should be selected to be in physiologic synchrony

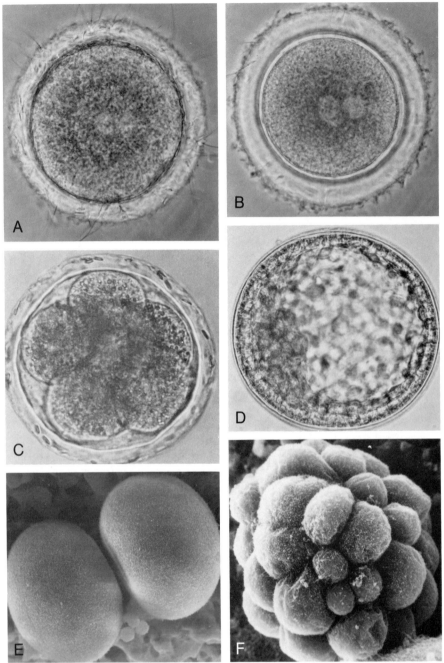

FIG. 23–13. *A,* Denuded and, *B,* untreated rabbit eggs with follicular cells about 5 hours after insemination with epididymal spermatozoa that had been exposed to a defined medium for 15 minutes and preincubated for 1 hour. Many more spermatozoa have penetrated into the perivitelline space of the denuded egg than into that of the egg with follicular cells. The eggs are slightly compressed under a coverslip and examined without staining under phase contrast. When they were examined after staining, second polar body, male and female pronuclei, and the penetrating sperm tail were clearly observed. *C.* Eight-cell sheep embryo recovered from the oviducts 3 days after end of estrus. *D.* Horse embryo, early blastocyst, recovered from the uterus 7 days after ovulation. *E, F.* Scanning electron micrographs of two-cell embryo (*E*) and morula (*F*) after removing the zona pellucida. (*A* and *B* courtesy of Professor Niaw et al., 1983; *C, D* courtesy of Professor N. Ogiri.)

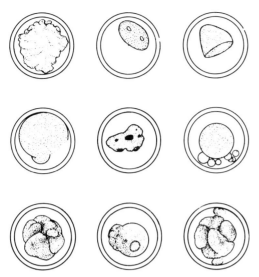

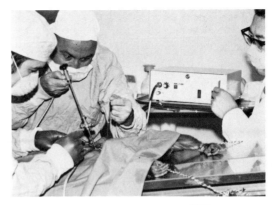

FIG. 23–14. Degenerating one-cell ova, which should not be used for routine embryo transfer.

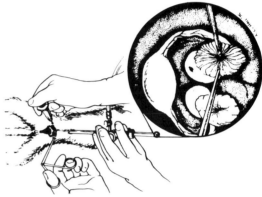

FIG. 23–15. (*Top*) Laparoscopy in the monkey. (*Bottom*) Laparoscopic embryo transfer procedure used with the squirrel monkey. (From Kuehl, T.J. and Dukelow, W.R. (1977). Methods in mammalian reproduction. J. Med. Primatol. *20*, 31.)

with the stage of development of the embryo. Thus, if embryos are frozen for 2 days, they should be transferred to recipients that were in estrus 2 days after the donor. Pregnancy losses from asynchronous transfers are probably due to the placement of embryos in an adverse environment or to an inability of asynchronous embryos to exert a luteotropic action on the CL of the recipient.

Reciprocal Interspecies Embryo Transfer

Reciprocal interspecies transfer of embryos (recovered surgically or nonsurgically) between horses and donkeys has been successful. Equine morulae, recovered surgically and kept in the ligated oviducts of three estrous rabbits for 40 to 49 hours, were successfully transferred surgically to the uterine horn ipsilateral to the CL in three recipient mares. Embryos recovered surgically from the oviduct or uterus of mares and transferred surgically into the corresponding location within recipients continued to develop; and five of seven embryos recovered nonsurgically were successfully transferred nonsurgically through the cervix (Oguri and Tsut-

sumi, 1982). Other interspecies embryo transfers are summarized in Table 23–11.

Maintenance of Pregnancy After Embryo Transfer

Pregnancy rates, the percentage of recipients pregnant, should not be confused with the percentage of embryos surviving. Under certain ideal conditions, up to 80% of the embryos survive to term following transfer to a synchronous recipient. The highest pregnancy rates in sheep, cattle, and goats are obtained with the transfer of one embryo into each uterine horn of the recipient. This frequently results in twins. In pigs and rabbits, 6 to 10 embryos should be transferred into each side to ob-

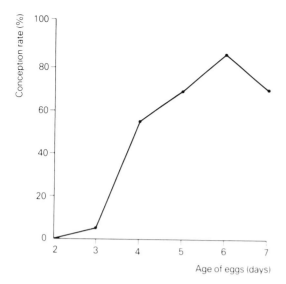

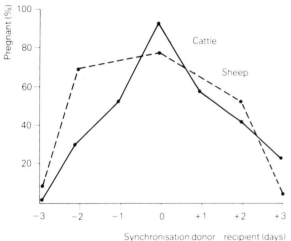

FIG. 23-16.   (*Top*) Optimum conception rates after embryo transplantation procedures in cattle are obtained with 6-day-old blastocysts. Selection of embryos to be transplanted undoubtedly contributes to the success rate at this stage. (*Bottom*) The importance of close synchrony in the estrous cycles of donor and recipient for a high conception rate after transplantation of embryos. (Hunter, R.H.F. (1982). Reproduction of Farm Animals. New York, Longman.)

tain a normal-sized litter because only about one-half of the embryos transferred are represented by viable young at birth.

Pregnancy and embryo survival rates that have been determined in early preg-nancy will usually be only slightly inflated relative to term pregnancy rates. Experiments were conducted by transferring embryos from young donor animals to aged recipients, from young to young, and from aged to young. The lowest percentage of embryonic survival was found when young embryos were transferred to aged mothers, indicating that poor implantation in aged females is due to a defective maternal environment.

Embryo Transfer Records

The following statistics should be compiled for embryo transfer records:

Number of eggs aspirated

Number of eggs/number of follicles aspirated (%)

Number of pregnancies/number of treatment cycle (%)

Number of cycles with endogenous LH surge (%)

Number of fertilized ova that cleaved

Number of clinical pregnancies/number replacement cycles (%)

Number of biochemical pregnancies as detected by sensitive method

Number of clinical abortions/number of clinical pregnancies (%)

IN VITRO FERTILIZATION

The first systematic studies of fertilization of rabbit eggs *in vitro* by spermatozoa recovered from the female tract were reported by Dauzier et al. (1954) and Thibault and Dauzier (1960, 1961). The development and application of IVF in farm animals has been reviewed extensively by Wright and Bondioli (1981). IVF is of practical significance to obtain large numbers of embryos for scientific investigations or for subsequent transfer to appropriate recipients (Table 23–12).

Collection and Capacitation of Sperm

Spermatozoa do not attain their full capacity for fertilization until after they are transported in the female reproductive tract. Sperm have to undergo further physiologic changes before they can pene-

TABLE 23–11. Transfer of Eggs Between Species

Donor	Recipient	Site of Transfer	Stage of Development or Age of Eggs at Transfer	Interval Between Transfer and Examination (Days)
Mouse	Rabbit	Oviduct	3½	3
	Rat	Ovarian capsule	1½, 2½, 3½	1–2
	Rat	Oviduct, uterus	2 cell, blastocyst	5–11
	Guinea pig	Uterus	3½	1–2
Rat	Mouse	Oviduct	2 to 8 cell	7–13
	Mouse	Uterus	6	1½
	Rabbit	Uterus	4½	1–2
	Rabbit	Oviduct	5, 7, to 11	2
	Golden hamster	Uterus	4 to 5 or pronuclear, morula	?
Golden hamster	Rat	Uterus	4 to 5 or pronuclear, morula	? or 2–3
Field vole	Mouse	Oviduct	2 and 8 cell	
Guinea pig	Mouse	Uterus	5	1–2
Rabbit	Rat	Uterus	1, 2, and 3	1–2
	Guinea pig	Uterus	1	1–2
	Mouse	Uterus	¼, 3	1–2
	Ferret	Uterus	1 cell, morula, blastocyst	2–4
	Cow	Uterus	2 to 3	½ or 2
Snowshoe hare	Rabbit	Oviduct	Pronuclear, 2–4 cell	6 or 13
Ferret	Rabbit	Oviduct	4	2–4
	Mink		6–7	5–23
Mink	Ferret	Uterus	6–8	6–25
Cow	Rabbit	Oviduct	4	5
Sheep	Goat		3 or 4	4–5
	Rabbit	Oviduct	8 cell	4
Goat	Sheep		5	Midterm
Pig	Rabbit	Oviduct	8, 32, 56, or 80 hrs after fertilization	1, 2, or 3
Squirrel	Rabbit	Oviduct	Follicular oocytes 10–12 hrs after hCG ± 24 hrs culture	2 or 3

(Courtesy of late Dr. C. Adams, Cambridge.)

TABLE 23–12. Species in which *In Vitro* Fertilization Has Been Accomplished*

Species	Fertilization *in Vitro*	Cleavage *in Vitro*	Birth of Young After Embryo Transfer
Mouse, rat, rabbit	+	+	+
Human	+	+	+
Cat	+	+/−	−
Hamster	+	−	−
Guinea pig, dog	+	−	−
Nonhuman primates	+/−	+/−	−
Cow, pig	+/−	−	−
Sheep, horse	−	−	−

*Accomplished (+); not reported or not accomplished (−); not routinely accomplished and/or not conclusively demonstrated (+/−). (Compiled by Bavister, 1982.)

trate the zona pellucida and fuse with the vitellus of the eggs (sperm capacitation) (Fig. 23–17). The development of defined conditions in which fertilization can take place outside the body has rapidly increased the depth of understanding of sperm capacitation and the sperm acrosome reaction. Most early experiments with IVF were unsuccessful because the sperm had not been capacitated, a term that refers to a modification of ejaculated sperm in the female reproductive tract, making them capable of fertilizing oocytes.

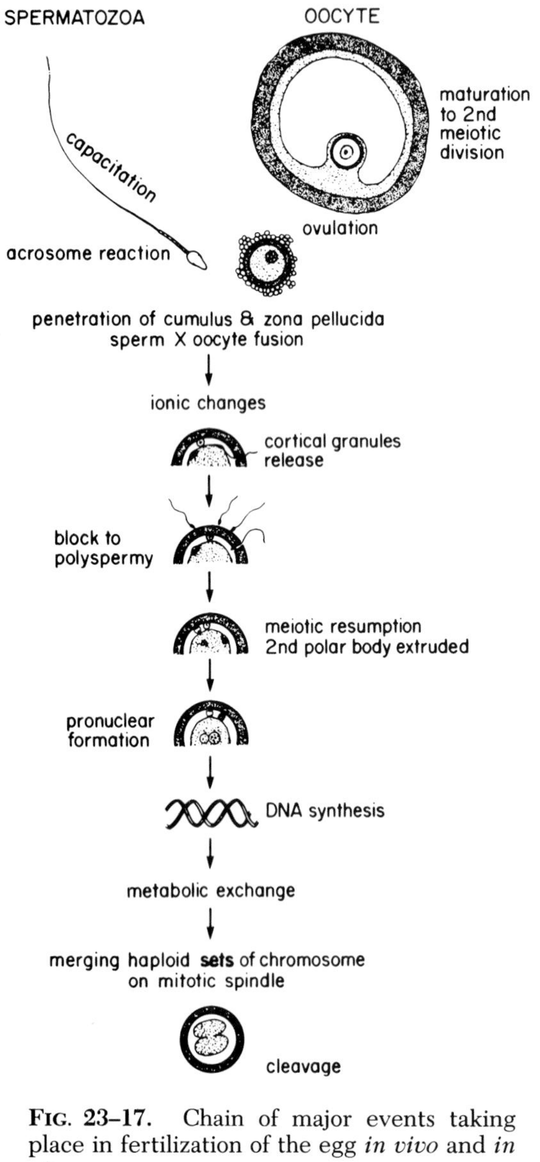

The molecular mechanism of capacitation is not known. One theory is that the membranes of the uncapacitated sperm cell are specifically stabilized to protect against damage in the female reproductive tract and that capacitation is the reversal of this stabilization. Another is that capacitation consists of the removal of inhibitors of acrosomal enzymes. In each species, capacitation is completed by the time most of the sperm come into contact with the oocytes. A probable explanation of capacitation invokes the decapacitation factor, which is thought to be produced in the epididymis or accessory sex glands of the male and bound to the sperm. Capacitation may involve the removal of the factor from the cell membrane of the sperm. Capacitated sperm are often obtained from the reproductive tract of a mated female. A common method is to flush medium through the uterus. The oviducts also contain capacitated sperm.

For some species, capacitation may be accomplished *in vitro*, although the mechanism as well as the duration of the process may differ from the *in vivo* phenomenon. Media of high ionic strength seem to promote *in vitro* capacitation.

Collection and Fertilization of Oocytes

Oocytes for IVF are usually obtained from the oviducts shortly after ovulation, but they may also be obtained from follicles or the surface of the ovary. While sperm can penetrate oocytes ranging in age from the immature primary stage before the breakdown of the nuclear membrane to aged oocytes recovered more than a day after ovulation, normal embryonic development does not result from the fertilization of oocytes at either extreme.

Spermatozoa readily become attached to the surface of the zona pellucida. The fertilizing sperm passes through this membrane, leaving a small slit that is noted

FIG. 23–17.   Chain of major events taking place in fertilization of the egg *in vivo* and *in vitro*.

many hours after penetration into the ova. Passage through the zona is rapid. The sperm undergoes remarkable changes with the ovum including (a) loss of sharpness of the outline of the sperm head and (b) appearance of the primary nucleoli within the enlarged sperm nucleus. The male pronucleus grows at a more rapid rate than that of the female pronucleus.

Several types of culture dishes have been used for IVF. The *in vitro* interactions between sperm and egg are shown for human (Fig. 23–18) and nonhuman primates.

In aged oocytes, the incidence of polyspermy is high. If the oocyte is too old, embryonic development is abnormal or fertilization may not take place at all. Unlike the sperm, the oocyte requires no exposure to the reproductive tract following release from the gonad to be fertile. Under some conditions, however, *in vitro* fertilization is enhanced by the presence of cells of the corona radiata and cumulus oophorus (Seidel et al., 1976).

The coculture of bovine morulae with bovine fibroblasts proved superior in supporting *in vitro* embryo hatching (Kuzan and Wright, 1982). The coculture of mouse embryos with other cell types reported that a higher percentage of mouse blastocysts hatched from the zona pellucida when cultured with a feeder layer of irradiated HeLa cells and other cell types.

In other systems, IVF proceeds normally when these cells have been removed mechanically or enzymatically with hyaluronidase.

In comparison to IVF, the percentage of oocytes fertilized *in vitro* is usually lower. In addition, fertilization may take longer to complete *in vitro* and the incidence of polyspermy may be increased.

Prerequisites and Criteria of IVF

There are several prerequisites for IVF:
1. Nuclear and cytoplasmic maturation of gametes in the gonads
2. Development of the fertilizability of gametes in the male and female reproductive tracts
3. An optimal number of fertilizable sperm with vigorous motility
4. A fertilizable ovum with a first polar body

Proof of IVF is the birth of normal young, genetically marked by means of the male parent and resulting from the transfer of the fertilized ova to a recipient female. As a result of the time and effort required to transfer embryos, however, other criteria are often used, such as penetration of sperm into the ooplasm, swelling of the sperm head, pronuclear formation, morphologically normal cleavage, blastocyst formation, demonstration of a Y chromosome in the embryo, breakdown of cortical granules, and evidence of a sperm tail in the ooplasm. None of these alone is sufficient proof of normal fertilization; parthenogenetic embryos, for example, also exhibit some of these traits.

GENETIC ENGINEERING

Fertilization involves the union of the DNA of the nucleus in the sperm head with the DNA in the nucleus of the ovum. The egg undergoes complex maturation changes known as *meiosis* before it is ready for fertilization. These changes begin during fetal life and are completed only after ovulation and sperm penetration. (Tables 23–13, 23–14)

Chromosomes and Genes

Chromosomal arrangements during mitosis and meiosis are illustrated in Figure 23–19. Normally, the ovum (X) is fertilized by sperm X or sperm Y. In abnormal cases of nondisjunction of oogenesis or spermatogenesis, fertilization may occur between an abnormal sperm and/or an abnormal egg resulting in various chromosomal anomalies (Tables 23–15 and 23–16). Structural anomalies of the chromosomes include translocation, deletions, rings, and inversions of chromosomes during either

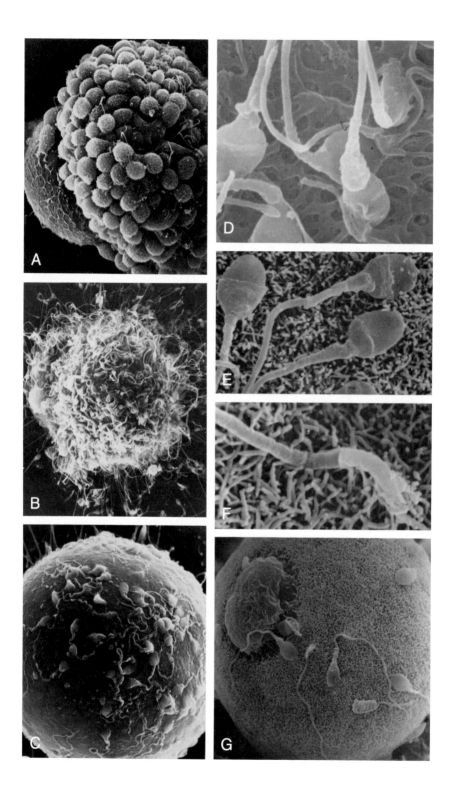

TABLE 23–13. Maturation of Oocytes and Sperm Capacitation for *In Vitro* Fertilization

Species	Oocyte Maturation* (Hours)	Sites of Sperm Capacitation	Sites of Fertilization
Cattle	20–30	Uterus (cattle, rabbit) Krebs-Ringer + BSA Oviduct or uterus of slaughtered cow or rabbit follicular fluid *In vitro* in high ionic-strength medium	Oviduct (rabbit, sheep, pig) *In vitro*
Sheep	24–28	Oviduct or uterus of ewe *In vitro* None	Oviduct of ewe *In vitro*
Pig	20–27	Oviduct or uterus in slaughtered sow Epididymal sperm in uterus or oviduct of slaughtered sow	Oviduct of sow *In vitro*

*Source of oocytes: ovarian follicle, oviduct, and matured *in vitro*.
BSA = bovine serum albumin.

mitosis or meiosis. Such anomalies affect individual autosomes or sex chromosomes.

The animal cell comprises a nucleus, protein-manufacturing units, and energy-production points. Spiraling double strands of atoms are the DNA (deoxyribonucleic acid), the master chemical of genes. The sequence or layout of those atoms contains all the instructions the cell needs to function. Recent advances in genetic engineering enable scientists to uncover, rearrange, and make copies, or clones, of genes. For example, each human cell contains some 100,000 genes. At least 22,000 of these genes have been isolated, and some of their specific functions have been identified.

Evaluation of Chromosomes of Ova

Morulae or blastocysts are incubated for 2 hours at 37°C in tissue culture (TC) medium 199 to which Colcemid (0.5 g/ml)

has been added. They are then placed in 0.9% sodium citrate in siliconized centrifuge tubes for 10 minutes and dissociated gently by aspiration with a siliconized Pasteur pipette. After further incubation for 10 minutes, the test tube is centrifuged at 800 rpm for 5 minutes, and the supernatant is removed and replaced with alcohol acetic fixative.

The preparations are stored overnight at 4°C, and after removal of the fixative by centrifugation, 45% aqueous acetic acid is added. The dissociated cells are resuspended following a second change of acetic acid, and small drops of the suspension are placed on a glass slide warmed to 56°C on a hot plate. The slides are then stained with carbol fuchsin.

Micromanipulation of Gametes, Embryos, and Zona Pellucida

Micromanipulation of embryos has shown that the embryos, in spite of a great

FIG. 23–18.   Scanning electron micrographs of human ova undergoing *in vitro* fertilization. *A.* Preovulatory oocyte partially surrounded by corona cells. Tails of spermatozoa are noted in between the corona cells. *B.* Some 100 spermatozoa may be noted on nonovulatory oocytes. *C.* Surface of the zona pellucida may appear smooth. This may facilitate observation of attached and penetrating spermatozoa. *D, E, F, G.* Sperm–egg interaction. Cytoplasmic processes of granulosa cells extend around sperm head. Most sperm lie flat on the zona pellucida, most bound sperm had lost their acrosomal caps, although some bound spermatozoa are under acrosomal reaction because the anterior part of sperm heads is vesiculated. Initially, the anterior part of the sperm head penetrates from the pore of zona almost tangentially. (*A, B, C,* courtesy of Professor P. Sundstrom of Sweden; *D, E, F, G,* courtesy of Professors H. Hoshiai, A. Tsuiki, K. Takahasi, and M. Suzuki of Japan.)

TABLE 23–14.   **Procedures and Physiologic Parameters of Gametes and Fertilization**

Stages and Procedures	Physiologic Parameters and Regulatory Mechanisms
Oocyte aspiration	Size of follicle Oocyte maturation, techniques, and timing Follicular fluid 　　Biochemistry 　　Hormone Cumulus mass Superovulation
Spermatozoa	Sperm maturity, motility, and concentration in media Sperm capacitation Acrosome reaction, changes in sperm surface Ion concentration and enzyme activity in milieu
In vitro fertilization	Quantity and quality of sperm in culture Sperm capacitation Basic culture medium Additives 　　Energy source 　　Sperm stimulants 　　Hormones 　　pH Gas phase (O_2 tension) Absence of seminal plasma Microscopic characteristics of fertilized ova
Criteria of *in vitro* fertilization	Penetration of spermatozoa within the vitellus Presence of sperm tail in the vitellus Presence of male and female pronuclei in the egg Presence of two polar bodies in the perivitelline space Cleavage and formation of two blastomeres with equal size, shape and no fragmentation
Embryo transfer	State of embryo Cleavage rate and regularity of blastomeres Developmental stage of endometrium Transfer technique

(McLaren, 1980)

reduction in their cell number, are able to develop through early cleavage (Willadsen and Polge, 1981) and to blastocyst formation (Ozil et al., 1982). The simple bisection of fully compacted late morulae or early blastocysts allows the production of identical twins in routine embryo transplantation procedures. Methods of producing identical twins, however, can only be fully explored in association with techniques of cryopreservation, which would permit transfer of each "half" of the same embryo at different times (Fig. 23–20). After the first irreversible cellular differentiation that occurs at the blastocyst stage, it is still possible to produce identical cattle twins by bisection of the day-8 blastocyst (Ozil, 1983).

Extensive investigations have been carried out on surface properties of the zona pellucida (Phillips and Shalgi, 1980), on the specificity of sperm–egg interactions (Yanagimachi, 1977), and on the mechanics of fertilization (Shalgi and Phillips, 1980). The transfer of pronuclei between eggs has been employed to assess changes induced in the development of embryos following an unusual pronuclear history. Eggs with two female pronuclei can result from various forms of parthenogenetic activation, or from the use of micromanipulation to remove and insert specific pronuclei into the oocytes. Gynogenetic embryos, those containing two female pronuclei, develop abnormally; this is especially evident in their extraembryonic tissues. Micromanipulation is also used to establish mammalian eggs containing two male pronuclei.

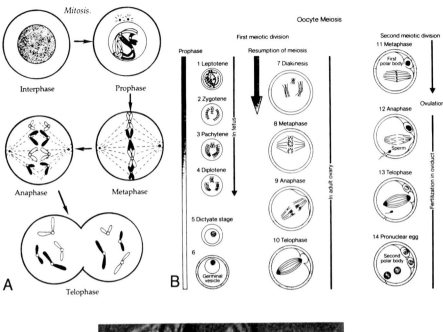

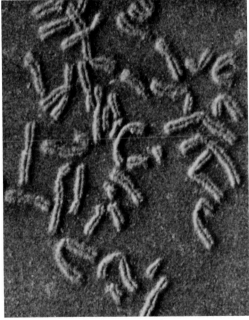

FIG. 23–19. Chromosome arrangement during mitosis and meiosis. *A.* Chromosome arrangement during mitosis. (Feingold, M. and Pashaya, H., 1983). *B.* Oocyte meiosis. For simplicity, only three pairs of chromosomes are depicted. Prophase stages (1 to 4) of the first meiotic division that occur in most mammals during fetal life. The meiotic process is arrested at the diplotene stage (first meiotic arrest), and the oocyte enters the dictyate stages (5 to 16). When meiosis is resumed, the first maturation division is completed (7 to 11). Ovulation occurs usually at the metaphase II stage (11), and the second meiotic division (12 to 14) takes place in the oviduct only following sperm penetration. (Tsafriri, A., et al., 1983). *C,* Scanning electron micrograph of chromosomes.

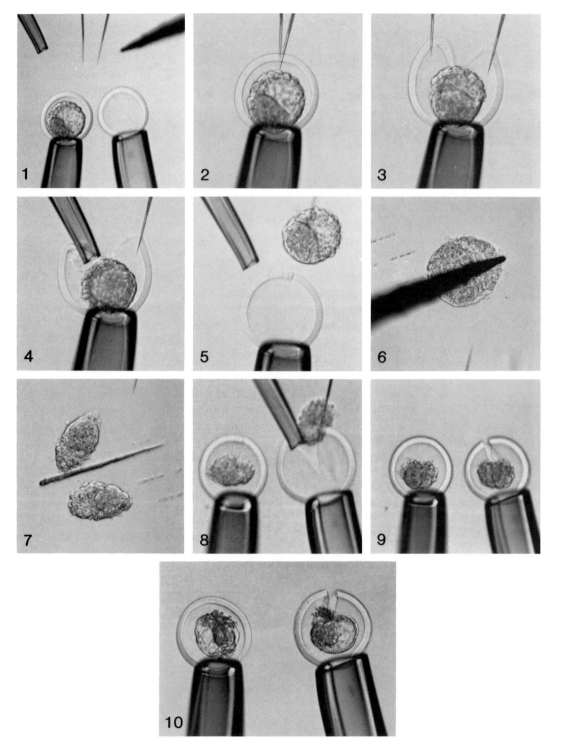

(Legend appears on facing page.)

TABLE 23–15. Types and Physiologic Mechanisms of Chromosome Anomalies

Types of chromosome anomalies	Monosomy	Absence of one chromosome
	Trisomy: single	One additional chromosome
	double	Two additional chromosomes
	Polyploidy	One or two additional haploid sets
	Structural anomaly of chromosomes	Unbalanced chromosome constitution
Physiologic mechanisms of chromosome anomalies	Errors during oogenesis causing chromosomally abnormal ova	
	Errors during spermatogenesis causing chromosomally abnormal sperm	
	Errors during early stages of cleavage of zygote	

TABLE 23–16. Normal and Abnormal Sex-Chromosome Constitutions Arising at Fertilization

		OVA		
		Normal	Nondisjunctive	
Normal		X	XX	O
	X	XX (= normal female)	XXX	XO
	Y	XY (= normal male)	XXY	YO
Sperm nondisjunction	XY	XXY		
	XX	XXX		
	YY	XYY		
	O	XO		

An O sperm or ovum is one that carries neither an X nor a Y chromosome. Nondisjunctive gametes arise through faulty sharing-out (nondisjunction) of the sex chromosomes. YO individuals probably are not viable; XXX individuals, in humans, are abnormal females. (McLaren, 1980)

Several techniques of embryo micromanipulation have been used to produce identical twins in cattle, sheep, and pigs (Willadsen, 1981, 1982, 1983; Willadsen and Polge, 1981). The success of the technique depends on the use of agar gel to seal incisions made in the zona pellucida during micromanipulation: the agar protects the blastomeres from damage by uterine secretions and leukocytes until the embryo has developed sufficiently to survive *in utero* without a zona (Fig. 23–21, Table 23–17).

Eggs are obtained by superovulation and denuded of cumulus cells with 0.1% hyaluronidase. Zona pellucidae are then

---

FIG. 23–20. Method of bisection of cow blastocysts by micromanipulation. *1*. Six microinstruments are placed in the optical field of an inverted microscope. Two micropipettes controlled by type-B micromanipulators hold the blastocyst and the empty zona pellucida by negative pressure. *2*. Instruments with a sharp tip in front of the blastocyst are controlled by a type-A micromanipulator. The micropipette on the left and the microscalpel on the right are controlled by a type-B micromanipulator. This equipment allows the bisection of 6 to 8 blastocysts per hour. (From Willadsen, S.M., (1982). Micromanipulation of embryos of the large domestic species. *In* Mammalian Egg Transfer. C.E. Adams (ed.). Boca Raton, FL, CRC Press.) *2, 3*. The two sharp microneedles cut the zona pellucida over as short a distance as possible along the middle. The blastocyst is subsequently rotated through 90° with the two microneedles to show the slit. *4, 5*. The micropipette is introduced through the slit inside the zona while a small volume of medium is injected to expel the embryo. *6, 7*. Bisection of the blastocyst is achieved using the microscalpel along the sagittal plane. *8, 9*. Using the suction of the micropipette, each "half" embryo is put back into an empty zona pellucida. *10*. "Half" (demi) embryos are then incubated at 37°C for 2 hours. They reconstitute their blastocele, and it is possible to distinguish again the inner cell mass in each "half" blastocyst. The cells destroyed during the bisection adhere to the outer surface of the "half" blastocyst. (From Ozil, J.P. (1983). Production of identical twins by bisection of blastocysts in the cow. J. Reprod. Fertil. *69*, 463.)

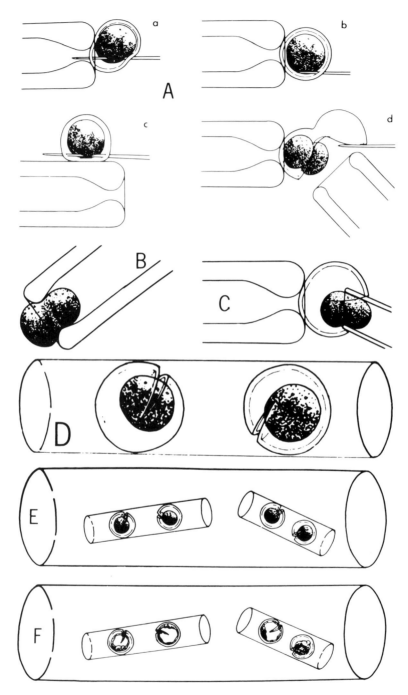

FIG. 23–21.   Micromanipulation of gametes and embryos. *A.* Removal of the zona pellucida. *B.* Separation of blastomeres. *C.* Insertion of single blastomeres into evacuated zona pellucida. *D.* First agar embedding. *E.* Agar chip before transfer to the sheep oviduct after recovery from the sheep. The position of the individual embryo within the chip allows it to be readily identified after culture. (Willadsen, 1982.)

TABLE 23–17.   Sperm–egg Interaction in the Presence of Vitellus (Intact Egg) and when the Vitellus Is Absent (Isolated Zona Pellucida)

Vitellus Absent (Isolated Zona)	Vitellus Present (Intact Egg)
Sperm protease(s) releases peptides ↓	Sperm protease(s) releases peptides ↓
Peptides diffuse through zona	Peptides diffuse through zona ↓
	"Central component" of peptide reacts with vitellus ↓
	Vitellus alters the peptide or a mechanism is triggered that releases a new peptide ↓
	Vitelline-dependent peptides diffuse outward towards sperm–zona interface ↓
	Sperm-activation/penetration inhibition mechanisms initiated ↓
Rapid binding is initiated ↓	Rapid binding is prevented, resulting in *attachment*, followed by binding
Rapid binding is completed ↓	
Penetration fails to occur	

(Adapted from Hartman, 1983)

isolated when eggs are drawn into a micropipette with an inner diameter of about 60 μm, and then the contents are expelled. The zonae are separated from the vitelli and washed several times (Hartman, 1983).

The blastomeres of two- to eight-cell horse embryos recovered surgically 1 to 3 days after ovulation from pony mares were mechanically separated and inserted, in various combinations, into evacuated pig zona pellucidae to make "half" (demi) and "quarter" micromanipulated embryos. These are then embedded in agar and cultured *in vivo* in the ligated oviducts of ewes for 3.5 to 5 days to allow development to the late morula–early blastocyst stage. Subsequent surgical or nonsurgical transfer of "half" and "quarters" embryos to mares resulted in pregnancies, including monozygotic pairs (Allen and Pashen, 1984).

USE AND LIMITATIONS OF EMBRYO TRANSFER AND RELATED TECHNIQUES

Embryo transfer is a useful technique that permits critical experimental approaches to problems in genetics, cytology, animal breeding, immunology, evolution, and the physiology and biochemistry of reproduction. For example, the technique can be used to evaluate the relative contributions of the aging oocyte and the aging reproductive tract to decreased reproduction in older animals (Maurer and Foote, 1971).

Successful embryo transfer depends on various factors including superovulation, estrus detection in the donor and recipients, insemination of the donor, recovery of embryos, short-term storage of embryos *in vitro*, embryo transfer, proper management of the recipient through parturition, and keeping the progeny healthy until useable or saleable. If even one of these steps is done poorly, the entire process may fail. When all treated donors are considered, the average number of calves produced per superovulation is between 3 and 4, even with the best technology. The median number is 2 and the mode, zero. Occasionally, litters of more than 20 calves are produced, but this occurs less than once in 100 attempts. The major contribution to this variability is the unpredictable response to superovulation; the second greatest problem is that many ova are unfertilized or abnormal. Because it is possible to induce superovulation in cows 4 or ble to induce superovulation in cows 4 or 5 times a year, more than 10 calves can be obtained per cow per year on the average.

Application

Embryo transfer can be used to rapidly increase rare blood lines, to obtain more offspring from valuable females, and to accelerate genetic progress by facilitating progeny testing of females and thus reducing the generation interval. Embryo transfer methods, however, are not nearly as effective as AI for making genetic progress (Land, 1977). One problem is that reproductive rates of donors are increased at the expense of decreased reproductive rates of the recipients because the females in the recipient pool frequently remain nonpregnant for prolonged periods until an embryo is transferred to them (Seidel and Seidel, 1978).

The transport of frozen embryos over long distances can be an inexpensive means of exporting livestock. Frozen bovine embryos were first transported successfully from New Zealand to Australia (Bilton and Moor, 1977).

Transferring either a single embryo into each uterine horn of an unmated cow or a second ovum to the horn contralateral to the CL of a recipient cow that conceived a few days earlier is more effective than mild superovulation for the production of twins in cattle (Rowson et al., 1971; Anderson, 1978).

In pig breeding, embryo transfer is of limited value. The transfer of supersized litters to unmated females or of additional embryos to previously bred recipients does not appreciably increase litter size. One important use of embryo transfer in swine, however, is the introduction of new genetic material into specific pathogen-free herds.

Superovulation is not very effective in horses. A single ovum, however, can usu-

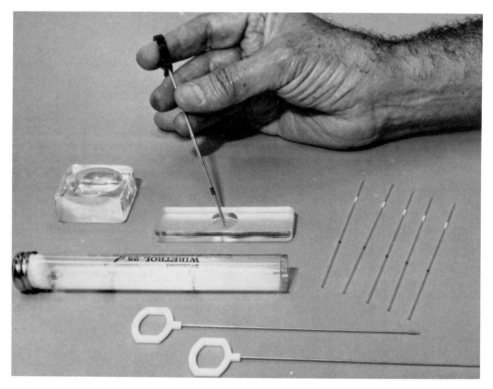

FIG. 23–22. Wiretrol for micropipetting: color-coded permanent calibration line permits one-hand operation and eliminates mouth aspiration of micropipetting.

ally be recovered nonsurgically during each estrous cycle 6 or 7 days after ovulation. Furthermore, nonsurgical transfer has been successful with mares (Oguri and Tsutsumi, 1974). It appears that embryo transfer may be especially useful for obtaining additional progeny from old, infertile brood mares.

Future Developments

Some progress has already been made with superovulation of prepuberal animals (Onuma et al., 1970; Wright et al., 1976; Trounson et al., 1977), although pregnancy rates from transferring calf embryos are low (Seidel et al., 1971). Another exciting area is the sexing of embryos, which will be of special significance but is expensive and time-consuming. About two thirds of older bovine embryos can be sexed successfully before transfer (Hare and Betteridge, 1978). The production of exact genetic copies of outstanding animals by cloning is also possible. Other problems remain to be solved before embryo transfer techniques reach a practical scale comparable to AI.

INSTRUMENTATION, WATER AND AIR FILTRATION, AND CULTURE MEDIA

Equipment and laboratory supplies for embryo transfer, IVF, and embryo manipulation are listed in Tables 23–18 to 23–20 and Figure 23–23.

Ultrapure Water

Distilled and bottled water leach new organics as little as 1 hour after storage. Unfortunately, storage problems are just one of the drawbacks to using distilled or bottled water. There are also the problems of higher operating and maintenance costs and contaminant carryover. Laboratory water purification has undergone dramatic changes in the 1980s. Chemists, life scientists, and medical technicians are now routinely concerned with impurity levels that were impossible to measure 10 years ago. Today, deionization, reverse osmosis, carbon absorption, and membrane

microfiltration are in some respects superior to distillation. Various systems of water ultrafiltration are now available commercially. These systems cost less than distilled or bottled water, and there is no contaminant carryover. Unlike stills, which require regular acid cleaning, ultrafiltration cartridges can be replaced in minutes.

Air Filtration

Lamina airflow is airflow in which the entire body of air within a designated space moves with uniform velocity in a single direction along parallel flow lines. Lamina-flow biologic safety cabinets are devices designed to minimize biohazards inherent in work with low- and moderate-risk biologic agents. Vertical lamina-flow containment hoods provide not only product protection by using a filtered downflow of air but also provide operator protection through a negative pressure air barrier created along the front opening. With proper aseptic conditions and good laboratory procedures, risk levels are substantially reduced.

CULTURE, CO-CULTURE, AND ORGAN CULTURE

Oviductal Secretions

The epithelial cells of the ovine and bovine oviduct secrete two classes of proteins. The first class is uniformly secreted throughout the estrous cycle and represents a small proportion of the total protein output, while the second class displays a cyclic pattern of secretion and is composed mainly of polypeptides. These two latter proteins, detected soon after estrus, remain in the oviduct fluid for the same time frame as the ova (Gandolfi et al., 1989). Oviductal levels of *de nova* synthesized proteins are highest during estrus and decline thereafter. Some 30 to 40 individual polypeptides are secreted, some of which are secreted at a greater rate during estrus. After ovulation, in spite of the surrounding cumulus and corona radiata cells, significant amounts of oviductal gly-

TABLE 23–18. Equipment and Laboratory Supplies for Embryo Transfer

Glassware	Petri dishes, pipettes, embryo dishes, thermos flask for short-term storage of embryos and assorted laboratory glass-/polyware	
Instruments and equipment	Instrument kits for recipients Refrigerator Deep freeze Laundry bin Water baths Microscope and spare bulbs Thermometers Hot air oven	CO_2 incubator Washing machine, dryer, autoclave, dry-heat sterilizer Distillation units to produce distilled ultrafiltered water Small gas sterilizer and refills Liquid nitrogen container with mobile base Instrument trolley Operating lamp
Biologic safety cabinets	Ventilated cabinets for personnel protection, with uncirculated inward flow of air away from the operator Ventilated cabinet for personnel and product protection with open front with inward airflow for personnel protection, HEPA-filtered mass recirculated airflow for product protection; exhaust air is filtered Closed-front ventilated cabinet, filtered with rubber gloves, with negative pressure of gas-tight construction	
Sterile and cleaning	Sterilization bags Sterile market indicator tape Laboratory coats, caps, and masks	Surgical gowns, caps, parturition gowns, and masks Hair clippers and spare blades Scrub brushes, scrub fluid dispensers

TABLE 23–19. Manipulation and Micromanipulation of Eggs and Morulae

Techniques	Definitions/Applications
Micromanipulation of zona pellucida and related techniques	Removal of excess pronuclei Zona drilling by mechanical force "Puncture" with acid Tryod, pronase, or trypsin solution with micropipette "Cracking" using two fine glass hooks controlled by micromanipulator "PZD" partial opening using mechanical force only, followed by microinsemination
Transfer of early germ cells	Transfer of male germ cells into PVS, chromosomes of male and female gametes undergo characteristics of species
Nuclear, cell and blastomere transfer	Transfer part of cell and especially nuclei or whole cell (fusion of cytoblast and karyoplasts with host cell is inhibited by electrofusion or Sendai virus)
Blastocyst biopsy	One or two blastomeres are removed (for preimplantation diagnosis of sex or genetic anomalies), allowing remaining embryos to develop into individual offspring
Cloning (nuclear substitution)	Nuclear transplant into enucleated egg, to enable continual propagation of particular gene, trait, and species (to preserve endangered species)
Transgenic animals	Cloned genes introduced into somatic cells or embryos (for analysis of molecular mechanisms of laboratory and farm animals)
Genetic	Haploid embryos from microsurgical removal of one pronucleus Haploid embryo from bisection of one-cell fertilized egg Microsurgical production of homozygous-diploid uniparental young Genetic analysis before implantation Nuclear transplantation from and in preimplantation embryo Microsurgical enucleation of tripronuclear zygote
Manipulation of gametes and embryos	Use of "cytochalasin B" microfilament inhibitor to inhibit cytokinesis Use of cytoskeletal inhibitors for pronuclear removal Prenatal diagnosis and gene therapy *In situ* hybridization and polymerase chain reaction (amplification of DNA sequence from single cell)

coprotein bind firmly to the porcine zona; however, the glycoproteins do not form a mucin coat, as seen with rabbit oviductal ova.

The mammalian oviduct has the ability to support the development of embryos across many species, indicating that many of the beneficial effects of the oviduct en-

TABLE 23–20. Assisted Reproductive Technology and Andrology (ARTA)

Assisted reproduction	*In vitro* fertilization and uterine embryo transfer (IVF-ET) Gamete intrafallopian transfer (GIFT) Pronuclear-stage tubal transfer (PROST) Zygote intrafallopian transfer (ZIFT) Tubal embryo-stage transfer, (embryos in premorula cleavage stages) (TEST) (TET) Surrogate motherhood (SM) Donation of oocytes of embryos (fresh or cryopreserved) Cryopreservation of oocytes or embryos; embryo banks Early pregnancy *in vitro* using artificially perfused uterus
Insemination	Intrauterine insemination (IUI) Intraperitoneal insemination (IPI)
Microseparation and micromanipulation	Drilling of zona pellucida Microinsemination sperm transfer into pervitelline space or partial zonal dissection or zona cracking Separation of an embryo into identical twins Isolation of blastomeres
Microremoval and microfusion	Removal of an accessory pronucleus Removal of one or more blastomeres (embryo biopsy) Removal of zona pellucida Fusion of 2-, 4-, 8-blastomere embryos and/or morulae Enucleation of blastomeres
Supporting techniques	Uterine blood flow Ultrasonography Pelvioscope surgery, microsurgery, and laser surgery Laparoscopic and transcervical procedures

vironment may actually be nonspecific with regard to species. Extensive investigations were conducted using the oviduct *in vivo* or *in vitro* (cell or organ culture). Pig early embryos (one- to 8-cell stage) cultured in "organ co-culture" in mouse excised oviducts, can develop to the morula and blastocyst stage (Krisher et al., 1989). The rate of this embryonic development of pig embryos is enhanced when the oviduct is taken from mice mated to fertile or vasectomized males. Embryos may be transferred directly in the oviduct, or they can be placed in agar chips before placement in the oviduct. Bovine embryos can develop in *in vivo* sheep and rabbit oviduct co-culture (Westhusin et al., 1989). Embryo viability was similar between both hosts; however, embryo recovery was slightly lower from the rabbit host as compared to the sheep.

Culture and Co-culture

Several culture and co-culture media have been used for *in vitro* physiologic maturation and subsequent cleavage at various degrees: modified Krebs-Ringer's bicarbonate, modified Dulbecco's, TC 199, modified Ham's F-10, Whitten medium, Eagle's basal medium with Hank's salts, and modified minimum essential medium (MEM) with Earl's salts.

In human IVF centers, animal tissues are used in human co-culture systems to evaluate pregnancy rates after embryo replacement. Fetal cattle uterine fibroblast monolayers are used to evaluate *in vitro* development and implantation of human embryos. Fetal uterine endometrial linings were obtained from healthy bovine fetuses and cells after several subcultures are used for co-culture. Human embryos co-cultured with cattle monolayers are transferred back to patients. The pregnancy rate is increased when human embryos co-cultured with human ampullary cells are replaced back into patients.

Macromolecular Supplementation

The preparation of serum added into maturation medium requires special attention. The serum obtained after coagu-

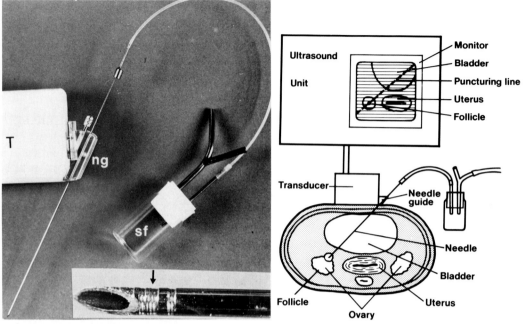

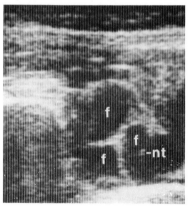

FIG. 23–23. (*Left*) Aspiration equipment for ultrasonically guided percutaneous follicle puncture. *T*, transducer; *ng*, needle guide; *sf*, sampling flask. (*Inset, left*) Needle tip with the shallow tracks (arrow) in the needle tip. (*Right*) Schematic illustration of the ultrasonically guided puncture technique. (*Bottom*) Illustration of ultrasonically guided puncture of a human follicle. The white echo inside the follicle (f) represents the needle tip (nt). (Courtesy of R. Wikland.)

lation of whole blood (delayed centrifuged [DC] serum) contains substances toxic to embryos. DC serum toxicity can be avoided completely by a serum preparation method that prevents the platelet-release reaction.

Several biologic culture media have been used for the manipulation of embryos (see Appendix). Usually, 50 mg of streptomycin sulfate and 100,000 IU of potassium penicillin G are added per liter, but other concentrations and other antibiotics and antifungal agents are frequently used as well. Media should be forced through a filter of 0.45 μm or smaller to remove bacteria.

Media may contain either bovine serum albumin (BSA) or blood serum (often from fetal calves) that has been inactivated by being held at 56°C for 30 minutes. BSA is usually added at 0.3 to 1%, but concentrations from 0.1% to 50% have been used. All media except the modified phosphate-buffered saline are bicarbonate-buffered and therefore require an atmosphere of 5% CO_2 to maintain proper pH. This is accomplished with a mixture of 5% CO_2 in air, or better, 5% CO_2, 5% O_2 and 90%

N_2. A CO_2 incubator or small, gassed, and airtight containers may be used. When media must be kept in an air environment (without CO_2) for long periods, 25 ml HEPES buffer is usually added and the NaCl decreased to maintain proper osmolality.

Phenol red, 1 to 20 mg/L is often added as a pH indicator. The pH of media may range from 7 to 8, but best results are obtained between 7.2 and 7.6. The osmolality may be adjusted from 250 to 320 mOsm/kg by varying the NaCl concentration. Osmolalities between 270 and 300 mOsm/kg are most commonly used for embryos. Water is the principal ingredient, and purity is important. Double distillation or glass distillation of deionized water is usually adequate.

Modified, balanced salt solutions such as Krebs-Ringer bicarbonate support *in vitro* fertilization. The acrosome reaction seems to occur much more readily in media containing serum albumin in the form of either heat-treated serum or bovine serum albumin (Bavister and Yanagimachi, 1977). It is also critical to provide an energy source, usually glucose or pyruvate, to support spermatozoal motility and the metabolism of the oocytes.

Development of early cleavage stage embryos is enhanced in the presence of oviduct epithelial cells, trophoblastic vesicles, uterine cells, or kidney cells. In some techniques, a whole chick embryo culture system is used: Embryos in agar chips are placed directly into the amniotic cavity of a developing chick embryo (Blakewood and Godke, 1989). Recovery of the agar chips is efficient, and embryonic development and viability are superior to that achieved *in vitro* for early cleavage stage goat and cattle embryos. In other techniques, bovine embryos (or blastomeres) are placed into hydrogel chambers, which are then placed into the peritoneal cavity of rodents.

Because most mammalian intercellular fluid environments function at pH 7.2 to 7.35, the commercial media solutions for embryo recovery and culture are adjusted within this range. Osmolarity is likewise monitored for each batch of media to maintain a constant quality control. The biologic media are prepared using sterile deionized and distilled water and processed through a 0.2 μm membrane filter. Bottle containers are sterilized in an autoclave with 260°F at 20 psi for 45 minutes. The object of these media is directed specifically to embryo maintenance and growth promotion ability. Media solutions are quality controlled at 24- to 32-hour embryo culture assays.

REFERENCES

Adams, C.E. (1983a). Egg transfer in carnivores and rodents, between species, and to extopic sites. *In* Mammalian Egg Transfer. Boca Raton, FL, CRC Press.

Adams, C.E. (1983b). Egg transfer in the rabbit. *In* Mammalian Egg Transfer. Boca Raton, FL, CRC Press.

Allen, W.R. (1984). Hormonal control of early pregnancy in the mare. Anim. Reprod. Sci. *7*, 284.

Allen, W.R. and Pashen, R.L. (1984). Production of monozygotic (identical twins) by embryo micromanipulation. J. Reprod. Fertil. *71*, 607.

Anderson, G.B. (1978). Methods of producing twins in cattle. Theriogenology *9*, 3.

Bavister, B.D. (1982). In vitro fertilization: principles, practice and potential. *In* In Vitro Fertilization and Embryo Transfer. E.S.E. Hafez and K. Semm (eds.). Lancaster, England, MTP Press.

Bavister, B.D. and Yanagimachi, R. (1977). The effects of sperm extracts and energy sources on the motility and acrosome reaction of hamster spermatozoa in vitro. Biol. Reprod. *16*, 228.

Beidl, A., Peters, H. and Hofstattler, R. (1922). Experimentelle studien uber die einnistung und weiter entwiclung des eies im uterus. Z. Gerburtsh. Gynak, *84*, 60.

Betterridge, K.J. (1977). Embryo Transfer in Farm Animals. Ottawa, Canada Dept. Agric. Monograph 16, 92 pp.

Bilton, R.J. and Moore, N.W. (1977). Successful transport of frozen cattle embryos from New Zealand to Australia. J. Reprod. Fertil. *50*, 363.

Blakewood, E.G. and Godke, R.A. (1989). A method using the chick embryo amnion for mammalian embryo culture. J. Tissue Culture Meth. *12*, 73–76.

Brackett, B.G., Killen, D.E. and Pearce, M.D. (1971). Cleavage of rabbit ova inseminated in vitro after removal of follicular cells and zonae pellucidae. Fertil. Steril. *22*, 816–828.

Brackett, B.G. (1973). Methods in Mammalian Reproduction. J.C. Daniel, Jr. (ed.). New York, Academic Press.

Britt, J.H. (1986). Induction and synchronization of ovulation. *Reproduction in Farm Animals.* 4th Ed. Philadelphia, Lea & Febiger.

Church, R.B. and Shea, B.F. (1977). The role of embryo transfer in cattle improvement programs. Can. J. Anim. Sci. *57*, 33.

Daniel, Jr., J.D. (1971). Methods in Mammalian Embryology. San Francisco, W.H. Freeman.

Dauzier, L., Thibault, C. and Wintenberger, S. (1954). La fecondation in vitro de l'oeuf de la lapine. C.R. Acad. Sci., Paris *238*, 844–845.

Dukelow, W.R. (1978). Methods in mammalian reproduction. Daniel, Jr., J.C. (ed.). New York, Academic Press.

Dukelow, W.R. (1983). Ovum recovery and embryo transfer in primates. *In* Mammalian Egg Transfer. C.E. Adams (ed.). Boca Raton, Florida, CRC Press.

Dziuk, P.J. (1971). Obtaining eggs and embryos from sheep and pigs. *In* Methods in Mammalian Embryology. J.C. Daniel, Jr. (ed.). San Francisco, W.H. Freeman.

Elsden, R.P., Hasler, J.F. and Seidel, G.E., Jr. (1976). Nonsurgical recovery of bovine eggs. Theriogenology *6*, 523.

Elsden, R.P., Nelson, L.D. and Seidel, G.E. Jr. (1978). Superovulating cows with follicle-stimulating hormone and pregnant mare serum gonadotrophin. Theriogenology *9*, 17.

Feingold, M. and Pashaya, H. (1983). Chapter 2. *In* The Chromosome, Genetics and Birth Defects in Clinical Practice. Boston, Little, Brown.

Fleming, A.D. (1982). Developmental capability of superovulated ova. *In* In-vitro Fertilization and Embryo Transfer. E.S.E. Hafez and K. Semm (eds.). Lancaster, England, MTP Press.

Foote, R.H. and Onuma, H. (1970). Superovulation, ovum collection, culture and transfer: a review. J. Dairy Sci. *53*, 1681.

Frachi, L.L. and Baker, T.G. (1973). Oogenesis and follicular growth. *In* Human Reproduction: Conception and Contraception. E.S.E. Hafez and T.N. Evans, (eds.). New York, Harper & Row.

Gandolfi, F., Brevini, T.A.L., Richardson, L., Brown, C.R. and Moor, R.M. (1989). Characterization of proteins secreted by sheep oviduct epithelial cells and their function in embryonic development. Development *106*, 303–312.

Gould, K.G. (1979). Fertilization in vitro of nonhuman primate ova: present status and rationale for further development of the technique. Report to the Ethics Advisory Board, HEW. Washington, DC, US Government Printing Office.

Gould, K.G. (1983). Ovum recovery and in-vitro fertilization in the chimpanzee. Fertil. Steril. *40*, 378–383.

Hare, W.C.D. and Betteridge, K.J. (1978). Relationship of embryo sexing to other methods of prenatal sex determination in farm animals: a review. Theriogenology *9*, 27.

Hartmann, J.F. (1983). Mammalian fertilization: gamete surface interactions in vitro. *In* Mechanism and Control of Animal Fertilization. New York, Academic Press.

Heape, W. (1890). Preliminary note on the transplantation and growth of mammalian ova within a uterine foster mother. Proc. Roy. Soc. (London) *48*, 457.

Hendricks, A.G. (1971). Embryology of the Baboon. Chicago, University of Chicago Press.

Hoshiai, H., Tsuiki, A., Takahashi, K. and Suzuki, M. (1984). Sperm-egg interactions by scanning electron microscopy. Arch. Androl. *12*, 146.

Hunter, R.H.F. (1982). Reproduction of Farm Animals. London, Longman.

Iritani, A. and Niwa, K. (1977). Capacitation of bull spermatozoa and fertilization in vitro of cattle follicular oocytes matured in culture. J. Reprod. Fertil. *50*, 119.

Iritani, A., Niwa, K. and Imai, H. (1978). In-vitro fertilization of pig follicular oocytes matured in culture. Biol. Reprod. *18* (Suppl. 1, 14a).

Jeffcoat, L.G. and Whitwell, K. (1976). Twinning as a cause of foetal and neonatal loss in Thoroughbred mares. J. Comp. Pathol. *83*, 91–96.

Jinno, M., Iizuka, B.A., Sandow, B.A. and Hodgen, G.D. (1990). In vitro maturation of oocytes assisted reproduction. Tech. Androl. (ARTA) *1*, 54–68.

Kanagawa, H., Inoue, T. and Ishikawa, T. (1982). Ovulation rate in beef cattle after repeated treatments with gonadotropins and prostaglandin. *In* In-Vitro Fertilization and Embryo Transfer. E.S.E. Hafez and K. Semm (eds.). Lancaster, England, MTP Press.

Katska, L. (1984). Comparison of two methods for recovery of ovarian oocytes from slaughter cattle. Anim. Reprod. Sci. *7*, 461–463.

Keuhl, T.J. and Dukelow, W.R. (1979). Maturation and in vitro fertilization of follicular oocytes of the squirrel monkey *(Saimiri sciureus)*. Biol. Reprod. *21*, 545.

Koos, R.D., Jaccarino, F.J., Magaril, R.A. and LeMaire, W.J. (1984). Perfusion of the rat ovary in vitro: methodology, induction of ovulation and pattern of steroidogenesis. Biol. Reprod. *31*, 1135–1141.

Krisher, R.L., Petters, R.M. and Johnson, B.H. (1989). Effect of oviductal condition on the development of one-cell porcine embryos in mouse or rat oviducts maintained in organ culture. Theriogenology *32*, 885–892.

Kuzan, F.B. and Wright, R.W., Jr. (1982). Observations of the development of bovine morulae on various cellular and noncellular substrata. J. Anim. Sci. *54*, 811–816.

Kvansnickii, A.V. (1951). Interbreed ova transplantation. Sovetsk. Zootech. *1*, 36.

Land, R.B. (1977). The genetics of breed improvement. *In* Embryo Transfer in Farm Animals. K.J. Betteridge (ed.). Ottawa, Canada, Dept. Agric. Monograph 16.

Marden, W.G.R. and Chang, M.C. (1952). Aerial transport of mammalian ova for transplantation. Science *115*, 705.

Maurer, R.R. and Foote, R.H. (1971). Maternal aging and embryonic mortality in the rabbit. (I.) Repeated superovulation, embryo culture, and transfer. J. Reprod. Fertil. *25*, 329–341.

McGaughey, R.W. and Polge, C. (1971). Cytogenetic analysis of pig oocytes matured in vitro. J. Exp. Zool. *176*, 383.

McLaren, A. (1980). Fertilization, cleavage and implantation. *In* Reproduction in Farm Animals. 4th Ed. E.S.E. Hafez (ed.). Philadelphia, Lea & Febiger.

Miller, B.G. and Armstrong, D.T. (1982). Infertility in superovulated immature rats: role of ovarian steroid hypersecretion. Biol. Reprod. *26*, 861–868.

Moor, R.M. and Trounson, A.O. (1977). Hormonal and follicular factors affecting maturation of sheep oocytes in vitro and their subsequent developmental capacity. J. Reprod. Fertil. *49*, 101.

Murray, F.A. (1978). Embryo transfer in large domestic mammals. *In* Methods in Mammalian Reproduction. J.C. Daniel, Jr. (ed.). New York, Academic Press.

Newcomb, R. and Rowson, L.E.A. (1975). Conception rate after uterine transfer of cow eggs in relation to sychronization of estrus and age of eggs. J. Reprod. Fertil. *43*, 539.

Nicholas, J.S. (1933). Development of transplanted rat eggs. Proc. Soc. Exp. Biol. Med. *30*, 1111.

Niwa, K., Hosoi, Y., O'Hara, K. and Iritani, A. (1983). Fertilization in vitro of rabbit eggs with or without follicular cells by epididymal spermatozoa capacitated in a chemically defined medium. Anim. Reprod. Sci. *6*, 143–149.

Oguri, N. and Tsutsumi, Y. (1974). Non-surgical egg transfer in mares. J. Reprod. Fertil. *42*, 313.

Oguri, N. and Tsutsumi, Y. (1982). Non-surgical transfer of equine embryos. *In* In Vitro Fertilization and Embryo Transfer. E.S.E. Hafez and K. Semm (eds.). Lancaster, England, MTP Press.

Onuma, H., Hahn, J. and Foote, R.H. (1970). Factors affecting superovulation, fertilization and recovery of superovulated ova in prepuberal cattle. J. Reprod. Fertil. *21*, 119.

Ozil, J.P., Heyman, Y. and Renard, J.P. (1982). Production of monozygotic twins by micromanipulation and cervical transfer in the cow. Vet. Rec. *110*, 126–127.

Ozil, J.P. (1983). Production of identical twins by bisection of blastocysts in the cow. J. Reprod. Fertil. *69*, 463.

Phillips, D.M. and Shalgi, R.M. (1980). Surface properties of the zona pellucida. J. Exp. Zool. *213*, 1–8.

Pincus, G.W. and Enzmann, E.V. (1935). The comparative behavior of mammalian eggs in vivo and in vitro. (I) The activation of ovarian eggs. J. Exp. Med. *62*, 665.

Quinlivan, T.D. (1980). Estrous synchronization and control of the estrous cycle. *In* Current Therapy in Theriogenology. D.A. Morrow (ed.). Philadelphia, W.B. Saunders.

Roche, J.F., Ireland, J. and Mawhinney, S. (1981). Control and induction of ovulation in cattle. J. Reprod. Fertil. Suppl. *30*, 211.

Rogers, B.J. (1978). Mammalian sperm capacitation and fertilization in vitro: a critique of methodology. Gamete Res. *1*, 165.

Rowson, L.E.A., Lawson, R.A.S. and Moor, R.M. (1971). Production of twins in cattle by egg transfer. J. Reprod. Fertil. *25*, 261.

Seidel, Jr., G.E., Bowen, R.A. and Kane, M.T. (1976). In vitro fertilization, culture, and transfer of rabbit ova. Fertil. Steril. *27*, 861.

Seidel, Jr., G.E., Larson, L.L., Spilman, C.H., Hahn, J. and Foote, R.H. (1971). Culture and transfer of calf ova. J. Dairy Sci. *54*, 923.

Seitz, H.M., Brackett, B.G. and Mastroianni, L. (1973). Fertilization. *In* Human Reproduction: Conception and Contraception. E.S.E. Hafez and T.N. Evans (eds.). New York, Harper & Row.

Shalgi, R. and Phillips, D.M. (1980). Mechanics of in-vitro fertilization in the hamster. Biol. Reprod. *23*, 433–444.

Shea, B.F., Hines, D.J., Lightfoot, D.E., Ollis, G.W. and Olson, S.M. (1976a). The transfer of bovine embryos. *In* Egg Transfer in Cattle. L.E.A. Rowson (ed.). Commission of the European Communities. EUR 5491, Luxembourg, pp. 145–152.

Sreenan, J.M. (1978). Non-surgical embryo transfer in the cow. Theriogenology *9*, 69.

Sreenan, M.J., Behan, D. and Mulvehill, P. (1975). Egg transfer in the cow: factors affecting pregnancy and twinning rates following bilateral transfer. J. Reprod. Fertil. *44*, 77.

Sugie, T. (1965). Successful transfer of a fertilized bovine egg by non-surgical techniques. J. Reprod. Fertil. *10*, 197.

Sugie, T., Soma, T., Tsunoda, Y. and Mizuochi, K. (1982). Embryo transfer in goat and sheep. *In* In-vitro Fertilization and Embryo Transfer. E.S.E. Hafez and K. Semm (eds.). Lancaster, England, MTP Press.

Sundstrom, P. (1984). Interaction of human gametes in vitro by scanning electron microscopy. Arch. Androl. *12*, 145.

Sundstrom, P. (1982). Interaction between spermatozoa and ovum in vitro. Ch. 24, *In* Atlas of Human Reproduction by Scanning Electron Microscopy. E.S.E. Hafez and O.P. Kenemans (eds.). Lancaster, England, MTP Press.

Thibault, C. and Dauzier, L. (1960). Fertilisines et fecondation in vitro de l'oeuf de la lapine. C.R. Acad. Sci. (Paris) *250*, 1358–1359.

Thibault, C. and Dauzier, L. (1961). Analyse des conditions de la fecondation in vitro de l'oeuf de la lapine. Ann. Biol. Anim. Biochim. Biophys. *1*, 227–294.

Trounson, A.O., Willadsen, S.M. and Moor, R.M. (1977). Reproductive function in prepubertal lambs: ovulation, embryo development and ovarian steroidogenesis. J. Reprod. Fertil. *49*, 69.

Trounson, A.O., Rowson, L.E.A. and Willadsen, S.M. (1978a). Non-surgical transfer of bovine embryo. Vet. Rec. *102*, 74.

Trounson, A.O., Shea, B.F., Ollis, G.W. and Jacobson, M.E. (1978b). Frozen storage and transfer of bovine embryos. J. Anim. Sci. *47*, 677.

Tsafriri, A., Bar-Ami, S. and Lindner, H.R. (1983). Control of the development of meiotic competence and of oocyte maturation in mammals. *In* Fertilization of the Human Egg In Vitro. Springer-Verlag, Berlin, Beier & Lindner.

Tsutsumi, Y. et al. (1976). J. Reprod. Fertil. *48*, 393.

Warwick, B.L. and Berry, R.O. (1949). Inter-generic and intra-specific embryo transfer. J. Hered. *40*, 287.

Wassarman, P.M. (1988). The mammalian ovum. *In* The Physiology of Reproduction, Vol. 1. E. Knobil and J.D. Neill (eds.). Raven Press, New York.

Westhusin, M.E., Slapak, J.R., Fuller, D.T. and Kraemer, D.C. (1989). Culture of agar-embedded one and two cell bovine embryos and embryos produced by nuclear transfer in the sheep and rabbit oviduct. Theriogenology *31*, 271.

Whittingham, D.G., Leibo, S.P. and Mazur, P. (1972). Survival of mouse embryos frozen to −196°C and −269°C. Science *178*, 411.

Willadsen, S.M. (1981). The developmental capacity of blastomeres from 4- to 8-cell sheep embryos. J. Embryol. Exp. Morp. *65*, 165–172.

Willadsen, S.M. (1982). Micromanipulation of embryos of the large domestic species. *In* Mammalian Egg Transfer. C.E. Adams (ed.). Boca Raton, FL, CRC Press.

Willadsen, S.M. (1983). Micromanipulation of embryos of the large domestic species. *In* Mammalian Egg Transfer. C.E. Adams (ed.). Boca Raton, FL, CRC Press.

Willadesen, S.M. and Polge, C. (1981). Attempts to produce monozygotic quadruplets in cattle by blastomere separation. Vet. Rec. *108*, 211–213.

Willett, E.L. et al. (1951). Successful transplantation of a fertilized bovine ovum. Science *113*, 247.

Wilmut, I. and Rowson, L.E.A. (1973). Experiments on the low-temperature preservation of cow embryos. Vet. Rec. *92*, 686.

Wright, Jr., R.W. et al. (1976). In vitro culture of embryos from adult and prepuberal ewes. J. Anim. Sci. *42*, 912.

Wright, Jr., R.W. and Bondioli, K.R. (1981). Aspects of in vitro fertilization and embryo culture in domestic animals. J. Anim. Sci. *53*, 701.

Xu, K.P., Greve, T., Callesen, H. and Hyttel, P. (1987). Pregnancy resulting from cattle oocytes matured and fertilized in vitro. J. Reprod. Fertil. *81*, 501–504.

Yanagimachi, R. (1981). Ch. 5. *In* Fertilization and Embryonic Development in Vitrol. L. Mastroianni, Jr. and J.D. Biffers (eds.). New York, Plenum Press.

Yanagimachi, R. (1977). Specificity of sperm–egg interaction. *In* Immunobiology of Gametes. M. Edidin and M.H. Jonson (eds.). London and New York, Cambridge University Press.

24

Preservation and Cryopreservation of Gametes and Embryos

E.S.E HAFEZ

The main advantage of cryopreservation of embryos instead of just the sperm or oocyte is that the embryo contains the complete genome, i.e., the quota of chromosomes for the individual, and it can be transferred to a foster mother of known or unknown genetic background without the risk of genetic change. Embryo cryopreservation enables animal breeding centers to carry a wider range of stocks and to store stocks not in immediate use, thereby saving space and money as well as affording protection against loss through fire, disease, and other hazards. Inbred strains, mutations, and special genetic combinations can be preserved; this is a valuable asset for advanced research in animal genetics. In addition, genetic pedigree standards can be established and checked for genetic drift in subsequent generations.

Since the pioneering efforts of Audrey Smith in 1952 concerning the effect of low temperature on further development of mammalian ova, much progress in embryo cryopreservation has occurred (Table 24-1). Cryopreservation of embryos of different mammalian species was tried with variable degrees of success. These differences are due to the varied response of certain stages of embryonic development to different biophysical and physiochemical parameters such as cooling media, the nature and concentration protocol of the cryoprotectant used, the type of programmable freezer, the thawing rate, and the

TABLE 24-1. First Successful Cryopreservation of Mammalian Embryos

Species	Author
Mouse	Whittingham et al., 1972, 1979; Kassai et al., 1980; Wood and Farrant, 1980
Rat	Whittingham, 1975a, 1975b
Rabbit	Bank and Maurer, 1974
Cattle	Wilmut and Rowson, 1973; Willadsen et al., 1978
Sheep	Willadsen et al., 1976; Willadsen, 1977
Goat	Bilton and Moore, 1976, 1979
Man	Trounson et al., 1982

dilution protocol of the concentration of the cryoprotectant after thawing. The transport of frozen embryos over long distances is an inexpensive way to export farm animals. The successful transport of frozen bovine embryos from New Zealand to Australia is one example (Bilton and Moore, 1976a, 1976b).

PRINCIPLES OF CRYOBIOLOGY

The biophysical principles that apply to cryopreservation of living cells and tissues also apply to cryopreservation of embryos. Embryos may be damaged during cryopreservation and/or thawing either by the formation of large intracellular ice crystals or by the increased intracellular concentration of solutes and accompanying changes that result from the dehydration of cells during cryopreservation (solution effects). Whereas fast freezing minimizes damage from solution effects, it leads to

503

the formation of large ice crystals that cause severe mechanical damage. On the other hand, while slow freezing prevents large ice crystal formation, it leads to increased damage from solution effects. Therefore, the optimal freezing rate for a given tissue depends on its relative tolerance to damage from ice crystals and toxicity from solution effects.

When a cell suspension is cooled below 0°C, extracellular ice crystals form, resulting in a concentration of the solutes in the remaining liquid water. The cell membrane acts as a barrier to prevent the spread of ice crystals into the intracellular compartments.

The ease of water transport depends on the membrane's permeability to water at any given temperature, the surface-volume ratio of the cell, and the freezing rate. If the cell is sufficiently permeable to water or the freezing rate is sufficiently low, pressure remains small and dehydration results as water moves out of the cell to freeze extracellularly. Although extracellular ice crystals deform the cell, extracellular ice does not rupture the plasma membrane and cause irreversible damage.

Adding cryoprotectants such as glycerol or dimethyl sulfoxide to the freezing medium results in freezing at lower temperatures. This probably retards dehydration of cells and the resultant harmful solution effects; thus, embryos may be cooled slowly enough to prevent the formation of large ice crystals.

The critical ranges of temperature of which low rates are necessary for optimal survival are from −4°C to −60°C during cooling and from −70°C to −20°C during rewarming. The injurious effects of intracellular ice are caused either by its growth and recrystallization during thawing or by the osmotic stress imposed on the cells when the intracellular ice melts.

Mammalian embryos can be preserved for prolonged periods in a state of suspended animation if they are able to withstand cryopreservation to temperatures at which no further biologic activity occurs.

Liquid nitrogen at −196°C satisfies this condition. The embryos of cattle, sheep, and mice can survive rapid thawing provided that slow cooling is terminated between −30°C and −50°C by direct transfer to liquid nitrogen at −196°C.

CRYOPRESERVATION OF EMBRYOS

Various techniques have been used for cryopreservation and thawing of cattle, sheep, swine, and horses (Table 24–2). Embryos selected for cryopreservation should be of the highest quality and at the correct stage of cleavage. They are handled with sterile techniques using a dissecting microscope. Embryos are transferred to sterile, freshly prepared culture media for microscopic classification and storage until use. If embryos are stored longer than 2 hours before transfer, they are transferred into fresh medium every 2 hours. The embryos are aspirated into pipettes with a small volume of medium (less than 0.2 ml) to prevent contamination of the fresh medium. The morphologic classifications of embryos are summarized in Table 24–3.

The embryos are handled gently to avoid any physical damage. Manipulation and evaluation are accomplished as quickly as possible to return the embryos to a stable culture environment. To gain experience with handling embryos, operators are trained to use commercially available micropipettes to pick up sephadix particles with a diameter similar to mammalian eggs. Pieces of debris, unfertilized ova, or degenerating ova can also be used for practice.

Embryo Containers

Embryos are stored in containers that are transparent, sealable, inert, convenient, and of small volume (less than 5 ml). Small, stoppered test tubes can be used, although they must be emptied into another container to locate the embryos under the stereoscope. The medium may be covered with a thin layer of paraffin oil to prevent evaporation, reduce bacterial contamination, and relate the rate of gas

TABLE 24–2. Summary of Precooling, Cooling, Seeding, Plunging, Storage, and Thawing of Embryos

Process	Techniques Employed
Collection of embryos	Selection and superovulation of donor, insemination during estrus
	Collection of embryos from female reproductive tract or ovaries (surgical, nonsurgical, or postmortem)
	Washing of embryos in sterile culture media
	Microscopic evaluation and classification of embryos
Cryoprotectant solutions	Gradual step-wise concentration of cryoprotectant (DMSO, glycerol, or ready-made cryoprotectant available commercially)
	Small volume should be freshly prepared
	Solutions to which serum is added are not stored more than 3–5 days, because protein denaturation occurs even under optimal temperatures
	Solutions are kept refrigerated or frozen until use
Precooling preparation	Embryos transferred in serial concentrations of cryoprotectants
	Straws attached to syringe using rubber adapter to aspirate medium/air bubbles and embryo/air bubbles
	Straws and canes labeled for future identification
	Straws heated or filled with phosphate-buffered saline
	Straws dipped in blue or red PVS at both ends
Cooling procedures	Slow cooling rate ranges from 0.5 to 1.6°C per minute
	Rapid cooling rate ranges from 17 to 30°C per minute
	Cooling rate −1°C/min. from ambient temperature to −7°C
	Cooling rate 0.3°C/min. to −35°C
	Cooling rate 0.1°C/min. to −38°C
Freezing, seeding, and plunging	Straws placed in freezer at −6°C and maintained for 10 minutes
	Forceps cooled in liquid nitrogen
	Straws grasped near embryos with cooled forceps until ice crystals form
	Seeded straw placed into programmable freezer and cooling regimen applied
	Thermos flask filled with liquid nitrogen
	Cane containing frozen embryos removed from freezer and plunged into liquid nitrogen
	Straws loaded in aluminum canes and stored in liquid nitrogen container at −196°C
Thawing	Thawing ranges from 20°C/min. in slow warming to 360–500°C for the rapid thawing; optimal temperature for cryopreservant thawing ranges between 20 and 37°C
	Temperature of a water bath adjusted to 37°C
	Color-marked canes identified and straws removed from cane to small canister containing liquid nitrogen; labels are checked before removing from liquid nitrogen
	Straws are held by neck, placed into 37°C water bath and gently swirled until ice disappears
	Embryos remain on bottom of vial and can be observed under microscope, counted, and removed with micropipette to avoid occasional loss of embryos experienced by washing embryos out of straw
	Straws are thawed for 4 seconds in 37°C water bath and removed when ice is melted
	Water is wiped from straws
Cryoprotectant removal	Heat seal or PVC plug cut from tips of straws
	Embryos washed through drops of serial dilutions of cryoprotectant mixture in a sterile petri dish (diameter of 35 mm)
	Embryos examined using a stereoscope to evaluate their quality

exchange between the medium and the atmosphere.

Culture and Storage Between 0 and 37°C

For experimental manipulations and storage between recovery and transfer, embryos are kept in culture medium at 37°C. The development of embryos *in vitro* is slowed to two thirds of the normal *in vivo* rate. Embryos frequently continue to develop for 2 to 3 days or more, although pregnancy rates are usually re-

TABLE 24–3. Morphologic Classification of Embryos Before and After Cryopreservation and Thawing

Parameters			Classification	
Stage of embryonic development	Unfertilized (UFO) 2–12 cell Early morula Morula Early blastocyst		Blastocyst Expanded blastocyst Hatched blastocyst Expanding hatched blastocyst	
Criteria for classification of embryos	Compactness of blastomeres Regularity of shape of the embryo Variation in cell size Color and texture of the cytoplasm Presence of vesicles		Presence of extruded cells Diameter Regularity of the zona pellucida Presence of cellular debris	
Quality of embryo	Excellent	Perfect embryo for its stage: Blastomeres are of similar size with even color and texture; they are neither very light nor very dark. Cytoplasm is not granular or unevenly distributed and contains some moderate-sized vesicles. Perivitelline space is empty and of regular diameter; zona pellucida is even and neither wrinkled nor collapsed.		
	Good	Trivial imperfections such as an oval zona, a few, small excluded blastomeres, and slight asymmetry		
	Fair	Definite but not severe problems such as moderate numbers of excluded blastomeres, small size, and small amounts of degeneration		
	Poor	Partly degenerate, vesiculated cells, greatly varying cell size, very small and/or similar problems		
	Very poor	Severely degenerate, probably not worth transferring, unfertilized, zona only, ghost-like, 3 cell, debris, bacteriologic contamination		
Artifacts	Air bubble, debris, empty zona pellucida, denuded oviductal epithelium			

duced if they are transferred after more than 24 hours *in vitro* (Davis and Day, 1978). Culture of bovine embryos from the one- to two-cell stage to the four-cell stage and from morulae to blastocysts has been successful. In sheep and swine, 4 to 32 embryos are cultured in relative culture media.

Embryos can be held in culture for several hours to a day between collection and transfer at ambient temperature (15° to 25°C. If they are cooled to 0° to 10°C or transferred to the ligated oviduct of a rabbit, they can be stored for several days with little reduction in viability (Hafez, 1971; Lawson et al., 1972; Boland et al., 1978). Porcine embryos are an exception and do not survive cooling below 15°C. Development of the embryos continues at a normal rate in the rabbit oviduct but is arrested during storage at 0° to 10°C.

For long-term storage and easy transportation, embryos in the late morula or early blastocyst stage may be cryopreserved at liquid nitrogen temperature.

Tissue Culture Medium. Tissue culture medium (TCM 199) or Dulbecco's phosphate-buffered saline (PBS) (which does not require 5% atmosphere) are suitable media and easy to use. TCM 199 with Hanks salts (without phenol red to facilitate locating the embryos) is used to flush out the embryos. Media for embryo storage contains: 25 mM HEPES buffer, 10 to 20% calf or steer serum, which has been Millipore-filtered and heat inactivated for 30 minutes at 56°C; these macromolecules prevent embryos from sticking to glass or plastic.

Embryo Cryopreservation Procedures

The medium used for cryopreservation is modified Dulbecco's PBS supplemented with bovine serum albumin or serum. Cryoprotectant is added in steps either at 0° or 20°C. Embryos are cooled rapidly to 0°C and at a rate of 1°C/min to −7°C, at which point freezing is initiated by adding a small crystal of ice to the medium (seeding). Seeding minimizes temperature fluctuations resulting from the heat of fusion. Embryos are then cooled very slowly (less than .3dgC/min) to about −33°C, and finally, placed into liquid nitrogen.

To prevent the enlargement of small, harmless ice crystals, embryos are thawed rapidly in a 25°C water bath; the cryoprotectant is then removed by stepwise dilution at room temperature. Pregnancy rates may be improved to some extent if embryos are cultured for several hours before transfer and if any morphologically abnormal ones are discarded.

The biophysical characteristics of the main cryoprotectants are shown in Table 24–4. The cooling and cryopreservation of bovine embryos are summarized in Table 24–5. The supplies, culture media, and cryopreservation records are listed in Table 24–6.

Extensive investigations have been conducted on the physiological, biochemical, and biophysical parameters of cryopreservation of semen, oocytes, and early embryos of farm animals (Tables 24–6 through 24–11; Figures 24–1 through 24–4). Also, various types of glassware and computerized freezers are commercially used for cryopreservation and storage of semen and embryos (Figures 24–1 through 24–4).

TABLE 24–5. Cooling, Freezing, and Thawing Procedure of Bovine Embryos

Two step addition of glycerol	(5%, 10%)
↓	Place at −6°C
−6°C	Hold for 5–10 minutes
↓	Seed
−33°C	0.3°C/min
Plunge into liquid nitrogen	
↓	
Thaw at 37 °C	
↓	
Evaluate and record results	
↓	
Dilute out cryoprotectant in 4 steps	*or* 2 steps with sucrose
7.5% glycerol in PBS with serum	
5.0% glycerol in PBS with serum	
2.5% glycerol in PBS with serum	*or* sucrose in PBS with serum
0% glycerol in PBS with serum	PBS with serum
↓	
Wash 3 times in PBS Evaluate and record results	

PBS = phosphate-buffered saline (Data from Elsden and Pickett, Personal Communication, 1984.)

Cryopreservation of Bovine Embryos

Extensive investigations on the cryopreservation of bovine embryos have been conducted by Drs. R. Peter Elsden,

TABLE 24–4. Some Biophysical Characteristics of Some Cryoprotectants

Parameters	DMSO	Glycerol	Ethylene glycol
Chemical formula	$(CH_3)_2SO_4$	$C_3H5(OH)_3$	$(CH_2)_2(OH)_2$
Molecular weight	78.13	92.10	62.07
Specific gravity (9/cm³ at 20°C)	1.10	1.25	1.11
Mass (gm/L)			
1.0 M	78.13	92.10	62.07
3.0 M	234.39	276.30	186.21
Volume (ml/L)			
1.0 M	71.00	73.70	55.90
3.0 M	213.10	221.10	167.70
Grade	Grade	Laboratory Grade	Laboratory Grade
Sigma Chemical Co.			
Catalog No.	D-5879	G-7757	E-9129

Specific gravity: the ratio of the weight of a given volume of a substance compared to the weight of the same volume of water at 0°C.

TABLE 24–6. Cryopreservation Record

	Cryopreservation form code
	Donor register
Container	Freezing date of cryopreservation
	Container number
	Score and registration number
	Day of embryo collection
	Number of cryopreserved embryos
	Cryoprotectant and concentration
Certificate	Medium used
	Cane code
	Storage tank (location)
	Cooling procedure
	Thawing procedure
	Embryo quality
	Date of collection of embryos
	Identification code
	Superovulation treatments
	PMSG, hCG prostaglandins
	Interval from hCG to recovery of embryo
Donor of embryo	Previous recovery of embryos
	Medium used to flush embryo
	Number, quality, and type of embryos recovered
	Cryoprotectant: glycerol or Dimethyl sulfoxide (DMSO)
	Cooling rate, cryopreservation technique
Cryopreservation	Storage in liquid nitrogen
	Thawing techniques
	Removal of cryoprotectant

hCG = human chorionic gonadotropin; PMSG = pregnant mare serum gonadotropin.

George E. Seidel, Jr., Tetsuo Takeda, and their associates at the Embryo Transfer Laboratory at Colorado State University. Their specific recommendations are as follows:

1. Start with good- to excellent-quality embryos recovered 6 to 8 days after donor estrus.

2. Put embryos through three washes of sterile Dulbecco's PBS + 10% *heat-treated* serum (steer serum, newborn calf serum, or fetal calf serum are all satisfactory). Standard antibiotic concentrations should be used; adding pyruvate and glucose is optional.

3. Place embryos into PBS + 10% serum + 5% glycerol for 5 minutes; then place them in PBS + 10% serum + 10% glycerol for 10 to 20 minutes. All of the preceding steps are done at room temperature. Embryos probably can be added to 10% glycerol without going through the 5% step, but currently Dr. Elsden and coworkers recommend two steps.

4. Place the embryos into prelabeled .25- or .5-ml French straws. (Avoid glass containers for optimal results.) The straw is filled halfway with freezing medium (PBS + 10% serum + 10% glycerol). An air bubble of 3 to 4 mm, is added followed by another column of freezing medium containing the embryo so that the straw is 90% full when the cotton end is wetted. Finally, add 1.5 to 2 mm of paraffin oil and seal the end. Elsden et al. use a heat seal, but other seals are satisfactory. The straw is then placed into the freezing machine with the heat-sealed end down so that the embryo sinks and rests on the paraffin oil. The amount of paraffin oil should not exceed 2 mm; physical damage may occur to the embryo with larger amounts of paraffin oil as a result of differing thermal expansion coefficients from PBS. Paraffin oil may not be necessary if straws are frozen in a horizontal position.

5. Cool straws to −5°C to −6°C at a rate of 2° to 4°C/min. Faster cooling to −5° to −6°C probably is not harmful.

6. Seed straws after they have been at −5° to −6°C for 5 minutes, and hold them at −5° to −6°C for an additional 10 minutes.

7. Cool straws from −6° to −30°C at .5°C/min. When straws reach −30°C, plunge them into liquid nitrogen immediately (within 2 to 3 minutes).

8. Thaw straws in a 37°C water bath for not longer than 20 seconds. Make the transfer from liquid nitrogen to the bath in 2 seconds or less. Use an intermediate vessel containing liquid nitrogen so that this step can be done within 2 seconds. After thawing, perform all steps at room temperature.

9. Glycerol may be removed in two ways. The standard method is to dilute it

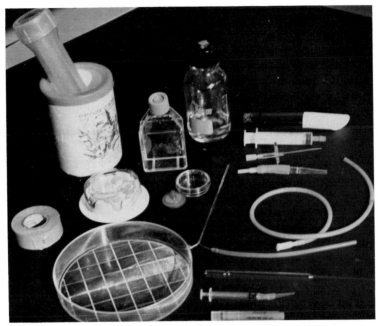

FIG. 24-1.   Glassware used for cryopreservation of embryos.

in six steps: PBS + 10% serum + 8.3% glycerol, and gradually decrease glycerol: 6.7%, 5%, 3.3%, 1.7% and finally 0%, taking 6 to 7 minutes per step. The alternative method uses four steps: 6% glycerol + 10.3% (.3M) sucrose, 3% glycerol + 10.3% sucrose, 10.3% sucrose (all in PBS + 10% serum), and then PBS + 10% serum with no sucrose or glycerol. Each step is for 6 to 7 minutes. Each dilution procedure leads to similar results, but the four-step method is faster.

10. Evaluate the embryo and transfer as soon as feasible, preferably within 30 minutes. Discard obviously degenerate embryos (should be less than 5% if procedures are done properly). If recipients are available, transfer the degenerate embryos anyway (nonsurgically). A few may develop into calves.

International Sales of Frozen Bovine Embryos

Frozen embryos of various cattle breeds and production standards are available. In dairy cattle, for example, Brown Swiss, Holstein, and Jersey embryos have 14,000 to 18,000 production and up to 305-day lactation. Frozen embryos are also available for various beef cattle breeds such as Angus, Beefmaster, Brangus, Brahman, Charolais, Chianina, Gelbvieh, Hereford, Limousin, Maine Anjou, Pinzgauer, Polled Hereford, Red Angus, Red Brangus, Salers, Santa Gertrudis, Simmental, and Texas Longhorn. Prices of frozen embryos are based on production records and pedigrees. Other breeds are available by custom order. Frozen embryos are sold with pedigree, health records, embryo certificates, and required breed registration forms.

The selection of embryo donor and sire matings has been governed by the parents' ability to significantly increase herd averages in the next generation. The use of embryos in developing nations can replace 25 to 30 years of breeding in one generation. Freezing facilitates handling and transporting embryos for transfer, making it superior to animal shipments between countries. Prospective buyers can obtain listings of embryos available from any country of origin throughout the

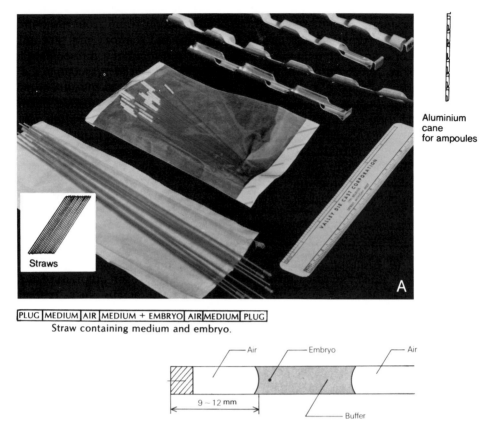

Aluminium
cane
for ampoules

Straws

A

| PLUG | MEDIUM | AIR | MEDIUM + EMBRYO | AIR | MEDIUM | PLUG |

Straw containing medium and embryo.

Air   Embryo   Air

9 ~ 12 mm

Buffer

FIG. 24–2.   Various types of straws, ampules, and aluminum canes used for cryopreservation and the methods used to transfer embryos to straws.

world from their local distribution affiliate. Experienced artificial insemination technicians can learn to thaw and inseminate frozen embryos with a minimum amount of training. This provides a more economical method of introducing superior stock through a manageable system.

Equipment, Glassware, and Accessories for Cryopreservation

The necessary equipment, glassware, and accessories for cryopreservation include the following:

Programmable freezer for cryopreservation of embryo
Refrigerator for media, solutions, and hormones
Liquid nitrogen tank with aluminum canes

Microscope and stereoscope
Laminar flow hood
Quantitative pipettes for preparation of cryoprotectant solutions
Catheters and pipettes for manipulation of embryos
Culture dishes of various sizes
Straws and ampules (Fig. 24–2) and selective sealer to seal ampules

Programmable Freezers

Electronically programmed machines are used to monitor the temperature over the critical phase of the cooling curve before the vials containing embryos are plunged into liquid nitrogen. Several types are completely self-contained and capable of obtaining controlled rates of cryopreservation with or without liquid

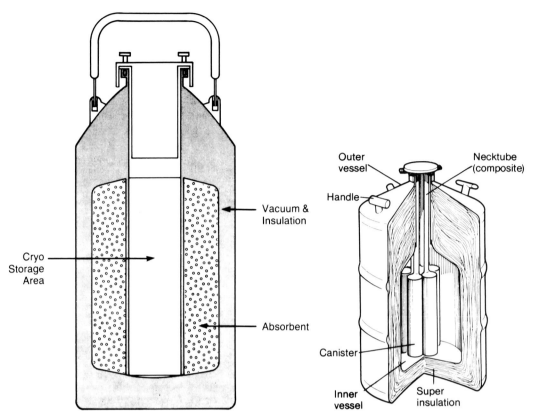

FIG. 24–3. Liquid nitrogen containers, showing inner construction and including storage area, absorbent, and vacuum and insulation. High-strength aluminum shell is both durable and lightweight.

nitrogen and without mechanical refrigeration devices or the use of conventional refrigerants. These are the three major systems:

1. Freezers with a cylindric chamber with circulating air cooled by microprocessor controlled thermoelectric cells
2. Freezers operated with liquid nitrogen
3. Freezers operated with alcohol

Some of these systems require only a 115-volt source for normal operation. The thermoelectric cells, which provide the cooling capability of the unit, operate on the basis of the Peltier effect. When two dissimilar metals are connected in series and an electric current is passed through

them, a thermal differential is established at each junction of the cell. The differential between the "warm" and "cool" side may be enhanced with the application of additional electrical amperage. The control over the rate of temperature reduction is achieved by a microprocessor that constantly monitors the actual chamber temperature and correlates the required current as indicated by the cooling program. Important features of cryopreservation units include the following:

1. Portability (thermoelectric devices are air cooled, which precludes the use of liquid nitrogen or any other compressed gas)
2. Low maintenance without mechanical refrigeration devices

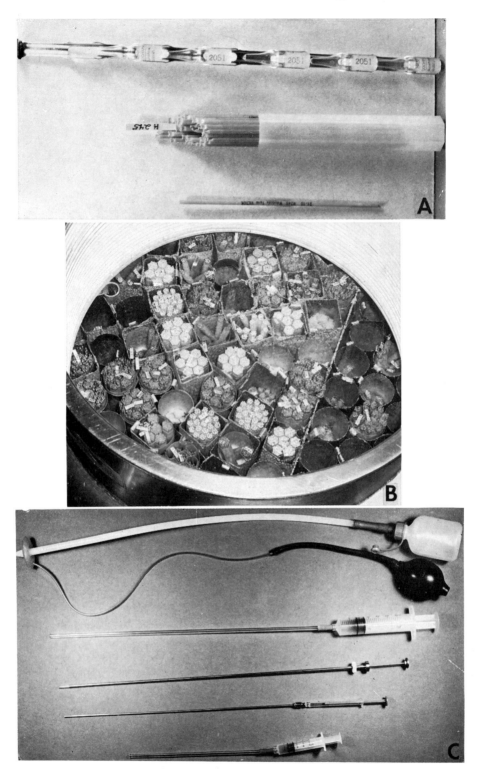

FIG. 24–4. *A.* A 0.5-ml straw and goblet holding 36 straws in comparison with a 1.0-ml ampule on a six-ampule cane. *B.* Storage of straws under liquid N_2 at $-196°C$. *C.* Insemination equipment for sows, mares, cows, ewes, and bitches (*top to bottom*).

3. Safety without danger of rapid gas volatilization or mechanical compressors
4. Warming capabilities (may be warmed rather than cooled by activating a protected button)
5. Digital thermometer for reliable monitoring and subsequent control of the cryogenic program

Thawing of Embryos

At thawing, the straws containing cryopreserved embryos are transferred from the storage tank of liquid nitrogen to a small container with a wide top and filled with liquid nitrogen. The label is then checked before thawing the straw. Straws are held by the neck, quickly placed in a 37°C water bath, and gently agitated in the water until the ice has disappeared. If care is taken, embryos remain on the bottom of the vial and can be observed easily under a microscope, counted, and removed with a micropipette. This technique avoids the occasional loss of embryos experienced when they are washed out of the vial. Straws can also be directly thawed in a 37°C water bath.

The serial dilution is started with the cryoprotectant solution; allow 10 minutes for each step. Then the embryos are placed in PBS + 20% fetal calf serum (FCS) for 30 minutes, and the surviving embryos are transferred. Embryos in straws are ejected and treated as mentioned or diluted in one or two steps within the straw. The various concentrations of cryoprotectants are separated by air bubbles. The embryo can be transferred from one solution to the next one by tapping the straw.

The optimum rate of thawing depends on the cryopreservation technique. A precise thawing curve must also be followed and the embryos rehydrated by bathing in progressively weaker solutions of the cryoprotectant. Using this technique, pregnancy rates of more than 50% can be obtained when freezing the best ova with poorer quality ova being transferred fresh.

Rapid warming limits the amount of growth of ice crystals in the frozen samples and often results in survival. If the samples have been frozen at a rate slow enough so that the cells are in osmotic equilibrium with the surrounding medium, the rate of warming need not be rapid. Embryos are sensitive to rapid warming, presumably as a result of the large transient osmotic stress that occurs during warming. This stress occurs as the ice is converted into free water, resulting in the transient exposure to a solution, which is hypertonic with respect to the inside of cells. Embryos must absorb water from their environment to remain in osmotic equilibrium and to return to their normal isotonic volume. Because most metabolic reactions are arrested or drastically slowed down during cryopreservation, they are especially susceptible to warming or dilution shock at this stage. For many cell types, it is important to have serum or other high molecular weight polymers in the thawing media to reduce any osmotic shock. When ice crystals are melted, the embryos are still exposed to multimolar concentrations of cryoprotectant that must be gradually diluted to return the embryos to the isotonic media.

Procedures to Test Embryo Survival

The main parameters used to evaluate embryo survival are based on the following: (a) morphological characteristics before and after freeze/thawing, (b) postthaw embryo survival, (c) percentage of embryos remaining viable in culture and (d) treatment × time interaction of *b* and *c*. A scoring system is recommended to grade the embryos after cryopreservation.

Several effective methods are used to evaluate survival after freezing, namely, morphologic appearance on thawing and development in culture; these are closely correlated with the ultimate survival of the frozen embryos. In species where morphologic examination and culture techniques are unreliable, other indirect methods are of value, i.e., transfer to interspecific oviducts and histologic examination. The development of the fluorescent dye test for the examination of these latter embryos would make assessment of viability much simpler. Consideration will be given to the development of metabolic tests for survival as well as more detailed ultrastructural studies of frozen embryos to ascertain the type and extent of damage after freezing and thawing. The main procedures to be used for embryos of farm animals follow:

1. Embryo viability after thawing is first assessed by testing the ability of the embryo to develop under conditions *in vitro* to the expanded blastocyst stage.
2. A second step includes the assessment of the frozen–thawed embryos' ability to develop into viable fetuses when blastocyst-stage embryos are transferred into pseudopregnant recipients.
3. Nonfrozen embryos are cultured to the blastocyst stage and then transferred to pseudopregnant recipients.
4. The survival of frozen–thawed embryos is compared to the survival of nonfrozen controls from the same animal.

Factors Affecting Post-Thaw Embryo Survival

Several maternal, technical, and operational factors influence the survival rate of embryos:

1. Physiologic and biophysical characteristics and developmental stage of embryos
2. Time interval and *in vitro* treatment from embryo collection to initiation of cryopreservation
3. Type of computerized freezers and program of cryopreservation
4. Osmotic shock during various steps of cryopreservation
5. Number of embryos in each straw and percentage of serum albumin in Dulbecco's PBS
6. Exposure of embryos to excessive light during microscopic examination
7. Osmotic and colloid osmotic pressures of fluids, prepared media, and cryoprotectants
8. Nature and extent of "seeding" and "plunging"
9. Microbiologic contaminants in glassware, freezer, and storage
10. Liquid nitrogen tank
11. Faults of the freezer, computer, or operator
12. Synchrony and nature of the recipient on embryo replacements (Schneider and Maurer, 1983)

Because all of these variables affect the embryo survival rate, the influence of each factor must be considered individually and in relation to the other factors.

Future Research

Future research is needed to improve pregnancy rates from the cryopreserved embryos of farm animals. Physiologic and cytologic techniques can be employed to evaluate post-thaw survival of embryos with emphasis on the rate of cryopreservation and thawing, the application of programmable freezers, the maturation of ova transferred into surrogate animal follicles, the optimum number of stepwise concentrations and of dilution of cryoprotectants, the criteria to evaluate the rate of embryo survival, and the possible effects of the culture of embryos before the cryopreservation effects of relative concentration of serum, culture media, and cryoprotectants (some batches of serum, culture media and embryos may be inferior), the relative functional role of blastocoelic fluid, zona pellucida, and right junctions between trophoblastic cells.

Cytogenetic techniques can be used for sexing of frozen–thawed embryos. Various biophysical and biochemical techniques can be used to assess molecular characteristics of membranes of blastomere, osmotic consequence of cryoprotectants' permeability, and relative significance of osmolarity and pH of the cryoprotectant medium during different stages of cryopreservation.

CRYOPRESERVATION OF SEMEN

The agents that comprise good extending media have the following functions: (a) provide nutrients as a source of energy, (b) protect against the harmful effect of rapid cooling, (c) provide a buffer to prevent harmful shifts in pH as lactic acid is formed, (d) maintain the proper osmotic pressure and electrolyte balance, (e) inhibit bacterial growth, (f) increase the volume of the semen so that it can be used for multiple inseminations and (g) protect the sperm cells during freezing (Berndtson and Pickett, 1978; Foote, 1975; Graham, 1978).

Semen Extenders

Pure substances and clean equipment should be used to exclude toxic materials from the sperm environment. Extenders should be prepared aseptically and stored for less than a week unless frozen. A simple carbohydrate, such as glucose, usually is added as a source of energy for the sperm. Both egg yolk and milk are used to protect against cold shock of the sperm cells as they are cooled from body temperature to 5°C. These substances also contain nutrients used by sperm. A variety of buffers may be used to maintain a nearly neutral pH and an osmotic pressure of approximately 300 milliosmoles, which is equivalent to that of semen, blood plasma, and milk. To inhibit the growth of microorganisms in semen, penicillin, streptomycin, polymyxin B, or other combinations of antibiotics that cover a broad bacterial spectrum are added. Similar procedures have been developed to cryopreserve embryos (Tables 24–7 and 24–8).

Bovine semen is usually diluted with egg yolk-citrate solution, homogenized whole milk, fresh and dried skim milk, coconut milk, or lactose solution. Semen has been successfully preserved in diluents

TABLE 24–7. Some Morphologic Changes in Embryos Following Cryopreservation and Thawing

Stage	Morphologic Changes After Freeze and Thaw
2–16 cell	Asymmetric appearance Uneven coloration of blastomeres Extruded blastomere Irregular blastomere Irregular cell mass
Morula	Extruded blastomere Extensive damage and reorganization Loss of cohesion (looseness) among blastomeres Loss of zona pellucida Lighter or darker color Presence of debris
Blastocyst	Vacuolated areas in cytoplasm (slight or extensive) Extruded blastomeres Collapsed Collapsed and re-expanded after thawing Reduction of size Early hatching
Zona pellucida	Cracked Rupture Loss of spheric smooth shape Oval in shape

based on the organic buffer, Tris (hydroxymethyl) aminomethane.

Buffer solutions such as phosphate or a 3.2% 2,9-trisodium citrate dihydrate adjusted to pH 6.9 by the addition to citric acid have been commonly used in combination with egg yolk. The addition of citric acid is unnecessary because the egg yolk component (20% by volume) has sufficient buffering capacity to return the pH to neutral. Skim milk is preferable to citrate diluents for ram semen. Tris is included only as the buffer component; other salts and sugars are necessary to maintain the osmolarity. Other organic buffers (Tricien, TES, MES, HEPES) offer a better alternative to citrate for buffering semen diluents especially in those species in which citrate is a poor medium.

There is a progressive increase in the use of boar semen that has been extended in a suitable diluent and used for artificial insemination in swine. Semen is diluted

TABLE 24–8.   Recommended Scoring System for Grading of Embryos After Cryopreservation and Thawing

Parameters	Characteristics	Estimated Scores
Blastomeres	1. Shape; size variability	15
	2. Number in relation to developmental stage (retardation), extruded material	
Vitellus	3. Homogeneity, granularity	20
(cytoplasm)	4. Color: dark, amber or grey (too dark, too light)	
Extruded debris	5. Extruded material or blastomeres	20
Cellular membranes	6. Intact plasma membrane of cytoplasm	15
	7. Vesicles with or without membranes or partially filled with lipid and glycogen	
Perivitelline space	8. Size in relation to developmental stage	10
Zona pellucida	9. Shape; integrity (intact)	10
Others	10. Miscellaneous anomalies	10
	Total score	100

Minor, major, unconsequential, and multiple anomalies are noted in mammalian embryos after cryopreservation.

In a computerized grading system of frozen–thawed embryos, based on the scores of anomalies, embryos may be categorized as "poor," "fair," "doubtful," "good," and "excellent."

and used the same day or stored for up to 6 days at temperatures ranging from 5 to 23°C. A storage temperature of 15 to 18°C is most successful for boar semen. Several extenders are used such as "Kiev" (also known as Guelph), the "Beltsville Liquid extender" (BL-1), the "Illinois Variable Temperature," and the "Zorlesco" (see Table 24–3). A storage and insemination volume of 100 ml is recommended for most extenders. Storage of semen extended in BL-1, however, is more successful using a 25-ml volume followed by dilution to 100 ml just before insemination.

The ultimate goal of semen preservation is to obtain pregnancies after artificial insemination as effectively as after natural mating. This depends on several factors apart from semen quality. Semen of farm animals was successfully cryopreserved more than 30 years ago; however, the techniques have been continually modified and improved. Semen cryopreservation formerly in solid carbon dioxide (dry ice at −79°C) has been replaced with liquid nitrogen (−196°C) with the advantage of a more stable condition of the cryopreserved semen. The application of cryopreservation procedures has been more successful in cattle than in other species of farm animals. The freezability (post-thaw survival of cryopreserved semen) varies between species and among individual males of the same species. These species and individual variations are related to the biophysical and biochemical characteristics of sperm membranes. The functional integrity of cryopreserved–thawed semen is evaluated by its capacity to fertilize the ovum and to sustain embryogenesis.

The survival of ejaculated spermatozoa in seminal plasma alone is limited to a few hours. To maintain spermatozoa for longer periods and to cool or cryopreserve semen, dilution with a protective solution is necessary. Different solutions have been used as diluents or extenders for semen, most of which are variations of a few principal formulae.

The preparation of egg yolk-citrate medium for cryopreservation of semen is time-consuming, particularly if it has to be prepared freshly for use. Egg yolk may be a prospective source of virus infections or allergic reactions. Thus, it is important to develop a new cryoprotectant that would be easier to handle and does not contain any egg yolk. Based on extensive investigations on sperm preservation medium (Mahadevan and Trounson, 1983) and findings on the use of kallikrein for enhancement of sperm motility. An instant cryoprotectant (ICP) has been commercially developed. Its effect on the cryopreservation of semen can be extended for 6 weeks.

Antibiotic preparations are added in diluents to control the proliferation of any microbiologic contaminants. A combination of penicillin (500 to 1000 IU/ml) and streptomycin (500 to 1000 μg/ml) provides a broad spectrum of antibacterial activity. The antibiotics are not toxic to spermatozoa. Newer antibiotics are added in low concentration and have no adverse effects on sperm; however, there is no evidence that any are more effective than the traditional penicillin–streptomycin combination.

Kallikrein and caffeine seem to stimulate sperm motility when added to semen after thawing. The action of caffeine is probably brought about by its stimulation of cyclic adenosine monophosphate (cAMP) levels in the sperm. Such additives are of doubtful value because they would be removed during sperm transport through the female reproductive tract.

Glycerol usually is added to protect sperm against the otherwise lethal effects of freezing. Dimethylsulfoxide (DMSO) and sugars such as lactose and raffinose also may be beneficial, as they serve as dehydrating agents.

Composition of Extenders. Practically all extenders for liquid or frozen semen have either egg yolk or heated milk or a combination of the two as basic ingredients. Egg yolk simply combined with sodium citrate or organic buffers and heated milk or skim milk have been used widely for bull semen, and with modifications for ram, buck, boar, and stallion semen.

For many years, the emphasis in artificial insemination (AI) programs was on the use of unfrozen semen. Numerous extender formulations were recommended (Salisbury et al., 1978). The ones used most widely were egg yolk buffered with sodium citrate or tris, or heated milk extenders for bull semen. These were adapted for use with other species. With the remarkable discovery by Polge and co-workers of the protective effect of glycerol during freezing, the emphasis shifted to the use of frozen semen.

Even with the best freezing techniques, more spermatozoa must be put into each breeding unit than with liquid (unfrozen) semen, because of the loss of some viable cells during freezing.

In areas where little refrigeration is available, semen may be stored at ambient temperatures. A carbonated egg-yolk extender called Illinois Variable Temperature extender (IVT) and coconut milk have given satisfactory fertility when semen was stored for up to a few days at moderate ambient temperatures. Most cattle are inseminated with frozen semen. This offers the user a wide variety of choice. It permits semen to be collected at one time and place and to be used anywhere, even after long periods of storage, provided that it is stored continuously at $-196°C$ with a good supply of liquid nitrogen. Thus, there need be no wastage of this semen. Examples of extenders for frozen semen are given in Table 24–9.

Pelleting extended bull semen and freezing it on solid carbon dioxide (dry ice) is practiced in a few countries. A sugar such as raffinose or 11% lactose may be used. Pellets offer an inexpensive way of preserving spermatozoa, but they are difficult to properly identify when large numbers of bulls are involved. However, in some species in which successful freezing of sperm cells is difficult, the pellet method has been the most successful. Goat semen can be frozen in skim milk with about 9 g of glucose per liter and 7% glycerol by volume (Corteel, 1977).

Ram semen frozen in the extender (Salamon, 1976) or in heated milk can be used successfully. However, it is not as fertile as when used undiluted or used unfrozen at low dilutions. Much of the semen used in countries where AI of sheep is practiced is not frozen. Boar semen has been difficult

TABLE 24–9. **Composition of Extenders with Egg Yolk for Frozen Semen**

| Ingredients* | For Frozen Semen (−196°C) | | | | | | |
| | Ampules or Straws | | | Pellet Freezing | | | |
	Bull	Bull	Buck	Bull	Ram	Boar	Stallion†
Sodium citrate dihydrate (g)	23.2	—	—	—	—	—	—
Tes-N-Tris (g)	—	—	—	—	—	12	—
Tris (gm)	—	24.2	24.2	—	36.3	2	—
Citric acid monohydrate (g)	—	13.4	13.4	—	19.9	—	—
Glucose or fructose (g)	—	10.0	10.0	—	5.0	32	50
Lactose (g)	—	—	—	—	—	—	3
Raffinose (g)	—	—	—	139	—	—	3
Casein (g)	—	—	—	—	—	—	—
Penicillin (units/ml)	1000	1000	1000	1000	1000	1000	1000
Streptomycin (µg/ml)	1000	1000	1000	1000	1000	1000	1000
Polymyxin B (units/ml)	500	500	—	500	—	—	—
Glycerol (ml)	70	70	80	47	50	10	50
Egg yolk (ml)	200	200	100	200	150	200	50
Orvus ES paste (ml)	—	—	—	—	—	5	—
Distilled water to final volume	1000	1000	1000	1000	1000	1000	1000

(Foote, 1980)

* Ingredients usually are dissolved in distilled water and then glycerol, more water and egg yolk are added to bring the final volume to 1 liter. Two buffers and extenders often are prepared, as the glycerol level in the initial medium mixed with sperm usually has a lower glycerol concentration than the extender in which sperm are frozen. Antibiotic levels also vary. See text for details.

† Also frozen in straws. Up to 0.5 g each of sodium phosphate and sodium-potassium tartrate is included in the medium, according to Japanese workers (Nishikawa et al., 1972). However, there is no completely satisfactory extender for freezing stallion semen.

to freeze satisfactorily. However, a variety of extenders has been developed (Larson, 1978). Glycerol is detrimental to boar fertility (Wilmut and Polge, 1977), and 2% by volume or less is included in the extended semen during freezing. Some frozen boar semen is available commercially. Much of the boar semen used for insemination in Europe is unfrozen, preserved for up to 3 days in a glucose-bicarbonate-yolk-extender gassed with CO_2.

Stallion semen also can be pelleted or frozen in straws. Egg yolk-tris and cream-gelatin extenders also have been used (Picket et al., 1975). Glycerol depresses the fertility of stallion semen; semen from some stallions freezes poorly, so the methods of freezing stallion semen are less than optimal (Sullivan, 1978). Nevertheless, commercial AI with frozen stallion semen has been successful.

Antibacterial agents are especially useful in controlling microorganisms present in extended semen stored at higher temperatures. It is important that proper antibiotics be used to control different types of organisms that may be encountered in different species. Glycerol may partially interfere with the inhibitory action of antibiotics on microorganisms. Vegetable dyes may be included in the extender at sufficient concentrations to distinctly color it. This will not harm the sperm and facilitates identification of semen from different males or breeds.

Semen Processing

The processing of semen through cooling it to 5°C is similar whether it is to be used frozen or unfrozen. Semen is collected at body temperature. Following collection, it should be kept warm (30°C) before extension to avoid cold shock. This can be done by placing semen and extender in a water bath kept at 30°C. An aliquot of semen should be removed for sample evaluation, and the remainder can be mixed with three to four parts of extender at 30°C. It is recommended that semen be held for 30 minutes at 30°C to increase the antibiotic action of the extender. The mixture is cooled gradually to 5°C for all species, except unfrozen boar semen, which usually is held at 15°C. Buck semen frequently is centrifuged first to prevent possible coagulation (Corteel, 1977). Cooling should be slow, taking at least 1 hour to cool the mixture from 30 to 5°C. Cooling usually is done with a surrounding water jacket to prevent cold shock.

Extension of Semen. Semen is extended at specified rates so that the volume of semen inseminated will contain sufficient spermatozoa to give high fertility without wasting many cells. The approximate extension rates possible with average ejaculates, appropriate sperm numbers to inseminate, and other relevant data under good management conditions are summarized in Table 24–10. The number of sperm cells required for insemination varies depending on the site of deposition. When extended semen can be placed through the cervix, the number of spermatozoa required is less than that for intracervical or vaginal insemination. When this variation and the range of sperm cell concentrations that occur in fresh semen are taken into consideration, the actual extension rates may be more extreme than those listed in Table 24–10.

Extension rates are higher with unfrozen semen than with frozen semen. Unfrozen bull semen can be extended 200 to 300 times with fewer than 5 million motile cells per insemination required for high fertility. Processing liquid semen after cooling to 5°C (or 15°C for boar semen) is simple. Tubes of extended semen should be nearly full to avoid excess air and agitation in shipment. They should be packaged in a manner that maintains the temperature constant and avoids exposure to light. With unfrozen bull, buck, ram, boar, and especially stallion semen, fertility declines within a few days of collection. It is recommended that semen be used the day of collection or the next day.

Glycerol Addition for Freezing Bull Semen. Glycerol is used almost universally as the cryoprotective agent for freezing semen. The amounts and methods of adding glycerol vary, depending on the extenders, freezing methods, and species (Table 24–10), and the recipes developed by individual laboratories (Foote, 1975; Graham, 1978).

Glycerol usually is added to semen after cooling to 5°C; however, it affords just as much protection when added just before freezing. The final amount varies from less than 5% in some yolk-sugar media to 10% in milk. Some add glycerol slowly by dripping or by adding small amounts over a period of 1 hour; others recommend a one-step addition. Extended semen normally is held for several hours at 5°C before

TABLE 24–10. Species' Characteristic Features of Cryopreservation of Semen

Species	Characteristic Features
Cattle	Semen was originally cryopreserved in 1-ml glass ampules; however, the introduction of pellet freezing and plastic straws has resulted in the use of smaller volumes of inseminated semen containing fewer spermatozoa, thus, more females can be inseminated from a single ejaculate.
Sheep	Semen cannot be diluted more than about tenfold without significant reduction in fertility, although motility at dilutions of up to 40-fold is not affected.
Pig	Artificial insemination of cryopreserved boar spermatozoa under usual management conditions results in lower fertility and a reduction in litter size. Lowered fertilizability of cryopreserved semen is caused by a reduced survival time of spermatozoa in the uterus, uterotubal junction, and oviducts compared to the survival of fresh spermatozoa.
Horse	Semen has been frozen in large ampules (2.5–10 ml), in pellets, in straws, and as a thin film in plastic bags. Cryopreserved semen is less fertile than undiluted fresh semen, but the success achieved so far, coupled with the relative lack of ultrastructural damage occurring with cryopreservation and thawing, is promising.

freezing. Tris buffers and the sugar buffers used with pellet freezing offer the advantage that glycerol can be included in the initial media used for cooling sperm. In most other extenders, sperm are damaged morphologically by adding glycerol at room temperature. With glycerol added to the initial extender, several laboratories using tris-buffered extender process semen before freezing in ambient temperature, avoiding the need for large cold rooms.

The semen-extender mixture is held for several hours before freezing to allow sperm cells to equilibrate with the extender (usually at 5°C). About 4 to 6 hours are optimal, depending on the medium used. Originally, this was thought to be partly necessary for equilibration of spermatozoa with glycerol. However, it is clear that little time, if any, is required for glycerol equilibration, and it can be added shortly before freezing. Other changes take place at 5°C that enhance sperm survival during freezing.

Bull spermatozoa are packaged in three ways: (a) polyvinyl chloride straws containing 0.25 to 0.5 ml of extended semen; (b) glass ampules containing 0.5 to 1 ml; (c) pellets containing approximately 0.1 to 0.2 ml. When the smaller volumes are frozen as a unit, the sperm concentration per milliliter is increased correspondingly, so that the total sperm per insemination dose is maintained. For example, semen frozen in 0.1-ml packages should have 10 times as many sperm per unit volume as semen frozen in 1.0-ml packages to contain the same total number of spermatozoa.

As the technology for freezing cattle semen was developed, glass ampules were used nearly exclusively. Ampules provide a sterile container that can be automatically labeled, filled, and sealed. The latter prevents any cross-contamination. Each ampule contains sufficient sperm for a single insemination. Six to eight ampules are attached to a metal cane (Fig. 24–2), which also carries the bull's identification.

Subsequently, polyvinyl chloride straws were developed by Cassou, patterned after Danish and Japanese straws used in earlier days of AI with liquid semen. The straw requires less storage space than the ampule, has slightly better freezing characteristics, and can be labeled, filled, and sealed automatically. Also, sperm can be transferred to the cow at the time of insemination with minimal loss of cells. The geometric configuration of a straw as a unit for the cryopreservation of bovine spermatozoa provides flexibility in freezing and thawing procedures. Faster thawing rates result in greater survival of sperm cryopreserved in straws. (Pace and Sullivan, 1978). Post-thaw survival of spermatozoa is affected by freezing rate, thawing rate, and concentration of glycerol.

Pelleted semen is prepared by pipetting about 0.1-ml drops of extended semen into hemispheric depressions made in a block of dry ice. Sperm survival is good following freezing. Pellets take little space when they are stored in bulk; they offer the cheapest storage method. The main disadvantage is the difficulty of placing bull identification on each pellet, although this has been done by incorporating a small printed paper disc during freezing. Cross-contamination by other spermatozoa or by microorganisms also is possible. Pellets can be placed in bulk containers that are labeled and then repackaged at low temperatures into individually labeled containers before field distribution. Another packaging technique is to place sperm directly into catheters used eventually for insemination, and to freeze these as breeding units.

Freezing Bull Semen. Mechanical freezers and freezers using dry ice, liquid air, liquid O_2, and liquid N_2 have all been tried successfully. Liquid N_2 has increased in popularity because it is also the refrigerant of choice for low-temperature, long-time storage of semen. Extended semen frozen as pellets, in straws, or in ampules is held at about 5°C before freezing. Straws usually are frozen in nitrogen vapor and stored at −196°C. Because of the large surface area of the straw and its thin wall, heat transfer is rapid and semen freezes rapidly, usually within a few minutes. Ampules often are frozen at about 3°C per minute to −15°C. At this point, the rate of freezing is increased until −150°C is reached. The ampules on canes then are transferred to liquid N₂ at −196°C. Pellets start to freeze within a few seconds after being placed on a block of dry ice. In a few minutes, they reach −79°C and are transferred quickly into containers immersed in liquid nitrogen at −196°C.

The exact nature of the freezing process—which allows spermatozoa under one set of conditions to be frozen rapidly (pellets) or moderately rapidly (straws) and under another set of conditions requires a slower rate (ampules)—is not understood. Freezing too rapidly may cause thermal shock and internal ice formation. Slow freezing causes salt concentrations to increase as water freezes out. This increase in osmotic pressure over a prolonged period of slow freezing may damage the proteins and lipoproteins of the sperm cells and the acrosome. The rate of freezing can affect ice crystal formation and this should be taken into account in selecting the thawing rate.

Storage of Frozen Semen. Frozen semen placed initially in dry ice and more recently in liquid nitrogen has been used successfully after more than 20 years of storage. With the lower temperature of liquid N₂, it should be possible to store frozen semen indefinitely. However, it is cheaper and genetically advantageous to use semen from outstanding sires promptly, rather than to store it for long periods.

A variety of efficient vacuum-sealed liquid N₂ refrigerators is available for storing frozen semen. These range in size from central units with a storage capacity of several hundred thousand 0.25-ml "ministraws" or 0.5-ml "midistraws" with an N₂ reserve that lasts about 6 months, to the common field units that hold up to several

thousand straws and an N₂ reservoir that lasts for up to 6 weeks. Ampules require more space; pellets stored in bulk occupy the least space. The large central storage units can hold up to 750,000 0.1-ml pellets and possibly provide economic banking of semen from young bulls in sampling programs. In some countries, after a large number of "breeding units" is frozen, the bulls are slaughtered, thereby decreasing total costs.

It is extremely important to check the liquid nitrogen refrigerator periodically to see that the nitrogen level is maintained. Loss of all liquid nitrogen, permitting the temperature to rise considerably, can result in killing the spermatozoa, even when the semen still appears to be frozen.

Thawing Bull Semen. Frozen semen should be held continuously at low temperatures until used. After thawing, frozen spermatozoa do not survive as long as unfrozen sperm, and they refreeze poorly. Therefore, one must be certain that the semen will be used soon once it has been thawed. Straws have been successfully thawed at temperatures ranging from that of ice water to 65°C or higher. At the higher thaw temperatures, the retention of normal acrosomes and the proportion of progressively motile sperm cells were higher. Thaw time must be controlled carefully to avoid killing the cells by overheating. It is recommended that under field conditions ampules be thawed in ice water; this takes about 8 minutes. Higher temperatures (37°C) may be superior for straws but may depend on the extender. Pellets are best thawed in a liquid medium at 40°C, but under practical field conditions, an ice-water thawing bath is easier to maintain and is satisfactory.

Frozen Semen of Other Farm Animals. The same general principles described for cattle semen appear to apply to handling frozen semen of other species (Table 24–11). However, AI with frozen semen has not been developed extensively on a commercial scale for these species. Either the semen has been more difficult

TABLE 24–11. Extension, Storage, and Insemination Requirements with Frozen Semen (Based on Average Conditions)

Parameters	All Frozen Semen				
	Cattle	Sheep	Goats*	Swine	Horses*
Storage temperature (C°)	−196	−196	−196	−196	−196
Storage time (years)	>1	>1	>1	>1	>1
Extension rate of 1 ml semen (ml)	10–75	5–10	10–25	4	2
Insemination dose					
Volume (ml)	.2–1	.05–.2†	.5	50	20–50
Motile sperm (10^6)	15	200	200	5000	1500‡
Best time to inseminate during estrus	9 hrs after onset to end of estrus	10–20 hrs after onset of estrus	12–36 hrs after onset of estrus	15–30 hrs after onset of estrus	Every second day, starting on day 2 of estrus
Site of semen deposition	Uterus and cervix	Uterus if possible	Uterus if possible	Cervix into uterus	Uterus
No. of breeding units per male					
Per ejaculate	300	15	15	10	5
Per week	1000	150	150	30	15
Conception on first insemination (% pregnant)	60	50	60	65	30–50

* Seasonal breeders; refers to artificial insemination during the normal breeding season.
† Small volumes with a high concentration of spermatozoa are preferable; sperm in extended semen should be reconcentrated by centrifugation.
‡ Based on three inseminations per estrus with 500 million motile sperm each insemination. Fewer sperm have been used with frozen semen, but it is doubtful if the number of sperm for best results is less than that required with fresh semen.

to freeze, resulting in lower fertility, or problems with the management of the females, including detection of estrus, have not made AI programs with frozen semen attractive or economic on an extensive basis.

Ram semen can be pelleted or frozen in straws with a milk, yolk-lactose, or yolk-tris extender. Semen collected during the normal breeding season freezes well. In the pellet method, the semen is cooled to 5°C, glycerol added as necessary, and the semen held for about 2 hours before freezing as 0.1-ml to 0.4-ml pellets on dry ice. Storage is in liquid nitrogen at −196°C. Pellets are thawed in a solution similar to the freezing extender but with glycerol and egg yolk omitted. Spermatozoa should be concentrated by centrifugation and a small volume containing the desired number of sperm cells (Table 24–10) inseminated, if possible, through the cervix. Fertility is considerably higher, and fewer spermatozoa are required with intrauterine insemination.

Buck (goat) spermatozoa also can be frozen with good survival when semen is collected during the breeding season. The semen is pre-extended, centrifuged, and resuspended in heated milk (Corteel, 1977) or yolk-tris media (Fougner, 1976). The centrifugation removes seminal plasma, which contains an enzyme that can cause coagulation. Following cooling, the semen is frozen in straws and stored at −196°C. Thawing should be done quickly, and intrauterine insemination is highly desirable, if possible.

Boar semen has been difficult to freeze, but there are several successful methods (Pursel and Johnson, 1975; Larsson, 1978). Sperm survival is improved by holding the raw semen for 2 hours to expose sperm cells to the seminal plasma. Then the cell concentration is increased by centrifugation, extender is added, and the extended semen is cooled to 5°C (Table 24–12). About 2% by volume of glycerol is added, and the semen pelleted as described previously. Following storage at −196°C,

TABLE 24–12. Composition of BL-1 and Kiev Extenders for Boar Semen

Ingredient*	Amount (g)	
	BL-1	Kiev
Glucose-1H$_2$O	29.7	60.0
Sodium citrate-2-H$_2$O	10.0	3.75
Sodium bicarbonate	2.0	1.20
EDTA	—	3.70
Potassium chloride	.3	—
Sodium penicillin G†	.6	.6
Dihydrostreptomycin	1.0	1.0

* Diluted to 1,000 ml in deionized water.
†1,000,000 IU.

enough pellets are rapidly thawed in a solution such as that given in Table 24–13 to provide the necessary sperm for insemination.

The success with which stallion semen can be frozen varies greatly. The Nagase type of yolk-lactose-glycerol or yolk-raffinose-glycerol extender (similar to the one given for bulls in Table 24–9), or a more complex extender (Nishikawa et al., 1972) can be used for straws as well. Only the sperm-rich fraction is collected, or much of the seminal plasma is removed by centrifugation. Semen is extended and cooled to 5°C. Stallion spermatozoa are sensitive to glycerol and this compound may be added just before freezing. Storage is at −196°C. The fertility of stallion semen is decreased by freezing.

Evaluation of Sperm Motility

Sperm motility is evaluated before cryopreservation and again after thawing. To evaluate sperm motility before cryopreservation, semen samples are diluted 1 : 20

TABLE 24–13. Thawing Solution for Boar Spermatozoa

Ingredients	Amount
Dextrose, anhydrous (g)	37
Sodium citrate, dihydrate (g)	6.
Sodium bicarbonate (g)	1.25
Disodium ethylenediamine tetra-acetate (g)	1.25
Potassium chloride (g)	0.75
Double distilled water to volume (ml)	1000.

(Adapted from Pursel and Johnson, 1975.)

in the same medium used for cryopreservation. The hemocytometer is filled then placed in a moist atmosphere for 3 minutes to stabilize before observation. The percentage of sperm with progressive forward motility, an important indicator of fertilizability, is evaluated. The number of spermatozoa with forward movement is divided by the total number of spermatozoa (motile and nonmotile) and multiplied by 100.

When cryopreserved semen is thawed, it is transferred from the liquid nitrogen tank to a controlled water bath at 37°C for 3 to 5 minutes or to an automatic thawing unit. Motility is estimated immediately after thawing and after a 30- or 60-minute incubation at 37°C. Sperm motility is compared after cryopreservation with motility before cryopreservation to evaluate the effect of cryoprotectant on the cryosurvival:

$$\text{Recovery Rate} = \frac{\text{Motility after freezing}}{\text{Initial motility before freezing}} \times 100$$

Semen Cryopreservation Damage

The following are semen abnormalities that may result from cryopreservation; also listed are methods of detecting these aberrations:

1. Certain sperm organelles, such as the acrosome, may show structural change.
2. Disruption of the acrosome is viewed by light microscopy of Giemsa-stained semen smears.
3. Degenerative changes may occur in the acrosome similar to those stained with the Giemsa stain, as judged by differential phase interference microscopy of unfixed sperm.
4. Breakages in the plasma membrane overlying the acrosome may result: The acrosome swells and subsequent rupture of the outer membrane is associated with the loss of acrosomal substance.
5. Mitochondria lose their internal structure and are more lightly stained than unfrozen controls. Remarkable species differences are apparent in response of spermatozoa to cryopreservation.
6. Leakage of sperm enzymes may be used to assay sperm damage. A decrease in one of two acid phosphatase isoenzymes in spermatozoa is associated with an increase of the same enzyme in the extracellular medium.
7. Methylene blue reduction, oxygen uptake, fructolysis, and pyruvate use of sperm as tests of sperm function.

REFERENCES

Berndtson, W.E. and Pickett, B.W. (1978). Techniques for the cryopreservation and field handling of bovine spermatozoa. *In* The Integrity of Frozen Spermatozoa. Washington, D.C., Conf. Natl. Acad. Sci. 53–57.

Bilton, R.J. and Moore, N.W. (1976a). In vitro culture, storage and transfer of goat embryos. Aust. J. Biol. Sci. *29*, 125–129.

Bilton, R.J. and Moore, N.W. (1976b). Proceedings: storage of cattle embryos. J. Reprod. Fertil. *46*, 537–538.

Bilton, R.J. and Moore, N.W. (1979). Factors affecting the viability of frozen stored cattle embryos. Aust. J. Biol. Sci. *32*, 101–107.

Corteel, J.M. (1977). Production, storage and insemination of goat semen. Proc. Symposium Management of Reproduction in Sheep and Goats. Am. Soc. of Anim. Sci. 41–57.

Davis, D.L. and Day, B.N. (1978). Cleavage and blastocyst formation by pig eggs in vitro. J. Anim. Sci. *46*, 1043.

Foote, R.W. (1975). Semen quality from the bull to the freezer: an assessment. Theriogenology *3*, 219.

Foote, R.W. (1980). Artificial insemination. *In* Reproduction in Farm Animals. E.S.E. Hafez (ed.). Philadelphia, PA, Lea & Febiger.

Fougner, U.A. (1976). Uterine insemination with frozen semen in goats. VIIIth Internat. Congr. Anim. Reprod. Artif. Insem. Krakow, *4*, 987.

Graham, E.F. (1978). Fundamentals of the preservation of spermatozoa. *In* The Integrity of Frozen Spermatozoa. Proc. Conf. Natl. Acad. Sci. Washington, D.C., 4–44.

Larsson, K. (1978). Deep-freezing of boar semen. Cryobiology *15*, 352.

Nishikawa, Y., Iritani, A. and Shinomiya, S. (1972). Studies on the protective effects of egg yolk and glycerol on the freezability of horse spermatozoa. VIIth Internat. Congr. Anim. Reprod. Artif. Insem., Munich, *1,* 1545.

Pace, M.M. and Sullivan, J.J. (1978). A biological comparison of the .5 ml ampule and .5 ml French straw systems for packaging bovine spermatozoa. NAAB Proc. 7th Tech. Conf. Artif. Insem. Reprod. 22–32.

Pickett, B.W., et al. (1975). Effect of seminal extenders on equine fertility. J. Anim. Sci. *40,* 1136.

Pursel, V.G. and Johnson, L.A. (1975). Freezing of boar spermatozoa: fertilizing capacity with concentrated semen and new thawing procedure. J. Anim. Sci. *40,* 99.

Salamon, S. (1976). Artificial Insemination of Sheep. University of Sidney, N.S.W., Australia.

Salisbury, G.W., VanDemark, N.L. and Lodge, J.R. (1978). Physiology of Reproduction and Artificial Insemination of Cattle. 2nd. Ed. San Francisco, W.H. Freeman.

Schneider, U. and Maurer, R.R. (1983). Factors affecting survival of frozen-thawed mouse embryos. Biol. Reprod. *29,* 121.

Sullivan, J.J. (1978). Characteristics and cryopreservation of stallion spermatozoa. Cryobiology *15,* 355.

Trounson, A.O., Woods, E. and Leeton, J.F. (1982). Freezing of embryos. An ethical obligation. Med. J. Aust. *2,* 332–333.

Wilmut, I. and Polge, C. (1977). The low temperature preservation of boar spermatozoa. (3) The fertilizing capacity of frozen and thawed semen. Cryobiology *14,* 483.

Glossary of Reproductive Biology*

Acrosome
Sac-like organelle on the anterior portion of the sperm head that contains several enzymes used during the penetration of egg membranes by the sperm.

Adhesion
Abnormal sticking together of tissues that should slip or slide freely over each other. Adhesions in the abdominal and pelvic cavities may occur after surgical operations, particularly if pus has spilled from a ruptured abscess.

Adipose tissue
Fatty connective tissue, commonly the part of the body where fat is stored.

Adrenalin
Proprietary name for epinephrine, the hormone produced by the inner portion, or medulla, of the adrenal gland.

Amnion
Innermost of the fetal membranes, forming the bag of waters that surrounds and protects the embryo.

Antibiotics
Chemical substances produced by certain living cells, such as bacteria, yeasts, and molds, which are antagonistic or damaging to certain other living cells, such as disease-producing bacteria. Different antibiotics may kill disease germs or prevent them from growing and multiplying.

Antibody
Protein in the blood modified by contact with a foreign substance (antigen) so that it exerts an antagonizing or neutralizing action against specific substances. Antibodies are chiefly associated with *γ-globulin* in the blood and are key elements of the immunity mechanisms of the body. The antibody–antigen reaction is protective.

Antigen
Any substance that stimulates the production of *antibodies*.

Antiprostaglandin
Drugs that prevent the formation of responsible chemical substances (prostaglandins).

Atresia
The closure or the failure of development of a normal opening or channel in the body.

Autoimmune disease
Several diseases of unknown cause may reflect a strange inability of the body to "recognize" itself, so that mechanisms that normally create immunity to foreign invaders somehow establish a specific sensitivity to certain of the body's own tissues.

Axon
A single long, fine fiber that conducts impulses away from the body of a nerve cell. Most axons are covered with a sheath of whitish material called *myelin.*

Azoospermia
Absence of sperm in the semen.

Biopsy
Removal of tissue from the living body for diagnosis. The tissue specimen may be subjected to biochemical tests; more often, it is set in a paraffin block, cut into thin slices, stained, and studied under a microscope.

Blastocyst
A hollow embryonic structure resulting from the accumulation of blastocoelic fluid within the expanding morula and found in the uterus from day 3 to 7 of gestation.

Cannula
A hollow tube for insertion into a body passage or cavity. Within the cannula there is usually a trocar, a sliding instrument with a pointed tip, designed to puncture a cavity and release fluid, after which

---

* Words in italics are also defined in glossary.

the trocar is withdrawn and fluid drains through the cannula.

Capacitation

Final maturation of spermatozoa in the female reproductive tract leading to fertilization of the egg.

Castration

Removal of the testicles or ovaries. Functional powers of the ovaries can be destroyed by radiation, sometimes necessary in treatment of disease; this is called non-surgical castration.

Catheter

A hollow tube for insertion through a narrow canal into a cavity to discharge fluids.

Centigrade (C)

A thermometer scale widely used in science and medicine in which water freezes at 0°C and boils at 100°C. To convert to Fahrenheit degrees, multiply degrees Centigrade by nine-fifths and add 32.

Chorion

The outermost of the fetal membranes. The fetal part of the placenta develops from it.

Chromosome

Threadlike bodies in the nucleus of a cell, they contain the *genes* and DNA. The chromosomes separate during a stage of cell division. Stained and prepared specimens can be studied under a microscope. Each parent contributes a chromosome to the pair. One of the pairs contains the sex chromosomes. A dam contributes the X (female-determining) chromosome to the pair, and a sire contributes either an X or a Y chromosome.

Cilia

Minute hairlike processes of specialized cells that beat rhythmically and keep debris-laden fluids flowing in one direction, for example, out of the lungs. The word also means eyelashes.

Cleavage

Fertilized ovum begins to divide. No increase in volume. **First cleavage:** plane passes through area where male and fe-

male pronuclei situated. **Second cleavage:** occurs at right angles. **Third cleavage:** occurs close to right angles. Division may not be perfectly synchronized. Divisions are mitotic. Each cell contains the diploid number of chromosomes (2n). Compaction occurs: cells become wedge-shaped. Fluid collects in intercellular spaces. Blastocoele appears.

Clitoris

Erectile sex organ of the female situated above the vagina; homologue of the penis.

Colostrum

The "first milk" secreted by the mammary gland shortly after birth. Colostrum is not "true" milk but a clear or slightly cloudy fluid containing fats and sugars that have a slight laxative effect on the newborn baby. Colostrum also contains immunoglobulins that pass on to the baby some of the immunities acquired by the mother; passive immunity thus transmitted is not long lasting.

Conception

Confusing term. Not recommended term, although others use it to refer to the onset of fertilization of the egg in the tube.

Conception (product of)

All structures developing from the blastocyst, including the fetus and the placental membranes and fluid.

Congenital malformations

Abnormalities present at birth.

Corpus luteum

The "yellow body" that develops from a follicle of the ovary after a ripened egg has been discharged. It produces progesterone, a hormone that prepares the lining of the uterus to receive a fertilized egg. If fertilization occurs, the corpus luteum enlarges and continues to produce pregnancy-sustaining hormone for several months. If conception does not occur, the corpus luteum degenerates.

Cranium
The skull, containing the brain.

Cremaster
Muscles that retract the testis.

Cryogenic fluid
A fluid or liquefied gas that remains unfrozen at very low temperatures.

Cryoprotective agent
Compounds such as dimethylsulfoxide or glycerol that are added to biologic solutions to minimize the deleterious effects of cryobiologic procedures.

Cryosurgery
The use of extreme cold to destroy or to freeze and later revive tissues. Instruments that precisely apply extreme cold to tissues are usually supercooled by liquid nitrogen.

Crypt
A cavity or pit such as a natural depression in the cervix.

Cryptorchidism
Failure of the testicles to descend into the scrotum during fetal development; the undescended testis remains in the abdominal cavity or groin.

Cyst
A normal or abnormal sac with a definite wall, containing liquid or semisolid material.

Cytology
Scientific study of the structure, elements, and functions of cells.

Cytoplasm
The substance of a cell outside of its nucleus. Transformations of energy, synthesis of proteins, and uncountable chemical exchanges that keep us alive occur incessantly in the cytoplasm.

Death (fetal)
Termination of fetal viability to the complete expulsion or extraction of a product of conception, irrespective of the duration of pregnancy.

Decalcification
The withdrawal of calcium from the bones where it had been deposited. It may be caused by an inadequate supply of calcium in the ration so that calcium has to be taken from the bones, or it may be caused by hormonal imbalances.

Decidua
That part of the lining of the uterus that is modified during pregnancy and cast off after delivery.

Dewar flask
An insulated flask used for holding cryogenic fluids. The flask contains an inner and outer layer usually separated by an evacuated space. The inner surface of the flask is usually coated with silver or aluminum to minimize heat loss.

Diagnosis
The art and science of identifying a disease; a prerequisite to treatment, hazardous if applied by the untrained in reckless self-diagnosis. Some diagnostic tools are as old as Hippocrates: history, symptoms, physical signs, thumping and listening, feeling, inspecting, and applying all the trained senses. Instruments amplify and transcribe minute currents of the heart, brain, and muscles.

Dizygotic
Developed at the same time from two fertilized eggs (fraternal twins).

DMSO
Dimethyl sulfoxide. A solvent that can penetrate intact skin or cell membrane and carry drugs or chemicals with it.

Dry Ice
Solid carbon dioxide with a temperature of $-77°C$. Used as a coolant either directly or mixed in alcohol such as ethanol and methanol.

Dysfunction
Abnormality or impairment of the normal activities of an organ or bodily process.

Dystocia
Painful or difficult labor or birth.

Dystrophy
Degeneration, wasting, and abnormal development.

Embryo
The conceptus from the time of implantation to the 2-, 4-, 8-, and 16-blastomeres, morula, blastocyst and implanted blastocyst until completed organogenesis. Later it is referred to as a fetus.

Epithelia
Cells that form the outer layer of the skin, i.e., those that line all the portions of the body that have contact with external air (eyes, ears, nose, throat, lungs), and tissues specialized for secretion such as the urogenital tract.

Estrogen
A hormone produced in the ovaries to stimulate growth of the inner lining of the uterus.

Fertilization
Penetration of the ovum by the spermatozoon and completed by the fusion of the female and male chromosomes with subsequent formation of male and female pronuclei and expulsion of the second polar body, syngamy leading to cleavage to two blastomeres.

Fetus (British: foetus)
Unborn offspring from completed organogenesis at the end of 8 weeks, until the completion of pregnancy. The term is applicable to unborn offspring from the date of implantation to the termination of pregnancy.

Fimbria
A fringelike structure; especially, fimbriae of the opening of the *oviducts,* close to the ovary. The fringelike projections are covered with cilia. The conversion of an unfrozen solution into the solid form.

Freezing
The conversion of an unfrozen solution into the solid form.

Freezing point
The temperature at which the solid and liquid phase of the media can exist in equilibrium.

Freezing point depression
The freezing point of a solution decreases as the molarity of all substances dissolved in that fluid increases. When salts or cryoprotective agents are added to water, the freezing point is depressed in proportion to the concentration of these agents.

FSH
Follicle-stimulating hormone.

Gamete
Egg or sperm.

Gene
Ultimate unit in transmission of hereditary characteristics contained in *chromosomes.*

Gestation (pregnancy; gravidity)
The period from implantation of the blastocyst in the endometrium until the termination of pregnancy.

Gonad
Primary sex glands, ovaries, or testes.

Graafian follicle
Round, transparent, ovarian follicle containing an immature egg. Under the influence of FSH of the pituitary gland, one of the blisters is stimulated to grow, and its egg matures in preparation for fertilization.

Gram-positive, Gram-negative
Classification of bacteria according to whether they do or do not accept a stain named for Hans Gram, a Danish bacteriologist. Different life processes and vulnerabilities of germs are reflected by their gram-positive or gram-negative characteristics.

Granulocyte
White blood cells containing granules that become conspicuous when dyed. They are manufactured in the red marrow of the bones. One of their functions is to digest and destroy invading bacteria.

Hemocytometer
A device for counting blood cells.

Hormone
Special chemicals made by the body that cause changes in the body.

Hyperplasia
Overgrowth of an organ or tissue from increased numbers of cells that are in normal patterns.

Hypertrophy
Increase in the size of an organ because of overgrowth of cells without an increase in the number of cells. The overgrowth of cells is in response to increased activity or functional demands.

Hypophysis.
The pituitary gland.

Hypothalamus
A part of the brain concerned with various functions such as appetite, procreation, sleep, body temperature. Closely associated with the pituitary gland.

Identical twin
Twins, always of the same sex and having the same heredity, developing from a single fertilized egg.

Implantation
The blastocyst adheres to, penetrates, and establishes nutritional support from maternal tissues, normally the endometrium.

In vitro
In glass; pertaining to studies done in test tubes or laboratory hardware, outside of the living body.

Insemination
Introduction of semen into the vagina by natural means or by artificial insemination.

Intracellular ice formation
The predominant deleterious effect to the survival of rapidly cooled cells. The ice crystals are believed to mechanically disrupt membranes and cellular organelles, leading to the loss of viability.

Intrauterine device (IUD)
A small device that is inserted and left inside the uterus to prevent pregnancy.

Labia
Lips or liplike organs. Labia majora: folds of skin on either side of the entrance of the vulva. Labia minora: folds of tissue covered with mucous membrane within the labia majora.

Laparoscopy
An operation in which the organs inside the body can be viewed through a lighted tube.

Lesion
Alteration of tissue or function due to injury or disease, e.g., pimple, fracture, abscess, scratch, or wart.

Leukocyte
White blood cells.

Leukocytosis
Abnormal increase in numbers of white blood cells. The cell count normally increases slightly after eating and in pregnancy, but the word implies an abnormal increase, often associated with bodily defenses against infection and inflammation.

Leydig cell
Interstitial cells of the testes that produce testosterone, the male hormone (and small amounts of female hormone). The cells are separate structures from those that produce spermatozoa. Thus, infertile males whose production of spermatozoa is impaired may produce adequate amounts of male hormone and be entirely potent.

LH
Luteinizing hormone of the pituitary gland. It causes a *graafian follicle* that has released a "ripened" egg to become a yellow body that produces progesterone, a hormone that helps to prepare the lining of the uterus for implantation of a fertilized egg.

Ligament
A band of tough, flexible fibrous tissue that connects bones or supports organs.

Liquid nitrogen
Liquefied nitrogen gas commonly used for cooling or storage in biologic samples. Its temperature is $-196°C$.

Monozygotic
Developed from a single fertilized egg, as identical twins.

Morula
A 16-, 32-, or 64-blastomere embryo resulting from cleavage of zygote, usually found in fallopian tube or uterus.

Osmosis
The phenomenon of transfer of materials through a semipermeable membrane that

separates two solutions, or between a solvent and a solution, tending to equalize their concentrations.

Osmotic effect
Alteration in the osmotic strength of the suspending media caused by conversion of water to ice or of ice to water. This results in a substantial flow of water across membranes of unfrozen cells, causing the cells to shrink or expand during freezing and thawing.

Oviduct
Tubes through which the egg is transported to the uterus and in which fertilization usually occurs.

Ovulation
Release of egg from the ovarian follicle.

Ovum
Egg cell. The ovum is the largest human cell, but it is barely discernible by the naked eye. It is about one fourth the size of the period at the end of this sentence. It is a round cell with a clear shell-like capsule, with the consistency of stiff jelly, weighing about a 50-billionth of an ounce—the "original weight" of every human being (the weight of the much smaller fertilizing sperm scarcely counts). Like the sperm, the ovum contains *chromosomes*, which at conception "pair off" with those of the sperm to give the embryo a normal complement of chromosomes. Although the ovum is about 90,000 times larger than the sperm, both contain the same number of genes.

Peristalsis
Wavelike movements created by constriction and relaxation, which propel materials along the tube. Encircling muscle contracts to squeeze material forward, while muscles in front of the material relax.

pH
Symbol expressing hydrogen ion concentration. Practically, it is a scale of the acidity or alkalinity of substances. The neutral point is pH 7; below 7, acidity increases and above 7, alkalinity increases.

Phagocyte
A white blood cell with properties of engulfing, digesting, and invading bacteria or other foreign particles.

Phimosis
Elongation and tightening of the foreskin of the penis, preventing retraction of the head of the organ.

Polyspermy
One or more supernumerary sperm form pronuclei. Pronuclei are reduced in size; this normally leads to triploidy.

Pregnancy
The period from implantation of the blastocyst until the expulsion of extraction of the fetus and placental membranes.

Programmed freezing
A sequence of automatically controlled cooling rates used for the preservation of cells in automatic or semiautomatic equipment.

Prostaglandin
Chemical made by the body that causes the muscle of the uterus to contract.

Purulent
Containing, exuding, or producing pus.

Rugae
Wrinkles, folds, elevations, ridges of tissue, as of the linings of the vagina.

Salpingitis
Inflammation of one or both oviducts, (fallopian tubes).

Scrotum
Pouch covering the testis.

Seeding
Artificial introduction of ice crystal nucleation in an aqueous sample. This is usually done to minimize the extent of supercooling allowed in the sample. It may be performed by either touching the surface of the sample with an ice crystal, with a cold probe or by mechanical vibration.

Seminal vesicle
Accessory glands of male reproductive systems; continuous with the prostate gland.

Septum
A partition or wall between two compartments or cavities.

Serum
The amber-colored fluid of blood that remains after the blood has coagulated and the clot has shrunk. It contains disease-fighting antibodies of the host.

Silastic
Form of silicone rubber.

Smear
Secretions or blood spread on a glass slide for examination under a microscope. Smears are often stained with various dyes to contrast details.

Speculum
An instrument for viewing the interior of a passage or body cavity, e.g., the vagina.

Spermatocele
A swelling of the *scrotum* caused by cystic dilation (fluid-filled sac) of the sperm-conducting tubules of the testis.

Steroid
Natural hormones or synthetic drugs whose molecules share a common skeleton of four rings of carbon atoms (the steroid nucleus) but which have different actions according to the attachment of other atoms. Several synthetic steroids developed by pharmaceutical research increase potency, enhance desired effects, minimize side effects, or otherwise improve the actions of a molecule by shifting, attaching, or detaching a few atoms.

Storage temperature
Temperature at which samples are held in the frozen stage before use. For biologic samples, storage to at least $-80°C$ is required and storage at liquid nitrogen temperature ($-196°C$) is highly recommended.

Straw
A thin glass or plastic tube often used for freezing embryos and sperm.

Stroma
The supporting tissue of an organ, as opposed to its active "producing" tissue.

Supercooling
Because ice seldom forms spontaneously at the freezing point of the solution and, in fact, the solution usually cools many degrees below its freezing point before spontaneous onset of ice formation, supercooling results.

Superovulation
An increase in ovulation rate over the characteristic for the species induced by the injection of various gonadotropins.

Syngamy
When male and female pronuclei come into contact, they begin to shrink and coalesce; at the time of first cleavage, two chromosome groups become visible, the maternal and paternal, and unite and form a single group.

Tattooing
Insertion of permanent colors into the skin through punctures, as by a needle.

Tendon
A band of tough white fibrous tissue that connects a muscle to a bone. Muscle fibers merge into one end of a tendon, the other end of which is attached to a bone.

Teratology
Science concerned with malformations and monstrosities.

Testosterone
Male hormone. A *steroid* hormone produced by cells of the testis independent from cells that produce spermatozoa.

Thermal shock
Injury occurring to cells as a result of change in temperature (in the absence of freezing or changes in the ionic strength of the media).

Thermocouple
A bimetallic wire that produces a temperature-dependent voltage at its junction; voltage change can be electronically processed to indicate sample temperature.

Tissue culture
The growing of cells in a suitable nutrient in flasks or test tubes outside of the body.

Trypsin
A protein-digesting enzyme produced by the pancreas gland.

TSH
Thyroid-stimulating hormone.

Ultrasound
Sound waves of high frequencies above the range of hearing. Ultrasonic devices of various and changing design have several veterinary and medical uses.

Umbilical cord
The long flexible tube that is attached to the placenta at one end and to the abdomen of the fetus at the other. It is the lifeline of the fetus. Through vessels of the cord, the fetus receives nutrients and disposes of wastes. The cord allows freedom of movement in the dark fluid in the amnion. The cord continues to function until it is tied and severed at birth.

Urea
A nitrogen-containing substance in blood and urine, formed mainly from nitrogen groups removed in the liver from the amino acids of protein foods. Some is formed from nitrogen released by the wear and tear of body tissues.

Ureter
The narrow tube through which urine from the kidneys passes into the bladder.

Urethra
The canal from the neck of the bladder to the outside through which urine passes.

Uric acid
A nitrogen-containing compound present in normal blood and urine. It is derived from substances in the nuclei of cells called purines.

Vaccine
Any bacterial or viral material for inoculation against a specific disease. Virus vaccines are of two types: live virus or killed virus vaccines. Live virus vaccines contain living viruses that are so weakened that they cannot cause significant disease but can still stimulate the body powerfully to make protective *antibodies* against a par-

ticular disease. Killed virus vaccines contain viruses treated by physical or chemical means to kill or inactivate them so they cannot cause disease but nevertheless can stimulate the immunity-producing mechanisms of the animal. Live virus vaccines are more potent and create longer lasting immunity than killed virus vaccines.

Vagina
A sheath. The female organ of copulation, a muscular canal that opens at the surface of the body and extends inward to the cervix of the uterus.

Vas deferens
The duct through which sperm are transported from the testis to the seminal vesicles and urethra.

Vasoconstrictor
A drug or natural body substance or mechanism that clamps down on small blood vessels, narrows their caliber, and reduces the volume of blood flowing through them. This action increases the amount of blood in the reservoirs of big expansible arteries and increases blood pressure until equilibrium.

Vasodilator
An agent that dilates small blood vessels so that more blood flows through them; blood pressure is usually lowered.

Vasomotor
Physiologic mechanisms that control dilation or constriction of walls of blood vessels and thus the volume of blood flowing through them. Impulses from centers in the brain go to muscle fibers in the walls of blood vessels over nerves of opposite action: constriction or dilation.

Viability
The ability of frozen and thawed gametes to function. Viability is usually expressed in the ability of the cells to reproduce, metabolize, exclude vital dyes, or carry out some other metabolic function. The viability of the frozen and thawed gametes must always be compared to the ability of unfrozen cells obtained at the same time to carry out the same function.

Villi
Minute fingerlike projection from the surface of a mucous membrane. The chorion, a placental membrane, contains millions of villi (chorionic villi) that increase the surface area.

Vitrification
Solidification of solution into glass-like state. Occurs at extremely high rates of cooling or extremely high pressures.

X chromosome
The female sex-determining chromosome; females have two of them, males only one.

See *chromosome*. The X chromosome is larger than the Y chromosome and contains some *genes* for which there are no complements on the Y chromosome.

Y chromosome
The male sex-determining chromosome. See *chromosome*.

Zygote
The fertilized ovum, after the penetration of spermatozoa in the vitellus, and the formation of the male and female pronuclei in syngamy, until the completion of the first cleavage and formation of the two-blastomere egg.

Glossary of Common Abbreviations

ACTH	adrenocorticotropic hormone
ADH	antidiuretic hormone
AFP	α-fetoprotein
AI	artificial insemination
AIDS	acquired immune deficiency syndrome (HIV)
AMH	anti-Müllerian hormone
AMP	adenosine monophosphate
ARC	AIDS-related complex
ATP	adenosine triphoshate
BBB	blood–brain barrier
BBT	basal body temperature
bFGF	basic fibroblast growth factor
BP	blood pressure
BSA	bovine serum albumin
cAMP	cyclic AMP
cDNA	DNA complementary to RNA
CDP	cytidine 5'-phosphate
CIC	circulating immune complexes
CL	corpus luteum (singular)
CRH	corticotropin-releasing hormone
CSF	colony-stimulating factor
CT	computed tomography
D&C	dilation and curettage
D&E	dilation and evacuation
DES	diethylstilbestrol
DHEA	dehydroepiandrosterone
DMB	diazobenzyloxymethyl
DMSO	dimethyl sulfoxide (Me$_2$SO)
DNA	deoxyribonucleic acid
EF	elongation factor
EGF	epidermal growth factor
ELISA	enzyme-linked immunosorbant assay
FCS	fetal calf serum
FGF	fibroblast growth factor
FHR	fetal heart rate
FRP	follicular regulating protein
FSH	follicle-stimulating hormone
FSH-RH	follicle-stimulating releasing hormone
GnRH	gonadotropin-releasing hormone
GH-RH	growth hormone-releasing hormone
GLC	gas-liquid chromatography
GM-CSF	granulocyte-macrophage colony stimulating factor
GTT	glucose tolerance test

hCB	human cord blood
hCG	human chorionic gonadotropin
hMG	human menopausal gonadotropin
hMT	human mammary tumor
HIV	human immunodeficiency virus
HMD	hyaline membrane disease
hPL	human placental lactogen
HPLC	high-pressure liquid chromatography
HSV	herpes simplex virus
IF	immunofluorescence techniques
IFN	interferon
Ig	immunoglobulin
IGFS	insulin-like growth factor serum
IM	intramuscular
IUGR	intrauterine growth retardation
IUGR-LBW	intrauterine growth retardation low birth weight
IV	intravenous
IVF	*in vitro* fertilization
kDa	kilodalton
LBW	low birth weight
LH	luteinizing hormone
LH-RH	luteinizing hormone-releasing hormone
LH-RF	luteinizing hormone-releasing factor
LI	luteinizing inhibitor
MIS	Müllerian-inhibiting substance
MRI	magnetic resonance imaging
mt	mitochondria
NA	neutralizing antibody
NGF	nerve-growth factor
NK	natural killer
PAF	platelet-activating factor
PAGE	polyacrylamide-gel electrophoresis
PBL	peripheral blood lymphocytes
PBS	phosphate-buffered saline
PDGF	platelet-derived growth factor
PG	prostaglandins
PGF_2	prostaglandin F_2
PIF	prolactin-inhibiting factor
PMSG	pregnant mare serum gonadotropin
PVS	perivitelline space
RNA	ribonucleic acid
RRA	radioreceptor assay
rRNA	ribosomal RNA
SMC	somatomedin-c
STH	somatotropic hormone
TBG	thyroxine-binding globulin
TDF	testis-determining factor
TGF	transforming growth factor
VIP	vasoactive intestinal peptide

UNITS

mg	milligram (10^{-3} g)
μg	microgram (10^{-6} g)
ng	nanogram (10^{-9} g)
pg	picogram (10^{-12} g)
IU	international unit

Appendix I

Chromosome Numbers of Bovinae, Equinae, and Caprinae Species

Common Name	Scientific Name	Chromosome Number (2N)	Fundamental Number
Domestic cattle	*Bos taurus*	60	62
Banteng	*Bos banteng*	60	62
Zebu	*Bos indicus*	60	62
Yak	*Bos grunniens*	60	62
European bison	*Bison bonasus*	60	62
American bison	*Bison bison*	60	62
Gaur	*Bos gaurus*	58	62
Nyala	*Tragelaphus angasi*	55	58
Congo buffalo	*Syncerus caffer nanus*	54	60
African buffalo	*Syncerus caffer caffer*	52	60
Asiatic buffalo	*Bubalus bubalis*	48	58
Anoa	*Anoa depressicornis*	48	60
Nilgai	*Boselaphus tragocamelus*	46	60
Four-horned antelope	*Tetracerus quadricornis*	38	38
Sitatunga	*Tragelaphus spekei*	30	58
Mongolian wild horse	*Equus przewalskii*	66	94
Domestic horse	*Equus caballus*	64	94
Donkey	*Equus asinus*	62	104
Nubian ass	*Equus asinus africans*	62	104
Mongolian wild ass	*Equus hemionus*	56	104
Tibetan wild ass	*Equus kiang*	56	104
Persian wild ass	*Equus onager*	56	104
Grevy zebra	*Equus grevyi*	46	78
African zebra	*Equus burchelli*	44	82
Grant zebra	*Equus burchelli boehmi*	44	82
Mountain zebra	*Equus zebra*	34(?)	60
Domestic goat	*Capra hircus*	60	60
Ibex	*Capra ibex*	60	60
Markhor	*Capra falconeri*	60	60
Saiga antelope	*Saiga tatarica*	60	60
Aoudad	*Ammotragus lervia*	58	60
Afghanistan sheep	*Ovis ammon cycloceros*	58	60
Kara-Tau sheep	*Ovis ammon nigimontana*	56	60
Domestic sheep	*Ovis aries*	54	60
Mouflon	*Ovis musimon*	54	60
Red sheep	*Ovis orientalis*	54	60(?)
Bighorn sheep	*Ovis canadensis*	54	60
Laristan sheep	*Ovis ammon laristanica*	54	60
Musk ox	*Ovibos moschatus*	48	60
Himalayan tahr	*Hemitragus jemlahias*	48	60
Rocky Mountain goat	*Oreamnos americanus*	42	60

Appendix II

Chromosome Numbers and Reproductive Ability in Equine, Bovine, and Caprine Hybrids

Species and Chromosome Number (2N)		Hybrids Chromosome Number (2N)	Reproductive Ability
Sire	Dam		
Mongolian wild horse, 66 (*E. przewalskii*)	Domestic horse, 64 (*E. caballus*)	65	Fertility (?)
Donkey, 62 (*E. asinus*)	Domestic horse, 64 (*E. caballus*)	63 (Mule)	Sterile
Domestic horse, 64 (*E. caballus*)	Donkey, 62 (*E. asinus*)	63 (Hinny)	Males are sterile, females are fertile, only in very exceptional cases
Nubian ass, 62 (*E. asinus africanus*)	Donkey, 62 (*E. asinus*)	62	Fertile
Mongolian wild ass, 56 (*E. hemionus*)	Donkey, 62 (*E. asinus*)	59	Fertile (?)
Grevy zebra, 46 (*E. grevyi*)	Domestic horse, 64 (*E. caballus*)	55 (Zebroid)	Sterile
African zebra, 44 (*E. burchelli*)	Donkey, 62 (*E. asinus*)	53 (Zebronkey)	Sterile
Donkey, 62 (*E. asinus*)	Mountain zebra, 34 (?) (*E. zebra*)	48	Sterile
American bison, 60 (*Bison bison*)	Zebu, 60 (*Bos indicus*)	60	Females are fertile
American bison, 60 (*Bison bison*)	Domestic cattle, 60 (*Bos taurus*)	60 (Cattalo)	Male F_1 are sterile
Domestic cattle, 60 (*Bos taurus*)	American bison, 60 (*Bison bison*)	60 (Cattalo)	Male F_1 are sterile
Domestic goat, 60 (*Capra hircus*)	Barbary sheep, 58 (*Ammotragus lorvia*)	59 (?)	Full-term fetuses, but no live hybrid
Domestic goat, 60 (*Capra hircus*)	Domestic sheep, 54 (*Ovis aries*)	57	Embryos are resorbed or aborted at 6 weeks pregnancy
Domestic sheep, 54 (*Ovis aries*)	Mouflon, 54 (*Ovis musimon*)	54	Fertile in both sexes
Bighorn sheep, 54 (*Ovis canadensis*)	Domestic sheep, 54 (*Ovis aries*)	54	Reduced fertility

Appendix III

Reproductive Diseases of Viral, Protozoan, and Bacterial Origin

Disease	Species	Etiology	Diagnosis Clinical	Diagnosis Other	Control
Epizootic bovine	Cattle	Unknown	Abortion in late pregnancy, lymphoid tissue lesions in fetus	Microscopic lesions of chronic inflammation	Change breeding season
Granular venereal disease	Cattle	Lymphoid reaction	Nodular vulvitis, balanitis	—	None
Infectious pustular vulvovaginitis (IPV)	Cattle	Bovine herpesvirus	Fibrinonecrotic vulvitis and vaginitis	Isolation of virus, serum neutralization test	Cessation of breeding, vaccination
Infectious bovine rhinotracheitis (IBR)	Cattle	Bovine herpesvirus	Respiratory disease, abortion	Isolation of virus, serum neutralization test	Vaccination
Bovine viral diarrhea (BVD)	Cattle	Virus	Abortion in early pregnancy, birth defects	Serum neutralization test	Vaccination
Catarrhal vaginitis	Cattle	Virus	Catarrhal vaginitis	Isolation of virus	None
Ulcerative dermatitis	Sheep	Virus	Ulceration of lips, legs, vulva and sheath	Lamb inoculation	Inspection of sale rams or rams purchased before breeding
Hog cholera	Swine	Virulent infection or modified live virus vaccination	Stillborn pigs, edematous dead pigs, weak pigs	History of pregnant sow vaccination or infection	Quarantine and slaughter of infected herds
SMEDI	Swine	Virus	Stillbirth mummified fetus, embryonic death, infertility	Virus isolation	Allow exposure before breeding, maintain closed herd
African swine fever	Swine	Virus	Disease resembling hog cholera, abortion in pregnant sows	Exposure to warthogs or other infected swine	Quarantine and slaughter of infected herds
Equine rhinopneumonitis	Horses	Equine herpesvirus I	Abortion in late pregnancy; respiratory disease in young	Focal necrosis of liver and edema of lungs in fetus, inclusion bodies, isolation of virus	Vaccination
Equine viral arteritis	Horses	Virus	Respiratory infection, cellulitis, abortion	Isolation of virus and serum neutralization test	Isolation of infected herds
Coital vesicular exanthema	Horses	Virus	Pustules on vulva, vagina, sheath, and penis	None	Isolation, cessation of breeding
Enzootic abortion	Sheep	Chlamydia	Abortion, fresh (not autolyzed)	Staining elementary bodies in placenta, complement-fixation test	Vaccination

Appendix III (cont'd)

Reproductive Diseases of Viral, Protozoan, and Bacterial Origin

Disease	Species	Etiology	Diagnosis		Control
			Clinical	Other	
Trichomoniasis	Cattle	*Trichomonas fetus*	Infertility, pyometra, and abortion in cows	Culture preputial cavity for trichomonads	Breeding rest, artificial insemination and treatment of bulls
Toxoplasmosis	Sheep Swine	*Toxoplasma gondii*	Encephalitis, abortion	Histopathology, dye test for antibodies	Isolation
Listeriosis	Cattle Sheep	*Listeria monocytogenes*	Nervous signs, circling, abortion	Isolation of bacterium	Avoid stress and feeding silage
Vibriosis	Cattle	*Campylobacter fetus* var. *venerealis*	Infertility	Mucus agglutination test, isolation, fluorescent antibody	Artificial insemination, vaccination
	Sheep	*Campylobacter fetus* var. *intestinalis*	Abortion	Isolation of bacterium	Vaccination
Leptospirosis	Cattle	*Leptospira pomona* *Leptospira hardjo*	Hemolytic anemia, abortion in late pregnancy, agalactia	Agglutination test	Vaccination, elimination of carriers with antibiotic treatment
	Swine	*Leptospira pomona* *Leptospira grippotyphosa* *Leptospira canicola*	Abortion in late pregnancy, birth of weak pigs	Isolation of *Leptospira*	
	Horses	*Leptospira pomona* *Leptospira grippotyphosa* *Leptospira icterohemorrhagiae*	Abortion in late pregnancy, periodic ophthalmia		
	Sheep	*Leptospira pomona*	Hemolytic anemia, abortion in late pregnancy		
Brucellosis	Cattle	*Brucella abortus*	Abortion in late pregnancy, sterility in bulls	Isolation of bacterium, serum and milk agglutination tests	Vaccination, test, and slaughter
	Swine	*Brucella suis*	Abortion, weak pigs, sterility in boars		
	Sheep Goat	*Brucella melitensis*	Abortion		
	Sheep	*Brucella ovis*	Epididymitis in rams, abortion		
	Dog	*Brucella canis*	Abortion		

(Afshar (1965). Vet. Bull. *35*, 165; Blood and Henderson (1963). Veterinary Medicine. 2nd Ed. Baltimore, Williams & Wilkins; Howarth (1960). Proc. U.S. Livestock Sanit. Assoc. *64*, 401.)

Appendix IV
Preparation of Physiologic Solutions

DULBECCO'S PHOSPHATE-BUFFERED SALINE (PBS)

To make 10 L:

CaCl$_2$·2H$_2$O	1.32 g	A
MgSO$_4$·7H$_2$O	1.21 g	
NaCl	80 g	
KCl	2 g	
Na$_2$HPO$_4$	11.5 g	
KH$_2$PO$_4$	2 g	B
Glucose	10 g	
Streptomycin sulfate	.5 g	
Na pyruvate	.36 g	
Na penicillin G	1,000,000 units	

A: May be weighed in advance and stored indefinitely in a sterile bottle under refrigeration.

B: May be weighed in advance and stored in sterile bottle under refrigeration for 1 month. Do not mix with CaCl$_2$ and MgSO$_4$ until just before use.

Before use:

1. Dissolve NaCl, KCl, Na$_2$HPO$_4$, KH$_2$PO$_4$, glucose, streptomycin, Na pyruvate, and penicillin in 8 L of deionized, distilled water.
2. Dissolve CaCl$_2$ and MgSO$_4$·7H$_2$O in 2 L of deionized, distilled water.
3. Add 2 L to 8 L with constant stirring. (Other methods of dissolving these ingredients often lead to formation of a precipitate.)
4. Add heat-treated bovine serum (1%) immediately prior to use for recovery of embryos and add 10% serum for storage of embryos.

Preparation of Stock Solutions

Two stock solutions are made:

1. Modified phosphate buffered saline	40 ml
Fetal calf serum (FCS)	10 ml
PBS + 20% FCS	50 ml
2. PBS + 20% FCS	45 ml
Glycerol	5 ml
Cooling medium (10% glycerol, v/v)	~50 ml

COMPOSITION OF SOME COMMON BUFFERS AND SOLUTIONS

Baker's solution:

Glucose	3 g
Na$_2$HPO$_4$	0.6 g
KH$_2$PO$_4$	0.01 g
NaCl	0.2 g

Add distilled water to 100 ml

Joel's solution:

80 ml of 5.42% dextrose in distilled water
20 ml of 0.125 NMgCl$_2$ in distilled water

Locke's solution:

CaCl$_2$	0.24 g
KCl	0.42 g
NaHCO$_3$	0.1 g
NaCl	9.0 g

Add distilled water to 100 ml

Physiologic saline:

NaCl	0.85 g

Add distilled water to 100 ml

Modified Ringer's buffer solution:

NaCl	120 mM
KCl	5 mM
KH$_2$PO$_4$	10 mM
MgSO$_4$H$_2$O	5 mM
Tris HCl	1 mM

Ringer-Locke's solution:

NaCl	9.5 g
KCl	0.075 g
CaCl$_2$	0.1 to 0.2 g
NaHCO$_3$	0.1 to 0.2 g
Glucose (optional)	1.0 g
Water	1000.0 g

Ringer-Tyrodes' solution:

NaCl	8.0 g
KCl	0.2 g
CaCl$_2$	0.2 g
MgSO$_4$	0.1 to 0.2 g
NaHCO$_3$	0.5 to 1.0 g
Glucose (optional)	1.0 g
Water	1000.0 ml

543

Scott's solution:

Sodium bicarbonate	3.5 g
Magnesium sulphate	20.0 g
Distilled water	1000 ml

The Scott's solution is to be used only when the ordinary tap water is "hard" and should be changed frequently, e.g., after rinsing 20 to 25 slides.

Hanks' BSS without bicarbonate (previously sterilized by autoclaving):

Penicillin	250 units/ml
Streptomycin	250 μg/ml
Kanamycin	100 μg/ml
or gentamycin	50 μg/ml
Amphotericin B	2.5 μg/ml

(All preparations sterile, store at $-20\,°C$.)

Dexamethasone 1 mg/ml (100×):

This comes already sterile in glass vials. To dissolve, add 5 ml of water by syringe to vial, remove, and dilute to give a concentration of 1 mg/ml. Aliquot and store at $-20\,°C$. Betamethasone and methylprednisolone may be prepared in the same way.

Penicillin (e.g., crystapen benzylpenicillin sodium):

1,000,000 units per vial

Use 4 vials and 400 ml Hanks' BSS

Prepare as for kanamycin; final concentration 10,000 units/ml

Phosphate Buffered Saline (PBS) (Dulbecco "A"):

Oxoid tablets, Code BR14a, 1 tablet per 100 ml distilled water

Dispense and then autoclave

Store at room temperature, pH 7.3, osmolality 280 mOsm/Kg

PBSB contains the calcium and magnesium and should be prepared and sterilized separately. Mix with PBSA, if required, immediately before use.

Appendix V
Preparation of Sperm Stains

PAPANICOLAOU STAINING

The Papanicolaou stain clearly distinguishes between basophilic and acidophilic cell components and allows a detailed examination of the nuclear chromatin pattern. This method, therefore, has been commonly used for routine diagnostic cytology. The Papanicolaou staining technique has also proved useful in the analysis of sperm morphology and in the examination of immature germinal cells.

1. Preparation of Specimen. The smear should be slightly air dried and then fixed in equal parts of ethanol (95%) and ether for 5 to 15 min.

2. Staining Procedure. Fixed smears should be stained according to the following procedure:

Ethanol 80%*	10 dips†
Ethanol 70%	10 dips
Ethanol 50%	10 dips
Distilled water	10 dips
Harris' or Mayer's hematoxylin	3 min exactly
Running water	3 to 5 min
Acid ethanol	2 dips
Running water	3 to 5 min
Scott's solution‡	4 min
Distilled water	1 dip
Ethanol 50%	10 dips
Ethanol 70%	10 dips
Ethanol 80%	10 dips
Ethanol 95%	10 dips
Orange G 6[4]	2 min
Ethanol 95%	10 dips
Ethanol 95%	10 dips
EA-50§	5 min
Ethanol 95%	5 dips
Ethanol 95%	5 dips
Ethanol 95%	5 dips
Ethanol 99.5%	2 min
Xylol (3 staining jars)	Approximately 1 min in each

Change xylol if it turns milky. Mount at once with Depex or any mounting medium.

---

* Check the acidity of water before preparing the different grades of ethanol. The pH should be 7.0.
† One dip corresponds to approximately 1 sec.
‡ Scott's solution is used when the ordinary tap water is "hard."

§ The prepared Papanicolaou stain (EA50 and OG 6) may be obtained commercially. The same companies usually manufacture the hematoxylin preparation. The commercially available stains are usually satisfactory, but the stains may be prepared in the laboratory at a substantial saving. The stains can be prepared as follows:

Eosin Y	10 g
Bismarck brown Y	10 g
Light-green SF, yellowish	10 g
Distilled water	300 ml
Ethanol 95%	2000 ml
Phosphotungstic acid	4 g
Saturated lithium carbonate solution (in distilled water)	0.5 ml

Belsey, M.A., Elliasson, R., Gallegos, A.J., Moghissi, K.S., Paulsen, C.A., and Prasad, M.R.N. (1980). Laboratory Manual for the Examination of Human Semen and Semen–Cervical Mucus Interaction. WHO Special Programme of Research, Development and Research Training in Human Reproduction. Singapore, Press Concern.

STOCK SOLUTIONS

Prepare separate 10% solutions of each of the stains as follows:

Eosin Y 10 g in 100 ml distilled water
Bismarck brown Y 10 g in 100 ml distilled water

Light-green SF 10 g in 100 ml distilled water

To prepare 200 ml of stain, mix the preceding stock solution as follows:

Eosin Y	50 ml
Bismarck brown Y	10 ml
Light-green SF	12.5 ml

Make up to 2000 ml with 95% ethanol; add 4 g phosphotungstic acid and 0.5 ml saturated lithium carbonate solution. Mix well and store solution at room temperature in dark-brown tightly capped bottles. The solution is stable for 2 to 3 months. Filter before using.

Constituents of OG6:

Orange G crystals	10 g
Distilled water	100 ml
Ethanol 95%	1000 ml
Phosphotungstic acid	0.15 g

Stock solution number I:

Prepare 10% aqueous solution as follows: Orange G crystal 10 g in 100 ml distilled water. Shake well and allow to stand in a dark-brown bottle at room temperature for 1 week before using.

Stock solution number II (Orange G, 0.5% solution):

Stock solution number 1	50 ml
Prepare with 95% ethanol to 1000 ml	

To prepare final solution of 1000 ml of the stain, add 0.15 g phosphotungstic acid to 1000 ml stock solution number II; mix well and store in dark-brown stoppered bottles at room temperature. Filter before using. The solution is stable for 2 to 3 months.

Harris hematoxylin without acetic acid:

Hematoxylin (dark crystals)	8 g
Ethanol 95%	80 ml
Aluminum ammonium sulphate	160 g
Distilled water	1600 ml
Mercuric oxide	6 g

To prepare the staining mixture, dissolve aluminum ammonium sulphate in distilled water by heating. Dissolve hematoxylin crystal in 95% ethanol. Add hematoxylin solution to ammonium sulphate solution. Heat the mixture to 95 °C. Remove from flame, and while stirring, slowly add the mercuric oxide. Solution will be dark purple in color. Immediately plunge the container in a cold-water bath and filter when the solution is cold. Store in dark-brown bottles at room temperature and let stand for 48 hours. Dilute the required amount with an equal part of distilled water and filter again.

Giemsa stain:

Layer undiluted methyl alcohol on the slide
Let stand for 10 min
Drain and let air dry
Cover the slide with Giemsa stain (17 drops of the stock Giemsa solution in enough distilled water to make the final volume 5 ml)
Let stand for 20 min
Rinse with distilled water

Meyer's hematoxylin stain:

Layer 10% formaldehyde on the slide
Let stand for 1 min
Rinse with distilled water
Stain for 2 min in Meyer's hematoxylin
Rinse in distilled water

Crystal violet-rose bengal stain:

Layer Chlorazene (chloramine-T) (5% in distilled water) on the slide
Let stand for 5 min
Rinse with 95% alcohol
Immerse in crystal violet (25% in distilled water)
Let stand for 8 min
Rinse with 95% alcohol
Immerse in rose bengal (1% in distilled water) for 8 sec
Rinse with distilled water

Bryan's sperm stain, Graham and Leishman's blood stain*:

Fix the slide in formalin (10% for 3 min, and subsequently in 95% ethanol for 3 min and in 70% ethanol for 3 min; change every third time)
Rinse with distilled water for 3 min and submerge in alphanaphthol for 4.5 min
Rinse with tap water for 15 min and add pyronine B for 2 min
Immerse 3 times in tap water
Add modified Bryan's stain for 15 min (description follows)
Immerse 3 times in 1% acetic acid
Wash with tap water for 1 min and add Leishman's blood stain for 5 minutes
Immerse 3 times in tap water and air dry

Modified Bryan's sperm stain:

Acetic acid 1%	1500 ml
Eosin yellow	0.5 g
Fast green	0.5 g
Naphthol yellow S	0.5 g

Mix thoroughly and store in stoppered bottle, the stain is filtered before use.

---

* Ulstein, M., Capell, P., Holmes, K. and Paulsen, C.A. (1976). Nonsymptomatic genital tract infection and male infertility. *In* Human Semen and Fertility Regulation in Men. St. Louis, Mosby.

Leishman's Blood Stain (Stock Solution):

Combine 0.5 g of eosinated methylene blue and 300 ml of absolute methyl alcohol (meOH).

Mix thoroughly and allow to age in the dark at room temperature for 7 days.

Place the stain in an incubator (35 to 37 °C) for 2 days.

The stock solution is now ready for use and should be stored in a tightly-stoppered dark bottle, away from heat and light.

Alternative blood stain stock solutions commercially available are Jenner's blood stain or Wright's blood stain. The timing involved with these stains must be varied at the "Leishman's" step in the procedure to achieve comparable results.

Buffer Solution: Combine 2 buffer tablets, pH 6.8, with 200 ml of distilled water. (If not used at once, recheck pH before use.)

Leishman's Blood Stain (Working Solution): Combine 10 ml formaldehyde solution with 90 ml of 95% E10H. (0.1 g of calcium acetate may be added per 200 ml of solution to ensure neutral pH of 7.0.)

Alcoholic Formalin: Combine 10 ml formaldehyde solution with 90 ml of 95% E10H; 0.1 g of calcium acetate may be added per 200 ml of solution to ensure neutral pH of 7.0.

Alphanaphthol: Dissolve 1 g alphanaphthol in 100 ml of 40% ethyl alcohol (E OH). Immediately before initial use, add 0.2 ml of 3% hydrogen peroxide solution.

Pyronine Y: Combine 1 g of pyronine, 4 ml aniline, and 96 ml of 40% EtOH.

Sodium citrate buffer: Mix 7 g sodium citrate with 1 L of 0.9 NaCl and adjust pH to 7.5.

Bryan/Leishman stain for seminal fluid morphology smears

Note: Use freshly made, air-dried smears from fresh samples on clean slides.

Alcohol formalin 10%	1 min	Fresh each time
Ethyl alcohol (EtOH) 80%	5 min	Change every third time*
EtOH 70%	5 min	Change every third time
EtOH 50%	5 min	Change every third time
Alphanaphthol	4 min	Change every 3 days

Add 0.4 ml of 3% hydrogen peroxide to 200 ml of alphanaphthol just before initial use; the solution is active for 3 days at room temperature.

Running tap water	15 min	Running slowly
Pyronine Y	4 min	Fresh each week
Running tap water	3 dips†	Running slowly
Sodium citrate buffer	3 min	pH 7.5; fresh each time
Distilled water	1 min	Fresh each time
Modified Bryan's stain	15 min	Fresh every other time
Acetic acid 1%	2 dips	Fresh each time
Running tap water	1 min	Running slowly
Buffer and Leishman's stain	30 min	Fresh each time

Filter Leishman's stock 50 ml, add pH 6.8 buffer 150 ml, filter again immediately before use.

Running tap water	1 to 2 dips	Running slowly
Air dry (do not blot)		

* Change after every 30 slides if a staining jar holding 10 slides is being used.
† Each dip should be approximately of 1 second duration.

SPECIAL CONSIDERATIONS

1. Pyronine Y, modified Bryan's and Leishman's stains should be filtered before initial use. In addition, the buffer and Leishman's working stain should be filtered before use to remove precipitating stain.

2. The final stain intensity can be increased by staining for a longer time in the buffered Leishman's stain or can be decreased by repeated washing. Check for the desired intensity with a microscope before mounting the slide.

3. Hydrogen peroxide deteriorates rapidly in the presence of light; thus, the stock 3% solution should be stored in an amber bottle in the dark.

4. The stock Leishman's stain should be aged before use by storing for 7 days at room temperature in the dark followed by incubation at 35 to 37 °C for 2 days in the dark. The aged solution is stable for a month if kept in a sealed container in the dark.

Appendix VI
Culture Media

Preparation of Culture Media for Mammalian Ova, Embryos, and Tissues

Ingredients (mg/l)	Brinster's Mouse Ova Culture Medium-3	Menezo's B-2 Medium	Eagle's Minimum Essential Medium*	Modified Dulbecco's PBS	Ham's Nutrient Mixture F-10	Synthetic Oviduct Fluid	Tissue-Culture Medium 199†	Whitten's Medium
Inorganic salts:								
NaCl	5546	5250	6800	8000	7400	6300	8000	5140
KCl	356	800	400	200	285	533	400	356
$CaCl_2$	189	—	200	100	33	190	140	—
$MgCl_2 \cdot 6H_2O$	—	—	—	100	—	100	—	—
$MgSO_4 \cdot 7H_2O$	294	200	200	—	153	—	200	294
$NaHCO_3$	2106	2500	2200	—	1200	2106	350	1900
Na_2HPO_4	—	61	—	1150	154	—	48	—
$NaH_2PO_4 \cdot H_2O$	—	—	140	—	—	—	—	—
KH_2PO_4	162	60	—	200	83	162	60	162
Carbohydrates:								
Glucose	1000	1,200	1000	1000	1100	270	1000	1000
Na pyruvate	56	250	—	36	110	36	—	36
Na lactate (DL)	2253	—	—	—	—	370	—	2416
$Ca (lactate)_2 \cdot 5H_2O$	—	664	—	—	—	—	—	527
Ribose	—	—	—	—	—	—	.5	—
Deoxyribose	—	—	—	—	—	—	.5	—
Amino acids	none	contains 23	contains 13	none	contains 20	none	contains 21	none
Vitamins	none	contains 1	contains 8	none	contains 10	none	contains 16	none
Nucleic acids and precursors	none	none	none	none	contains 2	none	contains 8	none
Trace elements	none	none	none	none	contains 3	none	contains 1	none
Other components:								
Bovine serum albumin	5000	10,000	varies	varies	varies	varies	varies	3000
Cholesterol	—	125	—	—	—	—	.2	—
Na acetate	—	50	—	—	—	—	50	—
Lipoic acid	—	—	—	—	.2	—	—	—
Tween 80	—	50	—	—	—	—	20	—
Glutathione	—	—	—	—	—	—	.05	—
α-tocopherol $PO_4(Na)$ $PO_4(Na)$	—	—	—	—	—	—	.01	—

* The formulation with Earle's salts.

† The formulation with Hank's salts.

GIBCO catalog (1976–1977), Grand Island, NY, Grand Island Biological Company.

Constituents of Complete Media Used for Culture of Embryos

Components	MEM* (Earle's salts), mg/L	Medium-199† (Earle's salts), mg/L
Inorganic salts		
$CaCl_2 \cdot 2H_2O$	200.00	200.00
$CuSO_4 \cdot 5H_2O$		
$FeSO_4 \cdot 7H_2O$		
KCl	400.00	400.00
KH_2PO_4		
$Fe(NO_3)_3 \cdot 9H_2O$		.72
$MgSO_4$ (anhyd.)	97.67	97.67
$MgSO_4 \cdot 7H_2O$		
NaCl	6,800.00	6,800.00
$NaHCO_3$		2,200.00
$NaH_2PO_4 \cdot H_2O$	140.00	140.00
$NaHPO_4 \cdot 7H_2O$		
$ZnSO_4 \cdot 7H_2O^c$		
Other components		
Glucose	1,000.00	1,000.00
Hypoxanthine		.300
Lipoic acid		
Phenol red	10.00	20.00
Na pyruvate		
Thymidine		
Amino acids		
L-alanine		50.00
L-arginine HCl	126.00	70.00
L-asparagine $\cdot H_2O$		
L-aspartic acid		60.00
L-cysteine		20.00
L-cysteine HCl $\cdot H_2O$	31.29	.110
L-glutamic acid		150.00
L-glutamine	292.00	100.00
Glycine		50.00
L-histidine HCl $\cdot H_2O$	42.00	21.88
L-hydroxyproline		10.00
L-isoleucine	52.00	40.00
L-leucine	52.00	120.00
L-lysine HCl	72.50	70.00
L-methionine	15.00	30.00
L-phenylalanine	32.00	50.00
L-proline		40.00
L-serine		50.00
L-threonine	48.00	60.00
L-tryptophan	10.00	20.00
L-tyrosine	52.10	40.00
L-valine	46.00	50.00
Vitamins		
Biotin		0.10
D-Ca pantothenate	1.00	0.10
Choline chloride	1.00	.500
Folic acid	1.00	.010
i-inositol	2.00	.050
Niacinamide	1.00	.025
Pyridoxine HCl	1.00	.025
Riboflavin	.10	.010
Thiamine HCl	1.00	.010
Vitamin B_{12}		

* MEM = minimum essential medium.

† Medium-199 contains numerous other components not found in the other three media.

(Compiled by R.W. Wright Jr. and K.R. Bondioli (1981). Aspects of in vitro fertilization and embryo culture in domestic animals. J. Anim. Sci. *53*, 701.)

Standard Egg Culture Medium
Biggers, Whitten, and Whittingham (BWW Medium) (Modified Kreb's Ringer's Solution)

Component	Molecular Weight	g/L	mM	Milliosmole
NaCl	58.4	5.540	94.59	189.19
KCl	74.6	0.356	4.78	9.56
Ca-Lactate-5H$_2$O	308.3	0.527	1.71	5.13
KH$_2$PO$_4$	136.1	0.162	1.19	2.38
MgSO$_4$·7H$_2$O	246.5	0.294	1.19	2.38
NaHCO$_3$	84.0	2.106	25.07	50.14
Na pyruvate	110.0	0.028	0.25	0.50
Na lactate	112.1	2.416	21.58	43.10
		(3.68 ml/L of syrup)		
Glucose	180.2	1.0	5.56	5.56
Crystalline bovine Albumin		1.0		
Antibiotic stock Solution*		1.0 ml		
Distilled water		1000 ml		
Total				308 (approximate osmolality of medium)†

* 100,000 IU/ml penicillin and 50 mg/ml streptomycin. This stock solution is kept frozen in 1-ml lots.
† pH of medium is 7.4–7.5 when equilibrated with 5% CO$_2$ in air.
Note: Human albumin is used in the medium for human gametes, and bovine albumin is used in the medium for hamster gametes and eggs of other species.

Osmolarities of Complete and Simple Culture Media Used for the Culture of Embryos from Farm Animals*†

		Medium Supplemented With			
		BSA, w/v‡		Fetal Calf Serum, v/v	
Item	No Supplement Mean ± SD	1% Mean ± SD	3% Mean ± SD	10% Mean ± SD	20% Mean ± SD
Complete medium§					
Ham's F-10	293 ± 5	303 ± 6	314 ± 6	306 ± 5	301 ± 4
MEM	289 ± 5	294 ± 3	298 ± 4	285 ± 4	286 ± 3
TCM-199	302 ± 6	304 ± 4	304 ± 4	291 ± 4	284 ± 3
Modified Ham's F-10	270 ± 6	—	—	—	—
Simple medium					
BMOC-3	316 ± 4	—	—	—	—
PBS	283 ± 3	284 ± 3	286 ± 4	281 ± 4	282 ± 3
SOF	276 ± 3	—	—	—	—
Whitten's	290 ± 3	—	—	—	—

* Means represent 10 measurements of each media in milliosmoles as determined by a vapor pressure osmometer.
† All media contained 1% (v/v) of antibiotic-antimycotic solution. Santa Clara, CA, Grand Island Biological Company.
‡ Bovine serum albumin, Fraction V.
§ MEM = Minimum Essential Medium; PBS = Phosphate Buffered Solution; SOF = Synthetic Oviduct Fluid.
(Adapted from Wright, R.W., Jr. and Bondioli, K.R. (1981). Aspects of in vitro fertilization and embryo culture in domestic animals. J. Anim. Sci. *53,* 701.)

Commercially Available* Culture Media for Manipulation and Cryopreservation of Gametes and Embryos

Media:	Serum:
Dulbecco's phosphate	Newborn calf serum (heat inactivated)
Buffered saline	Antibiotics/Antimycotics:
Dulbecco's phosphate buffered saline +	Antibiotic-Antimycotic, LYO
D-glucose 1000 mg/L	10,000 units penicillin/ml
Na pyruvate 36 mg/L	10,000 μg streptomycin/ml
Nutrient Mixture F-10	25 μg Fungizone/ml
(Ham's with)	Penicillin-streptomycin
(L-glutamine)	10,000 units penicillin/ml
	10,000 μg streptomycin/ml

* Cryo-Genetics, Inc., 3800A South Park Drive, Tyler, Texas 75703.

Concentration of Cryoprotectant vs. Freezing Point Temperature

Percentage of Cryoprotectant (DMSO or Glycerol)	Freezing Point Temperature
0	0° C
5	−2° C
7.5	−3° C
10	−4° C
12.5	−5° C
15	−6° C
20	−8° C
30	−12° C

Phase change, or *freezing point*, is defined as a process wherein a liquid is changed into a solid at constant temperature. Biologic samples, which are composed basically of water, have a freezing point temperature of 0° C when no other substances are added to the system. Adding a cryoprotective agent, such as dimethylsulfoxide (DMSO) or glycerol, will lower the freezing point temperature. CryoMed has observed this relationship between the percentage of cryoprotective agent added to a biologic specimen and the freezing point temperature.

Acetic Methanol:

Glacial acetic	1 part
Methanol	3 parts

Make up fresh each time used and keep at 4 °C

Balanced Salt Solutions (BSS):
Dissolve each constituent separately, adding $CaCl_2$ last and make up to 1 L. Adjust to pH 6.5
Hanks' BSS, no phenol red: use regular recipe but omit phenol red

Sterilize by autoclaving. Mark liquid level before autoclaving. Store at room temperature. Make up to mark with sterile deionized distilled water before use if necessary.

Streptomycin Sulphate (1 g per vial):
Take 2 ml from a bottle containing 100 ml sterile Hanks' BSS and add to 1 g vial of streptomycin.

When solution is complete, return 2 ml to 98 ml Hanks'.

Appendix VII
Cryoprotectants

Preparation of Cryoprotectants (Stock and Dilute Solutions)

Two stock solutions are prepared:
  A. Measure 54 ml PBS and add 6 ml of heat treated serum. This equals 60 ml of solution of 10% serum in PBS (solution A). Place in 25 cm² culture flask (orange cap).
  B. Measure 27 ml of PBS + 10% serum (solution A) and add 3 ml glycerol using a 14-gauge needle and 20-ml syringe. This equals 30 ml of a 10% cryoprotectant solution (solution B).

Place into black-capped tissue culture flask. Pass both solutions through a filter to sterilize.

Cryoprotectant Dilutions

PBS + Serum (ml) (Solution A)	PBS + Serum + Glycerol (ml) (Solution B)	Percentage of Diluent
0.0	4.0	10
1.0	3.0	7.5
2.0	2.0	.5
3.0	1.0	2.5

Preparation of 1.0 M Sucrose Solution
Sucrose 34.2 g
Add PBS until total volume of 100 ml
Use 6-ml syringe and 18-gauge needle

This solution is 1.0 M or 534.2% weight/volume. Mix solution for 30 min on stirring plate.

PREPARATION OF DILUTE SOLUTIONS

The following dilutions of cryoprotectant are made in culture medium using a 60-ml sterile syringe and 14-gauge hypodermic needle. Fifteen ml Vacutainer tubes are useful for holding the solutions.

Dilutions of Glycerol in PBS + 20% FCS Required for Freezing and Thawing

Modified PBS + 20% FCS Stock A	Modified PBS + 20% FCS + 10% Glycerol Stock B	Approx. % Glycerol
2 ml	10 ml	8.3%
4 ml	8 ml	6.7%
6 ml	6 ml	5.0%
8 ml	4 ml	3.3%
10 ml	2 ml	1.7%

Appendix VIII

Preparation of Trypsin for Zona-Free Hamster Ova

Trypsin diluent-buffered

Sodium chloride	6.0 g
Trisodium citrate	2.9 g
Tricine [N-Tris (hydroxy-methyl) methyl glycine]	1.79 g
Phenol red	0.005 g
Distilled water to	1000 ml

Stir ingredients until dissolved, adjust pH to 7.8

Filter through Whatman No. 1 filter paper

Dispense and autoclave

Osmolality = 290 mOsm/kg

Trypsin Stock (2.5% in 0.85% (0.14 M) NaCl)

Trypsin solutions can be bought commercially. Alternatively, to make up a 2.5% solution in 0.85% NaCl, stir for 1 hour at room temperature or 10 hours at 4° C. If trypsin does not dissolve completely, clarify by filtration through Whatman No. 1 filter paper.

Sterilize by filtration, aliquot and store at −20 °C.

Note: Trypsin is available as crude (e.g., Difco 1:250) or purified (e.g., Sigma (3× recrystallized) preparations. Crude preparations contain several other proteases that may be important in cell dissociation but may also be harmful to more sensitive cells. The usual practice is to use crude trypsin unless cell damage reduces viability or reduced growth is observed, then purified trypsin may be used. Pure trypsin has a higher specific activity and should therefore be used at a proportionally lower concentration, e.g., 0.05 or 0.01%.

Trypsin Verene Phosphate (TVP)

Trypsin (Difco 1 : 250)	25 mg (or 1 ml Flow or Gibco 2.5%)
Phosphate buffered saline (PBS)	98 ml
Disodium EDTA (2H$_2$O)	37 mg
Chick serum (Flow)	1 ml

Mix PBS and EDTA and autoclave, then add chick serum and trypsin.

If using powdered trypsin, sterilize by filtration before adding chick serum. Aliquot and store at −20° C.

Appendix IX
Kits Used for Immunomethods for Hormone Assays

Kit	Assay	Incubation	Testing Range
Aldosterone	Extraction	1 hr	0–1.28 ng/ml
Androstenedione	Extraction	30 min	0–12.8 ng/ml
Cortisol	Direct	30 min	0–64 μg/dl
DHEA-S DA	Direct	30 min	0–8000 ng/ml
Digoxin	Direct	15 min	0–8 ng/ml
Direct estradiol	Direct	1 hr	0–5120 pg/ml
Estradiol (extraction method)	Extraction	30 min	0–1280 pg/ml
Estriol	Extraction	30 min	0–32 ng/ml
FSH 4 H	Equilibrium	4 hrs	0–200 mIU/ml
Gastrins		1 hr	0–3200 pg/ml
β-phase quant hCG	Human standard	1 hr	0–200 mIU/ml
β-phase Pregnancy test	Human standard	1 hr	Qualitative
hGH		Overnight	0–50 ng/ml
17α-hydroxyprogesterone	Extraction	1 hr	0–20 ng/ml
Insulin		1 hr	0–200 μIU/ml
LH	Equilibrium	4 hrs	0–200 mIU/ml
Direct progesterone	Direct	1 hr	0–80 ng/ml
Progesterone (extraction method)	Extraction	1 hr	0–32 ng/ml
Prolactin	Equilibrium	3 hrs	0–100 ng/ml
Direct testosterone	Direct	30 min	0–25.6 ng/ml
Testosterone (extraction method)	Extraction	30 min	0–25.6 ng/ml
T_4 (thyroxine)		30 min	0–32 μg/dl
Free thyroxine	Sephadex sep.	30 min	1.0–2.3 ng/dl
T-3 (triiodothyronine)		1 hrs	0–800 ng/dl
T-3 uptake	Adsorbent sep.	10 min	25–36%
TSH Eq	Equilibrium	2 hrs	0–160 μIU/ml
TSH (sequential method)	Sequential	4 hrs	0–80 μIU/ml

* Normal range.

Available through Pantex: 21st St., Santa Monica, CA 90404. Phone: (213) 828-7423; (800) 421-6529. Telex: 652-412.

Index

Page numbers in *italics* indicate illustrations; numbers followed by "t" indicate tables.

Abortion, 274, 275t, 276
  chromosomal aberrations and, 304-305, *306-307*
  in horse, 381
    equine rhinopneumonitis and, 276-277
  induced, 274
  infections causing, 274, 276-277
    enzootic abortion of ewes and, 277
    epizootic bovine abortion and, 276
    equine rhinopneumonitis and, 276-277
  noninfectious, 274, 275t
  spontaneous, 274
Accessory glands, 11-12, *12*, *13*, 181-182, *182*
  biochemical constituents of seminal plasma and, 181-182
  comparative anatomy of, 1
  diseases of, fertilization failure and, 292, 293t
  function of, 12
Acrosomal phase, of spermiogenesis, 172
Acrosome, 166, *167*
ACTH, 71, 89
Activin, 179
  andrology and, 88
ADH (arginine vasopressin; vasopressin), 70
Adluminal compartment, of Sertoli cell junctions, 176
Adrenal glands, hormones of, 64t, 88-89
Age
  at puberty, reproductive cycles and, 99-100
  of dam, embryonic mortality and, 272
Aging
  anestrus due to, 264
  fertility and, *111*, 111t, 111-112
  of eggs, 162-163, *163*
AI. *See* Artificial insemination
Air filtration, 495
Albumin, andrology and, 88
Allantoic fluid, 227-228
  composition of, 228
  functions of, 227
  hydrallantois and, 282
  origin of, 227, 228t
  prepartum maternal behavior in sheep and, 251
  volume of, 227
Allantois, 218t
Amnion, 218t
Amnionic plaques, 228
Amniotic fluid, 227-228
  composition of, 228
  functions of, 227
  hydramnios and, 282
  origin of, 227, 228t
  prepartum maternal behavior in sheep and, 251
  volume of, 227
Ampulla, of oviduct, 30, *33*

Androgens, 82, *82*
  spermatogenesis and, *177*, 177-178
Andrology
  assisted reproduction technology and, 497t
  hormones and. *See* Hormones, andrology and
Anestrus, 261-265, 262t, *263*
  due to aging, 264
  during lactation, 262-264
  effect of male and, 247-248
  in mare, 379
  nutritional deficiencies and, 264
  ovarian or uterine abnormalities and, 264-265
  seasonal, 261-262
Aneuploidy, 299, 300t
Annular rings, 48, *50*, *51*
Annulus, 172
Antigen(s), histocompatibility (transplantation), 222
Antigenicity, of sperm, 183
Apex changes, ovulation and, 137
Arginine vasopressin (ADH; vasopressin), 70
ARTA (assisted reproduction technology and andrology), 497t
Artificial insemination (AI), 424-439
  estrus detection and, 430, 432
  factors affecting conception rate in, 436-437
  in poultry, 398-401, 437, *438*, 439
    fertility and hatchability and, 400, 400t
    semen collection, evaluation, and insemination and, 399-400
    semen production and, 400-401
  male infertility and, 294
  of superovulated donors, 469
  optimal insemination time and, 432, 435
  physical condition of males and, 425
  procedures for, 435-436, *436*
  semen collection and, 425-430
    artificial vagina for, 428, *430-433*
    electroejaculation and, 428-430
    frequency of, 426-428, 427t
    in poultry, 399-400
    massage method for, 430
    mounts and teasing procedures and, 425-426, *426*
Assisted reproduction. *See specific techniques*
Assisted reproduction technology and andrology (ARTA), 497t
Autoerotic behavior, 249
Autoimmunity, sperm and, 183-186, *185*
Autosomes, 298

Barker syndrome, in horse, 381
Basal compartment, of Sertoli cell junctions, 175
Bioassays, of hormones, 65
Bisexuality, embryonic, 20, 23t

Blastocyst
elongation of, 202-203, *203*, *204*
formation of, *201*, 201-202
hatching of, 202
Blastoderm, 385
Blastodisc, 385
Blastokinin, 44
Blastolemmase, 202
Blastomeres, 195
Blood flow. *See* Circulation
Blood-testis barrier, 174-178
cellular junctions and, 174-176
myoid layer and, 175, *176*
Sertoli cell, 175-176
Boar. *See also* Pig
hormone regulation in, *346*, *347*, *348*, 349-350
lack of libido in, 290
semen collection and
electroejaculation and, 430, *434*
frequency of, 428
semen cryopreservation and, 523, 523t
sperm production in, 350
bPSPD (pregnancy-specific protein B), pregnancy diagnosis and, 453-454
Breeding
of buffalo, 326
of cattle, 320, 321t
of sheep and goats, 336t, 336-337
frequency of, 339-340
Breeding season, 105-111
factors regulating, 109-111
endocrine and neuroendocrine mechanisms and, 109-111, *110*
in males, 108-109, 332, 361
nature of, 105-106, *106*, *107*
of buffalo, 325
of cattle, 316
of horses, 361-362
female, 361-362
male, 361
of sheep and goats, 330-332
advancing, 338
female, 330-332, *332*, *333*
male, 332
photoperiodism and temperature and, 106-108, *108*
Breeding techniques. *See also specific techniques*
for poultry, 398
male fertilization failure and, 294
reproductive failure and
in mare, 381-382
in stallion, 383
Buffalo, 324-328
estrous cycles of, 325
breeding season and, 325
cyclic changes and, 325
estrus and ovulation and, 325
gestation and parturition in, 326-327
puberty in, 324-325
puerperium in, 327-327t
ovarian activity during, 327
reproductive performance of, 327-328
increasing, 328
reproductive efficiency and, 327-328
sperm production and release in, 325-326
breeding and, 326
Bulbospongiosus muscles, 11, 12

Bulbourethral glands, comparative anatomy of, 1
Bull. *See* Male(s); *specific male animals*

Cap phase, of spermiogenesis, 172
Caput epididymis, 8
Cardiovascular system, perinatal adaptations of, 232-233
Cattle, 315-324
breeding and, 320, 321t
breeding season and, 316
cryopreservation of embryos of, international sales of frozen embryos and, 509-510
estrous cycle in
cyclic changes and, 316-319, *317*, 318t
detection of estrus and, 316, 318t
gestation and parturition in, 320-321
diagnosis of pregnancy and, 450
maternal recognition of pregnancy and, 210
maternal behavior in, 254
suckling and, 254, *255*
maternal recognition of pregnancy in, 210
ovulation and, 319, 319t
puberty in, 315-316
female, 315
male, 315-316
puerperium and, 321
ovarian function during, 321
uterine involution during, 321
reproductive performance of, 321-324
general fertility and, 322
improving, 322-324, *323*
measures of reproductive efficiency and, 321-322, 322t
sperm production and release and, 319-320
white heifer disease in, 268
Cauda epididymis, 8
Cervix uteri, *48-51*, 48-52
cervical mucus and, 50-51, *52*
sperm transport and, 150-151
changes during pregnancy, 215
dilation of, 229-230
functions of, 51-52
during pregnancy, 52
sperm transport and, 51-52
physiologic changes in, 48-50
sperm transport in, 147, 150-151
cervical mucus and, 150-151
sperm penetration in cervical mucus and, 151
stroma of, 48-50
Chicken. *See* Poultry
Chimerism, 299, 300t
sterility and infertility and, 304
Chorion, 218t
Chorionic villi, 217
Chromatid body, 172
Chromosomal aberrations, 299-301
nomenclature for, 300-301
numerical, 299, 300t
reproductive failure and, 303-310
congenital malformations and, 303-304
hybrids and, 309-310, 310t
intersexuality and, 305, 309
prenatal mortality and, 304-305, *306-307*
sterility and infertility and, 304
structural, 299-300, *300-302*

Chromosomes, 298, *298. See also* Chromosomal aberrations; Genetics; Sex chromosomes
  genetic engineering and, 485, 487, *489*, 491t
    evaluation of chromosomes of ova and, 487
  homologous, 298
Circulation. *See also* Vasculature
  fetal, *226*, 226-227
  ovarian, prenatal development and, 23-24, 26
  placental, 219-220
    microcirculation and, 220, *220*
    uterine blood flow and, 219-220
  to corpus luteum, 28-29, *30*
CLE (corpus luteum extract), 90t
Cleavage, 194-201
  genome expression and, 198-199
  normal time course of, 195-197, *196, 197*
  parthenogenesis and, 199-200
  rates of, 197-198
  twinning and embryo manipulation and, 200-201
Climate, sexual behavior and, 247
Clitoris, 54
Cloudburst, 265
Clover, fertilization failure and, 268-269, *269*
Clutch, poultry egg production and, 394-395
Co-culture media, 497
Colony-stimulating factor (CSF), 90t
Conception
  in pig, 355
  in sheep and goats, 336-337
  rate of
    gamete transport and, 161-162
    in artificial insemination, factors affecting, 436-437
Conceptus
  growth of, in pig, 355-356
  interaction with uterine environment, 206-207
Congenital malformations. *See also* Chromosomal aberrations
  reproductive failure and, 303-304
Convulsive foal syndrome, 381
Coolidge effect, 246
Copulation. *See also* Mating
  frequency of, 242, 244t
  inability to copulate and, 290-292
    failure to achieve intromission and, 290-291, *291*
    failure to ejaculate and, 291-292
    failure to mount and, 290
Corona radiata, 115t
Corpus albicans, 26t, 27
Corpus cavernosum penis, 12
Corpus epididymis, 8
Corpus hemorrhagicum, 26t
Corpus luteum, 26t, 26-29
  blood flow to, 28-*29, 30*
  development of, 27, *27*
  estrous cycle regulation and, 101-102
  in horse, 367, *367, 368*
  luteolysis and, 28
  pregnancy and, 29
    maternal recognition of, 29
  regression of, 27-28, *27-29*
Corpus luteum extract (CLE), 90t
Corpus luteum spurium, 29
Corpus luteum verum, 29
Corpus spongiosum glandis, 14
Corpus spongiosum penis, 12

Corpus vascularis paracloacalis, 394
Corticosteroid(s). *See also specific corticosteroids*
Corticosteroids, 88-89
Corticotropin-releasing hormone (CRH), 73
Coumestrol, 80, *81*
Cow. *See* Female(s); *specific female animals*
CRH (corticotropin-releasing hormone), 73
Crura, 12
Cryopreservation, 503t, 503-524
  of embryos, 504-515, 505t, 506t
    culture and storage between 0° and 37°C and, 505-506
    embryo containers for, 504-505
    equipment, glassware, and accessories for, 510
    factors affecting post-thaw embryo survival and, 514
    future research directions for, 514-515
    international sales of frozen bovine embryos and, 509-510
    procedures for, 506-507, 507t, 508t, *509-512*, 515t, 516t, 518t, 519t, 522t
    procedures for testing embryo survival and, 513-514
    programmable freezers for, 510-511, 513
    thawing of embryos and, 513
    tissue culture medium for, 506
  of semen, 515-524
    evaluation of sperm motility and, 523-524
    extension of semen and, 519
    glycerol addition for, 519-520
    semen damage and, 524
    semen extenders and, 515-518
    semen processing and, 518-521, 523
    storage of frozen semen and, 521
  principles of, 503-504
Cryptorchidism, 287-288
CSF (colony-stimulating factor), 90t
Culture media, 497
  for embryo cryopreservation, 506
  macromolecular supplementation and, 497-499
Cumulus cells, regulatory and physiology parameters of, 116t
Cyclopentanoperhydrophenanthrene nucleus, 78

Dam. *See* Female(s); *specific female animals*
Death
  neonatal. *See* Neonate, death of
  prenatal. *See also* Female reproductive failure, prenatal mortality and
    embryonic, 270t, 270-273, *274*
      causes of, *271*, 271-273
    fetal, 379. *See also* Abortion
Decidualization, 204
Deletion, chromosomal, 299, 300t
DES (diethylstilbestrol), 80, *81*
Dictyate nucleus, 130
Diestrus, prolonged, 265
Diethylstilbestrol (DES), 80, *81*
Diploid number of chromosomes, 298
Diplotene, 169
Ductus deferens, 3
  anatomy of, 9-11, *10*
Dystocia, *280*, 280-281, *281*
  fetal, 280
  fetopelvic disproportion and, 280-281
  maternal, 280

EAE (enzootic abortion of ewes), 277
Early pregnancy factor (EPF), pregnancy diagnosis and, 453, *456*
EBA (epizootic bovine abortion; foothill abortion), clinical signs of, 276
EGF (epidermal growth factor), 90t
EGF-like peptides, 90t
Egg(s). *See also* Oocyte(s)
abnormal, fertilization failure and, 267
aging of, 162-163, *163*
evaluation of chromosomes of, 487
fertilizable life of, 162-163, *163*
fertilization and. *See* Fertilization
fusion with sperm, *192*, 192-193
loss of, 163
maturation of, 124, *126*, 126-131, *127*
oocyte growth and, 126-127, 128t-129t, 130
oocyte preparation for fertilization and, 130-131, *130-133*
micromanipulation of, 496t
of horse, *370*, 370-371
of poultry, 385-388, *386*, 386t
fertility and hatchability of, 400, 400t
formation of, 387-388, 394-395
physiology related to fertilization, 144, 144t
transport of, 156-162, 157t, *158-161*, 470
in mare, 370-371
in poultry, 392
locking and unlocking of ova and, 160
neural mechanisms and pharmacologic response and, 159-160, 162t
oviductal contraction and, 158-159, 161t
sperm transport and conception rate and, 161-162
transuterine migration of, 163
Egg pick-up, 156
ovulation and, 142
Ejaculation, 16, 18, 242
disturbances of, 289-292
in stallion, 382
inability to copulate and, 290-292
lack of libido and, 289-290
electroejaculation and, 428-430
failure to ejaculate and, 291-292
neural mechanisms of, 244-245, *245, 246*
of stallions, 363-364
Electroejaculation, semen collection and, 428-430
Embryo(s). *See also* Prenatal development
cryopreservation of. *See* Cryopreservation, of embryos
development of, 201-206
blastocyst elongation and, 202-203, *203, 204*
blastocyst formation and, *201*, 201-202
blastocyst hatching and, 202
implantation and, 46-47, 91, 204-206, *205*
in oviduct, 164
intrauterine migration and spacing and, 203-204
zona hatching and, 202
in vitro maturation of, 475, 477-478
micromanipulation of, 487-488, *490*, 491-492, *492*
morphologic classification before and after cryopreservation and thawing, 506t
mortality of, 270t, 270-273, *274*
causes of, *271*, 271-273
survival of, in pig, 355
Embryo manipulation, 200-201
Embryo transfer, 478-479, 481-482, 493-495

application of, 494-495
equipment and supplies for, 495-499, 496t
future developments in, 495
interspecies, reciprocal, 481, 483t
nonsurgical, 478-479
pregnancy maintenance following, 481-482
record keeping for, 482
selection and preparation of recipients for, 479
surgical, 479, *481*
synchronization of estrus between donor and recipient and, 479, 481, *482*
Embryology, of female reproductive tract. *See* Female reproductive anatomy, embryology and
Embryonic bisexuality, 20, 23t
Emission, 16, 18
Endocrinology. *See also* Hormones; *specific hormones, hormone types, endocrine glands, and naimlas*
techniques in, 59t
Endogenous opioid peptides (EOPs), 89, 179
Endometrial cups, 218
Endometrial cysts, in mare, 380
Endometrial glands, 43-44
Endometritis, 284
Endorphin, 89
Energy metabolism, perinatal adaptation of, 233
Environmental factors
fetal growth and, 225
length of gestation and, 214
sexual behavior and, 246-247
enhancing effect of new stimulus animal and, 246
nonspecific stimuli and, 246
presence of other animals and, 246-247
season and climate and, 247
Enzootic abortion of ewes (EAE), 277
EOPs (endogenous opioid peptides), 89, 179
EPF (early pregnancy factor), pregnancy diagnosis and, 453, *456*
Epidermal growth factor (EGF), 90t
Epididymal region, in poultry, 394
Epididymis, 3
anatomy of, 8-9, *9*
caput, 8
cauda, 8
corpus, 8
sperm transport in, 179
development of fertilizing potential and, 180
mechanisms of, 179
Epizootic bovine abortion (EBA; foothill abortion), 276
clinical signs of, 276
Equine rhinopneumonitis (equine herpesvirus I infection; viral abortion), 276-277
Erection, 14-16, *16*
neural mechanisms of, 244-245, *245, 246*
Estradiol, 80
Estrogens, 80-81
clinical applications of, 80-81, *81*
estrous cycle regulation and, 101
functions of, 80
Estrone sulphate, pregnancy diagnosis and, 459
Estrous cycles, *100*, 100-105, 101t, *191. See also* Anestrus; Estrus; Ovulation
endocrine regulation of, 100-102, *102*
in buffalo, 325
breeding season and, 325
cyclic changes and, 325
estrus and ovulation and, 325

in horse. *See* Mare, estrous cycle in
in pig, 351-354
  ovarian morphology and hormone secretion and, *348*, 351-354
in sheep and goats, 334-335
  length of, 334-335
postpartum estrus and ovulation and. *See* Estrus, postpartum; Ovulation, postpartum
synchronization of
  embryo transfer and, 479, 481, *482*
  in mare, 369-370
  ovulation and, 461-466, 463t-465t, *466, 467*
  sperm transport and, 154-155
Estrus. *See also* Anestrus; Estrous cycles
  anovulatory, 266
  detection of, 430, 432
  duration of, 242
  in buffalo, 325
  in cattle, detection of, 316, 318t
  in mare, 365, 367
    induction of, 369-371
    split, 379
    synchronization of, 369-370
  in sheep and goats, 335
    duration of, 335
    male influence on, 335
    signs of, 335
  postpartum, 102-105, 103t, 234-235
    endocrine factors in, 103-104, *104*
    in mare, 378
    in pig, 358
    suckling and lactation and, 104-105, *105*
  prolonged, 249, 265
  prolonged diestrus and, 265
  silent, 266
  split, 249, 265
    in mare, 379
  synchronization of. *See* Estrous cycles, synchronization of
Euploidy, 299
Ewe. *See also* Sheep
  breeding season of, 330-332, *332, 333*
  enzootic abortion of ewes and, 277
  estrous cycle in, 334-335
    duration of estrus and, 335
    length of, 334-335
    male influence on estrus and, 335
    signs of estrus and, 335
  litter size in, 340
  maternal behavior in, 251-253
    aberrant, 252
    lambing and, 251
    postpartum, 251-252
    prepartum, 251
    suckling and, 252-253, *253*
  mutual recognition by ewes and lambs and, 252-253, *253*
  ovulation in, 335-336
    rate of, 335-336, *336*
  parturition in, 337-338
  pregnancy in, 337, 337t
    diagnosis of, 450, 452
  puberty in, 332-333, *334*, 334t
  puerperium in, 338-339
External genitalia. *See specific organs*
Eye, of foal, 381

Feedback mechanisms, hormonal, 62, 64
  stimulatory, 64
Female(s). *See also* Estrous cycles; Estrus; Ovulation; Parturition; Pregnancy; *specific organs and female animals*
  age of, embryonic mortality and, 272
  anestrous, effect of male on, 247-248
  epizootic bovine abortion and, 276
    clinical signs of, 276
  fertilization failure in. *See* Female fertilization failure
  maternal behavior in. *See* Reproductive behavior, maternal
  maternal recognition of pregnancy in, 210
  new, effect on male sexual behavior, 246
  nutrition of, embryonic mortality and, 272
  repeat breeder, embryonic mortality and, 273, *274*
  reproductive anatomy of. *See* Female reproductive anatomy
  reproductive failure in. *See* Anestrus; Female reproductive failure
  sexual behavior in. *See also* Sexual behavior
    endocrine mechanisms of, 84
    sequence of, 239-240
Female fertilization failure, 267-269, 268t
  abnormal eggs and, 267
  abnormal sperm and, 267-268
  structural barriers to fertilization and, 268-269, *269*
Female reproductive anatomy, 20-54, *21*
  cervix uteri and, *48-51*, 48-52
    cervical stroma and physiologic changes and, 48-50
    functions of, 51-52
    mucus and, 50-51, *52*
  embryology and, 20-21, *22*, 23t
    of gonads, 20
    of reproductive ducts, 20-21
    of urogenital sinus, 21
  external genitalia and, 54
  ovary and, 21-29
    corpus luteum and, 26-29
    ovariectomy and, 26
    prenatal development of, 21-24, 23t, *24*, 25t-26t, 26
  oviduct and, 30-40, *31*, 32t, *33-37*, 38t, *39, 40*
    function of, 35-36, 38
    mucosa of, 31-35
    musculature and ligaments and, 39-40
  uterus and, 40, *41-43*, 42-48, *46, 47*
    contraction of, 44-45
    endometrial glands and uterine fluid and, 43-44
    function of, 45-48
    metabolism of, 45
    vasculature of, 43
  vagina and, 52-54, *53*
    functions of, 54
    physiologic responses of, 53
Female reproductive failure, *261*, 261-284
  anestrus and. *See* Anestrus
  atypical fertilization and, 269, 270t
  dystocia and, *280*, 280-281, *281*
    fetal, 280
    fetopelvic disproportion and, 280-281
    maternal, 280
  estrus and, atypical, 265-266
  fertilization failure and, 267-269, 268t
    abnormal eggs and, 267
    abnormal sperm and, 267-268

Female reproductive failure (cont.)
  fertilization failure and (cont.)
    structural barriers to fertilization and, 268-269, *269*
  hydramnios and hydrallantois and, 282
  multiple pregnancy and, 282
  ovulatory failure and, 266-267, *267*
  perinatal and neonatal mortality and, 277-280, *278*, 279t
    in horse, 381
  placental retention and, 281-282
  prenatal mortality and, 269-277
    abortion and, 274, 275t, 276
    causes of, *271*, 271-273
    embryonic, 270t, 270-273
    enzootic abortion of ewes and, 277
    epizootic bovine abortion and, 276
    equine rhinopneumonitis and, 276-277
    fetal mummification and, 277
    repeat breeders and, 273, *274*
  prolonged gestation and, 282, 283t, 284
  uterine infections and, 284
Fertility. *See also* Female fertilization failure; Infertility; Male fertilization failure
  aging and, *111*, 111t, 111-112
  of poultry eggs, 400, 400t
  semen evaluation and, 405, 407-409, *407-409*, 409t
    appearance and volume and, 405, 407
    sperm concentration and, 407-409
  sperm transport and, *154*, 154-155
    estrous synchronization and, 154-155
Fertilization, 188-194
  atypical, 269, 270t
  failure of. *See* Female fertilization failure; Male fertilization failure
  fertilizing ability of sperm and, 420-423
    hamster test and, *418*, 420
    hypo-osmotic swelling test and, 420t, 421, 421t, *422*, 423
    induced agglutination of sperm and, 423
  fusion of gametes and, *192*, 192-193
  gamete physiology related to, 144t, 144-145
  in vitro. See In vitro fertilization
  interaction of sperm and ovum and, 188, 190t, 190-194
    block to polyspermy and, 193
    development of pronuclei and syngamy and, 193-194
    gamete fusion and, *192*, 192-193
    interspecies fertilization and, 194
    sperm attachment and, 191, *191*
    sperm-oocyte encounter and, 190-191
    sperm penetration and, 191-192
  interspecies, 194. *See also* Hybridization
  oocyte preparation for, 130-131, *130-133*
  ovum maturation and, 188
  sperm maturation and, 188
    capacitation and, 188, *189*
  storage of, 393
Fetal membranes, placenta and, 217, *218*, 218t
Fetal mummification, 277
Fetopelvic disproportion, 280-281
Fetus. *See also* Prenatal development
  as allograft, 222-223, *223*
  dystocia and, 280
  fetal mummification and, 277
  initiation of parturition and, 230, *231*

  length of gestation and, 213
  mortality of. *See also* Abortion
    in horses, 379
  perinatal adaptations of, 232-233
    cardiovascular, 232-233
    energy metabolism after birth and, 233
    immune status and, 233
    lung maturation and, 233
    thermoregulatory, 233
Fibroblast growth factor (FGF), 90t
Fimbriae, 30, *33*
Foal heat, 378
Follicle(s), 25t. *See also* Folliculogenesis; Gametogenesis
  atresia of, 133, 135, *135*
    factors affecting, 133, 135
  graafian, 25t
  growing, 25t
  growth of, 114, 117, 121-124, *122*, *123*
    during follicular and luteal phases, 121-124, *125*
    in poultry, 387-388, *389*, *390*
    steroidogenesis and, 121, *124*, *125*
  morphologic, physiologic, and biochemical aspects of, 115t
  preovulatory, 25t-26t
  primary, 25t
  primordial, 115t
  regulatory and physiology parameters of components of, 116t-117t
  secondary, 25t, 115t
  tertiary (vesicular), 25t, 115t
  wall of, 115t
Follicle-stimulating hormone (FSH), 67-70
  estrous cycle and, in mare, 367-368
  follicle growth and, 121-124, *122*, *123*, *125*, *126*
  in vitro effects of, 69-70
  preovulatory release of, 69
  spermatogenesis and, *177*, 177-178
  tonic release of, 67, 69
Follicle-stimulating releasing hormone (FSH-RH), 72
Follicular fluid, 115t, 117-121
  biochemical composition of, 117-118, 120t
  functions of, 118-121
Follicular phase, 101-102
  follicle growth during, 121-124, *126*
Folliculogenesis, 114-121, 115t-117t, *118*, *119*. *See also* Gametogenesis
  follicle growth and, 114, 117
  follicular fluid and, 115t, 117-121
    biochemical composition of, 117-118, 120t
    functions of, 118-121
  puberty and, 99
  recruitment and selection of follicles and, 117
Foothill abortion (EBA; epizootic bovine abortion), 276
  clinical signs of, 276
Foreign bodies, uterus and, 47-48
Freemartinism, 265, 309, *309*
  cellular theory of, 309
  hormonal theory of, 309
Freezers, programmable, 510-511, 513
FSH. *See* Follicle-stimulating hormone
FSH-RH (follicle-stimulating releasing hormone), 72

Gametes. *See* Egg(s); Sperm
Gametogenesis. *See also* Folliculogenesis; Spermatogenesis
  in poultry, 387-388, *389*, *390*

puberty and, 97, 99
Gas exchange, placental, 221
Genes, 298-299. *See also* Genetic factors; Genetics
  genetic engineering and, 485, 487, *489*, 491t
Genetic engineering, 485-493, 487t, 488t
  chromosomes and genes and, 485, 487, *489*, 491t
  equipment and supplies for, 495-499, 496t, 497t, *498*
  evaluation of chromosomes of ova and, 487
  micromanipulation of gametes, embryos, and zona
    pellucida and, 487-488, *490*, 491, *492*, 493, 493t
Genetic factors. *See also* Genetics
  fetal growth and, 225
  length of gestation and, 213-214
  sexual behavior and, 245-246, *247*
Genetics. *See also* Chromosomes; Genes; Genetic engineering; Genetic factors
  basic concepts of, 298-299
  chromosomal aberrations and, 299-301
  inherited traits and, 299
  of reproductive failure. *See* Reproductive failure, ge-
    netics of
Genistein, 80, *81*
Genitalia. *See specific organs*
Genome expression, cleavage and, 198-199
Germinal epithelium, 25t, 96
  prenatal development of, 23, *24*
Gestation. *See* Pregnancy
GH (growth hormone; Somatotropic hormone; STH),
  70
GH-Ih (growth hormone-inhibiting hormone; somatostatin), 73
Glucocorticoids, 89
Glycerol, semen cryopreservation and, 519-520
Glycolysis, spermatozoal, 183
GnRH (gonadotropin-releasing hormone), 71, 72, *76*,
  77
  spermatogenesis and, 177, *177*
Goat, 330t, 330-340
  breeding and conception in, 336t, 336-337
  breeding season in, advancing, 338
  breeding season of, 330-332
    advancing, 338
    female, 330-332, *332*, *333*
    male, 332
  estrous cycle in, 334-335
    duration of estrus and, 335
    length of, 334-335
    male influence on estrus and, 335
    signs of estrus and, 335
  litter size in, 340
  maternal behavior in, 254
  ovulation in, 335-336
    rate of, 335-336, *336*
  parturition in, 337-338
  pregnancy in, 337, 337t
    diagnosis of, 452
  puberty in, 332-334
    female, 332-333, *334*, 334t
    male, 334
  puerperium in, 338-339
  reproductive performance of, 339-340
    artificial regulation of reproduction and, 339-340
    reproductive efficiency and, 339
  semen cryopreservation and, 523
Golgi phase of spermiogenesis, 172
Gonad(s). *See specific organs*

Gonadal steroid hormones. *See specific hormones*; Steroid
  hormones
Gonadotropin(s). *See also specific hormones*
  in pregnancy, in mare, 375, 377
  ovulation and, 142
    neuroendocrine control of, 142
  pituitary, 67, 69-71
  pregnancy diagnosis and, *458*, 458-459
  prenatal and neonatal secretion of, reproductive cy-
    cles and, 94, *96*
Gonadotropin-releasing hormone (GnRH), 71, 72, *76*,
  77
  spermatogenesis and, 177, *177*
Gonocytes, 169
Granulosa cells, 115t
  ovulation and, 136-137, *139*
  regulatory and physiology parameters of, 116t
Growth factors, 89, 89t, 178-179
  implantation and gestation and, 91
  in uterine tissue and fluid, 206-207
  intraovarian regulators and, 91, *92*
Growth hormone (GH; somatotropic hormone; STH),
  70
Growth hormone-inhibiting hormone (GH-Ih; somatostatin), 73
Gubernaculum testes, 5

Hamster test, *418*, 420
Haploid number of chromosomes, 298
Hatchability, of poultry eggs, 400, 400t
hCG (human chorionic gonadotropin), 77t, 78
Heat stress
  embryonic mortality and, 272-273
  male fertilization failure and, 292
Hermaphrodites, true, 305
Heterogametic sex, 298
Hippomanes, 228
Histocompatibility antigens, 222
Homogametic sex, 298
Homosexuality, 248
Hormones, 59t-61t, 59-89. *See also specific hormones, hormone
  types, endocrine glands, and animals*
  andrology and, 87-88
    activin and inhibin and, 88
    Sertoli cells and Leydig cells and, 87-88
    transferrin, β_2 microglobulin, and albumin and, 88
  assays of, 65
  chemical composition of, 60t
  during pregnancy, in pig, *348*, 356-358
  egg production and, in poultry, 394-395
  embryonic mortality and, 271
  estrous cycle and
    in pig, *348*, 351-354
    regulation of, 100-102, *102*
  feedback mechanisms and, 62, 64
    stimulatory feedback and, 64
  fetal, fetal growth and, 226
  follicle growth and, 121, *124*, *125*
  freemartinism and, 309
  immunoendocrine aspects and, 64
  lactation and, 61-62
  mode of action of, 61t
  modes of transmission of, 61t
  molting and, in poultry, 397-398
  of pregnancy, 215-217

Hormones (cont.)
  of pregnancy (cont.)
    blood and urinary concentrations of, 215t, 215-217, *216*
    in mare, 375, 377
    maintenance of pregnancy and, 215, *215*
  of reproduction
    primary, 59-61, *62*, 63t, 64t
    secondary, 59-61, *62*, 63t, 64t, 88-89
    ovary and, in poultry, 395-396, *396*
    ovulatory cycle and, in poultry, 396-397, *397*
    placental, 63t, 64t, 77t, 77-78, 222, 454
    pregnancy diagnosis and, 454, 456-459
    puberty and, 61
    receptors for, 64-65, *66*, *67*
    sexual behavior and. *See* Sexual behavior, endocrine mechanisms of
    sperm transport and, 152
    spermatogenesis and, *177*, 177-178
    structure of, 60t
Horse, 361-383. *See also* Mare; Stallion
  Barker syndrome in, 381
  breeding season of, 361-362
    mare and, 361-362
    stallion and, 361
  foaling in, 377-378
    induced parturition and, 377-378
    postpartum estrus and, 378
  hybrids of, 378
  reproductive failure in. *See* Mare, reproductive failure in; Stallion, reproductive failure in
Human chorionic gonadotropin (hCG), 77t, 78
Hybridization
  in horse, 378
  interspecies fertilization and, 194
  reproductive failure and, 309-310, 310t
Hydrallantois, 282
Hydramnios, 282
Hypersexuality, 248
Hypo-osmotic swelling test, 420t, 421, 421t, *422*, 423
Hyposexuality, 248-249
Hypothalamus, *71*, 71-77
  function of, 71-72, 72t, *73-75*
  hormones of, 63t, 72-73, *76*, 76-77
    clinical uses of, 77
  mode of action of, 72

IFN (interferon), 90t
IGF. *See* Insulin-like growth factors; Intrafollicular growth factor; Intraovarian growth factor
IGF-I (insulin growth factor-r), 90t
Immune status, perinatal adaptation of, 233
Immunoendocrinology, 64
Immunologic factors
  incompatibility and, embryonic mortality and, 273
  male fertilization failure and, 294-295
  mother-fetus relationship and, fetus as allograft and, 222-223, *223*
Immunologic pregnancy diagnosis, 452, 455t
Immunologic responses, vaginal, 53
Implantation, 46-47, 204-206, *205*
  growth factors and, 91
Impotentia coeundi. *See* Libido, lack of
Infection(s). *See also specific infections*
  abortion caused by, 276-277
  fetal mummification and, 277

genital, in mare, 380
uterine, postpartum, 284
Infertility
  congenital malformations and, 304
  female. *See also* Female fertilization failure
  male. *See also* Male fertilization failure
    artificial insemination and, 294
Infundibulum, of oviduct, 30, *33*
Inherited abnormalities, of reproductive system, 301-303
  functional disorders and, 303
  morphologic defects and, 301-302, 303t
Inherited traits, 299
Inhibin, 83, 179
  andrology and, 88
In vitro fertilization, 482-485, 483t
  equipment and supplies for, 495-499, 496t, 497t, *498*
  oocyte collection and fertilization and, 484-485, *486*
  prerequisites and criteria of, 485
  sperm collection and capacitation for, 482, 484, *484*
Insulin growth factor-r (IGF-I), 90t
Insulin-like growth factors (IGF), 90t
  fetal growth and, 226
Interferon (IFN), 90t
Intersexuality, 305, 309
  freemartinism and, 309, *309*
    cellular theory of, 309
    hormonal theory of, 309
  pseudohermaphrodites and, 305, 308t, 309
  true hermaphrodites and, 305
Intrafollicular growth factor (IGF), 90t
Intraovarian growth factor (IGF), 91
Intrauterine devices (IUDs), 47-48
Intrauterine growth retardation, in horses, 380
Intromission, 16, 241-242, *243*
  failure to achieve, 290-291, *291*
Inversion, chromosomal, 299
Involution, postpartum, of uterus, 47, 234
  in cattle, 321
Ischiocavernosus muscles, 12
Isthmus, of oviduct, 30, 31, *33*
IUDs (intrauterine devices), 47-48

Labia majora, 54
Labia minora, 54
Labor. *See* Parturition
Laboratory animals, male reproductive anatomy of, *17*, 18, 18t
Lactation
  anestrus during, 262-264
  embryonic mortality and, 271-272
  endocrinology of, 61-62
  in pig, 358
    sow at weaning and, 358
  postpartum estrus and ovulation and, 104-105, *105*, 234-235
Lactoferrin (LF), 90t
Latebra, 385, *386*
Leptotene, 169
Leydig cells, andrology and, 88
LF (lactoferrin), 90t
LH. *See* Luteinizing hormone
LH-RH (luteinizing hormone-releasing hormone), 72, 73, *75*, 77
  estrous cycle regulation and, 100-101
Libido, lack of, in males, 289-290

Ligaments
  oviductal, 40
  pelvic, changes during pregnancy, 215
Ligamentum ovarii proprium, 156
Litter size
  in pig, *348*, 355
  in sheep and goats, 340
Lung maturation, parturition and, 233
Luteal phase, 101
  follicle growth during, 121-124, *126*
Luteinizing hormone (LH), 67-70
  estrous cycle and, in mare, 368-369
  follicle growth and, 121, *122*, *123*
    during luteal and follicular phases, 121-124, *126*
  in vitro effects of, 69-70
  preovulatory release of, 69
  spermatogenesis and, *177*, 177-178
  tonic release of, 67, 69
Luteinizing hormone-releasing hormone (LH-RH), 72, 73, *75*, 77
  estrous cycle regulation and, 100-101
Luteolysis
  corpus luteum and, 28
  uterine, 45-46

Macromolecular supplementation, 497-499
Male(s). *See also* Ejaculation; Semen; Sperm; *specific organs and male animals*
  breeding season in, 108-109, 332, 361
  fertility of. *See* Fertility
  lack of libido in, 289-290
  semen collection and
    electroejaculation and, 429-430
    frequency of, 427-428
  semen cryopreservation and
    freezing of semen and, 520-521
    glycerol addition for, 519-520
    semen storage and, 521
    thawing of semen and, 521
  sexual behavior in. *See also* Sexual behavior
    abnormal, in stallion, 382
    neural mechanisms of erection and ejaculation and, 244-245, *245*, *246*
    precoital stimulation and, 248
    sequence of, 239, 240t
Male fertilization failure, 292-295
  breeding techniques and, 294
    breeding management and, 294
    infertility and artificial insemination and, 294
  diseases of testes and accessory glands and, 292, 293t
  heat stress and, 292
  immunologic factors and, 294-295
Male pronucleus growth factor, 193
Male reproductive anatomy, 3-18, *4*. *See also specific organs*
  accessory glands and, 11-12, *12*, *13*
  development and, 4-6
    postnatal, 5-6
    prenatal, 4-5
    testicular descent and, 5, 5t
  epididymis and ductus deferens and, 3, 8-11, *9*, *10*
  in laboratory animals, *17*, 18, 18t
  penis and prepuce and, 12, 14-18
  testis and scrotum and, 3, 5, 5t, *6*, 6-8, *7*, 8t
Male reproductive failure, 287-296, *288*
  chromosomal aberrations and, 296
  congenital malformations and, 287-289

ejaculatory disturbances and, 289-292
  inability to copulate and, 290-292
  lack of libido and, 289-290
fertilization failure and. *See* Male fertilization failure
nutrition and, 295-296
Manchette, 172
Mare
  breeding season of, 361-362
  equine rhinopneumonitis in, abortion and, 276-277
  estrous cycle in, 365-371, 366t
    corpus luteum and, 367, *367*, *368*
    endocrine control of, 367-369
    estrus and, 365, 367, 369-370, 379
    induction of estrus and ovulation and, 369-371
    irregularities of, 378-379
  maternal behavior in, 254-255
  maternal recognition of pregnancy in, 210-211
  pregnancy in, 371-377
    developmental horizons and, 371, 372t, 373t
    diagnosis of, 371, 372t, 373t, 450, 450t
    endocrine profile and, 375, 377
    ovarian function and, 374
    placenta and, 374-375, *375*, *376*
    twinning and, 371-372, 374
  reproductive failure in, 378-382
    abortion and, 381
    anestrus and, 379
    breeding technique recommendations and, 381-382
    endometrial cysts and related pathologic conditions and, 380
    estrous irregularities and, 378-379
    excessive length of umbilical cord and, 380-381
    genital infections and, 380
    neonatal abnormalities and neonatal mortality and, 381
    ovarian neoplasms and, 379-380
    prenatal mortality and, 379
Massage method, for semen collection, 430
Masturbation, 249
Maternal behavior. *See* Reproductive behavior, maternal
Maternal factors, initiation of parturition and, 230
Maternal recognition of pregnancy. *See* Pregnancy, maternal recognition of
Mating, 240, *242*. *See also* Copulation; Sexual behavior
  natural, in poultry, 398
Maturation phase of spermiogenesis, 172-173
Medullary cords, 20
Membrana granulosa, 25t
Metabolism
  fetal, 224-225
  of energy, perinatal adaptation of, 233
  spermatozoal, 182-183
    glycolysis and, 183
    respiration and, 183
  uterine, 45
Microbiologic flora, vaginal, 53
Microcotyledons, 374
β_2 Microglobulin, andrology and, 88
Mineral deficiencies, male infertility and, 296
Mineralocorticoids, 88-89
MIS (müllerian-inhibiting substance), 91, 178-179
  in pig, 344
Modulations, in seminiferous epithelium, 174
Molting, hormones and, in poultry, 397-398

Monosomic aneuploids, 299
Morphologic defects, of reproductive system, inherited, 301-302, 303t
Morula, 195
    micromanipulation of, 496t
Mosaicism, 299, 300t
    sterility and infertility and, 304
Mount(s), for semen collection, 425-426, *426*
Mounting, 240-241
    failure to mount and, 290
Mucus, cervical, 50-51, *52*
    sperm transport and, 150-151
Müllerian ducts, embryology of, 20-21
Müllerian-inhibiting substance (MIS), 91, 178-179
    in pig, 344
Musculature
    ovarian, 25t
    oviductal, 39-40
Myoid layer, blood-testis barrier and, 175, *176*

Natural mating, in poultry, 398
Neonatal maladjustment syndrome, in horse, 381
Neonate, 249. *See also* Suckling
    abnormalities of, in horse, 381
    death of, 279t, 279-280
        behavioral anomalies and thermoregulation and, 256-257
        female reproductive failure and, 277-280, *278*, 279t
        in horse, 381
        respiratory distress syndrome and, 279-280
Neoplasms, ovarian, in mare, 379-380
Neurophysins, 70
Nondisjunction, 299
Nonsteroidal plant estrogens, 80
Nuclear maturation, 136
Nutrients, placental transport of, 221-222
Nutrition
    fetal, 224-225
    male reproductive failure and, 295-296
        mineral deficiencies and, 296
        toxic agents and, 296
        underfeeding and, 295
        vitamin deficiencies and, 296
    of dam
        anestrus due to deficiencies in, 264
        embryonic mortality and, 272
        ovulation rate and, in pig, 354
Nymphomania, 265-266

Oocyte(s)
    collection and manipulation of, 470-473, *471*, 471t
        donor preparation for, 472-473
        for *in vitro* fertilization, 484-485, *486*
        nonsurgical methods of, 471-472, *474*, 476-478
        selection of ova for transfer and, 473, 475, 475t, *479-481*
        surgical methods of, 470-471, *472*, *473*
    fertilization and, sperm-oocyte encounter and, 190-191
    maturation of, 126-127, 128t-129t, 130, 477
        in vitro, 475
    regulatory and physiology parameters of, 116t
    ovulation and, 136, *137*, *138*
    preparation for fertilization, 130-131, *130-133*

oTP-1 (ovine trophoblast protein 1; type I conceptus interferon), maternal recognition of pregnancy and, 208-209
Ova. *See* Egg(s); Oocyte(s)
Ovarian hypoplasia, anestrus due to, 264-265
Ovary(ies), 21-29. *See also* Follicle(s); Folliculogenesis
    abnormalities of, anestrus due to, 264-265
    changes during pregnancy, 215
    cortex of, 25t
    cystic, 265, 266-267, *267*
    function of
        in mare, 374
        in poultry, 395-396
    hormones of, 63t
    hypoplasia of, 304, 304t
    medulla of, 25t
    morphology of, in pig, estrous cycle and, *348*, 351-354
    neoplasms of, in mare, 379-380
    of poultry, 395-396, *396*
        egg formation and, 387, *388*
    prenatal and neonatal physiology of, reproductive cycles and, 96, *97*, *98*
    prenatal development of, 21-24, 23t, *24*, 25t-26t, 26
        ovarian blood flow and, 23-24, 26
    removal of, 26
    stroma of, 25t
Oviduct, 30-40, *31*
    anatomy of, 30-35, 32t, *33-37*, 38t, *39*, *40*
        mucosa and, 31-35
    contraction of, egg transport and, 158-159, 161t
    egg transport in. *See* Egg(s), transport of
    embryonic development in, 164
    function of, 35-36, 38
        oviductal fluid and, 35-36, 38
    in poultry, 388-389, *390*, *391*, 391-393
        egg transport and oviposition and, 392
        infundibulum of, 388-389, 391-392
        sperm storage, transport, and fertilization and, 392-393
    mucosa of, 31-35
        ciliated cells of, 31-33
        innervation of, 33-35
        nonciliated cells of, 33
        vasculature of, 33
    musculature and ligaments of, 39-40
        contraction patterns and, 39-40
        prostaglandins and, 40
        utero-ovarian and related ligaments and, 40
    sperm transport in, 152
Oviductal fluid, 35-36, 38
    culture of, 495-497
Ovine trophoblast protein 1 (oTP-1; type I conceptus interferon), maternal recognition of pregnancy and, 208-209
Oviposition, in poultry, 392
Ovulation, 131, 133-143, *134*. *See also* Superovulation
    anomalies of, 143
    biochemical mechanisms of, 139, 141-142
        gonadotropins and, 142
        prostaglandins and, 141-142
        steroid secretion and, 139
    cellular events and, *136*, 136-137
        apex changes and, 137
        granulosa cells and, 136-137, *139*
        oocyte and, 136, *137*, *138*

theca cells and, 137
egg pick-up and, 142
follicular atresia and, 133, 135, *135*
factors affecting, 133, 135
in buffalo, 325
in cattle, 319, 319t
in mare, induction of, 369-371
in pig, *348*, 354
increasing rate of, 354
nutrition and rate of, 354
in sheep and goats, 335-336
rate of, 335-336, *336*
induction of, 461-466, 463t
during anestrus, 462, 464t, 464-466, 465t, *466*, *467*
gonadotropins and, 69
in vitro, 142-143
collection of preovulatory eggs and, 143
mechanisms of, 137-139, 140t, 141t
neuroendocrine control of ovulatory gonadotropic discharge and, 142
neuromuscular mechanisms of, 142
ovulatory cycle and, in poultry, 396-397, *397*
postpartum, 102-105, 103t
endocrine factors in, 103-104, *104*
in buffalo, 327
in cattle, 321
suckling and lactation and, 104-105, *105*
site of, 135-136
Ovulation fossa, 135
Ovulatory cycle, in poultry, 396-397, *397*
Ovum. *See* Egg(s); Oocyte(s)
Oxytocin, 70-72
functions of, 70-71

Pachytene, 169
PAF (platelet-activating factor), 90t, 91
Pancreas, hormones of, 64t
Parathyroid glands, 88
hormones of, 64t
Parthenogenesis, 199-200
Parturition, 228-233, 230-232
dystocia and, *280*, 280-281, *281*
fetal, 280
fetopelvic disproportion and, 280-281
maternal, 280
forces of delivery and, 231-232
in buffalo, 326-327
in cattle, 321
in mare, induced, 377-378
in sheep and goats, 337-338
induction of, 232
in mare, 377-378
initiation of, 228, 229t
fetal mechanisms and, 230, *231*
maternal mechanisms and, 230
labor and, 230-232
forces of delivery and, 231-232
stages of, 230, 232t
mechanics of, *229*, 229-230
dilation of cervix and, 229-230
myometrial contractions and, 229
perinatal adaptations and, 232-233
signs of, 228
stages of labor and, 230, 232t
uterus and, 47
PDGF (platelet-derived growth factor), 90t

Pelvic ligaments, changes during pregnancy, 215
Penis, 12, 14-18
corpus cavernosum, 12
corpus spongiosum, 12
emission and ejaculation and, 16, 18
erection and protrusion of, 14-16, *16*
neural mechanisms of, 244-245, *245*, *246*
structure of, 12, 14, *14*, *15*
Perinatal mortality, 277-279, *278*
PGF$_2$ (prostaglandin F$_{2\alpha}$)
estrous cycle regulation and, 101
maternal recognition of pregnancy and
in cow, 210
in mare, 210
in pig, 208-210
Photoperiodism, breeding season and, 106-108, *108*
endocrine and neuroendocrine mechanisms and, 109-111, *110*
PIF (prolactin-inhibiting factor), 71
Pig, 343-358. *See also* Boar; Sow
conception rate in, 355
embryo survival in, 355
sexual development and maturation of, 343-345, 344t, *346*, 347
Pituitary gland, 65-71, *68*
anterior, hormones of, 63t, 64t, 67, 69-71
posterior, hormones of, 63t, 64t, 70-71
vascular supply of, 65-67
PL (placental lactogen), 77t, 78
pregnancy diagnosis and, 455
Placenta, 217-223. *See also* Placental circulation; Placental transport; Umbilical cord
classification of, 217-219, 218t
by gross shape, 217-219, *219*
development of, 217
chorionic villi and, 217
fetal membranes and, 217, *218*, 218t
functions of, 220-222, *221*
endocrine, 222
transport as, 220-222
hormones of, 63t, 64t, 77t, 77-78, 222, 455
in horse, 374-375, *375*, *376*
placental barrier and, 374-375
mother-fetus immunologic relationship and, fetus as allograft and, 222-223, *223*
retained, 281-282
Placental barrier, 219
Placental circulation, 219-220
uterine blood flow and, 219-220
placental microcirculation and, 220, *220*
umbilical, 219
Placental lactogen (PL), 77t, 78
pregnancy diagnosis and, 455
Placental transport, 220-222
of gases, 221
of nutrients, 221-222
Placentophagy, 250
Plasma, seminal. *See* Seminal plasma
Platelet-activating factor (PAF), 90t, 91
Platelet-derived growth factor (PDGF), 90t
PMSG (pregnant mare serum gonadotropin), 77t, 77-78, 216, 375, 377
Polarization, 195-196
Polyploidy, 299, 300t
Polyspermy, 269
block to, 193

Poultry, 385-401
artificial insemination in, 398-401, 437, *438*, 439
fertility and hatchability and, 400, 400t
semen collection, evaluation, and insemination and, 399-400
semen production and, 400-401
breeding practices with, 398
eggs of, 385-388, *386*, 386t
formation of, 387-388
hormones in, 394-398
anatomy and function of ovary and, 395-396, *396*
initiation of egg production and, 394-395
male, 398
molting and, 397-398
ovulatory cycle and, 396-397, *397*
natural mating in, 398
oviduct of, 388-389, *390*, *391*, 391-393
egg transport and oviposition and, 392
infundibulum of, 388-389, 391-392
sperm storage, transport, and fertilization and, 392-393
semen of, 393
seminal plasma and sperm composition and, 393
spermatozoa morphology and, 393
testis and duct system of, 393-394, *395*
Pregnancy, 213-217. *See also* Embryo(s); Fertilization; Fetus; Parturition; Placenta; Pregnancy diagnosis; Prenatal development
cervix during, 52
corpus luteum and, 29
maternal recognition of pregnancy and, 29
growth factors and, 91
hormones of, 215-217
blood and urinary concentrations of, 215t, 215-217, *216*
in mare, 375, 377
maintenance of pregnancy and, 215, *215*
in buffalo, 326
in cattle, 320-321
diagnosis of, 450
maternal recognition of, 210
in ewe, 337, 337t
diagnosis of, 450, 452
in goat, 337, 337t
diagnosis of, 452
in mare. *See* Mare, pregnancy in
in sow. *See* Sow, pregnancy in
length of, 213t, 213-214, *214*
environmental factors affecting, 214
fetal factors affecting, 213
genetic factors affecting, 213-214
maternal factors affecting, 213
prolonged, 282, 283t, 284
maintenance of
after embryo transfer, 481-482
hormones and, 215, *215*
maternal physiology in, 214-217
hormones of pregnancy and, 215-217
maternal adaptations and, 217
reproductive organ changes and, 214-215
maternal recognition of, 29, 207-211
in all farm animals, 207
in cow, 210
in mare, 210-211
in pig, 207-210, *209*
multiple, 200-201, 282

abortion and, 276
in horse, 371-372, 374
pseudopregnancy and, 208, 265
uterus and, 47
Pregnancy diagnosis, 446-459
hormones in, 454, 456-459
immunologic, 452, 455t
in cattle, 450
in mare, 371, 372t, 373t, 450, 450t
in sow, 450, 452, *453*
pregnancy-associated substances in, 452-454
radiography in, 446
rectal examination in, 446, *447*, 448t
ultrasonography in, 447-452
B-mode real-time, *449*, 449-452
Doppler phenomenon and, 447-448
pulse-echo, *448*, 448-449
vaginal biopsy, 452, *454*
Pregnancy-specific protein B (bPSPB), pregnancy diagnosis and, 453-454
Pregnant mare serum gonadotropin (PMSG), 77t, 77-78, 216, 375, 377
Preleptotene, 169
Prenatal development, 224-228
fetal circulation and, *226*, 226-227
fetal fluids and, 227-228
composition of, 228
functions of, 227
origin of, 227, 228t
volume of, 227
fetal growth and, 225-226
factors affecting, 225, *226*
fetal hormones and, 226
growth rate and, 225
insulin-like growth factors and, 226
intrauterine growth retardation in horse and, 380
fetal nutrition and metabolism and, 224-225
of pig, 343-345, 344t, *346*, 347
periods of, 224, *224*
Preovulatory surge, 69
Prepuce, anatomy of, 14
Primordial germ cells, 169
Progesterone, 81
estrous cycle and
in mare, 369
regulation of, 101
pregnancy diagnosis and, 454, 456-458, *457*, 457t
Progestogens, 81-82
clinical applications of, 81-82
functions of, 81
Prolactin, 70
Prolactin-inhibiting factor (PIF), 71
Pronuclei, development of, 193-194
Prostaglandin(s), 85-87, 86t, *87*
clinical application of, 86-87
functions of, 85, *87*
oviductal contractility and, 40
ovulation and, 141-142
induction of, in mare, 370
Prostaglandin $F_{2\alpha}$ (PGF$_2$)
estrous cycle regulation and, 101
maternal recognition of pregnancy and
in cow, 210
in mare, 210
in pig, 208-210
Prostate gland, comparative anatomy of, 1

Protein(s), uterine, 44
Protein B, 77t, 78
Protrusion, of penis, 14-16, *16*
Pseudohermaphrodites, 305, 308t, 309
Pseudopregnancy, 208
  in pig, 265
Puberty
  endocrinology of, 61
  in buffalo, 324-325
  in cattle, 315-316
    female, 315
    male, 315-316
  in pig, female, 350-351
  in sheep and goats, 332-334
    female, 332-333, *334*, 334t
    male, 334
  reproductive cycles and, 96-97, 99-100
    age at puberty and, 99-100
    endocrine mechanisms of puberty and, 96-97
    gametogenesis and, 97, 99
Pubic symphysis, changes during pregnancy, 215
Puerperium, 233-235, *234*
  in buffalo, 327, 327t
    ovarian activity and, 327
  in cattle, 321
  in sheep and goats, 338-339
  ovarian function during, 321
  uterine involution and, 234, 321
Pyometra, 284

Radiography, in pregnancy diagnosis, 446
Radioimmunoassays, of hormones, 65
Ralgro (zeronal), 80, *81*
Ram. *See also* Sheep
  breeding season of, 332
  lack of libido in, 290
  puberty in, 334
  semen collection and
    electroejaculation and, 430
    frequency of, 428, 429t
RDS (respiratory distress syndrome), neonatal mortality and, 279-280
Rectal examination, in pregnancy diagnosis, 446, *447*, 448t
Refractoriness, 242
Relaxin, 82-83, 90t
  estrous cycle regulation and, 101
Repeat breeders, embryonic mortality and, 273, *274*
Reproductive behavior, *237*, 237-257. *See also* Sexual behavior
  maternal, 249-256, 250t. *See also* Pregnancy, maternal recognition of
    farrowing and, 255
    in cattle, 254
    in goats, 254
    in horses, 254-255
    in pigs, 255-257
    in sheep, 251-253
    parent-young interactions and, 249-251
    postpartum, 251-252, 255-256
    prepartum, 251, 255
    suckling and, 249, 252-253, *253*, 254, *255*, 256, 256t
  neonatal, 249
    behavioral anomalies, thermoregulation, and neonatal mortality and, 256-257
    suckling and, 249, 252-253, *253*, 254, *255*, 256, 256t

Reproductive cycles, 94-112, *95*. *See also* Breeding season; Estrous cycles; *specific animals*
  aging and fertility and, *111*, 111t, 111-112
  prenatal and neonatal physiology and, 94, 96
    gonadotropins and, 94, *96*
    gonads and, 94, 96
  puberty and, 96-97, 99-100
    age at, 99-100
    endocrine mechanisms of, 96-97
    gametogenesis and, 97, 99
Reproductive ducts. *See also* Ductus deferens; Oviduct
  female, embryology of, 20-21
  in poultry, 393-394, *395*
Reproductive efficiency. *See also* Artificial insemination; Embryo transfer; Ovulation, induction of; Pregnancy diagnosis; Semen evaluation; Superovulation
  genetic engineering and, 485-493, 487t, 488t
    chromosomes and genes and, 485, 487, *489*, 491t
    evaluation of chromosomes of ova and, 487
    micromanipulation of gametes, embryos, and zona pellucida and, 487-488, *490*, 491, *492*, 493, 493t
  in vitro fertilization and, 482-485, 483t
    oocyte collection and fertilization and, 484-485, *486*
    prerequisites and criteria of, 485
    sperm collection and capacitation for, 482, 484, *484*
  of buffalo, 327-328
  of cattle, 321-322, 322t
  of sheep and goats, 339
  ovulation induction and synchronization and, 461-466, 463t
    during anestrus, 462, 464t, 464-466, 465t, *466*, *467*
  X- and Y-chromosome-bearing spermatozoa and, 440-444
    biology of spermatozoa and, 440-441
    future research directions for, 444
    sperm separation techniques and, 441-444, 443t
Reproductive failure
  anomalies of ovulation and, 143
  fertilization failure and. *See* Female fertilization failure; Male fertilization failure
  genetics of, 298-301
    chromosomal aberrations and. *See* Chromosomal aberrations, reproductive failure and
    inherited abnormalities of reproductive system and, 301-303
  in females. *See* Female reproductive failure
  in horses. *See* Mare, reproductive failure in; Stallion, reproductive failure in
  in males. *See* Male fertilization failure; Male reproductive failure; Stallion, reproductive failure in
Reproductive performance
  of buffalo, 327-328
    increasing, 328
    reproductive efficiency and, 327-328
  of cattle, 321-324
    general fertility and, 322
    improving, 322-324, *323*
    measures of reproductive efficiency and, 321-322, 322t
  of sheep and goats, 339-340
    artificial regulation of reproduction and, 339-340
    reproductive efficiency and, 339
Residual body, 173

Respiration, spermatozoal, 183
Respiratory distress syndrome (RDS), neonatal mortality and, 279-280
Retractor penis muscles, 14

Saline infusion, estrus induction by, in mare, 369
Scrotum. *See also* Testes
　anatomy of, *6,* 6-8, *7*
Season
　breeding. *See* Breeding season
　sexual behavior and, 247
Semen, 165, 165t. *See also* Ejaculation; Sperm
　collection of
　　for artificial insemination. *See* Artificial insemination
　　for *in vitro* fertilization, 482, 484, *484*
　cryopreservation of. *See* Cryopreservation, of semen
　embryonic mortality and, 273
　emission of, 16, 18
　evaluation of. *See* Semen evaluation
　in vitro evaluation of quality of, 183t, 184t, 186
　of poultry
　　morphology of, 393
　　production of, 400-401
　poor semen characteristics and, in stallion, 382-383
　production of, of stallions, 362-363, 364t, *365*
Semen evaluation, 405-423, 406t
　fertility and, 405, 407-409, *407-409,* 409t
　　appearance and volume and, 405, 407
　　sperm concentration and, 407-409
　fertilizing ability of sperm and, 420-423
　　hamster test and, *418,* 420
　　hypo-osmotic swelling test and, 420t, 421, 421t, *422,* 423
　　induced agglutination of sperm and, 423
　sperm morphology and, 409-414, *411, 412*
　　inherited sperm defects and, 411-413
　　live/dead sperm and, 413-414
　　supravital triple-staining technique and, *413,* 413-414
　sperm motility and, *414,* 414-420
　　factors affecting, 414, *415*
　　patterns of, 414-415, *415-417*
　　techniques for measurement of, 415-420
Semen extenders, 515-518, 519
　composition of, 517-518
Seminal plasma, 181
　composition of
　　biochemical constituents and, 181-182
　　in poultry, 393
　sperm motility in, measurement of, 416-419, *417*
Seminiferous epithelium, 169-178, *170*
　blood-testis barrier and, 174-178
　　cellular junctions and, 174-176
　　fluid secretions and, 176-177
　cycle of, 173
　spermatocytogenesis and, 169-170, *171*
　spermatogenesis and
　　duration of, 173-174
　　endocrine control of, *177,* 177-178
　spermatogenic wave and, 174, *175*
　spermatogonia and, 169
　spermiation and, 173, *174*
　spermiogenesis and, 170, 172-173
　wave of, 174, *175*
Seminiferous tubules, 8t, 20

Sequence, poultry egg production and, 394-395
Sertoli cell(s), 8t
　andrology and, 87-88
Sertoli cell junctions, 175-176
Sex
　heterogametic, 298
　homogametic, 298
　intersexuality and. *See* Intersexuality
Sex chromosomes, 298
　of sperm, 168-169, 440-444
　　biology of spermatozoa and, 440-441
　　future research directions for, 444
　　sperm separation techniques and, 441-444, 443t
Sexual behavior, 238-242
　abnormal, 248-249
　　in stallion, 382
　endocrine mechanisms of, 83-85
　　in females, 84
　　in males, 83-84
　　neural mechanisms and, 84-85
　　sex specificity of, 84
　factors affecting, 245-248
　　environmental, 246-247
　　experience as, 247-248
　　genetic, 245-246, *247*
　　males and, 248
　mechanisms of, 242-245, *243, 245*
　　cortex and sensory capacities and, 244
　　endocrine, 83-85
　　neural mechanisms of erection and ejaculation and, 244-245, *245, 246*
　psychosocial aspects of reproduction and, 238-239, *239*
　sequence of, 239-242, 240t, *241*
　　duration of estrus and, 242
　　ejaculation and, 242
　　frequency of copulation and, 242, 244t
　　in females, 239-240
　　in males, 239, 240t
　　intromission and, 241-242, *243*
　　mating and, 240, *242*
　　mounting and, 240-241
　　refractoriness and, 242
Sexual season. *See* Breeding season
Sheep, 330t, 330-340. *See also* Ewe; Ram
　breeding and conception in, 336t, 336-337
　breeding season of, 330-332
　　advancing, 338
　　female, 330-332, *332, 333*
　　male, 332
　puberty in, 332-334
　　female, 332-333, *334,* 334t
　　male, 334
　reproductive performance of, 339-340
　　reproductive efficiency and, 339
Smooth muscle, ovarian, 25t
Somatostatin (GH-Ih; growth hormone-inhibiting hormone), 73
Somatropic hormone (GH; growth hormone; STH), 70
Sow. *See also* Pig
　estrous cycle in, 351-354
　　ovarian morphology and hormone secretion and, *348,* 351-354
　hormones and puberty in gilts and, 350-351
　lactation in, 358
　　sow at weaning and, 358

litter size in, *348*, 355
maternal behavior in, 255-256
  farrowing and, 255
  postpartum, 255-256
  prepartum, 255
  suckling and, 256, 256t
maternal recognition of pregnancy in, 207-210, *209*
ovulation rate in, *348*, 354
  increasing, 354
  nutrition and, 354
pregnancy in, 355-358
  diagnosis of, 450, 452, *453*
  growth of conceptuses and, 355-356
  hormones during, *348*, 356-358
  maternal recognition of, 207-210, *209*
  postpartum estrus and, 358
pseudopregnancy in, 265
Sperm, 165t, 165-169, *166. See also* Gametogenesis; Semen; Spermatogenesis
abnormal, fertilization failure and, 267-268
antigenicity of, 183
autoimmunity and, 183-186, *185*
capacitation of, 188, *189*
  for *in vitro* fertilization, 482, 484
composition of, 168
  in poultry, 393
fate in female tract, 181
fertilization and. *See* Fertilization
fertilizing ability of, 420-423
  hamster test and, *418*, 420
  hypo-osmotic swelling test and, 420t, 421, 421t, *422*, 423
  induced agglutination of sperm and, 423
fusion with egg, *192*, 192-193
hyperactivation of, 152, 154
induced agglutination of, 423
loss of, during transport, 155-156
maturation of, 179-180
  development of fertilizing potential and, 180
metabolism of, 182-183
  glycolysis and, 183
  respiration and, 183
morphology of, 165-168, 409-414, *411*, *412*
  acrosome and, 166, *167*
  inherited defects and, 411-413
  live/dead sperm and, 413-414
  sperm head and, 165-166, *167*
  sperm tail and, 166-168
  supravital triple-staining technique and, *413*, 413-414
motility of. *See* Sperm motility
physiology related to fertilization, 144t, 144-145
polyspermy and, 269
  block to, 193
production and release of
  in buffalo, 325-326
  in cattle, 319-320
production of, in pig, 350
sex chromosomes of, 168-169
storage of, 179-180, 393
  in poultry, 392-393
survival of, during transport, 155
transport of. *See* Sperm transport
unejaculated, disposal of, 180-181
X- and Y-chromosome-bearing, 440-441, 440-444
  biology of spermatozoa and, 440-441

cytogenetics of, 440-441, 441t, *442*
  future research directions for, 444
  karyotyping of sperm and, 441
  sperm plasmalemma and, 441
  sperm separation techniques and, 441-444, 443t
Sperm concentration, 407-409
  sperm count and, 407-409, *410*
Sperm motility, *414*, 414-420
  evaluation of, semen cryopreservation and, 523-524
  factors affecting, 414, *415*
  patterns of, 414-415, *415-417*
  techniques for measuring, 415-420
    motility in seminal plasma and biologic fluids and, 416-419, *417*
    photoelectric and electronic, 419-420
Sperm nucleus-decondensing factor, 193
Sperm reservoirs, colonization of, 146-147, *150*
Sperm separation, 441-444, 443t
  flow cytometry and sorting and, 442-444
  layered separation over albumin columns and, 442
  practical application of, 443-444
Sperm transport
  conception rate and, 161-162
  endocrine control of, 152
  epididymal, 179
    mechanisms of, 179
  fertility and, *154*, 154-155
    estrous synchronization and, 154-155
  hyperactivation of sperm and, 152, 154
  in cervix, 51-52, 147, 150-151
    mucus and, 150-151
    sperm penetration in cervical mucus and, 151
  in female tract, 145t, 145-156, *146-149*
    cervical, 51-52, 147, 150-151
    colonization of sperm reservoirs and, 146-147, *150*
    in oviduct, 152
    in uterus, 151-152, *153*
    rapid, 146, *150*
    slow, 147, *151*
    sperm distribution and, 45-147
  in oviduct, 152
  in uterus, 151-152
    spermophagy and, 151-152, *153*
  loss of spermatozoa and, 155-156
  sexual experience and, 247
  survival of spermatozoa and, 155
  uterine, 45
Spermatids, 8t, 169, 170
Spermatocele, 287
Spermatocytes
  primary, 8t
  secondary, 8t
Spermatocytogenesis, 169-170, *171*
Spermatogenesis. *See also* Gametogenesis
  duration of, 173-174
  endocrine control of, *177*, 177-178
  puberty and, 97, 99
Spermatogonia, 8t, 169
  spermatocytogenesis and, 169-170, *171*
Spermiation, 173, *174*
Spermiogenesis, 169, 170, 172-173
  acrosomal phase of, 172
  cap phase of, 172
  Golgi phase of, 172
  maturation phase of, 172-173
Spermophagy, sperm transport and, 151-152, *153*

Stallion
  breeding season of, 361
  ejaculation in, 363-364
  lack of libido in, 289
  reproductive failure in, 382-383
    abnormal sexual behavior and ejaculatory distur-
      bances and, 382
    breeding technique recommendations and, 383
    poor semen characteristics and, 382-383
  semen collection and, frequency of, 428
  semen cryopreservation and, 523
  semen production in, 362-363, 364t, 365
  sexual maturity in, 362, 363
Steer. See Cattle
Sterility. See Infertility
Steroid-binding globulin, 82
Steroid hormones, 78-83, 79. See also specific hormones
  in pregnancy, in mare, 375
  ovulation and, 139
Steroidogenesis, follicle growth and, 121, 124, 125
STH (GH; growth hormone; somatropic hormone), 70
Stillbirth, 277-279, 278
Suckling
  maternal and neonatal behavior and, 249
    in cattle, 254, 255
    in pigs, 256, 256t
    in sheep, 252-253, 253
  postpartum estrus and ovulation and, 104-105, 105,
    234-235
Superficial epithelium, 25t, 96
  prenatal development of, 23, 24
Superovulation, 466-470
  insemination and, 469
  methods of, 467, 468t, 469, 469
  repeated, 469-470
Swine. See Boar; Pig; Sow
Syncytium, 205
Syngamy, 193-194

Tandem fusion, 300t
TBG (thyroxine-binding globulin), 88
TDF (testis-determining factor), in pig, 343
Tdy (testis-determining Y chromosome), in pig, 343
Teasing procedures, for semen collection, 426
Temperature, breeding season and, 106-108, 108
Testes, 3
  anatomy of, 3, 5, 5t, 6, 6-8, 7, 8t
  blood-testis barrier and, 174-178
    cellular junctions and, 174-176, 176
  cryptorchidism and, 287-288
  descent of, 5, 5t
  diseases of, fertilization failure and, 292, 293t
  gubernaculum, 5
  hormones of, 63t
  hypoplasia of, 288-289, 303-304
  in poultry, 393-394, 395
  prenatal and neonatal physiology of, reproductive
    cycles and, 94, 96
  prenatal development of, 4-5
  thermoregulation of, 7-8
Testicular fluid, secretion of, 176-177
Testis-determining factor (TDF), in pig, 343
Testis-determining Y chromosome (Tdy), in pig, 343
Testosterone, 82, 82
  spermatogenesis and, 177, 177-178
TGF (transforming growth factor), 179

Theca cells, 115t
  ovulation and, 137
Thermal stress
  embryonic mortality and, 272-273
  male fertility failure and, 292
Thermoregulation
  of testes, 7-8
  parturition and, 233
Thyroid gland, hormones of, 64t, 88
Thyrotropin-releasing hormone (TRH), 73, 77
Thyroxine-binding globulin (TBG), 88
TNF (tumor necrosis factor), 90t
Toxic agents, male infertility and, 296
Traits, inherited, 299
Transferrin, andrology and, 88
Transforming growth factor (TGF), 179
Translocation, 300
  reciprocal, 300t
  Robertsonian, 300t
Transplantation antigens, 222
TRH (thyrotropin-releasing hormone), 73, 77
Trisomic aneuploids, 299
Trophoblast (trophoectoderm), 201
Tumor necrosis factor (TNF), 90t
Tunica albuginea
  female, 25t
  male, 8t
Turkey. See Poultry
Twinning, 200-201
  abortion and, 276
  in horse, 371-372, 374
Type I conceptus interferon (oTP-1; ovine trophoblast
    protein 1), maternal recognition of pregnancy and,
    208-209

Ultrapure water, 495
Ultrasonography, in pregnancy diagnosis, 447-452
  B-mode real-time ultrasonography and, 449, 449, 449-452
  Doppler phenomenon and, 447-448
  pulse-echo ultrasonography and, 448, 448-449
Umbilical arteries, placental circulation and, 219-220
Umbilical cord, 218t
  excessive length of, in horse, 380-381
Underfeeding, male infertility and, 295
Urethra, male, 3
Urethral glands, comparative anatomy of, 1
Urogenital sinus, embryology of, 21
Uterine fluid, 44
Uterine vessels, placental circulation and, 219-220
Uteroferrin, 44
Uterus, 40, 41-43, 42-48, 46, 47
  abnormalities of, anestrus due to, 264-265
  changes during pregnancy, 215
  contractions of, 44-45
    during parturition, 229
  distention of, anestrus due to, 265
  egg migration through, 163
  endometrial glands and uterine fluid and, 43-44
    uterine proteins and, 44
  environment of, interaction of conceptus with, 206-
    207
  function of, 45-48
    foreign bodies and IUDs and, 47-48
    implantation and gestation and, 46-47
    luteolytic mechanisms and, 45-46
    parturition and postpartum involution and, 47

sperm transport and, 45
hormones of, 63t
in poultry, 392
involution of, 47, 234
   in cattle, 321
metabolism of, 45
overcrowding in, embryonic mortality and, 272
postpartum infections of, 284
sperm transport in, 151-152
   sexual experience and, 247
   spermophagy and, 151-152, *153*
vasculature of, 43

Vagina, 52-54, *53*
   artificial, for semen collection, 428, *430-433*
   biopsy of, in pregnancy diagnosis, 452, *454*
   changes during pregnancy, 214
   contractions of, 53
   functions of, 54
   immunologic responses of, 53
   microbiologic flora of, 53
   vaginal fluid and, 53
Vaginal fluid, 53
Vasculature. *See also* Circulation
   of oviductal mucosa, 33

of pituitary, 65-67
of uterus, 43
Vasopressin (ADH; arginine vasopressin), 70, 72
Vesicular glands, comparative anatomy of, 1
Vestibule, 54
Viral abortion (equine herpesvirus I infection; equine
   rhinopneumonitis), 276-277
Vitamin deficiencies, male infertility and, 296
Vulva, changes during pregnancy, 214

Water, ultrapure, 495
White heifer disease, 268
Wolffian ducts, segmental aplasia of, 287

X-chromosomes. *See* Sex chromosomes

Y-chromosomes. *See* Sex chromosomes
Yolk sac, 218t

Zeronal (Ralgro), 80, *81*
Zona pellucida
   hatching of blastocyst from, 202
   micromanipulation of, 488, 491-492
   regulatory and physiology parameters of, 117t
Zygotene, 169